S0-FJI-250

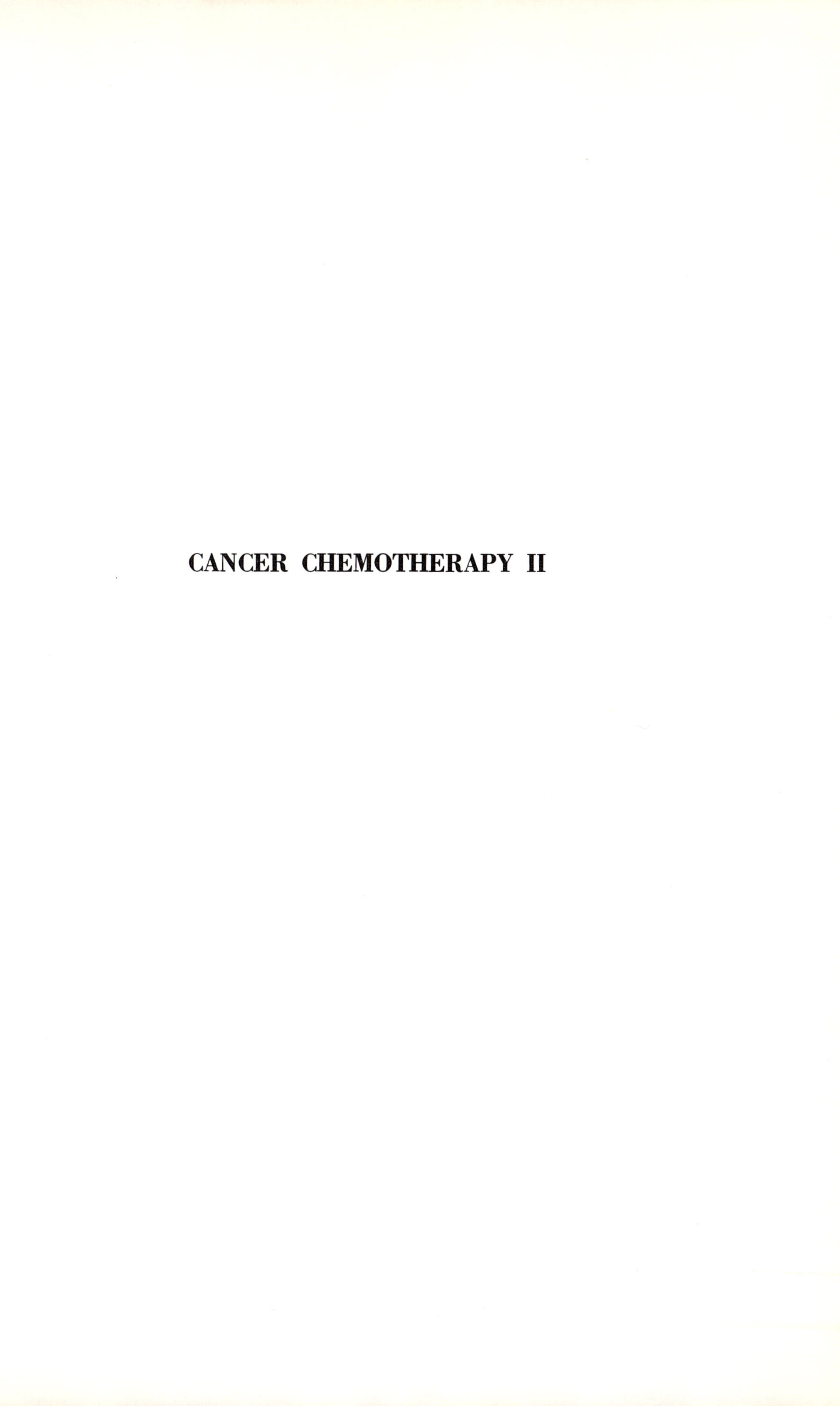

CANCER CHEMOTHERAPY II

CANCER CHEMOTHERAPY II

THE TWENTY-SECOND HAHNEMANN SYMPOSIUM

Edited by

ISADORE BRODSKY, M.D.

Professor, Department of Medicine
Director, Division of Hematology and Medical Oncology
Hahnemann Medical College and Hospital
Philadelphia, Pennsylvania

S. BENHAM KAHN, M.D.

Associate Professor, Department of Medicine
Associate Director, Division of Hematology and Medical Oncology
Hahnemann Medical College and Hospital
Philadelphia, Pennsylvania

Under the General Editorship of

JOHN H. MOYER, M.D.

Professor and Chairman, Department of Medicine
Hahnemann Medical College and Hospital
Philadelphia, Pennsylvania

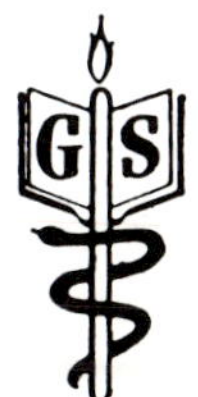

GRUNE & STRATTON, ***New York and London***

Grune & Stratton, Inc.
111 Fifth Avenue
New York, New York 10003

Library of Congress Catalog Card Number 73–164476
International Standard Book Number 0–8089–0691–7
Printed in the United States of America

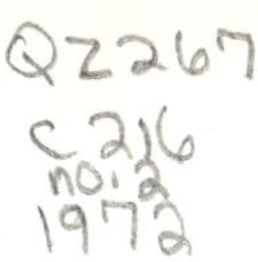

CONTENTS

III. Bone Marrow Physiology and Protection

IV. Hematologic Neoplasms

V. Regional Techniques

Contributors

AISENBERG, ALAN C., M.D.
Associate Professor of Medicine, Harvard Medical School, and Head, Medical Oncology, Massachusetts General Hospital, Boston, Mass.

ANTONIADES, JOHN, M.D.
Assistant Professor of Radiation Therapy and Nuclear Medicine, Hahnemann Medical College and Hospital, Philadelphia, Pa.

BAIG, MAHMOODULLAH, M.D.
Instructor in Medicine (Oncology), Division of Oncology, Department of Medicine, Georgetown University School of Medicine, Washington, D.C.

BERTINO, JOSEPH R., M.D.
Professor of Medicine and Pharmacology and Chief, Section of Oncology and Chemotherapy, Yale University School of Medicine, New Haven, Conn.

BODEY, GERALD P., M.D.
Assistant Professor of Medicine and Chief, Section of Clinical Microbiology, Department of Developmental Therapeutics, The University of Texas M. D. Anderson Hospital and Tumor Institute, Houston, Tex.

BOGGS, DANE R., M.D.
Professor of Medicine and Chief, Division of Hematology, Department of Medicine, University of Pittsburgh School of Medicine, Pittsburgh, Pa.

BRADY, LUTHER W., M.D.
Professor and Chairman, Department of Radiation Therapy and Nuclear Medicine, Hahnemann Medical College and Hospital, Philadelphia, Pa.

BRODSKY, ISADORE, M.D.
Professor of Medicine and Director, Division of Hematology and Medical Oncology, Department of Medicine, Hahnemann Medical College and Hospital, Philadelphia, Pa.

BURCHENAL, JOSEPH H., M.D.
Department of Medicine, Memorial Hospital for Cancer and Allied Diseases, and Division of Applied Therapy, Sloan-Kettering Institute for Cancer Research, New York, N.Y.

CAPIZZI, ROBERT L., M.D.
Major, MC USAR, Biomedical Laboratory, Edgewood Arsenal, Md.

CHANANA, ARJUN D., M.D.
Associate Professor of Pathology, State University of New York, Stony Brook, N.Y., and Head, Division of Experimental Pathology, Medical Department, Brookhaven National Laboratory, Upton, N.Y.

CHERVENICK, PAUL A., M.D.
Associate Professor of Medicine, Department of Medicine, University of Pittsburgh School of Medicine, Pittsburgh, Pa.

COHEN, HARVEY J., M.D.
Associate in Medicine, Duke University School of Medicine, Durham, N.C.

CONROY, JAMES F., D.O.
Senior Instructor in Medicine and Chief Fellow, Division of Hematology and Medical Oncology, Department of Medicine, Hahnemann Medical College and Hospital, Philadelphia, Pa.

CRONKITE, EUGENE P., M.D.
Professor of Medicine, State University of New York, Stony Brook, N.Y., and Chairman, Medical Department, Brookhaven National Laboratory, Upton, N.Y.

DEJONGH, DAVID S., M.D.
Assistant Professor of Pathology and Chief, Blood Bank, Department of Clinical Pathology, The University of Texas M. D. Anderson Hospital and Tumor Institute, Houston, Tex.

DIMITROV, NIKOLAY V., M.D.
Associate Professor of Medicine and Research Associate Professor of Biochemistry, Hahnemann Medical College and Hospital, Philadelphia, Pa.

DURANT, JOHN R., M.D.
Professor of Medicine and Director, Cancer Research and Training Program, University of Alabama School of Medicine, Birmingham, Ala.

ELION, GERTRUDE B., D.SC.
Head, Experimental Therapy, Burroughs Wellcome & Co., Research Triangle Park, N.C.

ERSLEV, ALLAN J., M.D.
Cardeza Research Professor of Medicine and Director, Cardeza Foundation, Department of Medicine, Jefferson Medical College, Thomas Jefferson University, Philadelphia, Pa.

EVANS, AUDREY E., M.D.
Associate Professor of Pediatrics, University of Pennsylvania School of Medicine, and Director of Oncology, Children's Hospital of Philadelphia, Philadelphia, Pa.

FAUST, DONALD S., M.D.
Associate Professor of Radiation Therapy and Nuclear Medicine, Hahnemann Medical College and Hospital, Philadelphia, Pa.

FREI, EMIL, III, M.D.
Professor of Medicine and Associate Director (Clinical Research), The University of Texas M. D. Anderson Hospital and Tumor Institute, Houston, Tex.

FREIREICH, EMIL J, M.D.
Professor of Medicine and Chief, Research Hematology, Department of Developmental Therapeutics, The University of Texas M. D. Anderson Hospital and Tumor Institute, Houston, Tex.

FUDENBERG, H. HUGH, M.D.
Professor of Medicine, University of California School of Medicine, San Francisco, and Professor of Bacteriology and Immunology, University of California School of Medicine, Berkeley, Ca.

GARDNER, FRANK H., M.D.
Professor of Medicine, University of Pennsylvania School of Medicine, Director of Medicine, and Director of Hematology Research Laboratory, Presbyterian-University of Pennsylvania Medical Center, Philadelphia, Pa.

GOLD, G. LENNARD, M.D.
Clinical Associate Professor of Medicine, Division of Oncology, Department of Medicine, Georgetown University School of Medicine, Washington, D.C.

GONICK, PAUL, M.D.
Associate Professor of Surgery and Director, Division of Urology, Hahnemann Medical College and Hospital, Philadelphia, Pa.

HALL, THOMAS C., M.D.
Director, Division of Oncology, and Professor of Medicine and Pharmacology, University of Rochester School of Medicine and Dentistry, Rochester, N.Y.

HANSZ, JANUSZ, M.D.
Hematology Research Fellow, Hahnemann Medical Service, Philadelphia General Hospital, Philadelphia, Pa.; presently on the staff of the Department of Medicine (Hematology), Medical School of Poznan, Poland.

HELM, FREDERICK, M.D.
Department of Dermatology, Roswell Park Memorial Institute, Buffalo, N.Y.

HENDERSON, EDWARD S., M.D.
Head, Leukemia Service, Medicine Branch, National Cancer Institute, National Institutes of Health, Bethesda, Md.

HITCHINGS, GEORGE H., PH.D.
Vice President, Burroughs Wellcome & Co., Research Triangle Park, N.C.

HOLTERMANN, OLE A., M.D., PH.D.
Department of Dermatology, Roswell Park Memorial Institute, Buffalo, N.Y.

JOHNS, DAVID G., M.D., PH.D.
Head, Section of Drug Metabolism, Laboratory of Chemical Pharmacology, National Cancer Institute, National Institutes of Health, Bethesda, Md.

KAHN, S. BENHAM, M.D.
Associate Professor of Medicine and Associate Director, Division of Hematology and Medical Oncology, Department of Medicine, Hahnemann Medical College and Hospital, Philadelphia, Pa.

KENNEDY, B. J., M.D.
Professor of Medicine and Director, Section of Oncology, Department of Medicine, University of Minnesota School of Medicine, Minneapolis, Minn.

KLEIN, EDMUND, M.D.
Chief, Department of Dermatology, Roswell Park Memorial Institute, Buffalo, N.Y.

KRAKOFF, IRWIN H., M.D.
Medical Oncology Service, Department of Medicine, Memorial Hospital for Cancer and Allied Diseases, and Division of Chemotherapy Research, Sloan-Kettering Institute for Cancer Research, New York, N.Y.

KREIS, WILLI, M.D., PH.D.
Division of Drug Resistance, Sloan-Kettering Institute for Cancer Research, New York, N.Y.

LACHER, MORTIMER J., M.D.
Clinical Assistant Professor of Medicine, Cornell University Medical College, Assistant Attending Physician, Memorial Hospital for Cancer and Allied Diseases, and Assistant Clinician, Sloan-Kettering Institute for Cancer Research, New York, N.Y.

LEVENTHAL, BRIGID G., M.D.
Senior Investigator, Leukemia Service, Medicine Branch, National Cancer Institute, National Institutes of Health, Bethesda, Md.

LEVIN, JACK, M.D.
Associate Professor of Medicine, The Johns Hopkins University School of Medicine and Hospital, Baltimore, Md., and John and Mary R. Markle Scholar in Academic Medicine.

LEVY, HILTON B., PH.D.
Head, Section of Molecular Virology, Laboratory of Viral Diseases, National Institute of Allergy and Infectious Diseases, National Institutes of Health, Bethesda, Md.

LUDLUM, DAVID B., PH.D., M.D.
Professor, Department of Cell Biology and Pharmacology, University of Maryland School of Medicine, Baltimore, Md.

MANCALL, ELLIOTT L., M.D.
Professor of Medicine (Neurology) and Director, Division of Neurology, Department of Medicine, Hahnemann Medical College and Hospital, Philadelphia, Pa.

MARSDEN, JOHN H., M.D.
Medical Research Division, Eli Lilly and Company, Indianapolis, Ind.

MASTRANGELO, MICHAEL J., M.D.
Instructor in Medicine, Division of Medical Oncology, Jefferson Medical College, Thomas Jefferson University, Philadelphia, Pa.

MILGROM, HALINA, M.D.
Department of Dermatology, Roswell Park Memorial Institute, Buffalo, N.Y.

MILLER, EDWARD, M.D.
Assistant Medical Director, Hoffmann-La Roche Inc., Nutley, N.J.

PRASASVINICHAI, SRIPRAYOON, M.D.
Assistant Professor of Radiation Therapy and Nuclear Medicine, Hahnemann Medical College and Hospital, Philadelphia, Pa.

RAI, KANTI R., M.D.
Long Island Jewish Medical Center, New Hyde Park, N.Y. and Brookhaven National Laboratory, Upton, N.Y.

REGELSON, WILLIAM, M.D.
Professor and Chairman, Division of Medical Oncology, Medical College of Virginia, Richmond, Va.

RUNDLES, RALPH WAYNE, M.D., PH.D.
Professor of Medicine and Chief, Division of Hematology and Oncology, Duke University School of Medicine, Durham, N.C.

SEMEL, CHESTER J., M.D.
Los Angeles, Ca.

SHNIDER, BRUCE I., M.D.
Professor of Medicine, Associate Dean, and Director, Division of Medical Oncology, Department of Medicine, Georgetown University School of Medicine, Washington, D.C.

STOLL, HOWARD L., M.D.
Department of Dermatology, Roswell Park Memorial Institute, Buffalo, N.Y.

STRAWITZ, JOSEPH G., M.D.
Associate Director, American Oncologic Hospital, and Assistant Professor, Department of Surgery, University of Pennsylvania School of Medicine, Philadelphia, Pa.

STREILEIN, J. WAYNE, M.D.
Associate Professor of Medical Genetics, University of Pennsylvania School of Medicine, Philadelphia, Pa.; presently Professor of Cell Biology and Associate Professor of Internal Medicine, University of Texas Southwestern Medical School at Dallas, Dallas, Tex.

SUHRLAND, LEIF G., M.D.
Professor of Medicine, Department of Medicine, College of Human Medicine, Michigan State University, East Lansing, Mich.

SULLIVAN, ROBERT D., M.D.
Los Angeles, Ca.

TORPIE, RICHARD J., M.D.
Assistant Professor of Radiation Therapy and Nuclear Medicine, Hahnemann Medical College and Hospital, Philadelphia, Pa.

WALKER, MARY J., M.S.
Department of Dermatology, Roswell Park Memorial Institute, Buffalo, N.Y.

WEISS, ARTHUR J., M.D.
Assistant Professor of Medicine, Division of Medical Oncology, Jefferson Medical College, Thomas Jefferson University, Philadelphia, Pa.

WHITECAR, JOHN P., JR., M.D.
Major, MC, Department of the Army, Brooke General Hospital, Brooke Army Medical Center, Fort Sam Houston, Tex.

WINKELMAN, A. CHARLES, M.D.
Assistant Professor of Medicine (Neurology), Division of Neurology, Department of Medicine, Hahnemann Medical College and Hospital, Philadelphia, Pa.

Preface

Additional knowledge has accumulated rapidly in cancer chemotherapy since our first symposium in 1965. Our purpose in conducting this second symposium on cancer chemotherapy was to update the first. Again our format has been to survey the field, presenting broad concepts but excluding controversy where it had not changed overall direction.

Several metastatic diseases other than malignant trophoblastic disease are now curable by chemotherapy. About 25 per cent of patients with Burkitt's lymphoma are cured by alkylating agents, whereas a smaller percentage of patients with metastatic testicular cancer and some patients with childhood lymphoblastic leukemia have been apparently cured by combination chemotherapy. Recently the demonstration that L-asparaginase, an enzyme, can inhibit certain leukemic cells while not impairing normal marrow cells has stimulated hope that a "magic bullet" for cancer might be found. However, as of this time the backbone of chemotherapy remains those agents whose cytotoxic capacity extends to normal cells as well as to tumor cells.

The use of combination chemotherapy in short repetitive courses, taking advantage of the fact that normal cells recover faster than malignant cells, has led to some spectacular results, especially in the therapy of Hodgkin's disease. Currently available data suggest that with this kind of treatment about 40 per cent of patients with Stage IV Hodgkin's disease will remain free of disease for 5 years.

The application of immunologic concepts to the therapy of malignancy has led to some interesting advances in cancer therapy. Patients with acute leukemia may have extended survival if prolonged stimulation of the immune system is undertaken with bacille Calmette-Guérin (BCG). The induction of interferon by nonspecific chemical agents is another approach in our efforts to bolster the body's reaction to the presence of malignant disease. These advances alone might mandate another text, yet none have basically changed our direction, although our path has been broadened and our energy revived.

This volume, like the first, groups the papers into five areas. First, the mechanism of action of the chemotherapeutic agents is covered in broad detail. This section has been expanded to include discussions of interferon, immunology, intermediary metabolism and hemostasis in relation to chemotherapy.

Second, the clinical management of the patient with neoplastic disease is extensively covered in ensuing chapters. Although they have recommended some dosages, most authors have stressed the concept of individualized courses, depending on such factors as the staging and aggressiveness of the tumor in specific patients. Again, since this form of therapy is for the most part palliative, treatment is approached with an investigative emphasis rather than with an established routine. This section has been expanded to include a clinical chemotherapeutic approach to brain tumor and skin cancer.

Third, an appreciation of bone marrow function and mechanisms for controlling marrow toxicity induced by use of these drugs is essential for the clinician. We have added a chapter on bone marrow transplantation. The chapters dealing with hematologic and infectious implications have been expanded.

Fourth, we have continued to emphasize the hematologic neoplasms, both because of our own interest in these diseases and because the currently available agents are effective in controlling these disorders as well as in producing profound toxic effects on the hematopoietic system. Chemotherapy of hematopoietic disease continues to serve as a yardstick by which success of solid tumor chemotherapy must be measured.

In the last segment, we cover regional techniques in the management of metastatic cancer. In this area we could not exclude the use of X-ray therapy in the management of Hodgkin's disease. Our purpose here was to establish appropriate criteria by which we could measure the results of chemotherapy of this disorder. The problem of how far to go with X-ray therapy in Hodgkin's disease remains unsolved, but it is our hope that the reader will be able to evaluate more objectively the continuously appearing reports involving various modes of therapy of this disease.

It is obvious that our greatest deficiencies in chemotherapy exist in the management of the extremely common neoplastic diseases, such as lung, breast, colon, and cervical carcinoma. However, the successes in the management of the hematologic neoplasms must serve as guidelines for continued investigations of newer approaches in the therapy of the common, presently resistant neoplasms. Therapeutic nihilism will lead to an abandonment of newer approaches and, what is even more tragic, an excuse for abandoning the patient. We feel confident that perhaps in the next volume we shall be able to report on chemotherapeutic modalities that may lead to the cure of these diseases.

Finally, we would like to stress what is well known to the oncologist but frequently confusing to the layman and even to general physicians: Cancer is not a single disease, and therapy must be individualized and broken down into component parts. The physician who truly recognizes his responsibility to his patient with metastatic disease will view even present-day cancer chemotherapy as one of the great advances of modern medicine.

The editors wish to thank Mrs. Sage Cordell, Mrs. Edith Schwager, Mrs. Kathleen Sullivan, Mrs. Rita Lavner, and Mrs. Marie Smith, who helped so much in the preparation of this symposium and this volume.

Grants from the U. S. Public Health Service, Hoffmann-La Roche Inc., and Wyeth Laboratories contributed to the financial support of this symposium and we gratefully acknowledge their assistance.

ISADORE BRODSKY, M.D.
S. BENHAM KAHN, M.D.

Philadelphia, Pa.

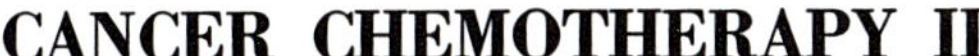

CANCER CHEMOTHERAPY II

I. MECHANISM OF ACTION OF CHEMOTHERAPEUTIC DRUGS

Mechanism of Action of Alkylating Agents

By DAVID B. LUDLUM, PH.D., M.D.

THE ALKYLATING AGENTS as a group contain some of our oldest effective drugs for the treatment of cancer. Although their mechanism of action has not been completely elucidated, it is known that they alkylate nucleic acids and interfere with DNA synthesis in vivo. Furthermore, these agents can be either mutagenic or carcinogenic under certain conditions. This suggests that an attack on the genetic apparatus, most likely DNA, is basic to their action.

Therefore, to limit this discussion to a manageable size, we shall consider reactions of alkylating agents with nucleic acids and nucleic acid models only, and not cover their reactions with other cellular constituents. In a review of this size, many careful investigations cannot even be mentioned, but most of these are covered in other recent reviews and collected works.[1-10]

We shall consider the relevant chemistry of alkylation, certain biologic effects of alkylation, and biochemical studies which utilize synthetic polynucleotides as models for nucleic acids. Throughout, we shall be particularly interested in studies which relate to the two major clinical deficiencies of these agents: their incomplete selectivity for neoplastic tissue, and the development of resistance.

CHEMISTRY OF ALKYLATION

Representative alkylating agents are shown in Figure 1. These compounds are attacked by nucleophilic sites on nucleic acids and other cellular constituents; this results in an addition of a portion of the alkylating agent to the nucleophilic site. Extensive studies by Brookes and Lawley[5,11,12] and other investigators have identified the base positions shown in Figure 2 as primary sites of reaction. The nucleosides shown in this figure are from RNA, but the corresponding positions are involved in DNA. Because of experimental difficulties, there is less agreement about the extent of alkylation of phosphate groups along the nucleic acid backbone; however, recent experiments with model compounds[13,14] have indicated that some phosphate alkylation probably occurs.

Considerable interest has centered on substitution of guanine in the 7 position, a reaction which frequently accounts for more than 90 per cent of the total alkylation. It has been suggested that the 7-substituted base might mispair with thymine or uracil in nucleic acid replication or transcription (see, however, the discussion below in "Biologic Effects of Alkylation"); alternatively, following depurination of DNA at this site, any base might be introduced opposite the empty location in subsequent replica-

From the Department of Cell Biology and Pharmacology, University of Maryland School of Medicine, Baltimore, Maryland.

Supported by the Markle Foundation, grant T-432 from the American Cancer Society and grant GM-16952 from the U.S. Public Health Service.

tive processes. More recently, certain genetic and biochemical studies have focused attention on the effects of alkylation at other sites, particularly the O-6 position of guanine[15] and the 3 position of cytosine.[16,17] Interest in reaction at these sites has been enhanced by the finding that agents with rather different biologic effects[18,19] may attack different base positions somewhat selectively under certain conditions.

It is an old observation that monofunctional agents generally have little therapeutic value, and that effective agents are found among compounds with two or more alkylating groups. These compounds can form crosslinks within a single molecule, or bind two macromolecules together with a relatively stable covalent bond. The existence of such links between the two strands of DNA may be demonstrated by the reversible denaturation of double-stranded DNA molecules.[20,21] Crosslinks seem to play an important role in explaining the action of many alkylating agents.

Apparent exceptions to the rule that clinically useful agents contain two or more

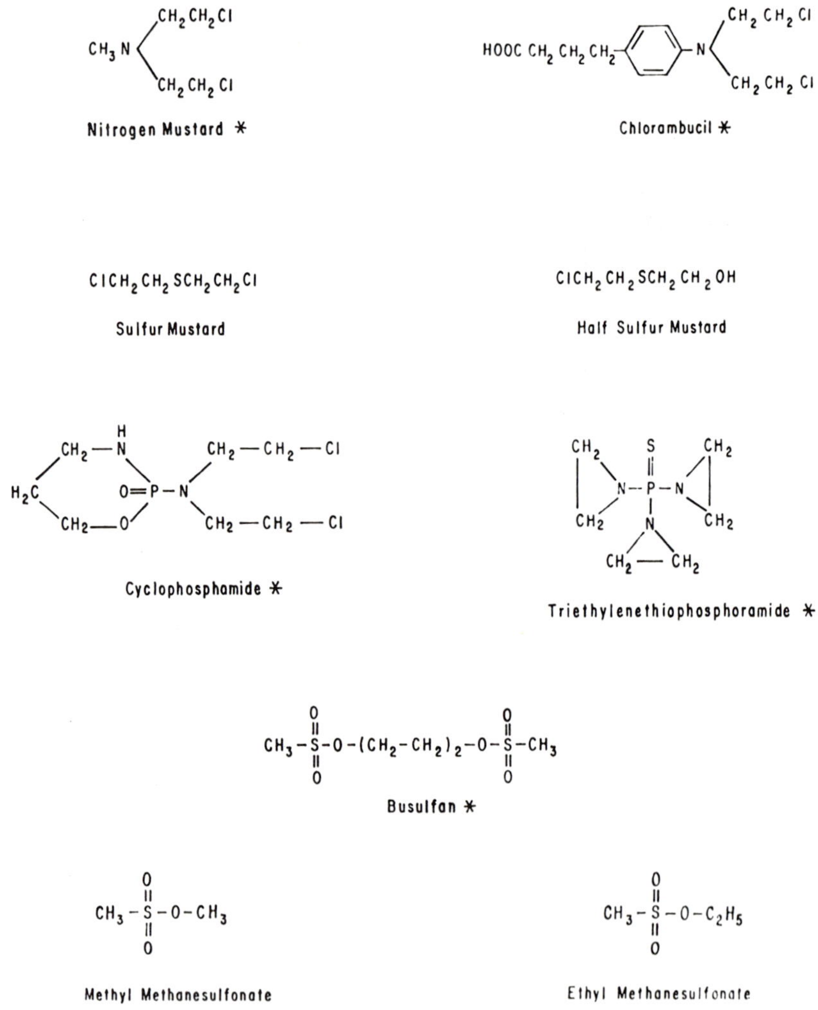

$CH_3N(CH_2CH_2Cl)_2$

Nitrogen Mustard *

$HOOC\,CH_2CH_2CH_2-C_6H_4-N(CH_2CH_2Cl)_2$

Chlorambucil *

$ClCH_2CH_2SCH_2CH_2Cl$

Sulfur Mustard

$ClCH_2CH_2SCH_2CH_2OH$

Half Sulfur Mustard

Cyclophosphamide *

Triethylenethiophosphoramide *

$CH_3-SO_2-O-(CH_2-CH_2)_2-O-SO_2-CH_3$

Busulfan *

$CH_3-SO_2-O-CH_3$

Methyl Methanesulfonate

$CH_3-SO_2-O-C_2H_5$

Ethyl Methanesulfonate

FIG. 1.—Representative alkylating agents. The compounds indicated by an asterisk are in clinical use; the rest are of theoretical interest only.

alkylating groups are CCNU, 1-(2-chloroethyl)-3-cyclohexyl-1-nitrosourea, and similar nitroso compounds which contain a single 2-chloroethyl group. However, it may be that the 2-chloroethyl group is transferred to a nucleophilic site and then acts as an alkylating group to produce a crosslink.

Although the main chemical features of alkylation have been elucidated, specific details of the process may be very important. Lawley and Brookes[12] have shown that the secondary structure of DNA influences the site of alkylation; studies with polynucleotides[22] have shown that this influence is very marked indeed. Changes in secondary structure during replication may well explain the special sensitivity of replicating cells to alkylation,[22,23] and more work should be done in this area.

Biologic Effects of Alkylation

Microorganisms, especially bacteriophages, are excellent models with which to study the lethal effects of alkylation. It has been shown[4,24,25] that bacteriophages which contain double-stranded nucleic acids are more sensitive to the action of difunctional agents than those which contain single-stranded material. This suggests that interstrand crosslinks are important in producing a lethal effect. However, even bacteriophages which contain single-stranded nucleic acids are more sensitive to difunctional than to monofunctional agents. This implies that intrastrand links are also important in explaining lethality. The studies described below suggest that somewhat different factors govern the lethality of different compounds; however, the clinically useful agents probably depend on crosslinking for their lethality.

Lawley and coworkers[21] have published a detailed study of the action of sulphur mustard and half mustard on the T7 coliphage, a virus which contains double-stranded DNA. At the mean lethal dose for immediate inactivation by mustard gas, there were about 1.3 moles of di-(guanin-7-yl-ethyl) sulfide and 7 moles of monoalkylation products per mole of DNA polymer, whereas at the mean lethal dose for half mustard there were 280 moles of monoalkylation products. These data indicate that formation of the crosslinked diguaninyl product is a particularly damaging event. Approxi-

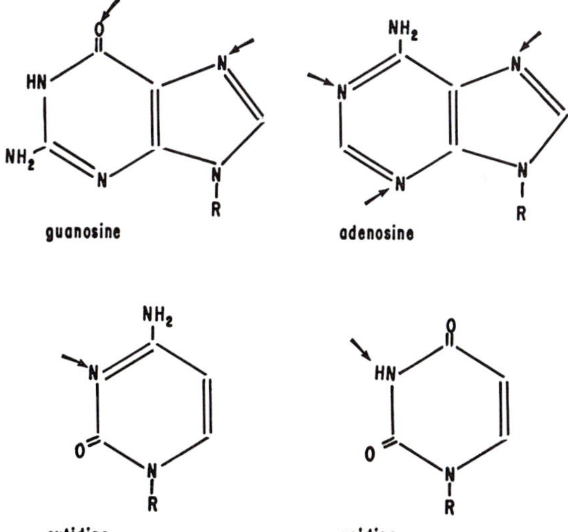

Fig. 2.—Reactive sites in nucleosides. The 7 position of guanosine is by far the most reactive.

mately one quarter of the diguaninyl molecules are associated with interstrand cross-links and the remainder with intrastrand links.

A relatively large number of alkylations were required for immediate inactivation by the monofunctional half mustard. Subsequent depurination and hydrolysis of DNA at alkylated base positions caused more extensive inactivation than alkylation itself.

Verly and Brakier[26] have studied the action of nitrogen mustard, ethyl methane-sulfonate, busulfan, and diepoxybutane on the same T7 phage. Crosslinks were again associated with lethality for nitrogen mustard; when survival was followed up after treatment with this agent, bonds between DNA strands first increased in number and then decreased.

On the other hand, treatment of T7 with ethyl methanesulfonate resulted in lethality which increased steadily after exposure, presumably due to depurination and hydrolysis. Surprisingly, when T7 was treated with the well-known difunctional agent, busulfan, there was no evidence for interstrand crosslinking. Intrastrand crosslinks were not ruled out, but the concentrations of busulfan and ethyl methanesulfonate required for equal lethality were similar. It thus appears that ethyl methanesulfonate and busulfan have a very similar action on T7 phage; some additional factor must operate to explain the difference between these two agents in higher organisms. The final agent studied, diepoxybutane, had a combined difunctional and monofunctional action.

When the effects of alkylating agents are studied in growing bacteria or mammalian cells, intracellular enzymes become extremely important in modifying the initial damage to DNA. These enzymes evidently recognize the alkylated base and remove it, an action which can either magnify the damage or open the way for subsequent repair.

Papirmeister and Davison[27] first demonstrated the loss of sulphur mustard alkylation products from the DNA of *Escherichia coli.* Bacteria which were treated with this agent and then incubated under certain conditions gradually regained their ability to synthesize DNA and to reproduce after an initial lag. Since sulphur mustard products were eliminated during this period, it was assumed that growth returned only after repair of damaged DNA.

Magnification of the original damage may occur if the alkylated DNA is subject to endonuclease attack without subsequent repair. Recent work by Papirmeister and coworkers[28] suggests that the DNA of T1 bacteriophage is sensitized to endonuclease attack by adenine rather than guanine alkylation.

Strauss and coworkers,[29] summarizing their extensive studies on the effects of DNA methylation, have shown that the transforming activity of *Bacillus subtilis* DNA can be greatly reduced after methylation by the action of cellular endonucleases. These nucleases attack some, but not all, heat-labile sites. Other enzymatic activities have been identified which can repair this damage. Depending on the intracellular environment, therefore, we can anticipate either increased sensitivity or resistance to the effects of alkylation.

Many different groups have studied the effects of alkylating agents on mammalian cells; Roberts and coworkers[30] have published the results of a detailed study of HeLa cells. Here again, the difunctional agent, sulphur mustard, is much more toxic than the monofunctional derivative; DNA synthesis again appears to be the cellular process most sensitive to alkylation. By using synchronous cultures, it was shown that cells in the late G_1 (postmitotic) or early S (DNA synthetic) phases are particularly sensitive to the effects of alkylation.

When cells are treated during these phases, there is an immediate inhibition of DNA synthesis and a delay in division and onset of the next (second) DNA synthetic cycle. However, it is evident that some recovery has occurred by the third synthetic cycle. This is attributed to repair of alkylated DNA, a process which is accompanied by release of alkylated products. Thus, the same general features of cytotoxicity appear to be present in both mammalian and bacterial cells.

The experiments described above are concerned, first, with the lethal action of alkylating agents, and then with the modifications of lethality which are imposed by cellular metabolism. Another approach, the genetic study of point mutations, yields useful information on the nature of the original DNA lesion produced by alkylating agents. Since the structure of the mutated DNA cannot be determined directly, the chemical identity of the altered base must be deduced from the altered gene product, or from genetic reversion data.

Tessman and coworkers[31] studied the effects of an ethylating agent, ethyl methanesulfonate, on a single-stranded DNA phage, S13. These data showed that changes in all four bases could occur, although one change appeared most frequently. They assigned this to a GC → AT transition, which seemed reasonable since guanine is, of course, the most readily alkylated base. The earlier data of Bautz and Freese,[32] as well as more recent studies by Osborn and coworkers,[33] support this hypothesis, but studies of amino acid replacement in the A protein of tryptophan synthetase[34] did not result in a clear-cut assignment. Thus, there is some uncertainty as to the base changes produced by alkylation, and the fact that all four bases can evidently be altered should be emphasized.

The problem of relating a particular alteration in nucleic acid structure to a specific biologic effect is greatly simplified by the use of synthetic polynucleotides.[35] These polymers may be prepared with a known composition and used in model biochemical systems to obtain direct information on the biologic effects of alkylation.

Systems which are available for such studies and which are part of the mechanism for transferring genetic information are shown in Table 1. Each of these systems utilizes the informational content of the polymer at the left to direct the synthesis of the polymer at the right. The template is incubated with the required enzyme or cell extract, and the performance of an unalkylated template is compared with the performance of an alkylated one. The genetic damage associated with a particular base substitution can then be observed directly.

Because of their greater availability, experiments with polyribonucleotides have progressed further than experiments with polydeoxyribonucleotides. However, the base-pairing properties of synthetic polydeoxyribonucleotides have, in general, resembled those of the ribose series. Accordingly, one would expect abnormal base pairing behavior in one series of polymers to be reflected in the other series.

TABLE 1.—*Models for Testing the Effects of Alkylating Agents on the Properties of Templates*

System	*Enzyme*
DNA → DNA	DNA polymerase
DNA → RNA	RNA polymerase
RNA → RNA	RNA polymerase
RNA → protein	Cell extract

TABLE 2.—*Incorporation of Nucleotides by Methylated Bases*

Base	*CMP*	*GMP*	*UMP*	*AMP*
Methylguanine	+	−	−*	−*
Methyladenine	−	−	NT	NT
Methylcytosine	−	−	+	+

Templates containing methylated bases were incubated with RNA polymerase and radioactive nucleoside triphosphates. Nucleotide incorporation was then determined on the TCA-insoluble product.

NT indicates that incorporation was not tested.

Abbreviations: Cytosine monophosphate = CMP; cytosine triphosphate = CTP; guanosine monophosphate = GMP; uridine monophosphate = UMP; adenosine monophosphate = AMP.

* Negative when the preferred substrate CTP was present.

Focusing on the substituted base found most frequently after treatment with methylating agents, Wilhelm and Ludlum[36] studied the ability of copolymers which contained 7-methylguanine to promote polypeptide synthesis. The experiments were designed to detect the incorporation of amino acids which would have been polymerized if 7-methylguanine mispaired like adenine. No evidence for such misincorporation was obtained; instead, the overall ability of the 7-methylguanine-containing templates to promote polypeptide synthesis was diminished.

More extensive studies have been performed with the enzyme RNA polymerase, which can utilize substituted RNA to direct the synthesis of daughter RNA strands.[17,37,38] The results of these experiments are shown in Table 2. It is evident, first of all, that 7-methylguanine retains the base pairing properties of guanine. Thus, cytosine monophosphate (CMP) is incorporated into the daughter strand opposite the substituted base. No other nucleotide is incorporated at detectable levels if the substrate for CMP incorporation, cytosine triphosphate (CTP), is present.

No evidence was obtained for misincorporation by 1-methyladenine either. However, 3-methylcytosine led to the surprising incorporation of either uridine monophosphate (UMP) or adenosine monophosphate (AMP). Although no molecular explanation for this misincorporation has yet been devised, it is worth noting that studies by Singer and Fraenkel-Conrat[16] emphasize the biologic importance of cytosine substitution as compared to guanine substitution. Thus, it may well be that the biologic significance of relatively minor alkylation products overshadows the biologic significance of guanine alkylation. It is probable that further studies in this area will pinpoint the most important base alterations and improve our understanding of the action of alkylating agents at a molecular level.

REFERENCES

1. Karnofsky, D. A. (Ed.): Comparative clinical and biological effects of alkylating agents. Ann. N.Y. Acad. Sci. 68:657, 1958.
2. Van Duuren, B. L. (Ed.): Biological effects of alkylating agents. Ann. N.Y. Acad. Sci. 163:589, 1969.
3. Ross, W. C. J.: Biological Alkylating Agents. London: Butterworth, 1962.
4. Loveless, A.: Genetic and Allied Effects of Alkylating Agents. University Park and London: Pennsylvania State University Press, 1966.
5. Lawley, P. D.: Effects of some chemical mutagens and carcinogens on nucleic acids. Progr. Nucl. Acid Res. 5:89, 1966.
6. Wheeler, G. P.: Studies related to the

mechanism of action of cytotoxic alkylating agents: A review. Cancer Res. 22:651, 1962.
7. Wheeler, G. P.: Studies related to mechanisms of resistance to biological alkylating agents. Cancer Res. 23:1334, 1963.
8. Kihlman, B. A.: Actions of Chemicals on Dividing Cells. Englewood Cliffs, N.J.: Prentice-Hall, 1966.
9. Warwick, G. P.: The mechanism of action of alkylating agents. Cancer Res. 23:1315, 1963.
10. Ochoa, M., Jr. and Hirschberg, E.: Alkylating agents. *In* Schnitzer, R. J. and Hawking, F. (Eds.): Experimental Chemotherapy, Vol. 5. New York and London: Academic Press, 1967, pp. 1–132.
11. Brookes, P. and Lawley, P. D.: The reaction of mono- and difunctional alkylating agents with nucleic acids. Biochem. J. 80: 496, 1961.
12. Lawley, P. D. and Brookes, P.: Further studies on the alkylation of nucleic acids and their constituent nucleotides. Biochem. J. 89:127, 1963.
13. Ludlum, D. B.: Reaction of nitrogen mustard with synthetic polynucleotides. Biochim. Biophys. Acta 119:630, 1966.
14. Rhaese, H.-J. and Freese, E.: Chemical analysis of DNA alterations. IV. Reactions of oligodeoxynucleotides with monofunctional alkylating agents leading to backbone breakage. Biochim. Biophys. Acta 190:418, 1969.
15. Loveless, A.: Possible relevance of O–6 alkylation of deoxyguanosine to the mutagenicity and carcinogenicity of nitrosamines and nitrosamides. Nature 223:206, 1969.
16. Singer, B. and Fraenkel-Conrat, H.: Chemical modification of viral ribonucleic acid. VIII. The chemical and biological effects of methylating agents and nitrosoguanidine on tobacco mosaic virus. Biochemistry 8:3266, 1969.
17. Ludlum, D. B. and Wilhelm, R. C.: Ribonucleic acid polymerase reactions with methylated polycytidylic acid templates. J. Biol. Chem. 243:2750, 1968.
18. Singer, B. and Fraenkel-Conrat, H.: Chemical modifications of viral ribonucleic acid. VII. The action of methylating agents and nitrosoguanidine on polynucleotides including tobacco mosaic virus ribonucleic acid. Biochemistry 8:3260, 1969.
19. Lawley, P. D. and Thatcher, C. J.: Methylation of deoxyribonucleic acid in cultured mammalian cells by N-methyl-N′-nitro-N-nitrosoguanidine. Biochem. J. 116:693, 1970.
20. Kohn, K. W., Spears, C. L. and Doty, P.: Inter-strand crosslinking of DNA by nitrogen mustard. J. Molec. Biol. 19:266, 1966.
21. Lawley, P. D., Lethbridge, J. H., Edwards, P. A. and Shooter, K. V.: Inactivation of bacteriophage T7 by mono- and difunctional sulphur mustards in relation to cross-linking and depurination of bacteriophage DNA. J. Molec. Biol. 39:181, 1969.
22. Ludlum, D. B.: Alkylation of polynucleotide complexes. Biochim. Biophys. Acta 95:674, 1965.
23. Cerdá-Olmedo, E., Hanawalt, P. C. and Guerola, N.: Mutagenesis of the replication point by nitrosoguanidine: Map and pattern of replication of the *Escherichia coli* chromosome. J. Molec. Biol. 33:705, 1968.
24. Yamamoto, N. and Naito, T.: Inactivation by nitrogen mustard of single- and double-stranded DNA and RNA bacteriophages. Science 150:1603, 1965.
25. Yamamoto, N., Naito, T. and Shimkin, M. B.: Mechanism of inactivation of DNA and RNA bacteriophages by alkylating agents *in vitro*. Cancer Res. 26:2301, 1966.
26. Verly, W. G. and Brakier, L.: The lethal action of monofunctional and bifunctional alkylating agents on T7 coliphage. Biochim. Biophys. Acta 174:674, 1969.
27. Papirmeister, B. and Davison, C. L.: Elimination of sulfur mustard-induced products from DNA of *Escherichia coli*. Biochem. Biophys. Res. Commun. 17:608, 1964.
28. Papirmeister, B., Dorsey, J. K., Davison, C. L. and Gross, C. L.: Sensitization of DNA to endonuclease by adenine alkylation and its biological significance. Fed. Proc. 29:726, 1970.
29. Strauss, B., Coyle, M. and Robbins, M.: Consequences of alkylation for the behavior of DNA. Ann. N.Y. Acad. Sci. 163:765, 1969.
30. Roberts, J. J., Brent, T. P. and Crathorn, A. R.: The mechanism of the cytotoxic action of alkylating agents on mammalian cells. *In* Campbell, P. N. (Ed.): The Interaction of Drugs and Subcellular Components in Animal Cells. London: Churchill, 1968, pp. 5–27.
31. Tessman, I., Poddar, R. K. and Kumar, S.: Identification of the altered bases in mutated single-stranded DNA. J. Molec. Biol. 9:352, 1964.

32. Bautz, E. and Freese, E.: On the mutagenic effect of alkylating agents. Proc. Nat. Acad. Sci. U.S.A. 46:1585, 1960.
33. Osborn, M., Person, S., Phillips, S. and Funk, F.: A determination of mutagen specificity in bacteria using nonsense mutants of bacteriophage T4. J. Molec. Biol. 26:437, 1967.
34. Yanofsky, C., Ito, J. and Horn, V.: Amino acid replacement and the genetic code. Sympos. Quant. Biol. 30:151, 1966.
35. Ludlum, D. B., Warner, R. C. and Wahba, A. J.: Alkylation of synthetic polynucleotides. Science 145:397, 1964.
36. Wilhelm, R. C. and Ludlum, D. B.: Coding properties of 7-methylguanine. Science 153:1403, 1966.
37. Ludlum, D. B.: The properties of 7-methylguanine-containing templates for ribonucleic acid polymerase. J. Biol. Chem. 245:477, 1970.
38. Ludlum, D. B.: Alkylated polycytidylic acid templates for RNA polymerase. Biochim. Biophys. Acta 213:142, 1970.

Folate Antagonists

By JOSEPH R. BERTINO, M.D. AND DAVID G. JOHNS, M.D., PH.D.

SINCE OUR REVIEW OF THIS SUBJECT in the previous volume of this series, several significant studies have appeared which have led to the improved use of folate antagonists in the clinic.[1-4] These developments, together with recent advances in our understanding of tumor biology, especially of the biology of human tumors, have resulted in further improvement in the chemotherapy of patients with disseminated malignancies.[5]

Elsewhere in this volume are discussed the uses of folate antagonists, in particular methotrexate (amethopterin), for the treatment of patients with malignant disease. Methotrexate is the drug of choice in the treatment of choriocarcinoma, where it can result in cure in a high percentage of patients.[6] Significant tumor regression has been obtained in acute lymphatic leukemia,[7] Burkitt's lymphoma,[8] carcinoma of the breast,[9] mycosis fungoides,[10] and epidermoid cancer of the head and neck.[2,11-13] The use of methotrexate in the treatment of non-neoplastic diseases such as psoriasis[14,15] and as an immunosuppressive agent[16] is increasing. In addition, other folate antagonists such as pyrimethamine and trimethoprim have been developed which have selective effects on parasitic diseases and on bacterial infections of man.[17]

In this chapter we attempt to relate the biochemistry and pharmacology of these compounds to their clinical application, with emphasis on more recent contributions. In particular, we discuss the use of folate antagonists in combination with other therapies, the use of leucovorin rescue, and studies of new folate antagonists which may have clinical value.

MECHANISM OF ACTION

The 2,4-diamino folate antagonists aminopterin, methotrexate, and dichloromethotrexate are powerful inhibitors of the enzyme dihydrofolate reductase (also called folate reductase)[18-20]; the change from the 2-amino-4-hydroxypteridine structure of the parent compound to the 2,4-diaminopteridine structure results in a great increase in binding to the enzyme.

Aminopterin and methotrexate bind extremely tightly, but reversibly, as shown by the finding that chromatography of the inhibited enzyme on DEAE cellulose or hydroxylapatite can dissociate the enzyme-inhibitor complex.[21] The binding of methotrexate to dihydrofolate reductase has been characterized as "stoichiometric" by Werkheiser[19] and under certain conditions (pH 5.9, low ionic strength), one molecule of methotrexate can inactivate one molecule of enzyme.[22] At pH 7.5 and higher, the binding of methotrexate to enzyme is less tight, and kinetic studies have shown that inhibition of the enzyme is competitive in nature with respect to the substrate, dihydrofolate.[20] Inhibition of this enzyme activity stops the synthesis of tetrahydrofolate, which in turn decreases the availability of N^5, N^{10}-methylenetetrahydrofolate, the

---

From the Departments of Pharmacology and Medicine, Yale University School of Medicine, New Haven, Connecticut, and the Laboratory of Chemical Pharmacology, National Cancer Institute, Bethesda, Maryland.

Supported by grants CA 08010, CA 08341, and CA 11334 from the U.S. Public Health Service, and by grant PRA 58 from the American Cancer Society.

coenzyme necessary for formation of thymidylate and thus for DNA synthesis. The lack of tetrahydrofolate could result also in inhibition of purine synthesis and thus of RNA as well as of DNA synthesis, and could also bring about inhibition of serine and methionine synthesis. In most cells studied, inhibition of thymidylate biosynthesis appears to be the key event leading to cell death.[23–25]

Additional sites of action of methotrexate have been proposed, in particular inhibition of thymidylate synthetase.[26] One strain of *Lactobacillus casei* resistant to methotrexate is characterized not only by an increase in the activity of the enzyme dihydrofolate reductase, but also by the enzyme thymidylate synthetase.[27] In leukocytes studied from patients with leukemia, an increase in thymidylate synthetase activity,[28] as well as of dihydrofolate reductase activity[29] may occur soon after therapy with methotrexate. An increase in the level of thymidylate synthetase activity could result not only from an increase in the rate of synthesis of this enzyme or a decrease in the rate of its degradation, but also from synchronization of the cell population by methotrexate in the early S (DNA synthesis) phase.[29] Since methotrexate kills cells which are in the S phase of the cycle,[30] this drug, like other inhibitors of DNA synthesis, kills cells more rapidly when it is present during the logarithmic or rapid growth phase of cell proliferation. It has much less effect on "plateau" growth or resting cells.[31] As a result of inhibition by methotrexate, cells are unable to complete DNA synthesis and unbalanced growth results. If the block is long enough and sufficiently complete, cell death will eventually occur.

Other inhibitors of DNA synthesis such as cytosine arabinoside and 5-fluorodeoxyuridine (FUDR) can also result in unbalanced growth, and all of these inhibitors can produce changes in the morphologic appearance of cells which have been characterized as being megaloblastic. Whereas cytosine arabinoside appears to inhibit only DNA synthesis, the fact that methotrexate may also inhibit RNA, and possibly protein synthesis as well as DNA synthesis, has led to some recent studies of great interest. Thus methotrexate inhibition not only of thymidylate biosynthesis, but also RNA synthesis and protein synthesis, could result in less unbalanced growth and possibly less cell kill. This appears to be true for at least one cell type grown in vitro, the L cell. When these cells were grown in the presence of a purine nucleoside, deoxyadenosine, thus allowing methotrexate to act as a "pure" DNA synthesis inhibitor, inhibition of logarithmic cell growth by methotrexate was more marked than when cells were grown in the absence of deoxyadenosine.[32] Thus, it has been postulated that methotrexate may limit its own killing ability in some cells by inhibiting not only DNA synthesis but also RNA and protein synthesis. In this circumstance the addition of a purine base has led to an increase in the ability of methotrexate to kill cells in vitro. The implications of this finding are of great importance. Combinations of methotrexate with other drugs that inhibit RNA or protein synthesis may be disadvantageous; indeed, asparaginase, an inhibitor of protein synthesis, has been shown to block the action of methotrexate when these drugs are used together.[33]

Metabolism, Distribution and Excretion of Folate Antagonists

Significant species differences exist in the metabolic handling of the folate antagonists. Furthermore, the folate antagonists differ among themselves in their susceptibility to metabolic alteration; as a general rule, the halogenated analogues are metabolized much more readily than are the non-halogenated analogues.

In the case of the non-halogenated analogue methotrexate (MTX), most of the drug appears in the urine in unchanged form in the first 48 hours after oral or parenteral administration to human subjects.[34-36] In typical experiments, urinary excretion of MTX during this initial period ranged from 56 per cent of the original administered dose at an MTX dose-level of 2.5 μg per kg,[35] to 83 per cent at a dose level of 10 mg per kg.[36] This initial excretion, however, represents primarily "surplus" drug, i.e., drug in excess of the amount required to bind the target enzyme dihydrofolate reductase; the therapeutically active fraction of the total administered dose is tightly bound by tissue dihydrofolate reductase. There is a detectable urinary excretion rate of 1 to 2 per cent of the retained dose per day for several weeks after a single dose;[35] a kinetic analysis of such a low continuous excretion rate suggests at least two possible explanations: slow release from tissue dihydrofolate reductase with subsequent kidney clearance; and slow appearance in the systemic circulation and hence low kidney clearance, as a result of enterohepatic circulation and intestinal reabsorption. It is likely that both these processes occur simultaneously, and it remains to be determined which predominates in its contribution to urinary excretion.

When urine samples from these later time periods are examined chromatographically, the presence of two MTX metabolites can be detected; in a typical experiment, these compounds, although constituting only a small fraction of the original administered dose, together accounted for 60 per cent of the drug being excreted at 19 days after administration, while unchanged MTX at this time amounted to only 38 per cent.[35] Similarly, in the mouse and rat, non-MTX radioactivity can be detected in urine and feces after administration of the labeled drug.[37,38] The identity of these MTX metabolites in rodents and in man has not been established; their chromatographic properties, however, are compatible with those of compounds lacking the glutamate moiety of MTX.[39] Sterilization of the intestinal tract of the mouse results in a significant decrease in the ratio of MTX metabolites to unchanged MTX in the urine and feces, indicating that gut bacteria acting on that fraction of the administered MTX which undergoes enterohepatic circulation might be responsible for the metabolic alteration observed.[37] The possible significance of these observations in the use of the drug in man have not been explored; this pathway, however, would appear to be of lesser quantitative importance in man than in the mouse or rat. This difference may arise because excretion of MTX by the biliary route appears to be less significant in man than in rodents.[36]

Certain species, notably the rabbit and the guinea pig, are able to catalyze the rapid oxidation of MTX to 7-hydroxyMTX;[40-42] the enzyme catalyzing this conversion has been identified as hepatic aldehyde oxidase (EC 1.2.3.1).[43] 7-HydroxyMTX is less than one-one hundredth as active as the parent compound as an inhibitor of dihydrofolate reductase;[42] this oxidation appears to account, therefore, for the unusually high resistance of the rabbit and the guinea pig to antifolate toxicity.[44] Although the enzyme aldehyde oxidase is present in human liver, it lacks the ability to utilize MTX as a substrate, and such a conversion does not take place to a measurable extent in man. Human liver aldehyde oxidase can, however, catalyze the 7-hydroxylation of the MTX analogue, dichloroMTX (DCM).[45]

DCM and the other halogenated analogues of MTX are much more susceptible to metabolic alteration than is the parent compound. Oliverio and Loo[46] showed that DCM undergoes metabolic alteration in mice and in human subjects, yielding 7-hydroxyDCM. A number of other halogenated analogues of MTX and aminopterin undergo a similar conversion when incubated with liver homogenates.[47] 7-Hydroxy-

DCM, like 7-hydroxyMTX, is a relatively weak inhibitor of dihydrofolate reductase, and it would appear likely that the low toxicity of DCM is at least partially a consequence of its rapid oxidation in vivo.[48] That this difference in rates of metabolism is not the sole explanation of the difference in DCM and MTX toxicity, however, is indicated by the observation that dogs, which are unable to metabolize either compound, exhibit 12 times as much tolerance to DCM as to MTX.[49]

Distribution

After administration to man or other mammalian species, MTX and other folate antagonists accumulate in highest concentration in the liver, kidneys, and spleen, where they can be shown to persist for several weeks.[50–52] The distribution of antifolates in man in vivo has been studied using 3′-iodoaminopterin labeled with the gamma emitter iodine-131; the distribution of the drug could then be followed by external scanning.[53] By this method, the accumulation of the drug in liver and kidney could be visualized; an additional finding of interest was the presence of considerable labeled drug in the sternal bone marrow.

The amount of MTX or aminopterin retained by a given tissue correlates well with the tissue level of dihydrofolate reductase, and it appears likely that this enzyme, with its extremely high affinity for folate antagonists, is responsible for the long-term tissue binding of the drug.[54] Additional evidence supporting this concept is the observation that other agents with affinity for this enzyme (e.g., pteroylglutamate, dihydropteroylglutamate) are effective in displacing bound MTX from tissues.[35] Werkheiser et al. have, in fact, suggested that aminopterin and MTX remain bound to the dihydrofolate reductase of the cell death, so that the rate of disappearance of bound MTX from tissues can be utilized as an index of the rate of cell turnover.[54,55] Since MTX binding to the enzyme, although tight, is readily reversible, however, it may be questioned whether such a label fulfills all the criteria for a valid cell protein label.

Although it would appear unlikely that other proteins are present in the cell which exhibit the extremely high affinity for MTX seen with dihydrofolate reductase, it is probable that binding between MTX and other proteins exists, and that such affinity contributes, in part, to the short-term and intermediate-term tissue retention of the drug. Silber et al.[56] have described an aminopterin-binding protein fraction distinct from dihydrofolate reductase in chicken liver extracts, and MTX-binding to non-dihydrofolate reductase tissue components has been reported by Condit and Yoshino[57] and Rothenberg and da Costa.[58]

Excretion

MTX is excreted in both the urine and the bile. In man, following intravenous doses in the therapeutic range (0.1–10 mg/kg), MTX appears mainly in the urine, with excretion in the feces representing only a minor route (2–5 per cent of the injected dose).[36] In the mouse, however, fecal excretion is more significant, with 12 to 40 per cent of the administered dose being excreted in this way.[59] In the rabbit, as indicated above, the disposition of the drug is anomalous, with virtually all of an intravenously administered dose being excreted in the urine as 7-hydroxyMTX, and with little or none of the unchanged drug being detectable.

Membrane Transport of Folate Antagonists

The investigation of MTX transport in mammalian cells was initiated in 1962 by

Fischer,[60] in the course of studies of MTX resistance in L5178Y murine leukemia cells. A clone of L5178Y cells was isolated which was resistant to MTX by virtue of defective transport of the drug: In MTX-sensitive cells, the intracellular level of MTX at equilibrium exceeded that of the medium by a factor of 2 to 3, while in resistant cells, the final MTX concentration was only 0.1 to 0.2 times that of the medium. In the sensitive cells, the intracellular MTX reached a concentration 10 times that which would be required to titrate the dihydrofolate reductase present. When the extracellular radioactive MTX was replaced by an equimolar level of nonradioactive MTX, a rapid displacement of intracellular radioactive MTX was observed. Folinic acid, 10 μM, inhibited the uptake of MTX by both sensitive and resistant cells.

Hakala[61,62] observed that with S-180 sarcoma cells, MTX influx was slow and proportional to concentration over a wide concentration range, a finding compatible with a process of free diffusion; a slight deviation from direct proportionality was noted at extremely high MTX concentrations. In addition, as with L5178Y cells, MTX uptake was slowed by folinic acid. These two latter observations would appear to indicate that the process is not one of simple diffusion, but rather of facilitated transport with a low affinity constant.

Werkheiser and his associates[63] have studied the uptake of MTX by MTX-resistant P-388 mouse leukemia cells. Good correlation was seen between the rate of entry of MTX and MTX sensitivity. Similarly, Kessel et al.[64] have shown that uptake of MTX correlates well with MTX sensitivity in a number of transplantable mouse leukemias including the P-388 and the L1210.

Kessel and Hall[65] have studied the uptake of MTX by L1210 cells and Ehrlich ascites cells, and Braganca and her coworkers[66,67] have studied the transport of aminopterin by aminopterin-sensitive and aminopterin-resistant Yoshida sarcoma cells. The primary mode of aminopterin resistance in Yoshida cells appeared to be defective transport of the drug. One of the resistant lines studied showed an increased level of dihydrofolate reductase; however, when the resistant cells were serially transplanted, the enzyme returned to normal levels although resistance and impaired aminopterin transport remained. These authors suggest that defective transport of antifolates by resistant cells may escape detection because, if dihydrofolate reductase is also elevated, transport may appear to be normal or increased unless precations are taken to distinguish clearly between the processes of transport and enzyme binding. In these studies, the resistant Yoshida cells could be shown to have an altered cell surface, being more resistant to lysis by snake venom lipases than were the sensitive cells.

In studies with L1210 cells, Sirotnak et al.[68] were able to detect intracellular MTX levels which, at equilibrium, exceeded extracellular levels by as much as 11 times, even after correction for the fraction of intracellular MTX bound to dihydrofolate reductase. Folate and dihydrofolate were shown to compete for the MTX uptake process, although a 100-fold excess over the MTX level was required for significant inhibition of uptake.

Goldman et al.[69] have studied both the unidirectional influx and efflux of MTX in L1210 cells grown in tissue culture. The transport process was temperature-sensitive, carrier-mediated, and uphill, and demonstrated Michaelis-Menten kinetics with a high degree of structural specificity. Folic acid and leucovorin (folinic acid, N^5-formyltetrahydrofolic acid) competed for MTX transport; addition of leucovorin to cells at the steady state resulted in counter transport of intracellular MTX. Leucovorin did not bring about the displacement of the intracellular MTX which was bound to dihydrofolate reductase, a result compatible with the observation that in vivo leucovorin is ineffective in displacing enzyme-bound MTX.[70]

As several of the studies cited above have shown, leucovorin competes for and inhibits the uptake of MTX. It would be anticipated, therefore, that the reverse process would also occur, i.e., that MTX would compete for the transport of leucovorin. Nahas et al.[71] have shown the uptake of labeled leucovorin by L1210 cells to be competitively inhibited by MTX ($K_I = 7.7\ \mu M$). Efflux of leucovorin was accelerated by MTX, while folic acid had no effect on either influx or efflux. It was suggested that leucovorin "rescue" of cells from the effects of MTX might be due not only to the repletion of intracellular pools of reduced folates, but also to the ability of leucovorin to inhibit the influx and accelerate the cellular efflux of MTX. This finding that MTX accelerates the efflux of leucovorin serves also to elucidate the early and well documented, but hitherto unexplained, observation, that the administration of either methotrexate or aminopterin results in a transient but significant increase in the urinary excretion of leucovorin in both man and experimental animals.[72,73]

Resistance to Folate Antagonists

Patients with neoplasms who are treated with folate antagonists may show little or no response, i.e., are naturally resistant, or may show partial or complete response, followed in most instances by the development of acquired drug resistance. An increase in dihydrofolate reductase, presumably due to decreased enzyme degradation,[29,74–76] together with poor transport, appears to provide a satisfactory explanation of the natural resistance to methotrexate observed in patients with acute myelocytic leukemia.[3,77] A binding protein capable of binding folic acid as well as methotrexate has been reported to be present in cells of some patients with chronic myelocytic leukemia; the relation of this finding to acquired drug resistance deserves further investigation.[58,78]

The biochemical mechanism of acquired resistance to methotrexate is less well understood. Some evidence has been presented that indicates that altered permeability of cells to methotrexate may explain certain instances of acquired resistance in patients with acute lymphatic leukemia,[79,80] but further work needs to be done in this difficult area.

Resistance to methotrexate in L5178Y cells occurred at a frequency of 8.0 in 10^6 cells, where the concentration of methotrexate was 7.2×10^{-8}M. Higher concentrations of drug were associated with a lower number of resistant mutants.[81] In experimental tumors, induced resistance to methotrexate is most often associated with an increase in dihydrofolate reductase, sometimes several hundredfold over the level of the sensitive parent line.[82–84] Occasional resistant lines have been characterized to contain normal levels of altered enzyme with a decreased affinity for methotrexate[85] or to transport methotrexate poorly, as described in the previous section.[60,63,66–68]

New Developments in Chemotherapy with Folate Antagonists

In this section we present a brief review of recent work with new folate antagonists or new approaches with known drugs.

New Folate Antagonists

Quinazoline antifolates. A new series of folate antagonists, the quinazoline antifolates, has been the subject of recent biochemical, pharmacologic, and preclinical study.[86–88] These compounds are related in structure to aminopterin and MTX, with the difference, however, that the 5- and 8-nitrogens of the pteridine ring system have been replaced by carbons.[89] Several of these compounds are as effective (as is MTX) as inhibitors of dihydrofolate reductase from L1210 mouse leukemia cells and from human myelocytic leukemia cells.[87,90] Below pH 7, the 5-chloro derivative of N-(*p*-(((2,4-diamino-6-quinazolinyl)methyl)amino)benzoyl)-L-glutamic acid, and its aspartyl analogue, like MTX, act as "stoichiometric" or "titrating" inhibitors of L1210 cell dihydrofolate reductase, i.e., inhibition is virtually complete at equimolar concentrations of inhibitor and enzyme. At alkaline pH, these compounds retain their activity as stoichiometric inhibitors, in contrast to MTX, which can be shown to be a reversible competitive inhibitor under these conditions.[91] Substitution of glutamate by aspartate does not result in a decrease in inhibitory activity, an unexpected result in view of earlier findings that a similar substitution in the 2,4-diaminopteridine series results in decreased activity.[92]

In vivo, several members of the quinazoline series are effective against L1210 mouse leukemia[86] and against dog lymphosarcoma.[93] The quinazoline antifolates are more effective than MTX in inhibiting the incorporation of deoxyuridine radioactivity into the DNA of L1210 mouse leukemia cells;[87] the basis for this difference has not been established. The quinazoline antifolate N-(*p*-(((2,4-diamino-5-chloro-6-quinazolinyl)-methyl)amino)benzoyl)-L-aspartic acid, significantly inhibited the uptake of ^{3}H-MTX by L1210 cells, an observation compatible with a shared mechanism of transport for the two compounds, although the possibility of additional modes of cell entry for the quinazolines has not been excluded.[87] The quinazoline antifolates are more effective than is MTX as an inhibitor of thymidylate synthetase; in this respect, the 2-amino-4-hydroxy-quinazolines are much more active than is the 2,4-diamino series.[94]

Pyrimidine and triazine folate antagonists. It has long been recognized that certain 2,4-diamino-pyrimidines and triazines are inhibitors of dihydrofolate reductase,[95–98] and the studies by Baker and his colleagues have resulted in the design of several new potent inhibitors of mammalian dihydrofolate reductase which are based on these purine and triazine ring structures.[99,100] These newer agents were developed as a consequence of investigations which led to the finding that the L1210 dihydrofolate reductase had a hydrophobic region which interacted with certain of these compounds, thus leading to a great increase in binding energy of the inhibitor to the enzyme.[97] It is also clear now that the differential effects of certain inhibitors on dihydrofolate reductase from various species, demonstrated by Burchall and Hitchings[101] and Baker and Ho,[102] derive from differences in this hydrophobic binding region, rather than differences in the active site of enzymes. As a result of these differences which have already led to the development of new antibacterial folate antagonists with little toxicity in man,[103] Baker has continued his search for differences in neoplastic and normal dihydrofolate reductases, using the mouse liver, spleen, intestine and the L1210 tumor as models. Differences in the metabolism of some of these compounds by these tissues has been elucidated,[104–106] but thus far no significant differences in binding energies of these compounds for the enzyme from leukemic tissues and normal tissues has been found. However, these differences, if present, may be small, and their demonstration could require purification and complete amino acid sequencing of dihydrofolate reductase from these sources.

Despite these difficulties, several triazine folate antagonists have been synthesized that are highly active when tested against the Walker 256 carcinoma in vivo, and further preclinical (and perhaps clinical) studies with these compounds are warranted.[107,108]

New Uses for Folate Antagonists

Dichloromethotrexate as an intra-arterial agent. 3′,5′Dichloromethotrexate (DCM), although not in general clinical use, appears to be as effective therapeutically as methotrexate (MTX) in man,[109] and considerably more effective than MTX in certain mouse leukemias.[110] Since DCM, unlike MTX, undergoes partial metabolic inactivation in man,[111] being converted to 7-hydroxyDCM by hepatic aldehyde oxidase, the possibility exists that larger doses of DCM than would be feasible with MTX could be delivered by regional perfusion to the tumor site, before the level of systemic toxicity is reached. In a recent study,[111] DCM was administered to 12 patients with cancer of the head and neck by continuous infusion via the external carotid artery, at a dose level of 10 mg per day for 7 to 10 days. Objective therapeutic response was noted in 8 of 10 patients with epidermoid carcinoma. Two patients with basal cell carcinoma and adenocarcinoma of the parotid gland showed no response. Although all patients developed local toxicity in 7 to 18 days, only two patients showed systemic toxicity at the dosages used.

On similar grounds, DCM would also appear to be of possible value in the treatment of primary hepatic carcinoma, where continuous infusion of MTX via the hepatic artery is currently the chemotherapeutic regimen of choice.[112] In preliminary clinical trials, however, DCM appears to offer no advantage over MTX in the treatment of this form of cancer.[113]

Leucovorin "rescue." Leucovorin, a reduced stable folate coenzyme, can act as an antidote for methotrexate inhibition by bypassing the block imposed by methotrexate. Recent studies of leucovorin uptake have also shown that leucovorin can block methotrexate uptake by competing with the latter for the same uptake mechanism.[71] Early studies of Goldin and coworkers,[114] recently extended,[115] using L1210 leukemia clearly demonstrate that leucovorin, if used at the correct interval after methotrexate administration, can actually improve the therapeutic index of methotrexate. This concept of leucovorin rescue has been extended to the clinic, and an increase in the therapeutic index of methotrexate appears to have been obtained in patients with acute leukemia,[1,3] malignant lymphoma,[116,117] epidermoid carcinoma of the head and neck[4,12] and mycosis fungoides,[118] but not in patients with acute myelocytic leukemia[3] or psoriasis.[119]

The exact reasons why leucovorin improves the therapeutic index of methotrexate in experimental animals and perhaps in man is not entirely clear, but it may relate to differences in the kinetics of growth of normal and tumor tissues, as well as to biochemical differences between these tissues. If the tumor cells are characterized by a short generation time, with few cells in the resting or G_0 state, several logs of cell kill may be expected from exposure to high intermittent courses of methotrexate; these cells may not be rescued by leucovorin if this antidote is delayed for an appropriate period of time. Normal bone marrow and mucosa stem cells, primarily in a resting or G_0 stage, will be much less affected by the short exposure to methotrexate, since they will be "rescued" by subsequent leucovorin. Some evidence also exists that small doses of leucovorin may actually increase methotrexate effects by providing enough folate coenzymes for purine but not for thymidylate biosynthesis.[32] It is also possible that leucovorin may not block methotrexate action completely in certain cells, if methotrexate has more than one site of action.[120]

Recent studies in man, using radiolabeled leucovorin, have demonstrated that this compound is absorbed readily, and rapidly enters the reduced folate coenzyme pool.[121,122] Thus leucovorin may be given orally and has been demonstrated to be effective when given by this route in both animals and man.[117,123]

Folate Deficiency

The use of folate deficiency induced by dietary restriction for treatment of human malignancy has not received much attention, since the advent of potent folate antagonists which are capable of more rapidly causing the folate deficiency state. Heinle and Welch, in a study over 20 years ago, did demonstrate this effect of a folate deficient diet in a patient with leukemia.[124] Recent studies of Rosen et al.[125,126] with the Walker 256 carcinoma demonstrated that this tumor is sensitive to folate depletion produced by dietary means, but not to methotrexate therapy. This led to renewed interest in this form of therapy, but treatment of seven patients with a folate deficient diet for several months demonstrated the difficulties in carrying out such therapy; patient acceptance was poor and folate deficiency takes several months to accomplish.[127] No significant tumor responses were seen in this group of patients treated. With these difficulties in mind, our laboratory has reinvestigated this problem using an enzyme capable of hydrolyzing folate coenzymes in order to cause rapid folate depletion.[128] The therapeutic usefulness of this enzyme is now under investigation.

References

1. Djerassi, I.: Methotrexate infusions and intensive supportive care in the management of children with acute lymphocytic leukemia: Follow-up report. Cancer Res. 27:2564, 1967.
2. Lane, M., Moore, J. E., III, Levin, H. and Smith, F. E.: Methotrexate therapy for squamous cell carcinoma of the head and neck. J.A.M.A. 204:561, 1968.
3. Hryniuk, W. M. and Bertino, J. R.: The treatment of leukemia with large doses of methotrexate and folinic acid: Clinical-biochemical correlates. J. Clin. Invest. 48:2140, 1969.
4. Schwarzenberg, L., Mathé, G., Hayat, M., DeVassal, F., Amiel, J. L., et al.: Une nouvelle combination de methotrexate et l'acide folinique pour le traitement des cancers. Presse Med. 77:385, 1969.
5. Bertino, J. R. and Johns, D. G.: Folate antagonists. Ann. Rev. Med. 18:27, 1967.
6. Hertz, R., Lewis, J., Jr. and Lipsett, M. B.: Five years' experience with the chemotherapy of metastatic choriocarcinoma and related trophoblastic tumors in women. Amer. J. Obstet. Gynec. 82:631, 1961.
7. "Acute Leukemia Group B": New treatment schedule with improved survival in childhood leukemia: Intermittent parenteral versus daily oral administration of methotrexate for maintenance of induced remission. J.A.M.A. 194:75, 1961.
8. Burkitt, D. P. and Burchenal, J. H. (Eds.): Treatment of Burkitt's Tumor. New York: Springer Verlag, 1966.
9. Vogler, W. R., Furtado, V. P. and Huguley, C. M., Jr.: Methotrexate for advanced cancer of the breast. Cancer 21:26, 1968.
10. Wright, J. C., Gumport, S. L. and Golomb, F. M.: Remissions produced with the use of methotrexate in patients with mycosis fungoides. Cancer Chem. Rep. 9:11, 1960.
11. Leone, L. A., Albala, M. M. and Rege, V. B.: Treatment of carcinoma of the head and neck with intravenous methotrexate. Cancer 21:828, 1968.
12. Capizzi, R. L., DeConti, R. C., Marsh, J. C. and Bertino, J. R.: Methotrexate therapy of head and neck cancer: Improvement in therapeutic index by the use of leucovorin "rescue". Cancer Res. 30:1782, 1970.
13. Nervi, C., Arcangeli, G., Casale, C., Cortese, M., Guadagni, A., et al.: A reappraisal of intra-arterial chemotherapy. Cancer 26:577, 1970.
14. Van Scott, E. S., Auerbach, R. and Wein-

stein, G. D.: Parenteral methotrexate in psoriasis. Arch. Derm. 89:550, 1964.
15. McDonald, C. J. and Bertino, J. R.: Parenteral methotrexate for psoriasis. Lancet 1:864, 1968.
16. Capizzi, R. L. and Bertino, J. R.: Methotrexate therapy of Wegener's granulomatosis. Ann. Intern. Med. 74:74, 1971.
17. Hitchings, G. A.: Folate antagonists as antibacterial and antiprotozoal agents. Ann. N.Y. Acad. Sci. (in press, 1971).
18. Osborne, M. J., Freeman, M. and Huennekens, F. M.: Inhibition of dihydrofolic reductase by aminopterin and amethopterin. Proc. Soc. Exp. Biol. Med. 97:429, 1958.
19. Werkheiser, W. C.: Specific binding of 4-amino folic acid analogues by folic acid reductase. J. Biol. Chem. 236:888, 1961.
20. Bertino, J. R., Booth, B. A., Cashmore, A., Bieber, A. L. and Sartorelli, A. C.: Studies of the inhibition of dihydrofolate reductase by the folate antagonists. J. Biol. Chem. 239:479, 1964.
21. Huennekens, F. M.: The role of dihydrofolic reductase in the metabolism of one-carbon units. Biochemistry 2:151, 1963.
22. Perkins, J. P. and Bertino, J. R.: Dihydrofolate reductase from the L1210R murine lymphoma. Fluorimetric measurements of the interaction of the enzyme with coenzymes, substrates and inhibitors. Biochemistry 5:1005, 1966.
23. Bertino, J. R.: The mechanism of action of the folate antagonists in man. Cancer Res. 23:1286, 1963.
24. Wells, W. and Winzler, R. J.: Metabolism of human leukocytes *in vitro*. III. Incorporation of formate-C^{14} into cellular components of leukemic human leukocytes. Cancer Res. 19:1086, 1959.
25. Totter, J. R.: Incorporation of isotopic format into the thymine of bone marrow DNA *in vitro*. J. Amer. Chem. Soc. 76:2196, 1954.
26. Borsa, J. and Whitmore, G. F.: Studies relating to the mode of action of methotrexate. III. Inhibition of thymidylate synthetase in tissue culture cells and in cell-free systems. Molec. Pharmacol. 5:318, 1969.
27. Crusberg, T. C., Leary, R. and Kisliuk, R. L.: Properties of thymidylate synthetase from dichloromethotrexate-resistant *Lactobacillus casei*. J. Biol. Chem. 245:5292, 1970.
28. Roberts, D., Hall, T. C. and Rosenthal, D.: Coordinated changes in biochemical patterns. The effect of cytosine arabinoside and methotrexate on leukocytes from patients with acute granulocytic leukemia. Cancer Res. 29:571, 1969.
29. Bertino, J. R., Cashmore, A., Fink, M., Calabresi, P. and Lefkowitz, E.: The "induction" of leukocyte and erythrocyte dihydrofolate reductase by methotrexate. Clin. Pharmacol. Ther. 6:763, 1965.
30. Bruce, W. R., Meeker, B. C. and Valeriote, F. A.: Comparison of the sensitivity of normal hematopoietic and transplanted lymphoma colony forming cells to chemotherapeutic agents administered *in vivo*. J. Nat. Cancer Inst. 37:233, 1966.
31. Hryniuk, W. M., Fischer, G. A. and Bertino, J. R.: S phase cells of resting and log cultures: Qualitative and quantitative responses to methotrexate. Molec. Pharmacol. 5:577, 1969.
32. Borsa, J. and Whitmore, G.: Cell killing studies on the mode of action of methotrexate (MTX) on L-cells *in vitro*. Cancer Res. 29:737, 1969.
33. Capizzi, R. L., Summers, W. P. and Bertino, J. R.: Antagonism of the antineoplastic effect of methotrexate by L-asparaginase or L-asparagine deprivation. Proc. Amer. Ass. Cancer Res. 11:14, 1970.
34. Freeman, M. V.: The fluorometric measurement of the absorption, distribution, and excretion of single doses of 4-amino-10-methylpteroylglutamic acid (amethopterin) in man. J. Pharmacol. Exp. Ther. 122:154, 1958.
35. Johns, D. G., Hollingsworth, J. W., Cashmore, A. R., Plenderleith, I. H. and Bertino, J. R.: Methotrexate displacement in man. J. Clin. Invest. 43:621, 1964.
36. Henderson, E. S., Adamson, R. H. and Oliverio, V. T.: The metabolic fate of tritiated methotrexate. II. Absorption and excretion in man. Cancer Res. 25:1018, 1965.
37. Zaharko, D. S., Bruckner, H., and Oliverio, V. T.: Antibiotics alter methotrexate metabolism and excretion. Science 166:887, 1969.
38. Zaharko, D. S. and Oliverio, V. T.: Reinvestigation of methotrexate metabolism in rodents. Biochem. Pharmacol. (in press, 1970).
39. Oliverio, V. T.: Personal communication.
40. Johns, D. G., Iannotti, A. T., Sartorelli, A. C., Booth, B. A. and Bertino, J. R.: Enzymic oxidation of methotrexate and aminopterin. Life Sci. 3:1383, 1964.
41. Redetzki, H. M., Redetzki, J. E. and Elias, A. L.: Resistance of the rabbit to metho-

trexate: Isolation of a drug metabolite with decreased cytotoxicity. Biochem. Pharmacol. 15:425, 1966.
42. Johns, D. G., and Loo, T. L.: Metabolite of 4-amino-4-deoxy-N^{10}-methylpteroylglutamic acid (methotrexate). J. Pharm. Sci. 56:356, 1967.
43. Johns, D. G., Iannotti, A. T., Sartorelli, A. C., Booth, B. A. and Bertino, J. R.: The identity of rabbit-liver methotrexate oxidase. Biochim. Biophys. Acta 105:380, 1965.
44. Minnich, V., Moore, C. V., Smith, D. E. and Elliott, G. V.: Studies on the acute toxic effects of 4-aminopteroylglutamic acid in dogs, guinea pigs, and rabbits. Arch. Path. 50:787, 1950.
45. Cleveland, J. C., Johns, D. G., Farnham, G. and Bertino, J. R.: Arterial infusion of dichloromethotrexate in cancer of the head and neck: A clinico-pharmacologic study. Curr. Topics Surg. Res. 1:113, 1969.
46. Oliverio, V. T. and Loo, T. L.: Separation and isolation of metabolites of folic acid antagonists. Proc. Amer. Ass. Cancer Res. 3:140, 1960.
47. Loo, T. L. and Adamson, R. H.: The enzymic oxidation of certain folic acid antagonists. Biochem. Pharmacol. 11:170, 1962.
48. Misra, D. K., Adamson, R. H., Loo, T. L. and Oliverio, V. T.: Inhibition of dihydrofolate reductase by dichloromethotrexate and its metabolite. Life Sci. 2:407, 1963.
49. Rall, D. P., Pallotta, A. J. and Elsea, J. R.: Comparative toxicity of amethopterin, 3′-monochloromethopterin, and 3′,5′-dichloroamethopterin in rats and dogs. Proc. Amer. Ass. Cancer Res. 3:54, 1959.
50. Charache, S., Condit, P. T. and Humphreys, S. R.: Studies of the folic acid vitamins. IV. The persistence of amethopterin in mammalian tissues. Cancer 13:236, 1960.
51. Fountain, J. R., Hutchison, D. J., Waring, G. B. and Burchenal, J. H.: Persistence of amethopterin in normal mouse tissues. Proc. Soc. Exp. Biol. Med. 83:396, 1953.
52. Anderson, L. L., Collins, G. J., Ojima, Y. and Sullivan, R. D.: A study of the distribution of methotrexate in human tissues and tumors. Cancer Res. 30:1344, 1970.
53. Johns, D. G., Spencer, R. P., Chang, P. K. and Bertino, J. R.: ^{131}I-3′-Iodoaminopterin: A gamma-labeled active-site-directed enzyme inhibitor. J. Nucl. Med. 9:530, 1968.
54. Werkheiser, W. C.: The relation of folic acid reductase to aminopterin toxicity. J. Pharmacol. Exp. Ther. 137:167, 1962.
55. Darzynkiewicz, A., Rogers, A. W., Barnard, E. A., Wang, D.-H. and Werkheiser, W. C.: Autoradiography with tritiated methotrexate and the cellular distribution of folate reductase. Science 151:1528, 1966.
56. Silber, R., Huennekens, F. M. and Gabrio, B. W.: Studies on the interaction of tritium-labeled aminopterin with dihydrofolic reductase. Arch. Biochem. Biophys. 100:525, 1963.
57. Condit, P. T. and Yoshino, T.: Isolation and properties of two binding sites of methotrexate (MTX) in the mouse. Proc. Amer. Ass. Cancer Res. 10:15, 1969.
58. Rothenberg, S. P. and da Costa, M.: Characterization of a folic acid-binding factor in leukemic cells. J. Clin. Invest. 49:82a, 1970 (abstract).
59. Henderson, E. S., Adamson, R. H., Denham, C. and Oliverio, V. T.: The metabolic fate of tritiated methotrexate. I. Absorption, excretion, and distribution in mice, rats, dogs, and monkeys. Cancer Res. 25:1008, 1965.
60. Fischer, G. A.: Defective transport of amethopterin (methotrexate) as a mechanism of resistance to the antimetabolite in L5178Y leukemic cells. Biochem. Pharmacol. 11:1233, 1962.
61. Hakala, M. T.: On the role of drug penetration in amethopterin resistance of sarcoma-180 cells *in vitro*. Biochim. Biophys. Acta 102:198, 1965.
62. Hakala, M. T.: On the nature of permeability of sarcoma-180 cells to amethopterin *in vitro*. Biochim. Biophys. Acta 102:210, 1965.
63. Werkheiser, W. C., Law, L. W., Roosa, R. A. and Nichol, C.A.: Further evidence that selective uptake modifies cellular response to the 4-amino folate antagonists. Proc. Amer. Ass. Cancer Res. 4:71, 1963.
64. Kessel, D., Hall, T. C., Roberts, D. and Wodinsky, I.: Uptake as a determinant of methotrexate response in mouse leukemias. Science 150:752, 1965.
65. Kessel, D. and Hall, T. C.: Amethopterin transport in Ehrlich ascites carcinoma and L1210 cells. Cancer Res. 27:1539, 1967.
66. Braganca, B. M., Divekar, A. Y. and Vaidya, N. R.: Defective transport of aminopterin in relation to development of resistance in Yoshida sarcoma cells. Biochim. Biophys. Acta 135:937, 1967.
67. Divekar, A. Y., Vaidya, N. R. and Braganca, B. M.: Active transport of aminopterin in

Yoshida sarcoma cells. Biochim. Biophys. Acta 135:927, 1967.
68. Sirotnak, F. M., Kurita, S. and Hutchison, D. J.: On the nature of a transport alteration determining resistance to amethopterin in the L1210 leukemia. Cancer Res. 28:75, 1968.
69. Goldman, I. D., Lichtenstein, N. S. and Oliverio, V. T.: Carrier-mediated transport of the folic acid analogue methotrexate in the L1210 leukemia cells. J. Biol. Chem. 243:5007, 1968.
70. Johns, D. G., Hollingsworth, J. W., Cashmore, A. R., Plenderleith, I. H. and Bertino, J. R.: Methotrexate displacement in man. J. Clin. Invest. 43:621, 1964.
71. Nahas, A., Nixon, P. F. and Bertino, J. R.: Uptake of 5-formyl-tetrahydrofolate by L1210 mouse leukemia cells and its effect on uptake of methotrexate. Proc. Amer. Ass. Cancer Res. 10:64, 1969.
72. Li, M. C., Nixon, W. E. and Freeman, M. V.: Increase of urinary citrovorum factor activity in patients receiving methotrexate (amethopterin). Proc. Soc. Exp. Biol. Med. 97:29, 1958.
73. Nichol, C. A. and Welch, A. D.: On the mechanism of action of aminopterin. Proc. Soc. Exp. Biol. Med. 74:403, 1950.
74. Hillcoat, B. L., Swett, V. and Bertino, J. R.: Increase of dihydrofolate reductase activity in cultured mammalian cells after exposure to methotrexate. Proc. Nat. Acad. Sci. U.S.A. 58:1632, 1967.
75. Wilmanns, W.: Determination, characteristics and significance of dihydrofolic acid reductase in the white blood corpuscles of leukemic patients. Klin. Wschr. 40:533, 1962.
76. Grignani, F., Martelli, M. F. and Tonato, M.: Dihydrofolic reductase in human blood cells. II. Enzyme activity after amethopterin and actinomycin C administration. Enzym. Biol. 8:363, 1967.
77. Bertino, J. R., Hillcoat, B. L. and Johns, D. G.: Folate antagonists: Some biochemical and pharmacological considerations. Fed. Proc. 26:893, 1967.
78. Rothenberg, S.: A macromolecular factor in some leukemic cells which binds folic acid. Proc. Soc. Exp. Biol. Med. 133:428, 1970.
79. Kessel, D., Hall, T. C. and Roberts, D.: Modes of uptake of methotrexate by normal and leukemic leukocytes *in vitro*, and their relation to drug response. Cancer Res. 28:564, 1968.
80. Bertino, J. R.: Current studies of the folate antagonists in patients with acute leukemia. Cancer Res. 25:1614, 1965.
81. Fischer, G. A.: Resistance to folate antagonists. Ann. N.Y. Acad. Sci. (in press, 1971).
82. Fischer, G. A.: Increased levels of folic acid reductase as a mechanism of resistance to amethopterin in leukemic cells. Biochem. Pharmacol. 7:75, 1961.
83. Hakala, M. T., Zakrzewski, S. F. and Nichol, C. A.: Relation of folic acid reductase of amethopterin resistance in cultured mammalian cells. J. Biol. Chem. 236:952, 1961.
84. Misra, D. R., Humphreys, S. P., Friedkin, M., Goldin, A. and Crawford, E. J.: Increased dihydrofolate reductase activity as a possible basis of drug resistance in leukemia. Nature 189:39, 1961.
85. Greenberg, D. M.: Personal communication.
86. Hutchison, D. J.: Quinazoline antifolates: Biologic activities. Cancer Chemother. Rep., Part I, 52:697, 1968.
87. Johns, D. G., Capizzi, R. L., Nahas, A., Cashmore, A. R. and Bertino, J. R.: Quinazoline antifolates as inhibitors of dihydrofolate reductase from human leukemia cells. Biochem. Pharmacol. 19:1528, 1970.
88. Hutchison, D. J., Bjerregaard, M. R. and Schmid, F. A.: Quinazoline antifolates: Dosage schedules and maximal antileukemic activities. Proc. Amer. Ass. Cancer Res. 11:39, 1970.
89. Davoll, J.: U.S. Patent 3,472,851 (1969).
90. Hutchison, D. J., Sirotnak, F. M. and Albrecht, A. M.: Dihydrofolate reductase inhibition by the 2,4-diaminoquinazoline antifolates. Proc. Amer. Ass. Cancer Res. 10:41, 1969.
91. Bertino, J. R., Cashmore, A. R. and Johns, D. G.: Unpublished data.
92. Mead, J. A. R., Greenberg, N. H. and Schrecker, A. W.: The pharmacological and biochemical activity of 4-amino-4-deoxy-10-methyl-pteroylaspartic acid. Biochem. Pharmacol. 14:105, 1965.
93. Fölsch, E., Abboud, G., Gralla, E. and Bertino, J. R.: Studies with a 2,4-diamino-5-chloro-quinazoline antifolate: *In vitro* and *in vivo* correlates in normal and lymphosarcoma dogs. Ann. N.Y. Acad. Sci. (in press, 1971).
94. Bird, O. D., Vaitkus, J. W. and Clarke, J.: 2-Amino-4-hydroxyquinazolines as inhibi-

tors of thymidylate synthetase. Molec. Pharmacol. 6:573, 1970.

95. Timmis, G. M., Felton, D. G., Collier, H. O. S. and Huskinson, P. L.: 5-Arylazo-2,4,6-triaminopyrimidine. J. Pharm. Pharmacol. 9:46, 1957.
96. Modest, E. J., Schlein, H. N. and Foley, G. F.: Antimetabolite activity of 5-arylazopyrimidines. J. Pharm. Pharmacol. 9:68, 1957.
97. Modest, E. J.: Chemical and biological studies on 1,2,-dihydro-5-triazines. II. Three-component synthesis. J. Org. Chem. 21:1, 1956.
98. Hitchings, G. H., Falco, E. A., Elion, G. B., Singer, S., Waring, G. B., et al.: 2,4-Diaminopyrimidines as antagonists of folic acid and folinic acid. Arch. Biochem. Biophys. 40:479, 1952.
99. Baker, B. R. and Lourens, G. J.: Irreversible enzyme inhibitors. CV. Differential irreversible inhibition of vertebrate dihydro folic reductase by derivatives of 4,6-diamino - 1,2 - dihydro - 2,2 - dimethyl - 1 - phenyl-*s*-triazines substituted with a terminal sulfonyl fluoride. J. Med. Chem. 10:1113, 1967.
100. Baker, B. R. and Janson, E. E.: Irreversible enzyme inhibitors. CLV. Active-site-directed irreversible inhibitors of dihydrofolic reductase derived from 1-[4-(w-aminoalkoxy) - 3 - chlorophenyl] - 4,6 - diamino-1,2-dihydro-2,2-dimethyl-*s*-triazines bearing a terminal sulfonyl fluoride. J. Med. Chem. 12:672, 1969.
101. Burchall, J. J. and Hitchings, G. H.: Inhibitor binding analysis of dihydrofolate reductoses from various species. J. Molec. Pharmacol. 1:126, 1965.
102. Baker, B. R. and Ho, B. T.: Differential inhibition of dihydrofolate reductase from different species. J. Pharm. Sci. 53:1137, 1964.
103. Bushby, S. R. M. and Hitchings, G. H.: Trimethoprim, a sulphonamide potentiator. Brit. J. Pharmacol. 33:72, 1968.
104. Fölsch, E. and Bertino, J. R.: Inactivation by mouse serum of a tightly bound inhibitor of dihydrofolate reductase. Molec. Pharmacol. 6:95, 1970.
105. Baker, B. R. and Vermeulen, M. J.: Irreversible enzyme inhibitors. CLXXVII. Active-site-directed irreversible inhibitors of dihydrofolate reductase derived from 4,6 - diamino - 1,2 - dihydro - 2,2 - dimethyl - 1 - (phenyl - alkylphenyl) - *s* - triazines. II. J. Med. Chem. 13:1154, 1970.
106. Baker, B. R. and Ashton, W. T.: Irreversible enzyme inhibitors. CLXXVIII. Active-site-directed irreversible inhibitors of dihydrofolate reductase derived from 1 - (4 - benzyloxy - 3 - chlorophenyl) - 4,6 - diamino - 2,2 - dihydro - 2,2 - dimethyl - *s* - triazine with a terminal sulfonyl fluoride. J. Med. Chem. 13:1161, 1970.
107. Fölsch, E., Cashmore, A., Gralla, E., Percy, D., Johns, D. G., et al.: 2,4-Diaminoquinazoline and 4,6-diaminotriazine antifolates: Biochemical and clinical studies with human leukemias and canine lymphosarcomas. Int. Cancer Congress (in press, 1970).
108. Baker, B. R., Vermeulen, N. M. J., Ashton, W. T. and Ryan, A. J.: Irreversible enzyme inhibitors. CLXXIII. Cure of Walker 256 ascites by reversible and irreversible inhibitors of dihydrofolate reductase derived from 1-(substituted phenyl) -4,6 - diamino - 1,2-dihydro - 2,2 - dimethyl-*s*-triazine. J. Med. Chem. 13:1130, 1970.
109. Frei, E., III, Spurr, C. L., Brindley, C. O., Selawry, O., Holland, J. F., et al.: Clinical studies of dichloromethotrexate (NSC 29630). Clin. Pharmacol. Ther. 6:160, 1965.
110. Goldin, A., Venditti, J. M., Humphreys, S. R. and Mantel, N.: Comparison of the relative effectiveness of folic acid congeners against advanced leukemia in mice. J. Nat. Cancer Inst. 19:1133, 1957.
111. Cleveland, J. C., Johns, D. G., Farnham, G. and Bertino, J. R.: Arterial infusion of dichloromethotrexate in cancer of the head and neck: A clinical-pharmacologic study. Curr. Topics Surg. Res. 1:113, 1969.
112. Falkson, G. and Geddes, E. W.: Controlled clinical trials in patients with primary liver cancer. Proc. Amer. Ass. Cancer Res. 11:25, 1970.
113. Vogel, C. L.: Personal communication.
114. Goldin, A., Mantel, N., Greenhouse, S. W., Venditti, J. M. and Humphreys, S. R.: Effect of delayed administration of CF on the antileukemic effectiveness of aminopterin in mice. Cancer Res. 14:43, 1954.
115. Goldin, A., Venditti, J. M., Kline, I. and Mantel, N.: Eradication of leukaemic cells (L1210) by methotrexate and methotrexate plus citrovorum factor. Nature 212:1548, 1966.
116. Djerassi, I., Royer, G., Treat, C. and Carim, H.: Management of childhood lymphosarcoma and reticulum cell sarcoma with high dose intermittent methotrexate

and citrovorum factor. Proc. Amer. Ass. Cancer Res. 9:18, 1968.

117. Levitt, M., DeConti, R. C., Marsh, J. C., Mitchell, M. S. and Bertino, J. R.: Combination therapy of reticulum cell sarcoma. J. Clin. Invest. (in press, 1971).

118. McDonald, C. J. and Bertino, J. R.: Unpublished observations.

119. Cipriano, A. D., Selsky, L. M. and Bertino, J. R.: Failure of leucovorin "rescue" in methotrexate treatment of psoriasis. Arch. Derm. 101:651, 1970.

120. Borsa, J. and Whitmore, G. F.: Studies relating to the mode of action of methotrexate. II. Studies of the sites of action in L-cells *in vitro*. Molec. Pharmacol. 5:303, 1969.

121. Nixon, P. F. and Bertino, J. R.: Absorption and utilization of oral 5-formyltetrahydrofolate. Fed. Proc. 29:610, 1970.

122. Baker, H., Frank, O., Feingold, S., Ziffer, H., Gellene, R. A., et al.: The fate of orally and parenterally administered folates. Amer. J. Clin. Nutr. 17:88, 1965.

123. Sandberg, J. S. and Goldin, A.: The use of leucovorin orally in normal and leukemic L1210 mice to prevent the toxicity of gastrointestinal lesions caused by high doses of methotrexate. Cancer Res. 30:1276, 1970.

124. Heinle, R. W. and Welch, A. D.: Experiments with pteroylglutamic acid and pteroylglutamic acid deficiency in human leukemia. J. Clin. Invest. 27:539, 1948.

125. Rosen, F., Sotobayashi, H. and Nichol, C. A.: Different effects of folic acid deficiency and treatment with amethopterin on the growth of several rat tumors. Proc. Amer. Assoc. Cancer Res. 5:54, 1964.

126. Rosen, F. and Nichol, C. A.: Inhibition of the growth of an amethopterin-refractory tumor by dietary restriction of folic acid. Cancer Res. 22:495, 1962.

127. Gailani, S. D., Carey, R. W., Holland, J. F. and O'Malley, J. A.: Studies of folate deficiency in patients with neoplastic diseases. Cancer Res. 30:327, 1970.

128. Bertino, J. R., O'Brien, P. and McCullough, J. L.: Inhibition of growth of leukemia cells by enzymic folate depletion. Science 172:161, 1971.

Mechanisms of Action of Purine and Pyrimidine Analogues*

By GEORGE H. HITCHINGS, PH.D. AND GERTRUDE B. ELION, D.SC.

IN THE CHEMOTHERAPEUTIC SENSE, the "mechanism of action" of an agent is the manner in which it exerts a selective effect. To be useful in chemotherapy, the drug must somehow be more damaging to the parasite or parasitic tissue than to any critically important tissue of the host. It is the goal of the biochemical chemotherapist to define this selectivity in biochemical—eventually enzymatic—terms. To date, this has been possible for only a limited number of agents, such as sulfonamides,[1] selective inhibitors of dihydrofolate reductase,[1-3] and penicillin.[4] It is not true of any agent used in cancer chemotherapy. What has been accomplished in cancer chemotherapy is the first step—the identification of loci of actions.[5-8] What remains to be done is the integration of this and other information still to be sought into a comprehensive scheme that will provide concepts of the selective effects of these agents.

Selectivity can be based on structural differences in the physical sense, i.e., location of the cell, its vascularization, temperature, tension, surface area, the nature of neighboring cells, etc. Differential effects based on such physical factors are likely to be small and unpredictable, and are generally unsuitable material for further developments. Differential effects based on biochemical factors may include transport at the intestinal, cellular, or renal level, or differences in catabolic or anabolic enzymes. It is the anabolic reactions which, justifiably, have received the greatest share of attention and hold the most promise for systematic exploitation of biochemical differences among cell types.

The nucleotides are the functional units of the purines and pyrimidines. They are the substrates for the enzymes which interconvert the heterocyclic moieties and for the

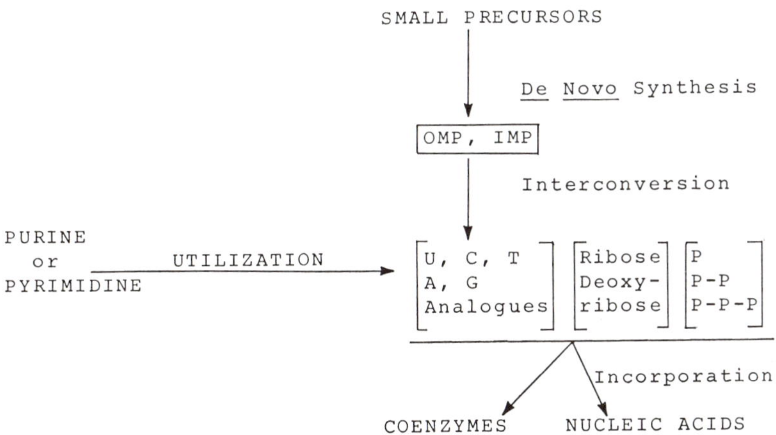

FIG. 1.—Scheme showing pathways for the formation and anabolism of nucleotides. In the central part of the scheme are shown the bases (uracil, cytosine, thymine, adenine and guanine), sugars, and phosphate derivatives (P = monophosphate, P-P = diphosphate, P-P-P = triphosphate).

From Burroughs Wellcome & Co., Research Triangle Park, North Carolina.

* *Reprinted, in slightly modified form, from Brodsky, I. and Kahn, S. B. (Eds.): Cancer Chemotherapy. New York: Grune & Stratton, Inc., 1967, pp. 26–36.*

polymerases which yield nucleic acids; in addition, they are components of various coenzymes. The formation of a nucleotide is essential to the activity of most, and perhaps all, of the base analogues. The most important evidence supporting this came from studies of resistant cells in which the specific pyrophosphorylase, requisite to the conversion of the base analogue to its nucleotide, had been deleted.[8,9] Although other mechanisms of resistance are possible, cells exhibiting such a deletion are universally indifferent to the analogue.

Figure 1 presents a generalized scheme for the biosynthesis of nucleotides and nucleic acids. In the purine series, the purine ring is built up, 1 to 3 atoms at a time, from phosphoribosylamine, and the nucleotide of hypoxanthine, inosinic acid (IMP), is the first structure which contains a purine as such. The first pyrimidine to be formed is orotic acid. It is converted to its ribonucleotide (OMP), which yields uridylic acid by decarboxylation. The formation of orotidylic acid by the reaction of the free heterocycle with phosphoribosylpyrophosphate, as catalyzed by a specific enzyme, illustrates the most important method of incorporation of all the free bases. A secondary route, more applicable to pyrimidines than to purines, is via the intermediate formation of a nucleoside and the phosphorylation of it by an appropriate kinase.

The two nucleotides, inosinic acid and uridylic acid, are analogous in that each serves as the precursor, in transformation reactions, for all the other nucleotides of the series. These reactions include alterations of the functional groups, reduction of the ribose to deoxyribose, and the coupling of additional phosphate residues through kinase reactions, producing, in all, about 40 nucleotides.

It is obviously impossible to present a balanced and comprehensive discussion of both purine and pyrimidine analogues within the evident space limitations of this volume. However, by concentrating attention on one outstanding member of each series, 5-fluorouracil and 6-mercaptopurine, respectively, it is hoped to bring out most of the principles involved.

The interconversion reactions of the pyrimidines are illustrated in Figure 2, which also serves to illustrate the participation of fluorouracil in anabolic reactions. Fluorouracil is incorporated rather extensively into the RNA of various species.[10,11] The formation of fluorouridine mono-, di- and triphosphates is thereby implied. The interference by fluorouracil with the incorporation of formate into the methyl group of thymine suggested interference with thymidylate synthetase.[8,11,12] The fluoro analogue of the substrate, deoxyuridylate, seemed the most probable inhibitor of this reaction; this supposition received support when fluorodeoxyuridine was synthesized

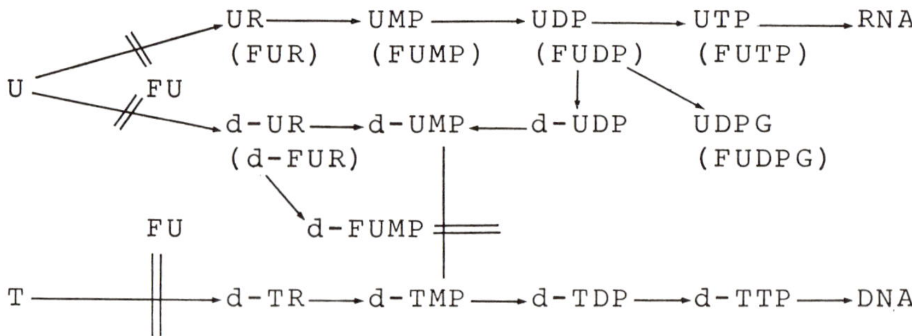

FIG. 2.—Scheme for pyrimidine interconversions involving uracil (U), 5-fluorouracil (FU), and thymine (T). Double lines indicate sites of inhibition.

and found to be some 4 orders of magnitude more potent than fluorouracil in inhibiting this reaction.[11] The identification of thymidylate synthetase as the most important locus of action of fluorouracil received support from studies on a resistant line of the Ehrlich ascites tumor in vitro[13] and in vivo[14] and from the demonstration by Lindner[15] that DNA synthesis was inhibited in ascites cells in mice treated with fluorouracil.

The incorporation of fluorouracil into ribonucleic acid might have been expected to interfere with the reading of the genetic code at several levels. However, polyfluorouridylate serves as a template for phenylalanine polymerizations as well as does polyuridylate, and fluorouracil can be incorporated into tobacco mosaic virus RNA with little obvious effect on its growth or infectivity. On the other hand, fluorouracil appears to block the induction of β-galactosidase, probably by its incorporation into a spurious messenger RNA, which results in the synthesis of a nonsense protein.[16–18] It is evident that the role of fluorouracil-containing RNA needs clarification, but it seems plausible at this point that analogue-containing RNA's may function normally in some situations and fail to function in others. The fact that fluorouridine is more toxic and less effective against tumors than fluorouracil[19] suggests that incorporation of the analogue into RNA is an undesirable reaction.

If one accepts the postulate that inhibition of thymidylate synthetase is the principal locus responsible for antitumor activity, how can one interpret the selective toxicity of fluorouracil? Some element of differential rate of cellular multiplication[20] probably is involved. It is true with fluorouracil, as it is with antimetabolites in general, that the more rapidly dividing cells are the more sensitive. However, the antitumor spectrum of fluorouracil does not fit this pattern very well, since the most sensitive tumors may be relatively slow-growing solid tumors rather than the leukemias. Heidelberger has put forward another suggestion, namely, that the degradation of the drug is slower and less complete in the tumor than in the normal cell.[11,21] Fluorouracil is rapidly and extensively degraded by normal tissues, and fluorodeoxyuridine is rapidly converted to FU in animal and human tissues. The possibility of inhibiting these degradative reactions has been and is being explored.[11] Successful solutions to these problems would almost certainly increase the potency of both drugs, but if, in fact, the selective toxicity depends on differential degradation, the chemotherapeutic index might as easily be worsened as improved.

The other 5-halogenouracils may be mentioned in passing. Neither bromouracil nor iodouracil is incorporated well by mammalian tissues, whether because of extensive degradation or because they are poor substrates for the necessary anabolic reactions. However, when the deoxynucleosides are provided, these substances do appear to be substrates for the kinases necessary for their conversion to the deoxynucleoside triphosphates, for both of them appear in DNA (Fig. 3).[5,6,8] The bromo- and iodo-

```
d-TR ──────→ d-TMP ──/──→ d-TDP ──/──→ d-TTP
                                              ↘
                                               DNA
                                              ↗
d-BrUR ────→ d-BrUMP ────→ d-BrUDP ────→ d-BrUTP
(BUDR)
(IUDR)
```

FIG. 3.—Anabolic pathways of incorporation of thymidine (d-TR), 5-bromodeoxyuridine (d-BrUR, BUDR) and 5-iododeoxyuridine (IUDR) into DNA. Dotted lines show loci of inhibition by the bromo analogues in the thymine nucleotide pathway.

derivatives provide quite a striking contrast to fluorodeoxyuridine, which is not incorporated into DNA.[22] This discrimination presumably reflects the same substrate specificity by which deoxyuridine is distinguished from thymidine by the kinases. The results with the halogenopyrimidines suggest that the diameter of the group in the pyrimidine-5 position may be a highly important recognition factor. It is interesting to speculate that a group of sufficient size may bring about an allosteric change in the enzyme that results in its activation.

Some of the reactions in which 6-mercaptopurine participates are illustrated in Figure 4. The first of these is its competition with hypoxanthine (Hx) for inosinic acid pyrophosphorylase[23] and its transformation to thioinosinic acid. Thioinosinic acid inhibits the formation of adenylic acid at two points, the conversion of inosinate to adenylosuccinate (SAMP)[24–26] and the conversion of adenylosuccinate to adenylic acid.[26–28] It inhibits the oxidation of inosinic to xanthylic acid (XMP),[24,29,30] and thus interferes with the formation of guanylic acid and may itself participate in these reactions. It is possible that thioinosinate is converted to di- and triphosphates which interfere with the formation of coenzymes and nucleic acids, and may participate in similar reactions to form analogue variants of these.

Mercaptopurine also inhibits the biosynthesis of purines from small molecule precursors such as glycine, formate, and phosphate.[8,31–33] The present view is that this represents a pseudo feedback inhibition by thioinosinic acid on the first step of purine biosynthesis, the conversion of phosphoribosylpyrophosphate to phosphoribosylamine.[34–36]

At one time or another, each of these and additional loci[38] have been put forward as *the* mechanism of action of 6-mercaptopurine. It is pertinent at this point to examine these reactions at the molecular level in an attempt to evaluate their possible relative contributions to the inhibition of tumor growth in vivo. Table 1 lists some of the enzymes that are inhibited by mercaptopurine in one of its forms, together with the binding constants for substrate (Km) and inhibitor (Ki). Studies on the pharmacokinetics of mercaptopurine[40–44] showed that plasma and tissue concentrations of the drug (total of all forms) following maximum tolerated doses might reach levels of a few micrograms per milliliters (as mercaptopurine), equivalent to about 10^{-5}M.[40,41] Many factors, in addition to the binding constants, will determine whether a given inhibition will be important to the economy of the cell as a whole. These include the relative importance of the reaction itself, the enzymatic activity or enzyme concentration, and the relative pool size of substrate and inhibitor. Several of the reactions listed can be eliminated on the ground that inhibition occurs only at concentrations of

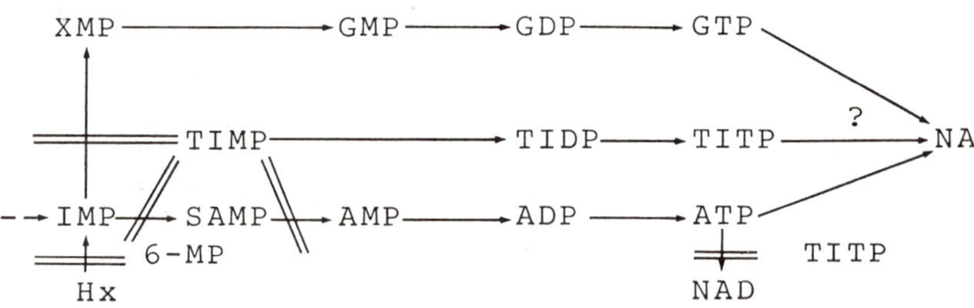

FIG. 4.—Scheme for purine interconversions and the loci of action of 6-mercaptopurine (6-MP), thioinosinic acid (TIMP), thioinosine diphosphate (TIDP) and thioinosine triphosphate (TITP). Double lines indicate inhibition.

TABLE 1.—*Enzymes Inhibited by 6-Mercaptopurine and Its Nucleotides**

Enzyme	*Source*	*Substrate*	K_m	*Inhibitor*	K_i	*Ref.*
SAMP synthetase	Ehrlich ascites	IMP	3×10^{-5}	TIMP	3×10^{-4}	26
IMP dehydrogenase	Ehrlich ascites	IMP	1.4×10^{-5}	TIMP	3.6×10^{-6}	30
IMP pyrophosphorylase	Ehrlich ascites	Hx	11×10^{-6}	6-MP	8.3×10^{-6}	23
Polynucleotide phosphorylase	Micrococcus lysodeikticus	ADP	(1.7×10^{-3})†	TIDP	(3.3×10^{-5})†	37
Glutamine-PRPP amidotransferase	Pigeon liver			TIMP	4.4×10^{-5}	36
NMN-adenylyl transferase	Hog liver	ATP	7.4×10^{-5}	TITP	3×10^{-4}	26
FAH_4 formate activating	Rat liver Human leukocytes	ATP	5×10^{-4}	6-MP	$3–25 \times 10^{-3}$	39

* Abbreviations: In addition to the abbreviations accepted as standard by the Journal of Biological Chemistry, the following have been used: SAMP = adenylosuccinate, 6-MP = 6-mercaptopurine, Hx = hypoxanthine, TIMP = 6-thioinosinic acid (6-mercaptopurine ribonucleotide), TIDP = 6-thioinosine diphosphate, TITP = 6-thioinosine triphosphate, and FAH_4 = tetrahydrofolate.
† 50% inhibition.

inhibitor much higher than those obtainable in vivo. This would be true of the formate-activating enzyme and particularly of SAMP-lyase, where the binding of substrate is a hundredfold greater than that of the inhibitor and the pool size of the metabolite is significantly large, especially in some tumors.[45] Inosinic acid pyrophosphorylase and polynucleotide phosphorylase are enzymes that probably are not critical to cell survival. The synthesis of coenzyme I (NAD, DPN) (Table 1, line 6) is inhibited by thioinosinetriphosphate (TITP), and the binding constants of substrate and inhibitor are similar. However, the formation of TITP in vivo has not been shown, and, in any case, its concentration is certainly several orders of magnitude lower than that of the substrate. Three enzymes deserve more detailed consideration. Inosinate dehydrogenase (Table 1, line 2) is sensitive to concentrations of thioinosinate which may be within the range attainable in vivo. Moreover, the intracellular concentration of inosinate is low, and it is less tightly bound than the inhibitor. Although adenylosuccinate synthetase does not bind the inhibitor as tightly as the substrate, it is possible that the inhibitor: substrate ratio may be within the inhibitory range in vivo. Inhibition of these enzymes would interfere with the transformation of inosinate to guanylate and adenylate, respectively. Each of these and glutamine-phosphoribosylpyrophosphate amidotransferase (Table 1, line 5) has been put forward as the principal site of action of 6-mercaptopurine, and each view has found some support in experiments at the cellular level and in vivo.

The incorporations of formate, glycine, and phosphate into nucleic acid purines are inhibited in mercaptopurine-treated cells and whole animals.[31–33,46,47] This could reflect inhibition of the transformations of inosinate to adenylate and guanylate or inhibition at some earlier step in purine biosynthesis. LePage and colleagues[34,48,49] and Wyngaarden and coworkers[36,50] have shown that feedback inhibition by mercaptopurine ribonucleotide does occur at the first step of purine biosynthesis, and the latter have shown that this reaction is more sensitive to thioinosinate than to adenylate or guanylate. Bennett et al.[35] feel that feedback inhibition is the primary site of action of mercaptopurine (ribonucleotide), since interference with the incorporation of formate and glycine occurred at levels of the drug much lower than those required to

TABLE 2.—*Chemotherapeutic Effectiveness and Feedback Inhibition in Tumors Treated with Thiopurines*

	Survival Time = Days			*Decrease in FGAR, %*	
Tumor	*Control*	*TG*	*6-MP*	*TG*	*6-MP*
Mecca lymphosarcoma	9.9	10.3	10.0	83	81
6C3H3D	13.1	13.0	12.9	64	28
Ehrlich ascites	15.9	22.0	20.5	80	48
S180	14.5	22.0	26.0	45	96
Adca. 755	11.6	17.0	23.0	76	62
TA3	8.0	14.5	23.0	84	65

TG = thioguanine, 6-MP = 6-mercaptopurine, FGAR = formylglycinamideribotide. Doses for survival time tests: TG = 0.5 mg/kg, 6-MP = 15 mg/kg, twice daily for 6 days. Doses for feedback inhibition studies: single doses of TG = 10 mg/kg, 6-MP = 15 mg/kg. (Data from LePage and Jones.[34])

show inhibition of incorporation of aminoimidazolecarboxamide or preformed purines into the nucleic acids. On the other hand, there is a considerable body of evidence which suggests that feedback inhibition by mercaptopurine is not critically important to tumor inhibition. Thus, Greenlees and LePage[49] found inhibition of the incorporation of glycine into the nucleic acid purines of 4 tumors treated with mercaptopurine, but only 2 of the tumors were inhibited. Le Page and Jones,[34] using thioguanine, found that the 2 least sensitive of 6 tumors showed as much suppression of FGAR accumulation as the most sensitive tumors or greater (Table 2). Similarly, the effects of mercaptopurine on formate incorporation were much the same in mercaptopurine-sensitive and resistant[51] lines of adenocarcinoma 755 (Table 3). Henderson[47] and Sartorelli[52] have both summarized discrepancies between the feedback and tumor-inhibitory activities of related thiopurines, and have directed attention to systems in which reversals of mercaptopurine inhibition could be related specifically either to adenine or guanine derivatives. Salser and Balis[25,45] noted differences in metabolite and enzyme activities between sarcoma 180 and host liver, which would make the tumor the more sensitive of the two to inhibition of interconversion steps. It may be pertinent also to point out[47] that the de novo pathway of purine biosynthesis can be blocked completely by azaserine,[53] but its action is potentiated by mercaptopurine and a number of additional purine analogues.[52,54,55] This is obviously inconsistent with

TABLE 3.—*Effect of 6-Mercaptopurine on the Incorporation of Formate into the DNA of Sensitive and Resistant Lines of Adenocarcinoma 755**
Inhibition of Formate Incorporation, %

	Ca. 755/+	*Ca. 755/MP*[59]
DNA	29.5	29.5
DNA Adenine	30.5	23.0
DNA Guanine	29	59.0

* Groups of C57BL mice bearing 20-day old tumors, Ca. 755/+ (6-MP-sensitive), or Ca. 755/MP (6-MP-resistant), were injected i.p. with 0.25 mg. sodium formate-C^{14} (3.2×10^7 cpm/mg) per mouse. The experimental animals (6 mice per group) received, in addition, 1 mg (= 50 mg/kg) of 6-MP. Control and experimental mice were sacrificed after 17 hours, tumors were excised and the DNA was isolated by the method of Kirby. The specific activity of the whole DNA was determined on the basis of the ultraviolet absorption spectrum and counts. The DNA was then hydrolyzed in 0.1*N* HCl for 1 hour in a boiling water bath and the adenine and guanine fractions were isolated from a Dowex-50 (H+) column. Results are given as the per cent decrease in the specific activities of the various fractions in the experimental groups as compared with the control groups.

the concept that the purine analogues act primarily on synthesis de novo, and rather strongly suggests that effects on the utilization of exogenous purines and purine interconversions may play an important role in tumor inhibition.

Still unmentioned is a considerable volume of work showing that mercaptopurine interferes with glycolysis.[8,56,57] To date, it has not been possible to relate this information to that dealing with nucleotides, although plausibly a connection with adenine nucleotides might be found if sought. Similarly, mercaptopurine interferes with the function of coenzyme A,[8,58] presumably through restriction of available adenylate or through formation of a spurious coenzyme A; but no probing into the mechanism of this interference has been reported. A curious dichotomy seems to exist separating, absolutely, glycolysis from nucleotide biochemistry.

A survey of loci of action of mercaptopurine results in more confusion than enlightenment if one is looking for definitive answers. It may be that some as yet undiscovered locus of action will be found, and this discovery will at once solve both problems, i.e., define the most sensitive site of action and satisfactorily explain the selective toxicity of the drug. This seems unlikely at the present writing. Perhaps one way of reconciling some of the divergences would be to assume that any one of several enzymatic reactions may be inhibited to a critical level in a given biologic system, depending on the balance of enzymic activities and enzyme specificity, pool size of metabolites, and other factors. It seems possible also that with so many enzyme inhibitions bordering on critical levels, synergisms among these may exist, e.g., feedback inhibition by thioinosinic acid may produce more favorable metabolite:antimetabolite ratios at other sites and so, in essence, mercaptopurine may serve the role of several sequential blockers. Additional comparative biochemistry is required in which comparisons are made of tumor with host tissues and sensitive with insensitive tumors. In striving to evaluate the present position, we should not lose sight of the fact that a great deal of ingenious and sophisticated biochemical knowledge already is in hand. This knowledge should serve well as a basis for further advances. We can discern in the effects of synergistic combinations the beginnings of practical applications of this knowledge, suggesting that still further advances are foreseeable.

References

1. Hitchings, G. H. and Burchall, J. J.: Inhibition of folate biosynthesis and function as a basis for chemotherapy. *In* Nord, F. F. (Ed.): Advances in Enzymology, Vol. XXVII. New York: Interscience, 1965, pp. 418–468.
2. Hitchings, G. H.: Antimetabolites and chemotherapy: Integration of biochemistry and molecular manipulation. *In* Plattner, P. A. (Ed.): Chemotherapy of Cancer. New York: Elsevier, 1964, pp. 77–87.
3. Burchall, J. J. and Hitchings, G. H.: Inhibitor binding analysis of dihydrofolate reductases from various species. J. Molec. Pharmacol. 1:126, 1965.
4. Burchall, J. J., Ferone, R. and Hitchings, G. H.: Antibacterial chemotherapy. Ann. Rev. Pharmacol. 5:53, 1965.
5. Handschumacher, R. E. and Welch, A. D.: Agents which influence nucleic acid metabolism. *In* Chargaff, E. and Davidson, J. N. (Eds.): The Nucleic Acids, Vol. 3. New York: Academic Press, 1960, pp. 453–526.
6. Brockman, R. W. and Anderson, E. P.: Pyrimidine analogs. *In* Hochster, R. M. and Quastel, J. H. (Eds.): Metabolic Inhibitors, Vol. 1. New York: Academic Press, 1963, pp. 239–285.
7. Hitchings, G. H. and Elion, G. B.: Purine analogues. *In* Hochster, R. M. and Quastel, J. H. (Eds.): Metabolic Inhibitors, Vol. 1. New York: Academic Press, 1963, pp. 215–237.
8. Elion, G. B. and Hitchings, G. H.: Metabolic basis for the actions of purines and pyrimidines. *In* Goldin, A. and Hawking, F.

(Eds.): Advances in Chemotherapy, Vol. 2. New York: Academic Press, 1965, pp. 91–177.

9. Brockman, R. W.: Mechanisms of resistance to anticancer agents. *In* Haddow, A. and Weinhouse, S. (Eds.): Advances in Cancer Research, Vol. 7. New York: Academic Press, 1963, pp. 129–234.
10. Chaudhuri, N. K., Montag, B. J. and Heidelberger, C.: Studies on fluorinated pyrimidines. III. The metabolism of 5-fluorouracil-2-C^{14} and 5-fluoroorotic-2-C^{14} acid *in vivo*. Cancer Res. 18:318, 1958.
11. Heidelberger, C.: Biochemistry of 5-fluorouracil. *In* Plattner, P. H. (Ed.): Chemotherapy of Cancer. New York: Elsevier, 1964, pp. 88–98.
12. Bosch, L., Harbers, E. and Heidelberger, C.: Studies on fluorinated pyrimidines. V. Effects on nucleic acid metabolism *in vitro*. Cancer Res. 18:335, 1958.
13. Heidelberger, C., Kaldor, G., Mukherjee, K. L. and Danneberg, P. B.: Studies on fluorinated pyrimidines. IX: *In vitro* studies on tumor resistance. Cancer Res. 20:903, 1960.
14. Heidelberger, C., Ghobar, A., Baker, R. K. and Mukherjee, K. L.: Studies of fluorinated pyrimidines. X. *In vivo* studies on tumor resistance. Cancer Res. 20:897, 1960.
15. Lindner, A.: Cytochemical effects of 5-fluorouracil on sensitive and resistant Ehrlich ascites tumor cells. Cancer Res. 19:189, 1959.
16. Naono, S. and Gros, F.: Synthese par E. coli d'une phosphatase modifiée en présence d'un analogue pyrimidique. C. R. Acad. Sci. (Paris) 250:3889, 1960.
17. Bussard, A., Naono, S., Gros, F. and Monod, J.: Effets d'un analogue de l'uracle sur les propriétés d'une protéine enzymatique synthétisée en sa presence. C. R. Acad. Sci. (Paris) 250:4049, 1960.
18. Nakada, D. and Magasanik, B.: Catabolite repression and the induction of β-galactosidase. Biochim. Biophys. Acta 61:835, 1962.
19. Heidelberger, C., Griesbach, L., Cruz, C., Schnitzer, R. J. and Grunberg, E.: Fluorinated pyrimidines. VI. Effects of 5-fluorouridine and 5-fluoro-2′-deoxyuridine on transplanted tumors. Proc. Soc. Exp. Biol. Med. 97:470, 1958.
20. Hitchings, G. H., Elion, G. B., Falco, E. A., Russell, P. B. and VanderWerff, H.: Studies on analogs of purines and pyrimidines, Ann. N.Y. Acad. Sci. 52:1318, 1950.
21. Mukherjee, K. L. and Heidelberger, C.: Studies on fluorinated pyrimidines. IX. The degradation of 5-fluorouracil-6-C^{14}. J. Biol. Chem. 235:433, 1960.
22. Harbers, E., Chaudhuri, N. K. and Heidelberger, C.: Studies on fluorinated pyrimidines. VIII. Further biochemical and metabolic investigations. J. Biol. Chem. 234:1255, 1959.
23. Atkinson, M. R. and Murray, A. W.: Inhibition of purine phosphoribosyltransferases of Ehrlich ascites-tumour cells by 6-mercaptopurine. Biochem. J. 94:64, 1965.
24. Salser, J. S., Hutchison, D. J. and Balis, M. E.: Studies on the mechanism of action of 6-mercaptopurine in cell-free preparations. J. Biol. Chem. 235:429, 1960.
25. Salser, J. S. and Balis, M. E.: The mechanism of action of 6-mercaptopurine. I. Biochemical effects. Cancer Res. 25:539, 1965.
26. Atkinson, M. R., Morton, R. K. and Murray, A. W.: Inhibition of adenylosuccinate synthetase and adenylosuccinate lyase from Ehrlich ascites tumor cells by 6-thioinosine 5′-phosphate. Biochem. J. 92:398, 1964.
27. Hampton, A.: Studies of the action of adenylosuccinase with 6-thio analogues of adenylosuccinic acid. J. Biol. Chem. 237:529, 1962.
28. Bridger, W. A. and Cohen, L. H.: The mechanism of inhibition of adenylosuccinate lyase by 6-mercaptopurine nucleotide (thioinosinate). Biochim. Biophys. Acta 73:514, 1963.
29. Hampton, A.: Reactions of ribonucleotide derivatives of purine analogues at the catalytic site of inosine 5′-phosphate dehydrogenase. J. Biol. Chem. 238:3068, 1963.
30. Atkinson, M. R., Morton, R. K. and Murray, A. W.: Inhibition of inosine-5′-phosphate dehydrogenase from Ehrlich ascites-tumor cells by 6-thioinosine 5′-phosphate. Biochem. J. 89:167, 1963.
31. Skipper, H. E.: On the mechanism of action of 6-mercaptopurine. Ann. N.Y. Acad. Sci. 60:315, 1954.
32. LePage, G. A. and Greenlees, J. L.: Investigation of diverse systems for cancer chemotherapy screening; incorporation of glycine-2-C^{14} into ascites tumor-cell purines as a biological test system. Cancer Res. Suppl. 3:102, 1955.
33. Davidson, J. D. and Freeman, B. B.: The effects of antitumor drugs upon P^{32} incorporation into nucleic acids of mouse tumors. Cancer Res. 15:31, 1955.

34. LePage, G. A. and Jones, M.: Purinethiols as feedback inhibition of purine synthesis in ascites tumor cells. Cancer Res. 21:642, 1961.
35. Bennett, L. L., Jr., Simpson, L., Golden, J. and Barker, T. L.: The primary site of inhibition by 6-mercaptopurine on the purine biosynthetic pathway in some tumors in vivo. Cancer Res. 23:1574, 1963.
36. McCollister, R. J., Gilbert, W. R., Ashton, D. M. and Wyngaarden, J. B.: Pseudo-feedback inhibition of purine synthesis by 6-mercaptopurine ribonucleotide and other purine analogues. J. Biol. Chem. 239:1560, 1964.
37. Carbon, J. A.: The inhibition of poly-nucleotide phosphorylase by 6-mercapto-purine riboside 5′-diphosphate. Biochem. Biophys. Res. Comm. 7:366, 1962.
38. Atkinson, M. R., Jacobson, J. F., Morton, R. K. and Murray, A. W.: Nicotinamide 6-mercaptopurine dinucleotide and related compounds: Potential sources of 6-mercaptopurine nucleotide in chemotherapy. Nature 196:35, 1962.
39. Unger, K. W. and Silber, R.: Studies on the formate activating enzyme: Kinetics of 6-mercaptopurine inhibition and stabilization of the enzyme. Biochim. Biophys. Acta 89:167, 1964.
40. Elion, G. B., Bieber, S. and Hitchings, G. H.: The fate of 6-mercaptopurine in mice. Ann. N.Y. Acad. Sci. 60:297, 1954.
41. Hamilton, L. and Elion, G. B.: The fate of 6-mercaptopurine in man. Ann. N.Y. Acad. Sci. 60:304, 1954.
42. Elion, G. B., Callahan, S., Nathan, H., Bieber, S., Rundles, R. W. and Hitchings, G. H.: Potentiation by inhibition of drug degradation: 6-substituted purines and xanthine oxidase. Biochem. Pharmacol. 12:85, 1963.
43. Elion, G. B., Callahan, S., Rundles, R. W. and Hitchings, G. H.: Relationship between metabolic fates and antitumor activities of thiopurines. Cancer Res. 23:1207, 1963.
44. Elion, G. B., Callahan, S. W., Hitchings, G. H., Rundles, R. W. and Laszlo, J.: Experimental, clinical, and metabolic studies of thiopurines. Cancer Chemother. Rep. 16:197, 1962.
45. Salser, J. S. and Balis, M. E.: The mechanism of action of 6-mercaptopurine. II. Basis for specificity. Cancer Res. 25:544, 1965.
46. Heidelberger, C. and Keller, R. A.: Investigation of diverse systems for cancer chemotherapy screening; effects of 29 compounds on nucleic acid and protein biosynthesis in slices of Flexner-Jobling carcinoma and rat spleen. Cancer Res. Suppl. 3:106, 1955.
47. Henderson, J. F.: Effects of anticancer drugs on biochemical control mechanisms. *In* Homburger, F. (Ed.): Progress in Experimental Tumor Research, Vol. VI. New York: Hafner, 1965, pp. 84–125.
48. LePage, G. A. and Jones, M.: Further studies on the mechanism of action of 6-thioguanine. Cancer Res. 21:1590, 1961.
49. Greenlees, J. and LePage, G. A.: Purine biosynthesis and inhibitors in ascites cell tumors. Cancer Res. 16:808, 1956.
50. Wyngaarden, J. B. and Ashton, D. M.: The regulation of activity of phosphoribosylpyrophosphate amidotransferase by purine ribonucleotides: A potential feedback control of purine biosynthesis. J. Biol. Chem. 234:1492, 1959.
51. Bieber, S. and Pomales, R.: The uptake of purines and formate into the DNA of 6-MP-sensitive and resistant strains of CA755. Proc. Am. Ass. Cancer Res. 3:304, 1962.
52. Sartorelli, A. C.: Approaches to the combination chemotherapy of transplantable neoplasms. *In* Homburger, F. (Ed.): Progress in Experimental Tumor Research. Vol. VI. New York: Hafner Publishing Co., 1965, pp. 228–288.
53. Fernandes, J. F., LePage, G. A. and Lindner, A.: The influence of azaserine and 6-mercaptopurine on the *in vivo* metabolism of ascites tumor cells. Cancer Res. 16:154, 1956.
54. Mantel, N.: An experimental design in combination chemotherapy. Ann. N.Y. Acad. Sci. 76:909, 1958. Discussion. Ibid. pp. 915–931.
55. Goldin, A., Humphreys, S. R., Venditti, J. M. and Mantel, M.: Factors influencing synergism: Relation to screening methodology. Ann. N.Y. Acad. Sci. 76:932, 1958.
56. Mihich, E., Clarke, D. A. and Philips, F. S.: Effects of 6-mercaptopurine on respiration, anaerobic glycolysis and succinodehydrogenase activity in normal and tumor tissues. Proc. Soc. Exp. Biol. Med. 92:758, 1956.
57. Laszlo, J., Stengle, J., Wight, K. and Burk, D.: Effect of chemotherapeutic agents on metabolism of human acute leukemia cells *in vitro*. Proc. Soc. Exp. Biol. Med. 97:127, 1958.
58. Garattini, S. and Paoletti, R.: 6-Mercaptopurine inhibits acetylation of sulfanil-

amide *in vivo.* G. Ital. Chemioter. 3:55, 1956.

59. Bieber, S., Dietrich, L. S., Elion, G. B., Hitchings, G. H. and Martin, D. S.: The incorporation of 6-mercaptopurine-S^{35} into the nucleic acids of sensitive and nonsensitive transplantable mouse tumors. Cancer Res. 21:228, 1961.

Mechanism of Action of the *Vinca* Alkaloids

By John H. Marsden, M.D.

Although the *Vinca rosea* alkaloids have been used in the clinic for over a decade, the mechanism of action of these drugs is still unknown. The alkaloids vincristine and vinblastine are closely related structurally (Fig. 1); however, there are significant differences in their toxicity and their range of activity in both the laboratory and the clinic. Therefore, whether data for one compound may be applicable to the other is somewhat uncertain.

There have been two general avenues of investigation: one, biochemical observation of the effects of the drugs on cell respiration, nucleic acid synthesis and protein synthesis; and the other, examination of the ultrastructure of various cells after exposure to the compounds.

Effects on Respiration, Nucleic Acid, and Protein Synthesis

Some of the early work was done to assess the influence of these drugs on cell respiration. Johnson et al.,[1] working with vincristine and vinblastine on S-180 and Freund ascites tumor cells, showed there was no effect on cell respiration or on glycolysis. This observation was confirmed by Beer[2] in liver tissue from animals treated with vinblastine. Hunter[3] reported data which were at variance with these observations, but he was using thioguanine-resistant L1210 cells, a tumor which is not sensitive to the *Vinca* alkaloids.

It had previously been shown that metaphase arrest was evident in human cells exposed to the *Vinca* alkaloids in tissue culture;[4] and Johnson et al.[5] were able to block the antimitotic and antitumor effect of vinblastine on Osgood J96 human monocytic leukemia cells by adding coenzyme A, tryptophan, aspartic acid, glutamic acid, α-ketoglutaric acid, ornithine, arginine, or citrulline. The last six are amino acids and can be related to one another through metabolic pathways derived from glutamic acid. Cutts[6] was successful in demonstrating in vivo that tryptophan and glutamic acid could inhibit mitotic arrest in murine tumors treated with vinblastine.

Armstrong and associates[7] at the Lilly Laboratory for Clinical Research and Vaitkevicius et al.[8] at the Henry Ford Hospital administered large doses of glutamic or

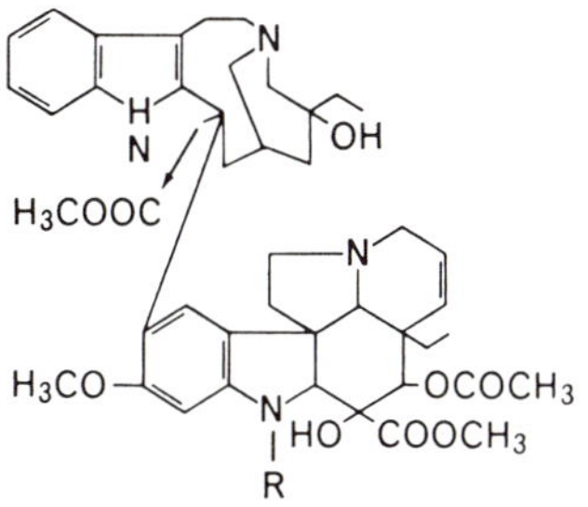

N
H
N
OH
H_3COOC
N
H_3CO
$OCOCH_3$
N
HO
$COOCH_3$
R

Fig. 1.—Structural formulae of vinblastine (VLB; vincaleukoblastine) ($R = CH_3$) and vincristine (leurocristine; VCR; LCR) ($R = CHO$.)

From the Medical Research Division, Eli Lilly and Company, Indianapolis, Indiana.

aspartic acid to patients being treated with vinblastine. The expected leukopenia did not occur.

Johnson et al. also observed that the acute toxicity of vincristine in mice could be decreased by subsequent administration of folinic acid but not of folic acid.[1] Neither of these two compounds, however, interferes with anti-P-1534 leukemia action of vincristine.

McGeer and McGeer[9] noted that the urinary excretion of 4-amino-5-imidazole-carboxamide was decreased after the administration of vinblastine; this suggested that purine synthesis was inhibited.

Extensive research has been done by Creasey and associates[10–16] on the relation of these alkaloids to alteration of protein and to nucleic acid production by the cells. The systems used for his study were a murine S-180 tumor and Ehrlich ascites carcinoma.

Johnson et al. reported that no alteration was seen in the production of DNA, RNA, or protein in S-180 cells exposed to either vincristine or vinblastine.[1] Other studies, however, showed that, although total RNA production was unchanged, a variation could be demonstrated in the subtypes of RNA in that the synthesis of soluble (or transfer) RNA was inhibited.[10,11]

Tissues which are not mitotically active were influenced by the *Vinca* alkaloids.[17] In mouse brain tissue, uptake of uridine-^{3}H was inhibited for all fractions of RNA. However, in this system soluble RNA was *least* inhibited by vincristine, in contrast to the situation in Ehrlich ascites carcinoma cells, in which soluble RNA was most inhibited.

It is important to note that although there was a decrease in DNA synthesis in vitro with vinblastine in high concentrations,[14] the uptake of ^{3}H-thymidine by mice in vivo was not evident. Colchicine and vincristine inhibited DNA formation in vivo and also inhibited the uptake of cytidine-^{3}H into DNA of human leukemic leukocytes. Van Lancker and coworkers[18,19] confirmed in vivo the suppression of DNA synthesis in rat spleen and bone marrow after administration of vinblastine.

At the University of British Columbia, Richards and Beer[20–22] have also made significant contributions in this field. Using thymus cell suspensions, they have demonstrated that the *Vinca* alkaloids as well as colchicine inhibit DNA synthesis. They further observed that incorporation of sodium formate-^{14}C and glycine-2-^{14}C into DNA was inhibited by vinblastine but that hypoxanthine and thymine were unaffected. Labeled adenine and guanine in DNA and RNA were only slightly decreased.

Richards[23] suggested that some effects of the *Vinca* alkaloids may be explained by the theory that these drugs are able to enter the cell at certain phases of the cell cycle. This theory was strengthened by the work of Madoc-Jones and Mauro,[24] who incubated HeLa cells and Chinese hamster cells with concentrations of vinblastine and vincristine which were higher than the levels needed to arrest mitosis. They observed that the cells were sensitive to vinblastine (0.3 μg/ml) in S and late G_1 phases, whereas they were sensitive to vincristine only in S phase. It should be pointed out, however, that these observations concerned very high drug concentrations as compared with in vivo drug levels. When time exposure was short, the cells in S phase continued at a normal rate to mitosis and were then irreversibly arrested. This was the case with either compound.

Some differences were demonstrated between normal and neoplastic cells in metabolic responses to these drugs.[25] Vincristine, for example, decreased RNA and protein synthesis in human neoplastic leukocytes but not in normal leukocytes. All classes of RNA were inhibited by vincristine. Further conflicting data are found in the observations of Wagner and Roizman,[26] who described the selective inhibition of synthesis and of processing of nucleolar RNA, as opposed to Creasey's observation of decreased synthesis of transfer RNA.

When one considers these conflicting data, several facts must be borne in mind. We are talking about two different drugs, even though they are closely related chemically. The in vitro and in vivo systems used were different. There were a number of variables, including drug concentration, duration of exposure, phase of cell cycle exposed, and methods of analysis. The mode of action might be explained if we could say conclusively that DNA or RNA or both were inhibited in concentrations of the *Vinca* alkaloids attainable in humans. This could be a logical explanation of the mechanism of tumor inhibition.

Obviously, the usual statement that the *Vinca* alkaloids arrest mitosis does not adequately explain the tumor inhibition. Other drugs, such as demecolcine (Colcemid), colchicine, and griseofulvin, also arrest mitosis but do not give the same clinical results, nor do they have the same range of toxicity as the *Vinca* alkaloids.

Creasey and associates[16] have postulated that the labile or stable protein-binding capability of the *Vinca* alkaloids rather than interference with nucleic acid synthesis may explain the arrest of the mitotic cycle.

The effect of various mitotic arresters on the spindle has been described. Malawista and Sato[27] have reported differences between these two *Vinca* alkaloids. Vinblastine produces a prompt, complete, and reversible dissolution of the mitotic spindle along with decrease in birefringence, whereas with vincristine birefringence is not abolished, spindle dissolution is delayed, and recovery is incomplete.

Noble and Beer[28] have made some interesting points regarding the dosage of and the tumor response to these drugs.

Effect on the Ultrastructure of the Cell

Palmer[4] and Cardinali et al.,[29] among others, have confirmed C-mitotic arrest produced by the *Vinca* alkaloids.

George et al.,[30–32] of St. Jude's Hospital in Memphis, Tennessee, were the first to describe the changes seen in the cellular ultrastructure after exposure to vincristine. In 1964, they demonstrated that HeLa cells showed a colchicine-type mitotic arrest after exposure to vincristine in as little as 0.001 μg/ml; at higher concentrations, this action was irreversible. Several changes were described. Spindle tubules were absent, centrioles continued to duplicate but did not appear to migrate to the spindle poles, and concentric membranes formed around the chromosomes. They suggested that vincristine and vinblastine interfere with the synthesis of spindle protein as well as with the organization of preformed spindle protein.

These investigators further observed that vincristine produced filaments in the cell which appeared to be closely related to the spindle tubules. Maturing nerve cells (nonmitotic) also demonstrated filaments in the breakdown of neurotubules. In mice given an intraperitoneal dose of vincristine, 5 mg/kg, severe alterations seen in the sensory nerves of the dorsal root ganglia included a decrease in neurotubules and an increase in the filamentous mass. The axonal neurotubules were more sensitive than those in the cell body.

Malawista and Bensch (at Yale) and Sato (at the University of Pennsylvania) reported in 1968[33] that, by using vinblastine (as the sulfate, 1×10^{-5} mole/liter) on *Pectinaria gouldi* oocytes, they could dissolve the spindle in six to twelve minutes; if the cells were then washed and perfused, recovery was complete in 40 to 60 minutes. Higher concentrations of vincristine were needed for spindle dissolution, and recovery was not complete. The investigators postulated that this difference might be due to variations in the ability of the compounds to enter the cell. Similar actions on the spindle were demonstrated with colchicine and griseofulvin.

These observers[34] demonstrated that the *Vinca* alkaloids caused crystallization of the microtubule protein in the same system, presumably by alteration of the charge or by a rearrangement of the protein.

At the Children's Cancer Research Foundation at Harvard, Krishan and associates[35–37] photographed the ultrastructural changes in Earle's L cells exposed to vinblastine in tissue culture. They confirmed the findings of George et al.[30] that the centrioles continued to divide and that many cells had multiple centrioles. The chromosomes, however, were randomly placed in the cell and were not oriented to the centriole. (In the C-mitosis of demecolcine this orientation is present.) It is also interesting to note that, in the cells exposed to vinblastine, no microtubules were seen in association with the centrioles or centromeres, whereas they were present in mitotic arrest produced by demecolcine. This may be evidence in favor of the need of microtubules for orientation of the chromosomes. When the arrested cells were washed, microtubules reappeared, especially near the centromeres. After the cells were washed, there was not a sudden burst of mitosis, but some cells proceeded promptly and others were delayed. The reason for this is unclear. Some of the cells with multiple centrioles divided into three or four daughter cells.

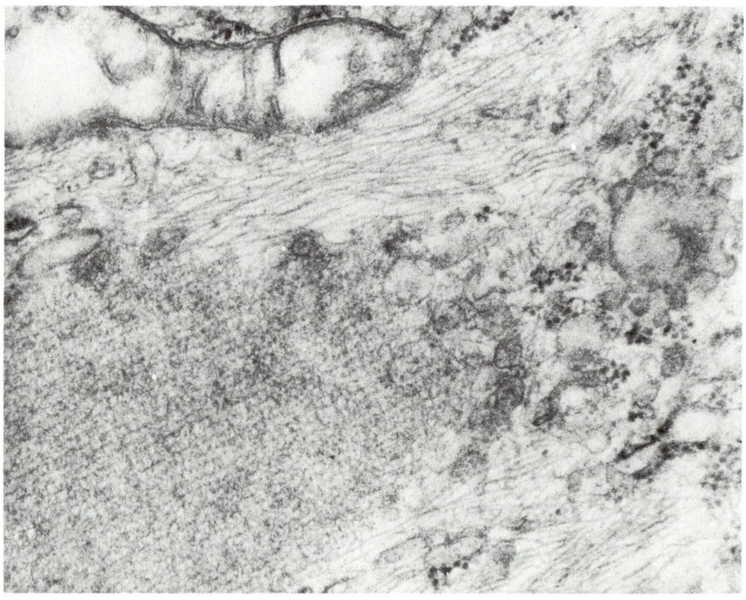

FIG. 2.—Electron microscopic view of a large vincristine-induced crystal and scattered filaments in the cytoplasm of a cell reincubated for 2 hours in fresh medium, illustrating continuity between filaments and crystal (×77,400). From Krishan and Hsu,[37] with permission of the Journal of Cell Biology (Rockefeller University Press).

Krishan also reported that, when Earle's L-929 fibroblasts were incubated for prolonged periods with nonlethal levels of vinblastine, great amounts of endoplasmic reticulum appeared in the enlarged multimicronucleated cells; this indicates active protein synthesis by the cell. Also seen were many annulated lamellae thought to be associated with nuclear/cytoplasmic exchange.

When the cells were incubated with high doses of vinblastine or vincristine, protein crystals were formed (Fig. 2). This crystallization was reversible. It is theorized that the microtubules, filamentous masses, and crystals are all from the same protein pool and are interchangeable. These findings are similar to observations in the neurotubules reported by George and coworkers.[30]

Observations by Lacy[38] on the release of insulin granules by the beta cells also provide us with information on the function of the microtubule. He has shown that it is vital in the movement of the beta granule within the cell. When the call for insulin is received, the beta granules are moved first to the cell surface and finally extruded. Such movement is the function of the microtubule and, indeed, can be prevented by colchicine or vincristine. This observation correlates well with the mitotic arrest of the dividing cell at metaphase. This is the time when movement within the cell is required for separation of the chromosomes and, finally, for cell division.

The effects of vinblastine, vincristine, and colchicine on the platelets have been described by White.[39] Again it was seen that the microtubules are abolished, which apparently allows the partial collapse of the discoid platelet. His experience showed that the platelet treated with the *Vinca* alkaloids maintained its ability to affect normal clot retraction. Incidentally, it was also seen that vinblastine and colchicine in high concentrations caused platelet destruction, whereas vincristine did not. It should be pointed out that the concentration necessary to cause microtubule loss in these cells was much higher than that of clinical doses.

Other ultrastructural changes in the platelet have been described by White,[40] especially in the dense tubular system when incubated with the *Vinca* alkaloids.

Hebden et al.[41] have described the binding of vinblastine in the platelets of rats. One and one-half hours after injection intraperitoneally into the rat, 2 per cent of the labeled material was in the circulation. Of this 2 per cent, 60 per cent was in the platelets and the remaining 40 per cent was about equally divided among the plasma, red blood cells, and white blood cells. Thus, about 75 per cent of the material was in the buffy coat. The vinblastine detected was unchanged in these cells and was easily removed by washing. Figure 3 demonstrates that the radioactive vinblastine was located in the platelets. The significance of this observation is not yet apparent, but it should be borne in mind when blood level measurements of the drug are attempted. This apparent affinity for platelets is particularly interesting when correlated with the work of Robertson and McCarthy[42] and of Hwang et al.,[43] who have reported thrombocytosis in patients receiving vinblastine.

The action of vinblastine in regenerative tissue was studied by Francoeur.[44] He observed regeneration of the tail structure of *Rana pipiens* larvae after amputation. It was previously reported that dactinomycin acted by inhibiting synthesis of those proteins dependent on DNA. The investigator compared this compound with vinblastine and found that although dactinomycin inhibited the total regenerative process (even growth of the entire animal), vinblastine did not. It selectively inhibited regeneration of mesodermal structures, i.e., notochord and muscle.

Francoeur and Wilber[45] observed an apparent arrest of development of blood

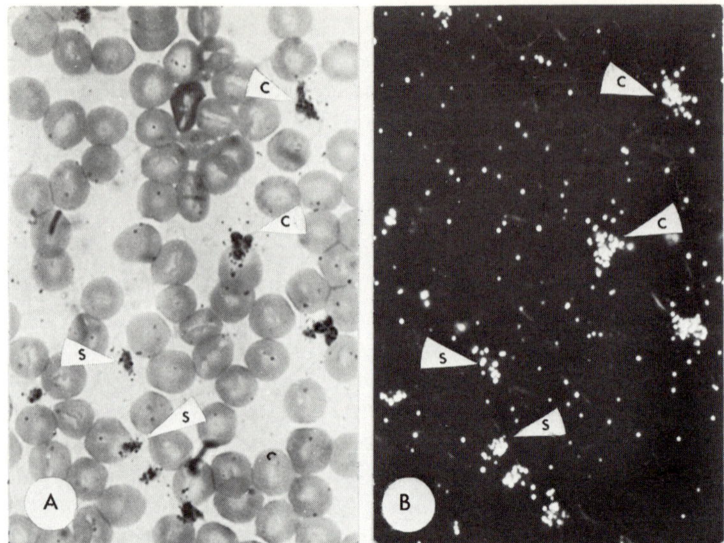

FIG. 3.—Autoradiogram of blood smear from rat given tritiated vinblastine (0.22 mg/kg). The blood was taken one and a half hours after intraperitoneal injection of the drug. A. Bright field, Wright-Giemsa stain, showing single platelets (S) and small clumps of platelets (C). B. Corresponding dark field showing silver grains associated with the single platelets and platelet clumps. From Hebden et al.,[41] with permission of Cancer Research.

islands in the regenerating amphibian tissue, so that it did not differentiate into blood vessels. (It had previously been theorized by others that an unrestricted development of blood supply is an essential factor in sustaining tumor growth.)

Moncrief and Heller[46] have proposed a theory of acylation as a mechanism of action of the *Vinca* alkaloids, as well as other chemotherapeutic agents.

COMMENT

This review makes it apparent that the precise mechanism of action of the *Vinca* alkaloids is not yet understood. A few deductions, however, can be made.

It seems likely that the mechanism of action of vinblastine and vincristine is similar but not necessarily identical. Certainly, both cause mitotic arrest, but it is hard to say how this accounts for the oncolytic effect. The fact that these compounds will cause crystallization of microtubule protein possibly explains the metaphase arrest but does not adequately explain the effect on cancer cells.

Observations of the ultrastructural changes reported by George and associates[30] and Krishan[35] would appear to correlate well with one another, but it is not possible to draw any conclusion from the conflicting results of biochemical experiments by the investigators mentioned previously.

Finally, one might ask what difference it makes. This could be a difficult question to answer were it well established that the dosages now being used are unequivocally the best, but we have some evidence that this may not be the case. The weekly dosage is hard to rationalize from a therapeutic standpoint, particularly in consideration of the cell cycle. When toxicity is considered, this schedule is more readily acceptable, since it has been shown that a specific amount of vincristine is more neurotoxic in small divided daily doses than in one weekly dose. The weekly dose of vinblastine also allows for leukopenia to be past the nadir before the next dose. Consequently, we have followed a weekly dosage in almost all clinical studies with these drugs.

Noble and Beer[28] have cited work in animals with tumors sensitive to vinblastine; there was marked variation in the response of the tumors to the timing of the doses.

These observations suggest that a greater understanding of the mechanism of action might lead to more effective dosage of these compounds and might also add to our understanding of cancer per se.

References

1. Johnson, I. S., Armstrong, J. G., Gorman, M. and Burnett, J. P., Jr.: The Vinca alkaloids: a new class of oncolytic agents. Cancer Res. 23:1390, 1963.
2. Beer, C. T.: Biochemical studies with vincaleukoblastine. Canad. Cancer Conf. 4:355, 1961.
3. Hunter, J. C.: Effects of vincaleukoblastine sulfate on metabolism of thioguanine-resistant L1210 leukemia cells. Biochem. Pharmacol. 12:283, 1963.
4. Palmer, C. G., Livengood, D., Warren, A. K., Simpson, P. J. and Johnson, I. S.: The action of vincaleukoblastine on mitosis *in vitro*. Exp. Cell Res. 20:198, 1960.
5. Johnson, I. S., Vlantis, J., Mattas, B. and Wright, H. F.: Anti-tumor principles derived from Vinca rosea Linn. II. Further studies of biological activities of vincaleukoblastine. Canad. Cancer Conf. 4:339, 1961.
6. Cutts, J. H.: Changes in mitosis in ascites tumors and normal bone marrow induced by vincaleukoblastine in vivo. Canad. Cancer Conf. 4:363, 1961.
7. Armstrong, J. G., Dyke, R. W., Fouts, P. J. and Gahimer, J. E.: Hodgkin's disease, carcinoma of the breast, and other tumors treated with vinblastine sulfate. Cancer Chemother. Rep. 18:49, 1962.
8. Vaitkevicius, V. K., Talley, R. W., Tucker, J. L., Jr. and Brennan, M. J.: Cytological and clinical observations during vincaleukoblastine therapy of disseminated cancer. Cancer 15:296, 1962.
9. McGeer, P. L. and McGeer, E. G.: Effect of amethopterin and vincaleukoblastine on urinary 4-amino-5-imidazolecarboxamide. Biochem. Pharmacol. 12:297, 1963.
10. Creasey, W. A. and Markiw, M. E.: Biochemical effects of the Vinca alkaloids. I. Effects of vinblastine on nucleic acid synthesis in mouse tumor cells. Biochem. Pharmacol. 13:135, 1964.
11. Creasey, W. A. and Markiw, M. E.: Biochemical effects of the Vinca alkaloids. II. A comparison of the effects of colchicine, vinblastine and vincristine on the synthesis of ribonucleic acids in Ehrlich ascites carcinoma cells. Biochim. Biophys. Acta 87:601, 1964.
12. Creasey, W. A. and Markiw, M. E.: Biochemical effects of the Vinca alkaloids. III. The synthesis of ribonucleic acid and the incorporation of amino acids in Ehrlich ascites cells in vitro. Biochim. Biophys. Acta 103:635, 1965.
13. Creasey, W. A.: Biochemical effects of the Vinca alkaloids. IV. Studies with vinleurosine. Biochem. Pharmacol. 18:227, 1968.
14. Creasey, W. A.: Modifications in biochemical pathways produced by the Vinca alkaloids. Cancer Chemother. Rep. 52:501, 1968.
15. Sartorelli, A. C. and Creasey, W. A.: Cancer chemotherapy. Ann. Rev. Pharmacol. 9:51, 1969.
16. Creasey, W. A., Bensch, K. G. and Malawista, S. E.: Binding of antimitotic agents as the basis for mitotic inhibition and anti-inflammatory action. Fed. Proc. 28:362, 1969.
17. Agustin, B. M. and Creasey, W. A.: Vinca alkaloids and the synthesis of RNA in mouse brain. Nature 215:965, 1967.
18. VanLancker, J. L., Flangas, A. L. and Allen, J.: Metabolic effects of vinblastine. I. The effect of vinblastine on nucleic acid synthesis in spleen and bone marrow. Lab. Invest. 15:1291, 1966.
19. Luyckx, A. and VanLancker, J. L.: Metabolic effects of vinblastine. II. The effect of vinblastine on deoxyribonucleic acid and ribonucleic acid synthesis of regenerating liver. Lab. Invest. 15:1301, 1966.
20. Richards, J. F. and Beer, C. T.: Some effects of Vinca alkaloids on nucleic acid metabolism. Lloydia 27:346, 1964.
21. Richards, J. F., Jones, R. G. W. and Beer, C. T.: Biochemical studies with the Vinca alkaloids. I. Effect on nucleic acid formation by isolated cell suspensions. Cancer Res. 26:876, 1966.
22. Jones, R. G. W., Richards, J. F. and Beer,

C. T.: Biochemical studies with the Vinca alkaloids. II. Effect of vinblastine on the biosynthesis of nucleic acids and their precursors in rat thymus cells. Cancer Res. 26:882, 1966.

23. Richards, J. F.: Biochemical studies with the *Vinca* alkaloids. Cancer Chemother. Rep. 52:463, 1968.
24. Madoc-Jones, H. and Mauro, F.: Interphase action of vinblastine and vincristine: Differences in their lethal action through the mitotic cycle of cultured mammalian cells. J. Cell. Physiol. 72:185, 1968.
25. Cline, M. J.: Effect of vincristine on synthesis of ribonucleic acid and protein in leukaemic leucocytes. Brit. J. Haemat. 14:21, 1968.
26. Wagner, E. K. and Roizman, B.: Effect of the Vinca alkaloids on RNA synthesis in human cells in vitro. Science 162:569, 1968.
27. Malawista, S. E. and Sato, H.: Vinblastine and griseofulvin reversibly disrupt the living mitotic spindle. Biol. Bull. 131:397, 1966. (Abstract).
28. Noble, R. L. and Beer, C. T.: Experimental observations concerning the mode of action of Vinca alkaloids. *In* Shedden, W. I. H. (Ed.): The Vinca Alkaloids in the Chemotherapy of Malignant Disease. Basingstoke, Eng.: Eli Lilly and Company, Ltd., 1969, p. 4.
29. Cardinali, G., Cardinali, G. and Blair, J.: The stathmokinetic effect of vincaleukoblastine on normal bone marrow and leukemic cells. Cancer Res. 21:1542, 1961.
30. George, P., Journey, L. J. and Goldstein, M. N.: Effect of vincristine on the fine structure of HeLa cells during mitosis. J. Nat. Cancer Inst. 35:355, 1965.
31. Journey, L. J., Burdman, J. and George, P.: Ultrastructural studies on tissue culture cells treated with vincristine (NSC-67574). Cancer Chemother. Rep. 52:509, 1968.
32. Journey, L. J., Burdman, J. and Whaley, A.: Electron microscopic study of spinal ganglia from vincristine-treated mice. J. Nat. Cancer Inst. 43:603, 1969.
33. Malawista, S. E., Sato, H. and Bensch, K. G.: Vinblastine and griseofulvin reversibly disrupt the living mitotic spindle. Science 160:770, 1968.
34. Bensch, K. G. and Malawista, S. E.: Microtubule crystals: A new biophysical phenomenon induced by Vinca alkaloids. Nature 218:1176, 1968.
35. Krishan, A.: Time-lapse and ultrastructure studies on the reversal of mitotic arrest induced by vinblastine sulfate in Earle's L cells. J. Nat. Cancer Inst. 41:581, 1968.
36. Krishan, A., Hsu, D. and Hutchins, P.: Hypertrophy of granular endoplasmic reticulum and annulate lamellae in Earle's L cells exposed to vinblastine sulfate. J. Cell Biol. 39:211, 1968.
37. Krishan, A. and Hsu, D.: Observations on the association of helical polyribosomes and filaments with vincristine-induced crystals in Earle's L-cell fibroblasts. J. Cell Biol. 43:553, 1969.
38. Lacy, P. E.: Beta-cell secretion—from the standpoint of a pathobiologist. Banting Memorial Lecture, Thirtieth Ann. Meeting of American Diabetes Ass., 1970.
39. White, J. G.: Effects of colchicine and Vinca alkaloids on human platelets. I. Influence on platelet microtubules and contractile function. Amer. J. Path. 53:281, 1968.
40. White, J. G.: Effects of colchicine and Vinca alkaloids on human platelets. II. Changes in the dense tubular system and formation of an unusual inclusion in incubated cells. Amer. J. Path. 53:447, 1968.
41. Hebden, H. F., Hadfield, J. R. and Beer, C. T.: The binding of vinblastine by platelets in the rat. Cancer Res. 30:1417, 1970.
42. Robertson, J. H. and McCarthy, G. M.: Periwinkle alkaloids and the platelet-count. Lancet 2:353, 1969.
43. Hwang, Y. F., Hamilton, H. E. and Sheets, R. F.: Vinblastine-induced thrombocytosis. Lancet 2:1075, 1969.
44. Francoeur, R. T.: General and selective inhibition of amphibian regeneration by vinblastine and dactinomycin. Oncology 22:218, 1968.
45. Francoeur, R. T. and Wilber, C. G.: Amphibian regeneration and the teratogenic effects of vinblastine. Oncology 22:302, 1968.
46. Moncrief, J. W. and Heller, K. S.: Acylation: A proposed mechanism of action for various oncolytic agents based on model chemical systems. Cancer Res. 27, Part I: 1500, 1967.

Antibiotics, L-Asparaginase and New Agents

By JOSEPH H. BURCHENAL, M.D. AND WILLI KREIS, M.D., PH.D.

DURING THE PAST 15 YEARS, there has been a large-scale screening of antibiotic filtrates for their activity against animal tumors both in vivo and in vitro. In these operations, a large number of active materials have been found but, because of duplication and difficulties in isolation, far fewer have come to clinical trial. Of the latter, those that have shown practical clinical activity have been even less. Because of the limitations of time and space, it is on this small select group that we would like to concentrate. The mechanisms of action of these clinically active compounds have been studied in isolated enzyme systems, in bacteria, in cell culture, or in normal or neoplastic tissues in the intact animal.

The first antitumor antibiotics on which mechanism of action studies were done were the glutamine antagonists, azaserine (*O*-diazoacetyl-L-serine) and DON (6-diazo-5-oxo-L-norleucine). These two naturally occurring diazo compounds were isolated from broth filtrates of *Streptomyces* and their chemical structures determined in 1954 by Fusari et al.[1] and in 1956 by Diom et al.[2] As can be seen from the formulae (Fig. 1), these compounds are closely related in structure to glutamine. They were shown by Stock et al.[3] and Clarke et al.[4] to have rather marked antitumor effect against sarcoma 180 and later against various strains of mouse leukemia[5,6] and experimental tumors in mice.[7–9] Original clinical studies of these compounds in 1954 and 1957[10,11] showed very little beneficial effect, but later studies by Karnofsky et al.[12,13] have demonstrated these compounds to be active and useful in the treatment of trophoblastic tumors. DON, particularly, appears to be practical in that it can be given by mouth and that doses which are essentially nontoxic produce permanent remissions in women with relatively slow-growing trophoblastic tumors. It appears to be definitely

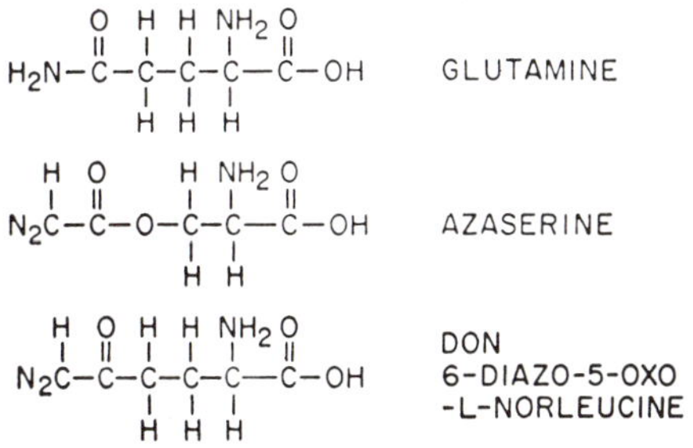

```
    O  H  H  NH2 O
    ‖  |  |  |   ‖
H2N-C--C--C--C---C-OH        GLUTAMINE
       |  |  |
       H  H  H

  H  O       H  NH2 O
  |  ‖       |  |   ‖
N2C--C--O----C--C---C-OH     AZASERINE
             |  |
             H  H

  H  O  H  H  NH2 O
  |  ‖  |  |  |   ‖          DON
N2C--C--C--C--C---C-OH       6-DIAZO-5-OXO
        |  |  |              -L-NORLEUCINE
        H  H  H
```

FIG. 1.—Formulae showing the close structural relation between glutamine and its antagonists, azaserine and 6-diazo-5-oxo-L-norleucine (DON). From Burchenal and Kreis: Mechanism of action of antibiotics and new agents. *In* Brodsky, I. and Kahn, S. B. (Eds.): Cancer Chemotherapy. New York: Grune & Stratton, Inc., 1967, with permission.

From the Divisions of Applied Therapy and Drug Resistance, Sloan-Kettering Institute for Cancer Research, and the Department of Medicine, Memorial Hospital for Cancer and Allied Diseases, New York, New York.

Supported in part by grants CA-08748 and CA-05826 from the National Cancer Institute, grant T-45 from the American Cancer Society, and the Hearst Foundation.

inferior to methotrexate or actinomycin D in the treatment of fulminating choriocarcinoma.[13]

In the metabolic pathway for the synthesis of purines, both azaserine and DON block the conversion of formylglycineamide ribotide (FGAR) to the corresponding formylglycineamidine ribotide (FGAM), a process involving glutamine and a phosphoribosyl-formyl glycineamidine synthetase. The antimetabolites are tightly bound to this enzyme, so that in an in vitro system, if they react with the enzyme prior to the addition of glutamine, they cannot be displaced.[14] The glutamine antagonists also act earlier in the metabolic pathway for the synthesis of the purine skeleton to block the reaction of 5-phosphoribosyl-1-pyrophosphate with glutamine to form 5-phosphoribosylamine. This system is not so sensitive to the antimetabolites as the preceding one.[15] DON also acts to prevent the transfer of the amide nitrogen of glutamine to uridylic acid to form cytidylic acid, and to xanthylic acid to form guanylic acid.[16]

Diazo-oxo-norvaline (DONV) was synthesized by Handschumacher et al.[17] in the hope that it would be an antagonist of asparagine and so be of value in combination with the enzyme asparaginase in the treatment of asparagine-dependent tumors and leukemias. Unfortunately, this compound binds irreversibly with asparaginase and so prevents its deamination of asparagine.[18] It has not so far been shown to be of therapeutic value.[19]

A congener, 5-chloro-4-oxo-2-aminopentanoic acid, synthesized by Khedouri et al.[20] and shown by them to be an inhibitor of asparagine synthetase,[21] has been shown by our group to potentiate the effects of asparaginase in sensitive mouse leukemias.[22]

Actinomycin, the first crystalline antibiotic obtained from a *Streptomyces*, was isolated by Waksman and Woodruff in 1940.[23] It was active against rodent tumors[24,25] and was shown by Schulte[26] to be the first antibiotic with activity against human tumors. The actinomycins have their greatest field of usefulness in Wilms' tumor in children, as shown by Farber et al.[27,28] and Tan[29]; in uterine choriocarcinomas, by Ross et al.[30]; in the lymphomas, by Schulte[26]; and in combination with methotrexate and chlorambucil in testicular tumors, by Li et al.[31] The structures of some of the actinomycins have been elucidated and different derivatives separated out or specifically synthesized by Brockmann et al.[32,33] Although they differ markedly in toxicity, there is no evidence that any one of them is definitely more effective in mouse leukemia than actinomycin D or has a different mechanism of action.[34]

Actinomycin D inhibits DNA-dependent RNA synthesis,[35-37] and this effect is reversed by the addition of an excess of native DNA.[38,39] In vitro, actinomycin combines with DNA.[40-44] The DNA-actinomycin complexes are unaffected by ionic strength, are preferentially formed with native rather than denatured DNA, and show absolute base-specificity for guanine.[45] It is suggested that this specificity is mediated by the amino group located in the minor groove of the DNA helix. In vitro, actinomycin inhibits RNA polymerase.[38,39] Studies in vivo with liver tissue[46-48] or ascites cells,[49] with cells in culture[35,40,50-52] or with isolated enzyme systems[36,39,42,53-57] all indicate the inhibition of RNA polymerization by the complexing of actinomycin with the DNA templates.

Mitomycin C is an antibiotic isolated from *Streptomyces caespitosus*.[58,59] It has a wide range of antitumor activity against transplantable mouse and rat tumors.[60] Broad clinical trials in Japan and in the United States have shown effects in lymphomas, chronic leukemias, and some forms of solid tumors.[61-64] It appears to be a useful agent for the treatment of chronic granulocytic leukemia and possibly also for carcinoma of the stomach, although the therapeutic role in the latter has not been definitely established. Studies on the structure of mitomycin C[65–68] have shown it to contain a quinone ring, a carbamate, and an aziridine ring, and at one time or another certain compounds containing any of these groups have been shown to have independent chemotherapeutic action in some animal tumors. The general spectrum of activity of mitomycin C, including toxicity, effects on experimental tumors, and clinical effects has suggested that it might be acting as an alkylating agent. Mitomycin, however, is much more active by weight than any known monofunctional alkylating agent, and Karnofsky and Clarkson have considered this simple explanation as unlikely.[69]

Mitomycin inhibits selectively DNA synthesis in bacteria[70–72] and mammalian cells in culture.[73] The early inhibition of DNA synthesis by mitomycin C is probably the result of a failure in the synthesis or utilization of precursors but not of a primary depolymerization of DNA.[74] The early inhibition of DNA synthesis precedes the inhibition of RNA synthesis and is accompanied by lowered mitotic activity. The finding that RNA is not affected initially indicates that the inhibition of DNA synthesis is not caused by a disturbance in the metabolism of precursors common to both DNA and RNA. The simultaneous inhibition of thymidine incorporation and of mitosis suggests that the primary action is on the final assembly of DNA.

Mithramycin is closely related chemically to olivomycin and chromomycin. Mithramycin was isolated from *Streptomyces* species in 1962,[75] chromomycin from *S. griseus* 7 in 1958,[76] and olivomycin from *S. olivoreticuli* 16749 in 1962.[77] All three are active against rodent tumors and have had beneficial effects in some human tumors as well. Mithramycin is now recommended for actinomycin D-resistant testicular tumors. Olivomycin is considerably less toxic and requires a larger dose than the other two.[78] In many spectrophotometric tests, the three drugs are indistinguishable, but by using a series of four solvent systems Gause[78] has been able to separate the three. Chromomycin A_3 has been reported to selectively inhibit the biosynthesis of RNA in mammalian cells grown in cell culture, human bone marrow cells, and human leukemic leukocytes, while the formation of DNA was not affected.[78,79] Olivomycin produces selective inhibition of the synthesis of RNA in the cells of Sarcoma 180 in the mouse.[80] Except for the Mg^{++} requirement the properties of chromomycin, mithramycin, and olivomycin, in respect to their binding to DNA in vitro, are similar to those of actinomycin. However, their tumor-inhibiting properties and their toxicity differ somewhat from those of the actinomycins.[78]

Daunomycin (daunorubicin) was isolated by DiMarco et al. in 1963 and was shown to have activity against certain animal tumors.[81–85] It has been studied clinically by Tan et al.[86,87] and Bernard et al.[88] and shown to produce remissions in acute leukemias. Daunomycin preferentially inhibits RNA synthesis both in the cell and in vitro in isolated enzyme systems.[89] It inhibits the template activity for RNA synthesis of all deoxynucleotide polymers. It also inhibits the template activity of poly A and poly I, but not that of poly U or poly C.[45] RNA synthesis is inhibited by daunomycin, regardless of the base composition of the DNA template, but seems to react preferentially with purine nucleotides[45] and resembles in this respect the action of proflavin.[90–92] Daunomycin suppresses RNA synthesis more than DNA synthesis and acts more like actinomycin D. If the specificity of the polymerases consists in their choice of different grooves in the DNA, then the differences of the action of proflavin C, actinomycin D, and daunomycin might be the results of the obstruction of different grooves by the nonintercalated part of the antibiotic.

ADRIAMYCIN

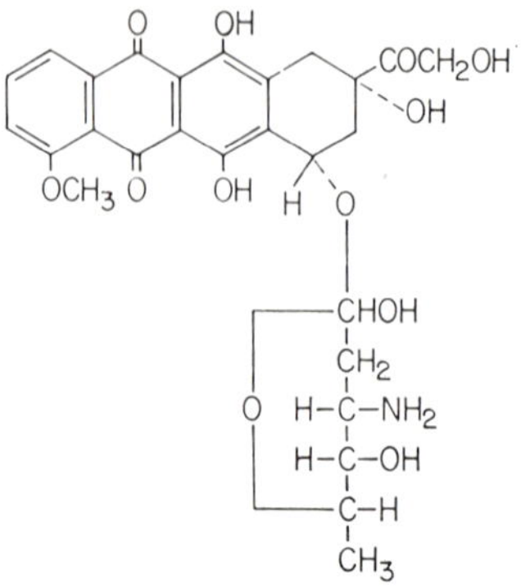

ROUTE OF ADMINISTRATION: IV

TOXICITY:	Bone marrow depression G.I. disturbances and ulcerations Alopecia - fever Local thrombophlebitis
MECHANISM OF ACTION:	Intercalates with DNA and inhibits DNA-dependent RNA synthesis

FIG. 2.—Structural formula of adriamycin.

Adriamycin, a closely related compound (Fig. 2), was isolated by DiMarco et al. in 1969[93] and shown to possess clinical activity in acute leukemia and particularly in tumors in children by Bonadonna and Monfardini[94] and by Tan et al.[95] Its mechanism of action is presumed to be similar to that of daunorubicin, but the development of oral ulcerations just before signs of marrow depression and the absence, so far, of cardiac toxicity suggest slight differences.

Bleomycin, a new antibiotic possessing antitumor activity, was isolated from *Streptomyces verticillus.*[96] Its importance lies in the virtual absence of depressant effects on the bone marrow[97] and a significant activity against epidermoid cancers in man.[98,99] The limiting toxicity is extensive damage to the skin[97] and the lung. The selectivity of therapeutic[98,99] and toxic effects upon epidermal tissues suggests preferential drug localization therein. This has been confirmed by drug distribution studies.[100,101] Despite the lack of marrow toxicity, this antibiotic has also produced a high percentage of remissions in patients with Hodgkin's disease when the tumor was resistant to the conventional agents.[102]

Biochemical studies of the effects of bleomycin upon bacteria and mammalian cells have shown the copper-free antibiotic to be more active than the chelate.[103] The drug inhibited synthesis of DNA under conditions where synthesis of RNA and protein was apparently unimpaired.[103–105] However, progression to mitosis was inhibited at drug concentrations that did not alter isotope incorporation into DNA, and by initial drug exposure late in G2.[104] Single strand scissions have also been demonstrated in DNA extracted from HeLa cells and *E. coli* following treatment of the intact cells with bleomycin.[106]

The rifamycin group of antibiotics has become of considerable theoretical interest recently with the discovery of Temin and Mizutani,[107] Baltimore,[108] Green et al.[109]

and Spiegelman et al.[110] that all oncogenic viruses so far tested possess a unique enzyme, RNA-directed DNA polymerase, not found in any non-oncogenic viruses (with the possible exception of two "slow" viruses). Gallo[111] has recently demonstrated that this enzyme is present in the cells of patients with acute lymphoblastic leukemia but not in PHA-transformed normal lymphocytes. Rifampicin, a member of this rifamycin group, is active against a broad spectrum of bacteria including mycobacteria, presumably by inhibiting DNA-directed RNA polymerase by reacting with the enzyme rather than with the template. Gallo[111] and Gurgo[112] have shown that, although rifampicin is inactive against the RNA-directed DNA polymerase in the leukemic cell, or of oncogenic viruses, at concentrations as high as 400 γ/ml, a close derivative, N-demethyl rifampicin, inhibits this enzyme at 40 γ/ml. No antileukemic or antitumor effects of this compound either in vitro or in vivo have as yet been reported.

Asparaginase has been shown to produce remissions in approximately 60 per cent of patients with acute lymphoblastic leukemia and 10 per cent of those with the acute myeloblastic type. It has not had significant reproducible activity in other types of leukemia or solid tumors. The remissions in acute leukemia are of short duration with a median duration of about three months, and resistance frequently develops rapidly. It is probable that asparaginase must be combined with other agents to realize its full therapeutic potential.[113–115] Fortunately, its antileukemic effects are potentiated by a large number of compounds of diverse mechanisms of action, such as actinomycin D, vincristine, daunomycin, adriamycin, arabinofuranosyl cytosine (Ara-C), thioguanine, and 5-hydroxypicolinaldehyde thiosemicarbazone (5-HP). A clinical evaluation of a sequential combination of vincristine, prednisone, daunomycin, Ara-C plus thioguanine, and asparaginase is under way.[116]

Asparaginase-sensitive leukemic cells in both mouse and man lack the enzyme asparagine synthetase and so must rely on an exogenous source of asparagine. The mechanism of action of asparaginase is the destruction of the plasma asparagine, thus depriving these cells of an amino acid essential for protein synthesis. DNA and RNA synthesis are also inhibited by asparaginase. Cells developing resistance to asparaginase contain large quantities of the enzyme asparagine synthetase, and the mechanism of most resistance is presumably the induction of this enzyme in the resistant cell.

1-β-D-arabinofuranosyl cytosine (Ara-C) was shown to have effects against animal tumors by Evans et al.,[117] and pilot studies by Talley et al.[118] demonstrated bone marrow depression. Ara-C has since been shown to produce remissions in both acute lymphoblastic and acute myeloblastic or monocytic leukemias.[119–121] The combination of Ara-C with a purine derivative is more effective in mouse leukemia than either compound by itself,[122] and the combination of Ara-C and thioguanine is now considered to be the most effective treatment for the acute myeloblastic and monocytic leukemias of man.[123,124]

Ara-C presumably acts to inhibit DNA polymerase[125] or by being directly incorporated into DNA.[126] Uchida and Kreis[127] have studied specificity and resistance to Ara-C in mouse leukemia. A comparison of the distribution of ^{3}H-Ara-C in different tissues of the host and the Ara-C-sensitive and Ara-C-resistant solid P815 tumors revealed a distinct, specific, and protracted accumulation of Ara-C in the sensitive tumor tissue. The other tissues show, as a rule, the usual exponential clearing of the radioactive material.[127]

Trichloroacetic acid extracts from the two tumors revealed after paper chromatographic separation a striking difference only in the amount of di- and triphosphates synthesized, which are produced abundantly in the sensitive cells but only to a minor degree in the resistant ones. The ratios of synthesis of Ara-C di- and triphosphates in sensitive versus resistant cells reaches levels of up to 20:1.

These same results were also found in the ascites form of the tumor.

When Ara-C-5′-monophosphate (Ara-CMP) is used as substrate instead of Ara-C, both crude cell extracts (P815 and P815/Ara-C) phosphorylate the monophosphate to the same extent to the di- and triphosphates (Fig. 3).[128] When the nucleoside kinase, extracted and highly purified from P815 cells, was added to the crude extract of the resistant cells, Ara-C was phosphorylated again to the di- and triphosphates. The extent of this phosphorylation was proportional to the amount of nucleoside kinase added and reached a plateau at the same level as for the sensitive extract. However, when the nucleoside kinase was added to the sensitive crude enzyme preparation, no further increase of the already significant synthesis of di- and triphosphate was found. Since, furthermore, no inhibitor of the nucleoside kinase was found in P815/Ara-C cells, and Ara-CMP was slowly broken down to Ara-C to the same degree in both sensitive and resistant cells, it was concluded that the inability of P815/Ara-C cells to convert Ara-C to Ara-CDP and Ara-CTP is due to the lack of an active nucleoside kinase.[128]

5-Hydroxypicolinaldehyde thiosemicarbazone,[129] an inhibitor of ribonucleotide reductase,[130] has a marked inhibitory effect against transplanted mouse leukemias L1210, L5178Y, and P815 as well as against variants made resistant to 6-mercaptopurine, methotrexate, Ara-C, vincristine, and 6-hydroxylaminopurine riboside (HAPR).[115,131] It is presumed to act as an inhibitor of ribonucleotide reductase by chelating the ferrous ions required for this enzymatic reaction.[129] This theoretical mechanism of action is supported by blockage of the antileukemic effect of 5-HP, both in vivo and in vitro, by ferrous sulfate or cobaltous chloride.[115] This compound has a strong synergistic activity with asparaginase against transplanted mouse leukemia.[115]

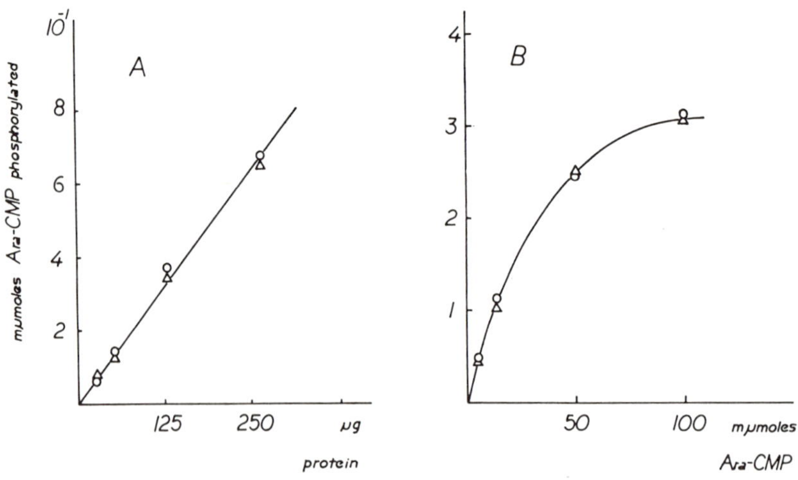

Fig. 3.—Phosphorylation of Ara-CMP in crude enzyme preparation from P815 cells (open circles) and P815/Ara-C cells (triangles). Ordinates A and B, amount of substrate phosphorylated. Abscissa A, protein concentration; B, substrate concentration (260 μg protein used). From Drahovsky and Kreis,[128] with permission.

In preliminary clinical trials, bone marrow improvement has been seen in patients with acute lymphoblastic leukemia.[132] This has been evidenced by a marked decrease in the percentage of blast cells and an increase in erythroid activity to as high as 75 per cent. Further clinical trials of this compound are in progress.

Procarbazine is a compound which was originally found to have antitumor activity in mice and rats[133] and which has since been shown to be a very active and useful compound in the treatment of Hodgkin's disease in man.[134,135] Its value has been particularly striking when used by DeVita et al.[136] in combination with vincristine, prednisone, and nitrogen mustard in 2-week courses repeated once each month for 6 months in stages III and IV Hodgkin's disease. Its mechanism of action is thought to be a selective transmethylation of the intact *N*-methyl group of procarbazine onto the 7 positions of guanine in the macromolecule, especially of transfer RNA. Possibly connected with this, a disturbance and inhibition of the normally occurring methylation takes place which precedes a distinct inhibition of the synthesis of transfer RNA. The absence of functional transfer RNA could cause the cessation of protein and consequently DNA and RNA synthesis.[137]

It is interesting that with almost all antitumor agents, the mechanism of action was studied after evidence of antitumor effect was found; in none, with the possible exception of the rifamycin derivatives, did studies on the mechanism of action of the drug lead to its trial against various forms of experimental cancer. With the rapid advances in molecular biology and other fundamental studies of a cancer cell, this trend may be reversed and from these fundamental studies will come discoveries of compounds active against cancer.

References

1. Fusari, S. A., Haskell, T. H., Frohardt, R. B. and Bartz, Q. R.: Azaserine, a new tumor-inhibitory substance: Structural studies. J. Amer. Chem. Soc. 76:2881, 1954.
2. Diom, H. W., Fusari, S. A., Jakubowski, Z. L., Zora, J. G. and Bartz, Q. R.: 6-Diazo-5-oxo-L-norleucine, a new tumor-inhibitory substance. II. Isolation and characterization. J. Amer. Chem. Soc. 78:3075, 1956.
3. Stock, C. C., Reilly, H. C., Buckley, S. M., Clarke, D. A. and Rhoads, C. P.: Azaserine, a new tumor-inhibitory substance: Studies with Crocker mouse sarcoma 180. Nature 173:71, 1954.
4. Clarke, D. A., Reilly, H. C. and Stock, C. C.: Comparative study of 6-diazo-5-oxo-L-norleucine and *O*-diazoacetyl-L-serine on sarcoma 180. Proc. Amer. Ass. Cancer Res. 2:100, 1956 (abstract).
5. Burchenal, J. H., Murphy, M. L., Yuceoglu, M. and Horsfall, M.: The effect of a new antimetabolite, *O*-diazoacetyl-L-serine, in mouse leukemia. Proc. Amer. Ass. Cancer Res. 1:7, 1954 (abstract).
6. Burchenal, J. H. and Dagg, M. K.: Effects of 6-diazo-5-oxo-L-norleucine and 2-ethylamino-thiadiazole on strains of transplanted mouse leukemia. Proc. Amer. Ass. Cancer Res. 2:97, 1956 (abstract).
7. Gellhorn, A. and Hirschberg, E. (Eds.): Investigation of diverse systems for cancer chemotherapy screening. Cancer Res. 15, Supplement 3, 1955.
8. Sugiura, K. and Schmid, M. S.: Effects of antibiotics on growth of variety of mouse and rat tumors. Proc. Amer. Ass. Cancer Res. 2:151, 1956 (abstract).
9. Sugiura, K. and Stock, C. C.: Effect of *O*-diazoacetyl-L-serine (azaserine) on growth of various mouse and rat tumors. Proc. Soc. Exp. Biol. Med. 88:127, 1955.
10. Ellison, R. R., Karnofsky, D. A., Sternberg, S. S., Murphy, M. L. and Burchenal, J. H.: Clinical trials of *O*-diazoacetyl-L-serine (azaserine) in neoplastic disease. Cancer 7:801, 1954.
11. Magill, G. B., Myers, W. P. L., Reilly, H. C., Putnam, R. C., Magill, J. W. et al.: Pharmacological and initial therapeutic observations on 6-diazo-5-oxo-L-norleucine (DON) in human neoplastic disease. Cancer 10:1138, 1957.
12. Karnofsky, D. A., Golbey, R. B. and Li, M. C.: Remissions induced in tropho-

blastic tumors by 6-diazo-5-oxo-L-norleucine (DON). Proc. Amer. Ass. Cancer Res. 5:33, 1964.
13. Karnofsky, D. A., Golbey, R. B. and Li, M. C.: Remissions induced in trophoblastic tumors by 6-diazo-5-oxo-L-norleucine (DON). *In* Holland, J. F. and Hreshchyshyn, M. M. (Eds.): Choriocarcinoma. (UICC Monograph, Vol. 3). New York: Springer Verlag, 1967, pp. 126–134.
14. Levenberg, B., Melnick, I. and Buchanan, J. M.: Biosynthesis of purines. XV. The effect of aza-L-serine and 6-diazo-5-oxo-L-norleucine on inosinic acid biosynthesis *de novo*. J. Biol. Chem. 225:163, 1957.
15. Goldthwait, D. A.: 5-Phosphoribosylamine, a precursor of glycinamide ribotide. J. Biol. Chem. 222:1051, 1956.
16. Anderson, E. P. and Law, L. W.: Biochemistry of cancer. Ann. Rev. Biochem. 29:577, 1960.
17. Handschumacher, R. E., Bates, C. J., Chang, P. K., Andrews, A. T. and Fischer, G. A.: 5-Diazo-4-oxo-L-norvaline: Reactive asparagine analog with biological specificity. Science 161:62, 1968.
18. Jackson, R. C. and Handschumacher, R. E.: *Escherichia coli* L-asparaginase. Catalytic activity and subunit structure. Biochemistry 9:3585, 1970.
19. Handschumacher, R. E.: Personal communication.
20. Khedouri, E., Anderson, P. M. and Meister, A.: Selective inactivation of the glutamine binding site to *Escherichia coli* carbamyl phosphate synthetase by 2-amino-4-oxo-5-chloropentanoic acid. Biochemistry 5:3552, 1966.
21. Horowitz, B. and Meister, A.: Asparagine synthetase from RADA1 leukemia cells. Proc. Int. Symp. on L-asparaginase, 1970 (in press).
22. Burchenal, J. H., Clarkson, B. D., Dowling, M. D., Jr., Gee, T., Haghbin, M. et al.: Experimental and clinical studies of L-asparaginase in combination therapy. Proc. Int. Symp. on L-asparaginase, 1970 (in press).
23. Waksman, S. A. and Woodruff, H. B.: Bacteriostatic and bactericidal substances produced by a soil actinomyces. Proc. Soc. Exp. Biol. Med. 45:609, 1940.
24. Reilly, H. C., Stock, C. C., Buckley, S. M. and Clarke, D. A.: The effect of antibiotics upon the growth of sarcoma 180 *in vivo*. Cancer Res. 13:684, 1953.
25. Hackmann, C.: Experimentelle Untersuchungen über die Wirkung von Actinomycin C (HBF 386) bei bösartigen Geschwülsten. Z. Krebsforsch. 58:607, 1952.
26. Schulte, G.: Erfahrungen mit neuen cytostatischen Mitteln bei Hämoblastosen und Carcinomen und die Abgrenzung ihrer Wirkungen gegen Roentgentherapie. Z. Krebsforsch. 58:500, 1952.
27. Farber, S., D'Angio, G., Evans, A. and Mitus, A.: Clinical studies on actinomycin D with special reference to Wilms' tumor in children. Ann. N.Y. Acad. Sci. 89:421, 1960.
28. Farber, S.: Current clinical and experimental studies in cancer chemotherapy. Cancer Chemother. Rep. 13:159, 1961.
29. Tan, C. T. C., Dargeon, H. W. and Burchenal, J. H.: The effects of actinomycin D on cancer in childhood. Pediatrics 24:544, 1959.
30. Ross, G., Stolbach, L. L. and Hertz, R.: Actinomycin D in the treatment of methotrexate resistant trophoblastic disease in women. Cancer Res. 22:1015, 1962.
31. Li, M. C., Whitmore, W. F., Golbey, R. and Grabstalt, H.: Effects of combined drug therapy on metastatic cancer of testis. J.A.M.A. 174:1291, 1960.
32. Brockmann, H., Bohnsack, G., Franck, B., Gröne, H., Muxfeldt, H., and Süling, C. H.: Zur Konstitution der Actinomycine. Angew. Chem. 68:70, 1956.
33. Brockmann, H.: Structural differences of the actinomycins and their derivatives. Ann. N.Y. Acad. Sci. 89:323, 1960.
34. Burchenal, J. H., Oettgen, H. F., Reppert, J. A. and Coley, V.: The effect of actinomycins and their derivatives on a spectrum of transplanted mouse leukemia. Ann. N.Y. Acad. Sci. 89:399, 1960.
35. Franklin, R. M.: The inhibition of ribonucleic acid synthesis in mammalian cells by actinomycin D. Biochim. Biophys. Acta 72:555, 1963.
36. Kahan, E., Kahan, F. M. and Hurwitz, J.: The role of deoxyribonucleic acid in ribonucleic acid synthesis. VI. Specificity of action of actinomycin D. J. Biol. Chem. 238:2491, 1963.
37. Reich, E.: Biochemistry of actinomycins. Cancer Res. 23:1428, 1963.
38. Goldberg, I. H. and Rabinowitz, M.: Actinomycin D inhibition of deoxyribonucleic acid-dependent synthesis of ribonucleic acid. Science 136:315, 1962.
39. Hurwitz, J., Furth, J. J., Malamy, M. and Alexander, M.: The role of deoxyribo-

nucleic acid in ribonucleic acid synthesis. III. The inhibition of the enzymatic synthesis of the ribonucleic acid and deoxyribonucleic acid by actinomycin D and proflavin. Proc. Nat. Acad. Sci. U.S.A. 48:1222, 1962.
40. Kawamata, J. and Imanishi, M.: Interaction of actinomycin with deoxyribonucleic acid. Nature 187:1112, 1960.
41. Kersten, W.: Interaction of actinomycin D with constituents of nucleic acids. Biochim. Biophys. Acta 47:610, 1961.
42. Kersten, W., Kersten, H. and Rauen, H. M.: Action of nucleic acids on the inhibition of growth by actinomycin of *Neurospora crassa*. Nature 187:60, 1960.
43. Kirk, J. M.: The mode of action of actinomycin D. Biochim. Biophys. Acta 42:167, 1960.
44. Rauen, H. M., Kersten, H. and Kersten, W.: Zur Wirkungsweise von Actinomycinen. Hoppe Seyler Z. Physiol. Chem. 321:139, 1960.
45. Ward, D. C., Reich, E. and Goldberg, I. H.: Base specificity in the interaction of polynucleotides with antibiotic drugs. Science 149:1259, 1965.
46. Schwartz, H. S., Dodergren, J. E., Garofalo, M. and Sternberg, S. S.: Actinomycin D: Effects on nucleic acid and protein metabolism in intact and regenerating liver of rats. Cancer Res. 25:307, 1965.
47. Merits, I.: Actinomycin inhibition of RNA synthesis in rat liver. Biochem. Biophys. Res. Commun. 10:254, 1963.
48. Revel, M. and Hiatt, H. H.: The stability of liver messenger RNA. Proc. Nat. Acad. Sci. U.S.A. 51:810, 1964.
49. Harbers, E. and Müller, W.: On the inhibition of RNA synthesis by actinomycin. Biochem. Biophys. Res. Commun. 7:107, 1962.
50. Baltimore, D. and Franklin, R. M.: The effect of Mengovirus infection on the activity of the DNA-dependent RNA polymerase of L-cells. Proc. Nat. Acad. Sci. U.S.A. 48:1383, 1962.
51. Blum, J. J. and Buetow, D. E.: Effects of actinomycin D on acetate-starved and logarithmically growing *Euglena gracilis*. Biochim. Biophys. Acta 68:625, 1963.
52. Levinthal, C., Keynan, A. and Higa, A.: Messenger RNA turnover and protein synthesis in *B. subtilis* inhibited by actinomycin D. Proc. Nat. Acad. Sci. U.S.A. 48:1631, 1962.
53. Cavalieri, L. F. and Nemchin, R. G.: The mode of action of actinomycin D with DNA. Biochim. Biophys. Acta 87:641, 1964.
54. Goldberg, I. H., Rabinowitz, M. and Reich, E.: Basis of actinomycin action. I. DNA binding and inhibition of RNA-polymerase synthetic reactions by actinomycin. Proc. Nat. Acad. Sci. U.S.A. 48:2094, 1962.
55. Hamilton, L. D., Fuller, W. and Reich, E.: X-ray diffraction and molecular model building studies of the interaction of actinomycin with nucleic acids. Nature 198:538, 1963.
56. Haselkorn, R.: Actinomycin D as a probe for nucleic acid secondary structure. Science 143:682, 1964.
57. Reich, E.: Actinomycin: Correlation of structure and function of its complexes with purines and DNA. Science 143:684, 1964.
58. Wakaki, S., Marumo, H., Tomioka, H., Shimizu, G., Kato, G., et al.: Isolation of new fractions of antitumor mitomycins. Antibiot. Chemother. 8:228, 1958.
59. Wakaki, S.: Recent advances in research on antitumor mitomycins. Cancer Chemother. Rep. 13:79, 1961.
60. Sugiura, K.: Antitumor activity of mitomycin C. Cancer Chemother. Rep. 13:51, 1961.
61. Jones, R., Jr.: Mitomycin D. A preliminary report of studies on human pharmacology and initial therapeutic trial. Cancer Chemother. Rep. 2:3, 1959.
62. Frank, W. and Osterberg, A. E.: Mitomycin C (NSC-26980)—an evaluation of the Japanese reports. Cancer Chemother. Rep. 9:114, 1960.
63. Osamura, S.: Present state of chemotherapy of chronic leukemia in Japan. Cancer Chemother. Rep. 13:145, 1961.
64. Evans, A. E.: Mitomycin C. Cancer Chemother. Rep. 14:1, 1961.
65. Lefemine, D. V., Dann, M., Barbatschi, F., Hausmann, W. K., Zbinovsky, V., et al.: Isolation and characterization of mitomycin and other antibiotics produced by *Streptomyces verticillatus*. J. Amer. Chem. Soc. 84:3184, 1962.
66. Webb, J. S., Cosulich, D. B., Mowat, J. H., Patrick, J. B., Broschard, R. W., et al.: Structures of mitomycins A, B and C and porfiromycin. J. Amer. Chem. Soc. 84: 3185, 1962 (Communications to Editor, Part I).
67. Webb, J. S., Cosulich, D. B., Mowat, J. H., Patrick, J. B., Broschard, R. W., et al.: Structures of mitomycins A, B and C, and porfiromycin. J. Amer. Chem. Soc. 84:

3187, 1962 (Communications to Editor, Part II).
68. Tulinsky, A.: The structure of mitomycin A. J. Amer. Chem. Soc. 84:3188, 1962.
69. Karnofsky, D. A. and Clarkson, B. D.: Cellular effects of anticancer drugs. Ann. Rev. Pharmacol. 3:357, 1963.
70. Shiba, S., Terawaki, A., Taguchi, T. and Kawamata, J.: Studies on the effect of mitomycin C on nucleic acid metabolism in *Escherichia coli* strain B. Biken J. 1:179, 1958.
71. Shiba, S., Terawaki, A., Taguchi, T. and Kawamata, J.: Selective inhibition of formation of deoxyribonucleic acid in Escherichia coli by mitomycin C. Nature 183:1056, 1959.
72. Reich, E., Shatkin, A. J. and Tatum, E. L.: Bacteriocidal action of mitomycin C. Biochim. Biophys. Acta 53:132, 1961.
73. Reich, E. and Franklin, R. M.: Effect of mitomycin C on the growth of some animal viruses. Proc. Nat. Acad. Sci. U.S.A. 47:1212, 1961.
74. Schwartz, H. S., Sternberg, S. S. and Philips, F. S.: Pharmacology of mitomycin C. IV. Effects *in vivo* on nucleic acid synthesis; comparison with actinomycin D. Cancer Res. 23:1125, 1963.
75. Rao, K. V., Cullen, W. P. and Sobin, B. A.: A new antibiotic with antitumor properties. Antibiot. Chemother. 12:182, 1962.
76. Tatsuoka, S., Nakazawa, K., Miyake, A., Kaziwara, K., Aramaki, Y., et al.: Isolation, anticancer activity and pharmacology of a new antibiotic chromomycin A_3. Gann Suppl. 49:23, 1958.
77. Gause, G. F., Ukholina, R. S. and Sveshinikova, M. A.: Olivomycin: a new antibiotic produced by *Actinomyces olivoreticuli.* Antibiotiki 7:34, 1962.
78. Gause, G. F.: Olivomycin, mithramycin, chromomycin: Three related cancerostatic antibiotics. *In* Goldin, A., Hawking, F. and Schnitzer, R. J. (Eds.): Advances in Chemotherapy, Vol. 2. New York: Academic Press, 1965, pp. 179–195.
79. Wakisaka, G., Uchino, H., Nakamura, T., Sotobayashi, H., Shirakawa, S., et al.: Selective inhibition of biosynthesis of ribonucleic acid in mammalian cells by chromomycin A_3. Nature 198:385, 1963.
80. Layashenko, V. A.: The effect of olivomycin on the content of nucleic acids in the transplantable mouse sarcoma 180. Antibiotiki 9:520, 1964.
81. DiMarco, A., Gaetani, M., Dorigotti, L., Soldati, M. and Bellini, O.: Experimental studies on the antitumor activity of daunomycin: A new antibiotic with new antitumor activity. Tumori 49:203, 1963.
82. DiMarco, A., Soldati, M., Fioretti, A. and Dasdia, T.: Studies on the activity of daunomycin, a new antitumor antibiotic, on normal and tumor cells growing "in vitro." Tumori 49:235, 1963.
83. Grein, A., Spalla, C., DiMarco, A. and Canevazzi, G.: Descrizione e classificazione di un Attinomicete (*Streptomyces peucetius sp. nova*) produttore di una sostanza ad attività antitumorale: La daunomicina. G. Microbiol. 11:109, 1963.
84. DiMarco, A., Gaetani, M., Orezzi, P., Scarpinato, B. M., Silvestrini, R., et al.: "Daunomycin," a new antibiotic of the rhodomycin group. Nature 201:706, 1964.
85. Dorigotti, L.: An electron-microscopic study of the changes produced by daunomycin on HeLa cells. Tumori 50:117, 1964.
86. Tan, C., Tasaka, H. and DiMarco, M.: Clinical studies of daunomycin C. Proc. Amer. Ass. Cancer Res. 6:64, 1965 (abstract).
87. Tan, C., Tasaka, H., Yu, K.-P., Murphy, M. L. and Karnofsky, D. A.: Daunomycin, an antitumor antibiotic, in the treatment of neoplastic disease: Clinical evaluation with special reference to childhood leukemia. Cancer 20:333, 1967.
88. Bernard, J., Jacquillat, C. L., Boiron, M., Najean, Y., Seligmann, M., et al.: Essai de traitement des leucémies aigues lymphoblastiques et myeloblastiques par un antibiotique nouveau: La rubidomycine (13057 RP). Presse Med. 75:19, 1967.
89. Hartmann, G., Goller, H., Koschel, K., Kersten, W. and Kersten, H.: Hemmung der DNA-abhängigen RNA- und DNA-Synthese durch Antibiotica. Biochem. Z. 341:126, 1964.
90. Peacocke, A. R. and Skerrett, J. N. H.: The interaction of aminoacridines with nucleic acids. Trans. Faraday Soc. 52:261, 1956.
91. Lerman, L. S.: Structural considerations in the interaction of DNA and acridines. J. Molec. Biol. 3:18, 1961.
92. Goldberg, I. H., Reich, E. and Rabinowitz, M.: Inhibition of ribonucleic acid-polymerase reactions by actinomycin and proflavine. Nature 199:44, 1963.
93. DiMarco, A., Gaetani, M. and Scarpinato, B.: Adriamycin (NSC-123,127): A new

antibiotic with antitumor activity. Cancer Chemother. Rep. 53:33, 1969.

94. Bonadonna, G. and Monfardini, S.: Therapeutic effects of adriamycin in the neoplastic disease of children and adults. Proc. Amer. Ass. Cancer Res. 11:10, 1970 (abstract).
95. Tan, C., Wollner, N., King, O. and Ilano, D.: Adriamycin, a new antibiotic, in treatment of childhood leukemia and other malignant neoplasms. Proc. Amer. Ass. Cancer Res. 11:79, 1970 (abstract).
96. Umezawa, H., Maeda, K., Takeuchi, T. and Okami, Y.: New antibiotics, bleomycin A and B. J. Antibiot. (Tokyo) 19:200, 1966.
97. Ishizuka, M., Takayama, H., Takeuchi, T. and Umezawa, H.: Activity and toxicity of bleomycin. J. Antibiot. (Tokyo) 20:15, 1967.
98. Ichikawa, T., Nakano, I. and Hirokawa, F.: Bleomycin treatment of the tumors of penis and scrotum. J. Urol. 102:699, 1969.
99. Takeda, K., Sagawa, Y. and Arakawa, T.: Therapeutic effect of bleomycin for skin tumors. Gann 61:207, 1970.
100. Ishizuka, M., Kimura, K., Iwanaga, J., Takeuchi, T. and Umezawa, H.: Biological studies on individual bleomycins. J. Antibiot. (Tokyo) 21:592, 1968.
101. Umezawa, H., Ishizuka, M., Hori, S., Chimura, H. and Takeuchi, T.: The distribution of ^{3}H-bleomycin in mouse tissue. J. Antibiot. (Tokyo) 21:638, 1968.
102. Yagoda, A., Krakoff, I., LaMonte, C. and Tan, C.: Clinical trial of bleomycin. Proc. Amer. Ass. Cancer Res. 12:37, 1971 (abstract).
103. Suzuki, H., Nagai, K., Yamaki, H., Tanaka, N. and Umezawa, H.: Mechanism of action of bleomycin. Studies with the growing culture of bacterial tumor cells. J. Antibiot. (Tokyo) 21:379, 1968.
104. Kunimoto, T., Hori, M. and Umezawa, H.: Modes of action of phleomycin, bleomycin and formycin on HeLa S3 cells in synchronized culture. J. Antibiot. (Tokyo) 20:277, 1967.
105. Ohnuma, T. and Holland, J. F.: Studies on the biochemical and biological activities of bleomycin. Proc. Amer. Ass. Cancer Res. 11:60, 1970.
106. Suzuki, H., Nagai, K., Yamaki, H., Tanaka, N. and Umezawa, H.: On the mechanism of action of bleomycin scission of DNA strands *in vitro* and *in vivo*. J. Antibiot. (Tokyo) 22:446, 1969.
107. Temin, H. M. and Mizutani, S.: RNA-dependent DNA polymerase in virions of Rous sarcoma virus. Nature 226:1211, 1970.
108. Baltimore, D.: Viral RNA-dependent DNA polymerase. Nature 226:1209, 1970.
109. Green, M., Rokutanda, M., Fujinaga, K., Ray, R. K., Rokutanda, H. and Gurgo, C.: Mechanism of carcinogenesis by RNA tumor virus. I. An RNA-dependent DNA polymerase in murine sarcoma viruses. Proc. Nat. Acad. Sci. U.S.A. 67:385, 1970.
110. Spiegelman, S., Burny, A., Das, M. R., Keydar, J., Schlom, J., et al.: Characterization of the products of RNA-directed DNA polymerase in oncogenic RNA viruses. Nature 227:563, 1970.
111. Gallo, R. C., Yang, S. S. and Ting, R. C.: RNA dependent DNA polymerase of human acute leukaemic cells. Nature 228: 927, 1970.
112. Gurgo, C., Ray, R. K., Thiry, L. and Green, M.: Inhibitors of the RNA and DNA dependent polymerase activities of RNA tumour viruses. Nature 229:111, 1971.
113. Oettgen, H. F.: Clinical evaluation of L-asparaginase. Proc. 10th Int. Cancer Cong. 1970. (In press.)
114. Burchenal, J. H.: Clinical evaluation and future prospects of asparaginase. *In* Mathé, G. (Ed.): Recent Results in Cancer Research, Vol. 30. Heidelberg: Springer-Verlag, 1970, pp. 20–27.
115. Burchenal, J. H., Clarkson, B. D., Dowling, M. D., Jr., Gee, T., Haghbin, M. and Tan, C. T. C.: Experimental and clinical studies of L-asparaginase in combination therapy. Proc. Int. Symp. on L-asparaginase, 1970 (in press).
116. Oettgen, H. F., Tallal, L., Tan, C. C., Murphy, M. L., Clarkson, B. D., et al.: Clinical experience with L-asparaginase. *In* Grundmann, E. and Oettgen, H. F. (Eds.): Recent Results in Cancer Research, Vol. 33. Heidelberg: Springer-Verlag, 1970, pp. 219–235.
117. Evans, J. S., Musser, E. A., Mengel, G. D., Forsblad, K. R. and Hunter, J. H.: Antitumor activity of 1-β-D-arabinofuranosylcytosine hydrochloride. Proc. Soc. Exp. Biol. Med. 106:350, 1961.
118. Talley, R. W. and Vaitkevicius, V. K.: Megaloblastosis produced by a cystosine antagonist, 1-β-D-arabinofuranosylcytosine. Blood 21:352, 1963.
119. Henderson, E. S. and Burke, P. J.: Clinical experience with cytosine arabinoside. Proc.

Amer. Ass. Cancer Res. 6:26, 1965 (abstract).

120. Loo, R. V., Brennan, M. J. and Talley, R. W.: Clinical pharmacology of cytosine arabinoside. Proc. Amer. Ass. Cancer Res. 6:41, 1965 (abstract).

121. Papac, R., Creasey, W. A., Calabresi, P. and Welch, A. D.: Clinical and pharmacological studies with 1-β-arabinofuranosylcytosine (cytosine arabinoside). Proc. Amer. Ass. Cancer Res. 6:50, 1965 (abstract).

122. Burchenal, J. H. and Dollinger, M. R.: Cytosine arabinoside (NSC-63878) in combination with 6-mercaptopurine (NSC-755), methotrexate (NSC-740), or 5-fluorouracil (NSC-19893) in L1210 mouse leukemia. Cancer Chemother. Rep. 51: 435, 1967.

123. Gee, T. S., Yu, K. P., Augustin, B. T., Krakoff, I. H. and Clarkson, B. D.: Combination therapy of adult acute leukemia with thioguanine (TG) and 1-β-D-arabinofuranosylcytosine (CA). Proc. Amer. Ass. Cancer Res. 9:23, 1968 (abstract).

124. Gee, T. S., Yu, K.-P. and Clarkson, B. D.: Treatment of adult acute leukemia with arabinosylcytosine and thioguanine. Cancer 23:1019, 1969.

125. Furth, J. J. and Cohen, S. S.: Inhibition of mammalian DNA polymerase by the 5′-triphosphate of 1-β-D-arabinofuranosylcytosine and the 5′-triphosphate of 9-β-D-arabinofuranosyladenine. Cancer Res. 28: 2061, 1968.

126. Silagi, S.: Metabolism of 1-β-D-arabinofuranosylcytosine in L cells. Cancer Res. 25:1446, 1965.

127. Uchida, K. and Kreis, W.: Studies on drug resistance. I. Distribution of 1-β-D-arabinofuranosylcytosine, cytidine and deoxycytidine in mice bearing Ara-C sensitive and resistant P815 neoplasms. Biochem. Pharmacol. 18:1115, 1969.

128. Drahovsky, D. and Kreis, W.: Studies on drug resistance. II. Kinase patterns in P815 neoplasms sensitive and resistant to 1-β-D-arabinofuranosylcytosine. Biochem. Pharmacol. 19:940, 1970.

129. Blanz, E. J., Jr. and French, F. A.: The carcinostatic activity of 5-hydroxy-2-formylpyridine thiosemicarbazone. Cancer Res. 28:2419, 1968.

130. Sartorelli, A. C.: Effect of chelating agents upon the synthesis of nucleic acids and protein: Inhibition of DNA synthesis by 1-formylisoquinoline thiosemicarbazone. Biochem. Biophys. Res. Com. 27:26, 1967.

131. Burchenal, J. H. and Dowling, M.: Potentiation of the antileukemic effect of 5-hydroxy-2-formylpyridine thiosemicarbazone (5-HP) by asparaginase (A-ase). Proc. Amer. Ass. Cancer Res. 11:13, 1970 (abstract).

132. Etcubanas, E., Tan, C., Wollner, N., Bethune, V., Krakoff, I. and Burchenal, J.: Preliminary clinical trials of 5-hydroxy-2-formylpyridine thiosemicarbazone (5-HP). Proc. Amer. Ass. Cancer Res. 12:38, 1971 (abstract).

133. Bollag, W. and Grunberg, E.: Tumor inhibitory effects of a new class of cytotoxic agents: Methylhydrazine derivatives. Experientia 19:130, 1963.

134. Martz, G., D'Alessandri, A., Keel, H. J. and Bollag, W.: Preliminary clinical results with a new antitumor agent RO 4-6467 (NSC-77213). Cancer Chemother. Rep. 33:5, 1963.

135. Brunner, K. W. and Young, C. W.: A methylhydrazine derivative in Hodgkin's disease and other malignant neoplasms. Ann. Intern. Med. 63:69, 1965.

136. DeVita, V. T., Serpick, A. and Carbone, P. P.: Combination therapy of advanced Hodgkin's disease (HD): The NCI program, a progress report. Proc. Amer. Ass. Cancer Res. 10:19, 1969 (abstract).

137. Kreis, W.: Metabolism of an antineoplastic methylhydrazine derivative in a P815 mouse neoplasm. Cancer Res. 30:82, 1970.

Interferon and Interferon Inducers in the Treatment of Neoplastic Diseases

By Hilton B. Levy, Ph.D.

Although investigators knew a number of years ago that interferon can inhibit malignant transformation by oncogenic viruses, only recently have they recognized that interferon and its inducers may have value in the treatment of malignant diseases.

Isaacs originally proposed that the interferon response is induced by the presence in a cell of foreign nucleic acid. The net effect of this response is, in effect, to reduce the damage brought about by the presence of this foreign nucleic acid, which usually would be viral nucleic acid. Isaacs' hypothesis was supported by some data showing that foreign nucleic acids do indeed lead to the production of some slight amount of interferon. His data were not very convincing, and general acceptance of this concept was consequently held in abeyance. The validity of this hypothesis has recently received support from the findings that certain double-stranded synthetic and natural ribonucleic acids, particularly polyinosinic:polycytidylic acid (poly I:poly C), can lead to the development by cells of a high level of resistance to virus replication and to the production of large amounts of interferon, both in vivo and in tissue culture.[1]

Several laboratories have reported that viral interference,[2] interferon,[3] and inter-

Table 1.—*Effect of Polyinosinic:Polycytidylic Acid (Poly I:Poly C) on Animal Tumors*

Tumor	*Increase in median Survival over Control* (%)
J96132 Reticulum cell sarcoma (subcutaneous)	130*
J96132 Reticulum cell sarcoma (ascites)	96*
Carcinosarcoma Walker 256	100
Reticulum cell sarcoma RCSL	89
Ehrlich ascites tumor	70
S91 Melanoma	55
Fibrosarcoma	52
B1237 Lymphoma (ascites)	45
L1210 Leukemia	42
Plasma cell YPC-1	39
B1237 Lymphoma (subcutaneous)	28
MT-1 Tumor (subcutaneous)	26
Reticulum cell sarcoma ovarian	20
Leukemia P388	16
Leukemia K1964	12

Treatment, in most cases, was 150–200 μg per mouse, 3 times weekly, by the intraperitoneal route. With the exception of the J96132 reticulum cell sarcoma, some Ehrlich ascites tumors, and a few Walker carcinosarcomas, all animals ultimately died.

* Mean day of death of the animals that died. About 30 per cent of all the animals treated have survived, although treatment was stopped at about day 50.

From the Section of Molecular Virology, Laboratory of Viral Diseases, National Institute of Allergy and Infectious Diseases, National Institutes of Health, Bethesda, Maryland.

feron inducers[4] can inhibit the growth of oncogenic viruses in tissue culture[5,6] and can alter the course of murine leukemias in animals.[7,8] It has also been shown that the double-stranded RNA polyinosinic:polycytidylic acid, which, among other things, is a good interferon inducer,[1] inhibits the growth of a large variety of tumors in animals.[9,10] Finally, exogenous interferon also inhibits some transplanted tumors that were induced originally by chemical carcinogenesis and not by viruses.[11] The purpose of this review is to consider some factors involved in these tumor inhibitions. The variety of tumors inhibited by poly I:poly C is indicated in Table 1. In addition, carcinogenesis by dimethylbenzanthracene (DMBA) plus croton oil or DMBA alone is strongly inhibited by suitable administration of poly I:poly C.[12]

For reasons of convenience, further discussion will center on the various actions of poly I:poly C. The mechanism of action of this compound appears to be complex. Poly I:poly C has been shown to be a potent inducer of interferon synthesis.[1] Gresser et al.[7] demonstrated that the murine leukemias, such as those induced by the Friend virus, are inhibited by exogenous interferon. Similarly, Wheelock[4] has shown that Friend virus leukemia is inhibited by the administration of statolon, an inducer of interferon. Sarma et al.[8] have shown the inhibition of the growth of the leukemia viruses in tissue culture by the interferon system. Interferon inducers can inhibit virus-induced cell transformation.[13,14] In addition, Gresser has shown that the growth of a dimethylbenzanthracene-induced tumor is also inhibited by interferon[15] (Fig. 1). In the animals bearing those tumors, interferon treatment brought about an increased

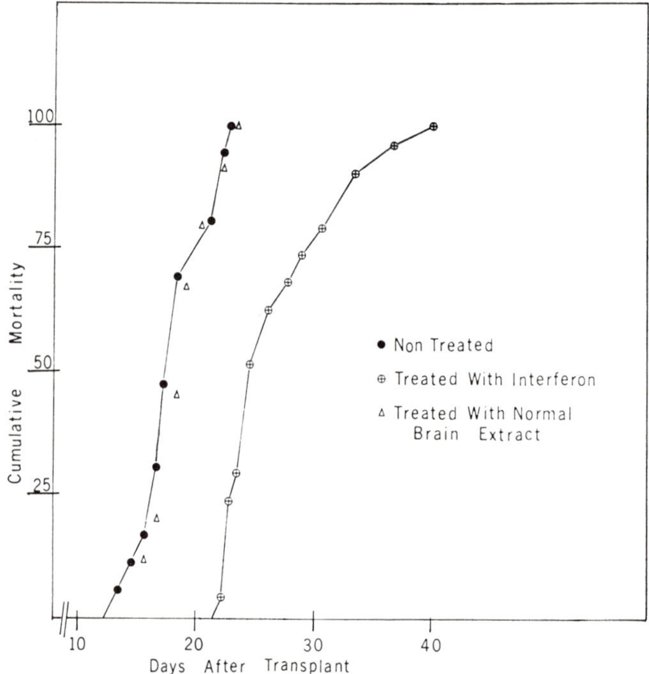

FIG. 1.—Increased survival in C57 black mice inoculated intraperitoneally with EL4 tumor cells and treated with interferon preparations. Reproduced through the courtesy of Dr. Gresser. From Gresser, I., Bourali, C., Lévy, J. P., et al.: Prolongation de la survie des souris inoculées avec des cellules tumorales et traitées avec des préparations d'interférons. C. R. Acad. Sci. 268:994, 1969.

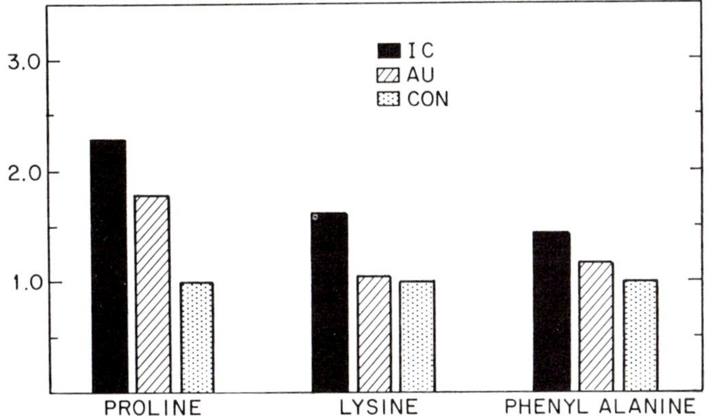

FIG. 2.—Effect of poly I: poly C and poly A: poly U on amino acid incorporation into primary mouse embryo cells. Primary mouse embryo cells were exposed for 16 hours to 100 μg/ml of the RNA in the presence of Eagle's Basal Medium (BME) +5 per cent fetal calf serum. The medium was changed to BME without serum for one hour and then the cells were exposed to the labeled amino acid for 30 minutes. Radioactivity was determined on the acid-insoluble portion of the cells. The ordinate represents specific activity normalized to a value of 1 for the controls. IC = polyinosinic: polycytidylic acid; poly I:poly C. AU = polyadenylic:polyuridylic acid; poly A:poly U. Con = controls.

phagocytosis of tumor cells. Gresser has shown that the growth of certain tumor cells in tissue culture is inhibited by interferon preparations, but the possibility remains that this inhibition may be due to impurities. Since poly I:poly C is a potent inducer of interferon in mice, it is likely that part of the antitumor action of the double-stranded RNA is through the interferon system.

A second aspect of the activity of poly I:poly C may be as a direct chemotherapeutic agent. Poly I:poly C is a double-stranded RNA, the homopolymers of which can code for the synthesis of polypeptides in a suitable cell-free test system. Poly C, for example, should code for the synthesis of polyproline. If the poly C component of poly I:poly C were responsible for the synthesis of polyproline in the cell one might imagine any number of cellular reactions to the presence of this "nonsense" protein. Poly I:poly C does stimulate the incorporation of proline into the proteins of L-cells but it also stimulates incorporation of a number of other amino acids for which it should not code. Further, polyadenylic-polyuridylic acid also stimulates proline incorporation, for which it does not code, and it does not stimulate phenylalanine incorporation, for which the poly U should code (Fig. 2). One can conclude that the double-stranded RNA's do stimulate amino acid incorporation into proteins in tissue culture but are not acting intracellularly as synthetic messenger RNA's. The nature of this stimulation is under study.

The compound also alters precursor incorporation into macromolecules in vivo. Poly I:poly C was injected into mice bearing any one of three different types of tumors. After 16 to 20 hours the mice received radioactive uridine, radioactive proline or both. The specific activities of the RNA and protein of the tumor and a number of normal organs were determined, and the effect of the poly I:poly C treatment on such specific activity was calculated. The drug inhibited the incorporation of the precursor into tumor macromolecules by 60 to 95 per cent. The effect on normal organs depended on the strain of mice studied, ranging from occasional enhancement or only slight effect in C57 black Kaplan mice (Fig. 3) to moderately strong inhibition in BALB/c mice (Fig. 4).

Considering the extent of inhibition seen, it was surprising that the tumor did not disappear more rapidly than it did and that the host did not manifest greater toxicity.

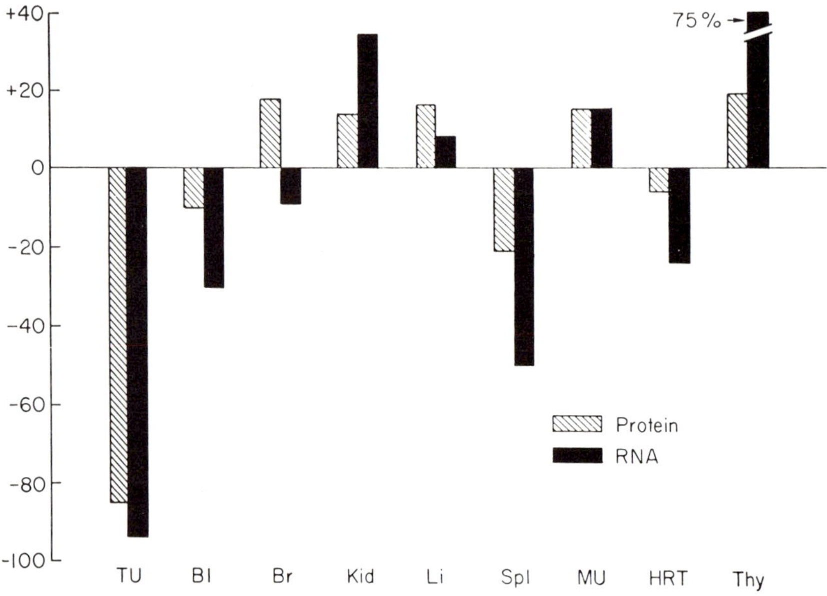

FIG. 3.—Effect of poly I:poly C on ^{14}C proline and ^{3}H-uridine incorporation into various organs of C57 black mice bearing reticulum cell sarcoma J96132. Three C57 black mice were treated with 200 μg/mouse of poly I:poly C intraperitoneally. Three mice served as controls. After 16 hours, the mice were exposed to 10 μCi ^{14}C proline and 100 μCi ^{3}H-uridine for 40 minutes, and the radioactivity incorporated into acid-insoluble components of the indicated organs was measured. The ordinate is the percentage of enhancement (+) or diminution (−) of specific activity of organs from animals treated with poly I:poly C as compared with controls.

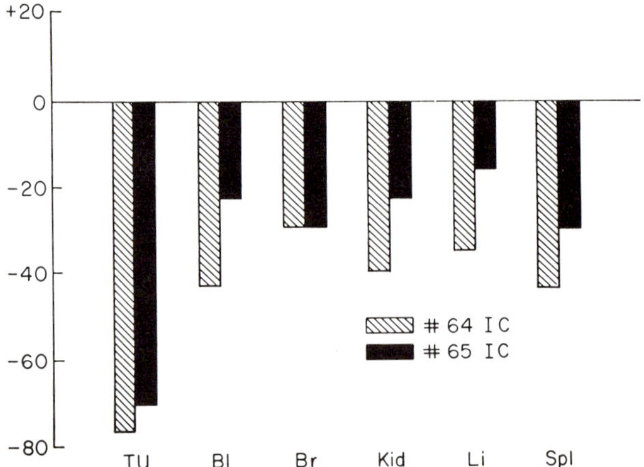

FIG. 4.—Effect of poly I:poly C on ^{14}C proline incorporation into various organs of BALB/c mice bearing MT-1 tumors. Same conditions as in Fig. 3.

The explanation became apparent from experiments in which multiple injections of the drug were given prior to injecting the radioactive precursors (Fig. 5). It can be seen that the tumor, as well as the normal organs, develops a hyporeactive state to the inhibitory action of the poly I:poly C, analogous to the decreasing production of interferon in response to repeated injections of the drug.

A third facet of the antitumor action of poly I:poly C is its ability to enhance cell-mediated defense mechanisms against foreign antigens. If spleen cells from adult mice are injected into newborn F1 hybrids, one of whose parents is of the same strain as the donor mice, the donor cells develop a graft-versus-host reaction which affects the recipient animals in a number of ways.[16] One of these ways is splenomegaly in the recipient.[17,18] The degree of spleen enlargement is a function of the activity and the logarithm of the number of donor cells. This test is useful in evaluating immunosuppressive drugs and antilymphocyte serum. The depressed reactivity of the spleen cells from such drug-treated donor animals results in less splenomegaly in the recipient than that obtained from spleen cells from untreated donors. When donor mice are given poly I:poly C, their subsequently removed spleen cells show enhanced immunologic reactivity against the foreign antigens in the recipient and result in increased

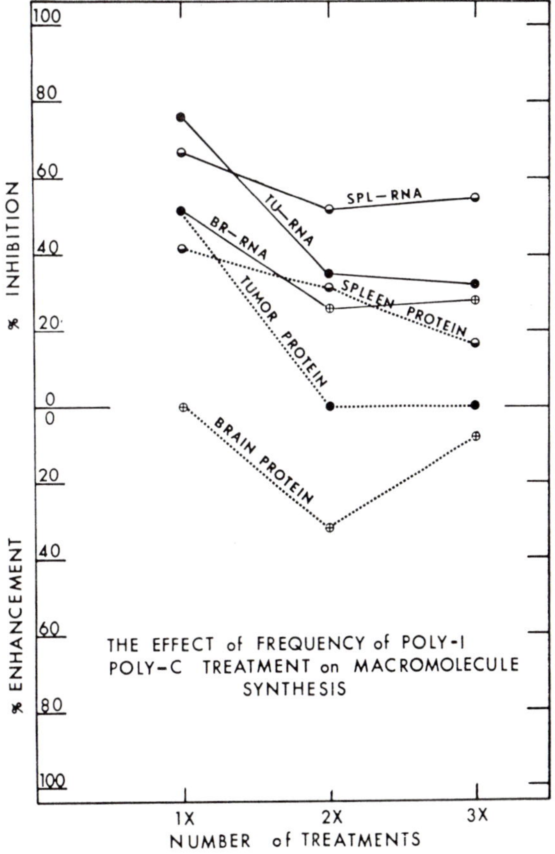

FIG. 5.—Effect of repeated injections of poly I: poly C on precursor incorporation. Same conditions as in Fig. 3, except that poly I: poly C was given once, twice, or three times, on alternate days.

splenomegaly[19,20] (Fig. 6). Comparison of the position of the two parallel lines obtained from injecting different numbers of cells reveals that poly I:poly C at 1 mg/mouse caused nearly a tripling of the effectiveness of the cells in the graft-versus-host reaction, while smaller amounts of poly I:poly C produced definite but less stimulation. Enzymatic hydrolysis of the poly I:poly C destroys its enhancing ability.

It is reasonable to think that enhancement by poly I:poly C of such cell-mediated rejection of foreign antigens could effectively act against the foreign antigens of the tumor, facilitating the rejection of the tumor. Indeed, the inhibition of macromolecule synthesis discussed earlier may be a manifestation of such cellular immunologic activity. This enhancement of immunologic reactivity by polynucleotides has been observed repeatedly.[21]

It appears, then, that there are at least three different aspects of the action of poly I:poly C that bear on the antitumor activity of the compound: the activity of the interferon induced, possible direct chemotherapeutic action, and enhancement of immunologic rejection mechanisms. The relative importance of each of these components and the interrelations among them will be discussed. Since exogenous interferon is effective in mice against some tumors, it is obvious that the interferon induced by poly I:poly C is important, but it is not understood how interferon inhibits tumors. It has been reported that interferon can inhibit cell growth in tissue culture,[22] but lack of such inhibition has also been reported.[23,24] Because all the testing has been done

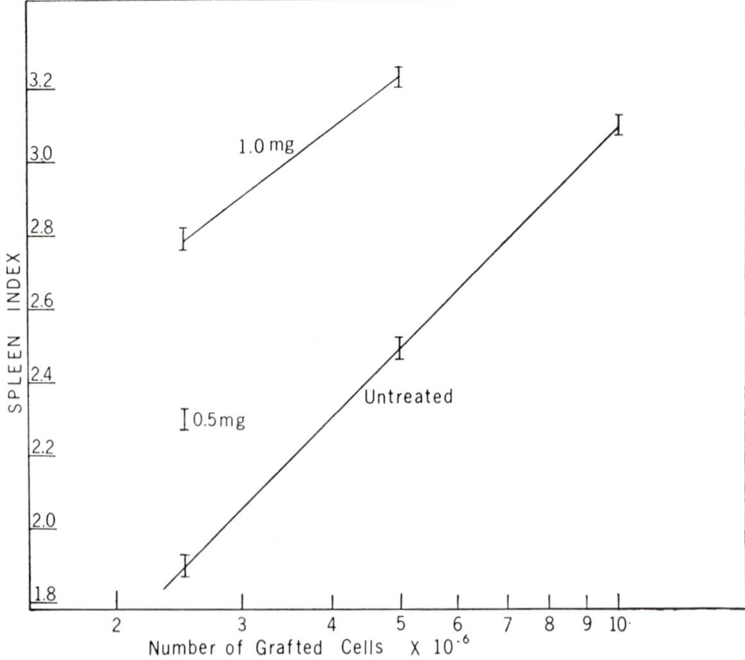

FIG. 6.—Effect of poly I:poly C on graft-versus-host reaction. BALB/c mice were inoculated intraperitoneally with the indicated amount of poly I:poly C. They were sacrificed 48 hours later and their spleens were removed and minced. The indicated number of spleen cells was inoculated into newborn F1 hybrids of BALB/c × C57 black mice. These animals and their spleens were weighed 9 days later and the spleen weight was normalized to body weight. The spleen index is the ratio of this normalized spleen weight to the normalized spleen weight of animals not inoculated with spleen cells.

with interferons of varying degrees of impurity, it is hard to exclude the possibility that the observed inhibitions have been due to impurities. It may be that in an animal, interferon treatment increases the immune reactivity of the host. We are currently testing this possibility. A number of reports have suggested a close association between the interferon system and the immunologic systems. For example, lymphocytes from animals (and man) immunized with a specific antigen respond, in tissue culture, to exposure to that antigen by producing interferon.[25–27] Lymphocytes on exposure to phytohemagglutinin change to lymphoblasts, which then produce interferon. This is the same type of cellular transformation that occurs when these cells are stimulated to produce antibodies. It is possible, therefore, that a coordinated relation may exist between initiation of antibody response and initiation of interferon production.

The ability of poly I:poly C to enhance cell-mediated graft-versus-host reaction could partially account for its ability to inhibit the growth of tumors containing foreign antigens. It is worth noting that polyadenylic:polyuridylic acid has been reported to be as good an adjuvant for the production of circulating antibodies as is poly I:poly C.[28] However, poly A:poly U is a much poorer inhibitor of tumor growth than poly I:poly C. It remains to be determined whether poly A:poly U enhances cell-mediated graft-versus-host reactions as well as does poly I:poly C. If it does, the implication would be that the immunologic rejection mechanisms may not be very important in tumor inhibition by poly I:poly C.

The inhibition of macromolecule synthesis observed in tumors of animals treated with poly I:poly C may be attributable to a direct chemotherapeutic action or may reflect the beginning of the immune-rejection mechanisms. We have seen that within two days after injection of poly I:poly C there is maximum stimulation of the graft-rejection capacity of the spleen cells of the treated animals. It might indeed be that the inhibition of macromolecule synthesis simply reflects the fact that these cells are dying from immune-rejection mechanisms. In any case, one to two days after treatment of mice bearing the reticulum cell sarcoma is begun, there is marked alteration in the histologic appearance of the tumor.

The effect of poly I:poly C on chemical carcinogenesis may throw some light on the mechanism of action.[12] Dimethylbenzanthracene (DMBA) can be used to induce tumors in mice by two different procedures. One very small application followed by repeated treatment of the skin with croton oil will also induce tumors. Poly I:poly C almost totally prevents the induction by the DMBA/croton oil system but only delays the production of tumors induced by DMBA alone. It has been shown that impairment of the host immunologic processes will increase chemical carcinogenesis.[29]

Two additional items are worth pointing out with particular reference to the possible use of poly I:poly C or interferon in the treatment of malignancies in man. One is the fact that the sera of certain species hydrolyze poly I:poly C to split products that are altered in their biologic properties.[30] The split products no longer have the pyrogenic capability of the intact poly I:poly C; they do not induce interferon synthesis[31] and do not have any antitumor activity.[32] Human serum is one such hydrolytic serum. This immediately poses the question as to whether in man poly I:poly C will be hydrolyzed before it can exert its full effects. Preliminary evidence with other species of animals that have hydrolytic sera indicates that poly I:poly C still can be strongly antiviral.[33]

The other point of importance deals with the toxicity of poly I:poly C. In monkeys and dogs, levels of 3 mg/kg are frequently fatal.[34] One milligram per kilogram is reasonably well tolerated and leads to the production of low levels of interferon. Toxicity is associated with intravascular coagulation in severe instances and with only transient elevation of serum transaminase levels and lactic dehydrogenase levels in mild instances. The levels that are lethal to mice approach 100 mg/kg, while levels that are effective in antitumor tests in mice are 5 to 10 mg/kg. On the basis of relative surface areas, 12 mg/kg in a mouse would be equivalent to 1 mg/kg in man.

In the so-called phase 1 part of a cooperative program with the National Cancer Institute, we have been treating patients with malignancies with poly I:poly C. So far the highest dose given to man has been about 0.4 mg/kg, roughly equivalent to 5 mg/kg in a mouse. The interferon response in man has been perhaps one-one hundredth of that in the mouse. The capacity of human serum to hydrolyze poly I: poly C may play a role here. The toxicity in man has been much less than anticipated, and we plan to try higher doses.

References

1. Field, A. D., Tytell, A. A., Lampson, G. P. and Hilleman, M. R.: Inducers of interferon and host resistance. II. Multistranded synthetic polynucleotide complexes. Proc. Nat. Acad. Sci. U.S.A. 58:1004, 1967.
2. Atanasiu, P. and Chany, C.: Action d'un interféron provenant de cellules malignes sur l'infection expérimentale du Hamster nouveau-né par le virus du polyome. C. R. Acad. Sci. 251:1687, 1960.
3. Gresser, I., Coppey, J., Falcoff, E. and Fontaine, D.: Action inhibitrice de l'interféron brut sur le développement de la leucémie de Friend chez la Souris. C. R. Acad. Sci. 263 (Series D): 586, 1966.
4. Wheelock, E. F.: Effect of statolon on Friend virus leukemia in mice. Proc. Soc. Exp. Biol. Med. 124:855, 1967.
5. Wheelock, E. F.: Interferon in established Friend virus leukemia. Proc. Soc. Exp. Biol. Med. 127:230, 1968.
6. Rhim, J. S., Greenawalt, C. and Huebner, R. J.: Synthetic double-stranded RNA: Inhibitory effect on murine leukaemia and sarcoma viruses in cell cultures. Nature 222:1166, 1969.
7. Gresser, I., Berman, L., De-Thé, G., Brouty-Boyé, D., Coppey, J. and Falcoff, E.: Interferon and murine leukemia. V. Effect of interferon preparations on the evolution of Rauscher disease in mice. J. Nat. Cancer Inst. 41:505, 1968.
8. Sarma, P. S., Shiu, G., Neubauer, R. H., Baron, S. and Huebner, R. J.: Virus-induced sarcoma of mice: Inhibition by a synthetic polyribonucleotide complex. Proc. Nat. Acad. Sci. 62:1046, 1969.
9. Levy, H. B., Law, L. W. and Rabson, A.: Inhibition of tumor growth by polyinosinic-polycytidylic acid. Proc. Amer. Ass. Cancer Res. 10:49, 1969 (abstract); idem, Proc. Nat. Acad. Sci. U.S.A. 62:357, 1969.
10. Zeleznick, L. D. and Bhuyan, B. K.: Treatment of leukemic mice with double-stranded polyribonucleotides. Proc. Soc. Exp. Biol. Med. 130:126, 1969.
11. Gresser, I., Bourali, C., Lévy, J. P., Fontaine-Brouty-Boyé, D. and Thomas, M. T.: Increased survival in mice inoculated with tumor cells and treated with interferon preparations. Proc. Nat. Acad. Sci. U.S.A. 63:51, 1969.
12. Gelboin, H. and Levy, H. B.: Effect of polyinosinic-polycytidylic acid on DMBA carcinogenesis. Science 167:205, 1970.
13. Peries, J., Canivet, M., Guillemain, G. and Boiron, M.: Inhibitory effect of interferon preparations on the development of foci of altered cells induced in vitro by mouse sarcoma virus. J. Gen. Virol. 3:465, 1968.
14. Rhim, J. S., Huebner, R. J. and Gisin, S.: Effect of statolon on acute and persistent murine leukemia and sarcoma virus infections. Proc. Soc. Exp. Biol. Med. 130:181, 1969.
15. Gresser, I.: Effect of interferon on mouse tumors. *In* Chany, C. and DeSomer, P. (Eds.): L'Interféron, 6th ed. Paris: Institut National de la Santé et de la Recherche, 1970.
16. Simonsen, M.: Graft versus host reactions. Progr. Allergy 6:349, 1962.
17. Simonsen, M.: The factor of immunization: Clonal selection theory investigated by spleen assays of graft-versus-host reaction. *In* Ciba Foundation Symposium on Trans-

plantation. London, Churchill, 1962, p. 185.
18. Mandel, M. A. and Asofsky, R.: The effects of heterologous anti-thymocyte sera in mice. J. Immunol. 100:1319, 1968.
19. Levy, H. B., Asofsky, R., Riley, F., Garapin, A., Cantor, H. and Adamson, R.: The mechanism of the antitumor action of poly I:poly C. Ann. N.Y. Acad. Sci. 173:640, 1970.
20. Cantor, H., Asofsky, R. and Levy, H. B.: Effect of polyinosinic:polycytidylic acid on graft versus host reaction. J. Immunol. 104:1035, 1970.
21. Braun, W., Nakano, M., Jaroskova, L., Yajima, Y. and Jiminez, R.: Nucleic acids in immunology. New York, Springer Verlag, 1968, p. 347.
22. Paucker, K., Cantell, K. and Henle, W.: Quantitative studies on viral interference in suspended L cells. III. Effect of interfering viruses and interferon on the growth rate of cells. Virology 17:324, 1962.
23. Baron, S., Merigan, T. C. and McKerlie, M. L.: Effect of crude and purified interferon on the growth of cells in tissue culture. Proc. Soc. Exp. Biol. Med. 121:50, 1966.
24. Levy, H. B. and Merigan, T. C.: Interferon and uninfected cells. Proc. Soc. Exp. Biol. Med. 121:53, 1966.
25. Glasgow, L. P.: Leukocytes and interferon in the host response to viral infections. J. Bacteriol. 91:2185, 1966.
26. Green, J. A., Cooperband, S. R. and Kibrick, S: Immune specific induction of interferon production in cultures of human blood lymphocytes. Science 164:1415, 1969.
27. Stinebring, W.: Personal communication.
28. Braun, W. and Nakano, M.: Antibody formation: Stimulation by polyadenylic and polycytidylic acids. Science 157:819, 1967.
29. Miller, J. F. A. P., Grant, G. A. and Roe, F. J. C.: Effect of thymectomy on the induction of skin tumours by 3,4-benzopyrene. Nature 199:920, 1963.
30. Nordlund, J., Wolff, S. and Levy, H. B.: Inhibition of biologic activity of poly I: poly C by human plasma. Proc. Soc. Exp. Biol. Med. 133:439, 1970.
31. Baron, S. and Levy, H. B.: Unpublished results.
32. Adamson, R., Nordlund, J., Wolff, S. and Levy, H. B.: Unpublished results.
33. Davis, W., Padgett, G., Merigan, T., Gorham, J. and Levy, H. B.: Unpublished results.
34. Homan, E., Adamson, R. and Levy, H. B.: Unpublished results.

Intermediary Metabolism and its Implications in Cancer Chemotherapy

By Nikolay V. Dimitrov, M.D. and Janusz Hansz, M.D.

The rapid development of research concerning cancer chemotherapy during the last two decades has introduced a variety of chemotherapeutic agents to the practicing physician. Experience with these drugs provided a great deal of information regarding their therapeutic value, selectivity, sensitivity and side effects. The action of such agents is based primarily on their metabolic interference, particularly the inhibition of certain steps of the intermediary metabolism related to the abnormal proliferation of the malignant cell.

Whereas the histologic characteristics of solid tumors depend upon the variety of cells and tissues (stroma and parenchyma), the hematologic malignancies (leukemias) are represented in most cases by a homogeneous population of cells. The morphologic diagnosis of acute leukemia has been the subject of much discussion and its morphologic classification remains a debatable issue. The introduction of many histochemical methods did not actually change the use of simple smear staining, which remains the most generally applied method for the diagnosis of leukemia. The varying effects of one drug or a combination of drugs on morphologically identical cells emphasized the necessity for a more accurate determination of the type of leukemic cell.

When the investigator is dealing with a homogeneous cell population, the metabolic pattern of such cells could serve as a more complete indicator of sensitivity, response and resistance to antileukemic agents. Extensive studies in this direction undertaken during the last decade provided important information regarding the correlation between changes in the biochemical profile of the cell and the effects of therapy.[1–5]

The first well-controlled study on the intermediary metabolism of normal and

Table 1.—*Glucose Metabolism*

Cell or condition	*Glucose utilization* (μ*moles/hr/*10^8)	*Glycogen turnover* (μ*moles/hr/*10^8)	*Pentose cycle* (%)
Normal neutrophil (10)*	4.0–5.0	0.25–0.30	1.5–2.5
Chronic granulocytic leukemia (5)	3.5–4.5	0.25–0.30	1.5–2.5
Chronic granulocytic leukemia, blastic crisis (14)	2.0–4.0	0.20–0.30	1.5–2.5
Acute granulocytic leukemia (8)	2.0–3.0	0.15–0.25	1.8–2.8
Normal lymphocyte (16)	0.28–0.50	0.004–0.030	1.2–1.7
Chronic lymphocytic leukemia (10)	0.15–0.40	0.006–0.026	1.3–2.1
Acute lymphocytic leukemia (6)	0.27–0.35	0.010–0.030	1.5–2.8
Lymphosarcoma cell leukemia (7)	0.14–0.36	0.012–0.030	1.5–2.8

From Stjernholm et al.,[7] with permission.
* The numbers in parentheses refer to the number of cases studied in each series.

From the Division of Hematology and Medical Oncology, Hahnemann Medical College and Hospital, and Philadelphia General Hospital, Philadelphia, Pennsylvania.

Supported by grant CA-11060 from the National Cancer Institute, U.S. Public Health Service.

leukemic leukocytes was done by Beck and Valentine.[6] These authors demonstrated that glycolysis was identical in normal polymorphonuclear leukocytes (PMN) and leukemic leukocytes from chronic granulocytic leukemia (CGL), confirming the fact that the biochemical differences are not attributable solely to cell immaturity. They also showed that glycolysis is higher in CGL than in chronic lymphocytic leukemia (CLL). This finding was later confirmed by several other investigators[7–9] and could be used as an index for differentiation between the lymphoid and the nonlymphoid origin of the cells. The metabolic differences among various blood cells have been extensively studied by Stjernholm and associates at Case Western Reserve University (Table 1).[10–13]

We investigated glucose utilization of 11 patients with acute monocytic leukemia (AMoL) with 91 to 98 per cent blasts before treatment and correlated the results with the effect of antileukemic therapy. As shown in Table 2, low glucose utilization and an absence of phagocytosis indicate resistance to therapy and a short survival time. All patients had the same therapeutic management.

Another interesting area of research is the metabolism of propionic acid. Lymphocytes from patients with acute lymphocytic leukemia (AcLL) utilized propionic acid via two different pathways.[11,14,15] Thus, the first type of lymphocytes obtained from patients with a normal or moderately elevated leukocyte count form lactic acid mainly via propionyl CoA–acrylyl CoA–lactyl CoA (direct pathway). The second type of lymphocytes forms lactic acid via the Krebs cycle (indirect pathway). This second metabolic pattern, identical to that of lymphosarcoma cell leukemia, indicated a poor therapeutic response. Acute granulocytic leukemia (AGL) and blastic crisis of CGL utilize propionic acid very actively.[15,16] CGL and normal PMN have identical metabolic patterns with regard to propionic acid. When utilization of propionic acid is increased in CGL without accompanying morphologic changes in the leukemic cells, a blastic crisis may be imminent.[16]

Amino acids are regarded as important metabolites for the leukemic cell. The active participation of the amino acids in cellular processes other than protein synthesis determines their significant role in the entire cell metabolism. The leukocyte is considered a metabolically active cell which has specific transport mechanisms.[17,18]

TABLE 2.—*Glucose Utilization and Phagocytosis in Acute Monocytic Leukemia*

Patient's Age	*Sex*	*Blasts (%)*	*Glucose utilization (μmoles/10⁸ cells/hr)*	*Phagocytic index**	*Therapy†*	*Remission*	*Survival time (wks)*
37	F	93	1.9	0	VAMP	Resistant	4
29	M	96	2.3	0	VAMP	Resistant	3
38	M	98	2.2	0	VAMP	Resistant	3
33	M	91	2.0	0	VAMP	Resistant	7
42	F	95	3.2	21	VAMP	Partial	11
36	F	92	3.4	18	VAMP	Partial	10
39	F	98	3.1	24	VAMP	Partial	17
35	M	98	4.2	87	VAMP	Complete	>54
40	F	93	3.8	83	VAMP	Complete	48
30	M	97	4.7	90	VAMP	Complete	39
28	M	93	4.3	94	VAMP	Complete	39

* The phagocytic index is expressed as percentage of polymorphonuclear leukocytes (PMN) containing 6 or more particles.
† Therapeutic agents: V = vincristine ; A = amethopterin (methotrexate); M = 6-mercaptopurine; P = prednisone.

TABLE 3.—*Asparagine Metabolism*

Diagnosis	*Patient's Age*	*Patient's Sex*	*Total utilization (mμmoles/10⁸ cells/hr)*	*Therapy**	*Remission*	*Survival time (wks)*
AcLL†	7	F	61.4	VACP	Complete	>91
AcLL	5	M	64.7	VAP	Complete	>84
AcLL	6	F	66.1	VAC	Complete	>87
AcLL	12	M	62.4	VAP	Complete	56
AcLL	4	M	136.8	VAP (Asp)	Partial	37
AcLL	9	F	141.2	VAP	Partial	34
LySa	49	M	127.4	MP	Partial	12
LySa	57	M	144.1	VAMP (Asp)	Partial	18
LySa	17	M	120.6	VAMPC	Resistant	9

* Therapeutic agents: V = vincristine; A = methotrexate (amethopterin); C = cytoxan; P = prednisone; M = 6-mercaptopurine; Asp = asparaginase.
† AcLL = acute lymphocytic leukemia; LySa = lymphosarcoma cell leukemia, with leukemic blood picture.

The leukemic cells, which have an abnormal proliferative capacity, compete actively with the normal cells of the body for the metabolic requirement of the amino acids. It has been shown that certain malignant cells require amino acids[19–21] and that depletion of these amino acids results in the death of the cell.[22–24] This finding has been wisely applied in the treatment of acute leukemia. Thus, the enzyme asparaginase hydrolyzes asparagine to aspartic acid and lowers the amount of asparagine available for the growth of leukemic cells.

Several tests have been developed to determine sensitivity to asparaginase and are used in many institutions.[3,20,24,25] (The results of the clinical applications of this enzyme are discussed in this volume in the chapter by Burchenal.) This interesting approach to antileukemic therapy left many questions unanswered. When the first encouraging results became available, we investigated the entire asparagine metabolism of leukemic and normal leukocytes. The metabolic pattern of asparagine in normal polymorphonuclear leukocytes and leukemic leukocytes from CGL, AGL and AMoL were not significantly different. However, the utilization of asparagine differs in lymphoproliferative disorders (Table 3). Lymphocytes from normal individuals and patients with uncomplicated chronic lymphocytic leukemia (CLL) possess identical metabolic patterns.[26] Leukocytes from patients with AcLL exhibit similar metabolic patterns and respond to conventional chemotherapy; this results in long-lasting remissions. Lymphosarcoma cell leukemia has a very high asparagine utilization and shows resistance or only a partial response to conventional chemotherapy. In some of these cases a partial remission has been achieved with asparaginase.

Whereas the treatment of children with AcLL during the last two decades is considered a major achievement, the successful treatment of the leukemias in adults remains a problem. Recent studies have demonstrated that serine is an essential amino acid for cultures of leukemic cells.[8] We investigated serine utilization by leukemic cells from patients with AGL and AMoL. Leukocytes from these two types of leukemia converted serine to CO_2 at a rate 5 to 10 times higher than the other types of leukemia and normal leukocytes (Table 4). Cells from blastic crisis in CGL exhibit production of CO_2 identical to that in AGL. Increased CO_2 production in CGL (above 1.5 mμmoles) indicates an imminent blastic crisis. When respiratory CO_2 exceeded 2.5 mμmoles, the leukemic cells became totally resistant to any therapeutic agent and the survival time of these patients ranged from 2 to 6 weeks. Leukemic cells from AMoL

TABLE 4.—*Serine Metabolism*

Patient's Sex	Age	Diagnosis	Blasts (%)	CO_2 (mμmoles/10^8 cells/hr)	Therapy*	Response	Survival time (wks)
F	69	AGL	73	4.58	VAMP	Resistant	3
M	44	AGL	88	5.31	CAR,† VP	Resistant	2
F	57	AGL	78	2.51	VAMP	Resistant	5
F	42	AMoL	95	4.58	VAMP	Resistant	3
M	38	AMoL	98	3.18	VAMP	Resistant	6
M	35	AMoL	98	0.71	VAMP	Complete remission	>54
F	58	BC	51	8.61	VAMP	Resistant	10
M	29	BC	42	4.04	CAR, VMP	Partial remission	17
M	52	CGL	1	0.33	None		
F	48	CGL	0	0.74	None		
Normal PMN (9 patients)				0.55 ± 0.16 (Mean ± S.D.)			

* See Table 3 for explanation of abbreviations.
† Other abbreviations: CAR = cytosar (cytosine arabinoside); PMN = polymorphonuclear leukocytes; AGL = acute granulocytic leukemia; AMoL = acute monocytic leukemia; BC = blastic crisis; CGL = chronic granulocytic leukemia.

with a low production of CO_2 responded very well to therapy and a long remission was achieved.

A fundamental problem in the treatment of leukemia is determining when the total leukemic cell kill has been achieved. This is especially difficult in AcLL and AMoL. In complete remission, when the total leukocyte and differential count is normalized, it is very difficult to isolate sufficient numbers of morphologically normal lymphocytes and monocytes. If these cells cannot be isolated for control studies, their presence can be indicated only by detecting the abnormal metabolic products which they produce. Unfortunately, such a method is not available at the moment. However, a more favorable situation exists for patients with AGL since the metabolic changes could be used as an index of the restoration of normally functioning polymorphonuclear leukocytes.

We have followed up four patients with AGL who achieved complete remission. Utilization of propionic acid was determined before therapy and after remission was complete (Table 5). Differential counts showed a shift to the left with the presence of 8 to 18 band forms. The bone marrow revealed 1 to 2 per cent blast cells. The metabolic pattern of propionic acid before therapy, during therapy and in complete

TABLE 5.—*Propionate Metabolism in Acute Granulocytic Leukemia*

Patient's Sex	Age	Blasts (%) Before therapy	In remission	Therapy*	Remission	PMN % in remission	Propionate utilization (mμmoles/10^8 cells/hr) Before therapy	In remission	Survival time (wks)
M	66	81	0	MP	Complete	73	28.3	20.1	34
F	59	92	0	MP	Complete	68	19.3	17.6	41
M	51	67	0	AMP	Complete	79	23.7	14.6	38
M	60	84	0	VAMP	Complete	77	31.8	22.4	29
Normal PMN							5.0–6.0		

* See Table 3 for explanation of abbreviations.

TABLE 6.—*Glucose Metabolism and Phagocytosis in Acute Granulocytic Leukemia—Complete Remission*

Patient's Sex	Age	PMN % in remission	Phagocytic index*	Glucose utilization (μmoles/10^8 cells/hr) Resting	Phagocyting†	Hexose monophosphate shunt (%) Resting	Phagocyting	Cause of death
M	66	73	22	3.7	3.5	2.2	2.6	Staph. septicemia; miliary tuberculosis.
F	59	68	49	4.1	4.3	2.7	2.7	Klebsiella septicemia; candidiasis.
M	60	77	30	3.0	3.0	1.9	2.5	Pneumococcal septicemia; candidiasis; brain hemorrhage.
Normal‡ (10 individuals)		(mean $\pm$ S.D.)	76.2 $\pm$ 7.2	5.8 $\pm$ 1.3	6.3 $\pm$ 1.2	2.3 $\pm$ 0.6	13.2 $\pm$ 3.6	

* The phagocytic index is expressed as percentage of polymorphonuclear leukocytes containing six or more particles.
† Latex polystyrene particles (0.81μ) were used as the phagocytic material.
‡ See Ref. 27.

remission was similar. Glucose utilization was low and very little stimulation of CO_2 was noticed after the addition of latex particles to the incubation medium (Table 6). In some experiments no metabolic response occurred during oxygen uptake or when these morphologically normal leukocytes were incubated with formic acid. All patients suffered repeated infections and died with fulminant septicemia. A postmortem examination of two of these patients with AGL revealed no leukemic infiltrates. The survival time of patients who achieved complete remission appears to be 8 to 13 months, as compared with the survival time of most of the other patients, 4 to 8 months. Such results indicate that restoration of the maturation line of myeloid elements in the bone marrow does not reveal the functional state of the stem cell which releases metabolically abnormal leukocytes.

This study indicates that the metabolic evaluation of polymorphonuclear leukocytes in remission is more indicative than morphology alone. These problems require further attention and investigation for a more complete understanding.

REFERENCES

1. Fischer, G. A.: Increased levels of folic reductase as a mechanism of resistance to amethopterin in leukemic cells. Biochem. Pharmacol. 7:75, 1961.
2. Bertino, J. R., Donohue, D. R., Gabrio, B. W., Silber, R., Alenty, A., et al.: Increased level of dihydrofolic reductase in leukocytes of patients treated with amethopterin. Nature 193:140, 1962.
3. Mashburn, L. T., Boyse, E. A., Old, L. J. and Campbell, H. A.: A comparison of concurrent and delayed tests for antitumor activity of L-asparaginase. Proc. Soc. Exp. Biol. Med. 124:568, 1967.
4. Prager, M. D. and Bachynsky, N.: Asparagine synthetase in normal and malignant tissues: Correlation with tumor sensitivity to asparaginase. Arch. Biochem. 127:645, 1968.
5. Kessel, D., Hall, T. C. and Roberts, D.: Modes of uptake of methotrexate by normal and leukemic leukocytes in vitro and their relation to drug response. Cancer Res. 28: 564, 1968.
6. Beck, W. S. and Valentine, W. N.: The aerobic carbohydrate metabolism of leukocytes in health and leukemia. I. Glycolysis and respiration. Cancer Res. 12:818, 1952.
7. Stjernholm, R. L., Dimitrov, N. V. and Zito, S.: Carbohydrate metabolism in leukocytes. XIII. Differentiation by metabolism of leukemic leukocytes into three

groups. J. Reticuloendothel. Soc. 7:539, 1970.
8. Seitz, I. F.: Biochemistry of normal and leukemic leukocytes, thrombocytes, and bone marrow cells. Advances Cancer Res. 9:303, 1965.
9. Seitz, J. F. and Luganova, I. S.: The biochemical identification of blood and bone marrow cells of patients with acute leukemia. Cancer Res. 28:2548, 1968.
10. Stjernholm, R. L.: Metabolism of glucose, acetate and propionate by human plasma cells. J. Bact. 93:1657, 1967.
11. Stjernholm, R. L.: The metabolism of human leukocytes. *In* Plenary Session Papers of Twelfth Congress of Int. Soc. of Hematology. New York: International Society of Hematology, 1968, pp. 175–186.
12. Stjernholm, R. L., Thomas, P. and Esmann, V.: Metabolism of the human eosinophil. J. Reticuloendothel. Soc. 6:300, 1969.
13. Stjernholm, R. L., Noble, E., Dimitrov, N. V., Morton, D. J. and Falor, E. H.: Carbohydrate metabolism in leukocytes. XII. Metabolism of the human lymphocyte. J. Reticuloendothel. Soc. 6:590, 1969.
14. Dimitrov, N. and Stjernholm, R. L.: Metabolic deviations in lymphoproliferative disorders. Blood 28:998, 1966.
15. Stjernholm, R. L., Noble, E. P., Dimitrov, N. V., Kellermeyer, R. W. and Falor, W. H.: Differentiation of normal and leukemic leukocytes into three groups by propionate metabolism. J. Reticuloendothel. Soc. 8:446, 1970.
16. Stjernholm, R. L. and Dimitrov, N. V.: Intermediary metabolism by leukemic granulocytes. *In* Abstracts of Int. Cong. of Biochemistry, Vol. J. Tokyo: International Congress of Biochemistry, 1967, p. 1054.
17. Yunis, A. A., Arimura, G. K. and Kipnis, D. M.: Amino acid transport in blood cells. I. Effect of cations on amino acid transport in human leukocytes. J. Lab. Clin. Med. 62:465, 1963.
18. Rosenberg, L. E. and Downing, S.: Transport of neutral and dibasic amino acids by human leukocytes: Absence of defect in cystinuria. J. Clin. Invest. 44:1382, 1965.
19. Foley, G. E., Barell, E. F., Adams, R. A. and Lazarus, H.: Nutritional requirements of human leukemic cells: Cystine requirements of diploid cell lines and their heteroploid variants. Exp. Cell Res. 57:129, 1969.
20. Sobin, L. H. and Kidd, J. G.: A metabolic difference between two lines of lymphoma 6C3HED cells in relation to asparagine. Proc. Soc. Exp. Biol. Med. 119:325, 1965.
21. Regan, J. D., Vodopick, H., Takeda, S., Lee, W. H. and Faulcon, F. M.: Serine requirement in leukemic and normal blood cells. Science 163:1452, 1969.
22. Broome, J. D.: Evidence that the L-asparaginase activity of guinea pig serum is responsible for its antilymphoma effects. Nature 191:1114, 1961.
23. Schrek, R., Dolowy, W. C. and Ammeraal, R. N.: L-asparaginase: Toxicity to normal and leukemic human lymphocytes. Science 155:229, 1967.
24. Oettgen, H. F., Old, L. J., Boyse, E. A., Campbell, H. A., Phillips, F. S., et al.: Inhibition of leukemias in man by L-asparaginase. Cancer Res. 27:2619, 1967.
25. Horowitz, B., Madras, B. K., Meister, A., Old, L. J. and Boyse, E. A.: Asparagine synthetase activity of mouse leukemias. Science 160:522, 1968.
26. Dimitrov, N. and Brodsky, I.: Asparagine metabolism in some lymphoproliferative disorders. Cancer Res. 30:1338, 1970.
27. Dimitrov, N. V., Douwes, F. R., Bartolotta, B., Nochumson, S. and Toth, M. A.: Studies of the metabolic activity of polymorphonuclear leukocytes in sickle cell anemia. Acta Hematol. (in press).

Immunologic Factors and Chemotherapy

By William Regelson, M.D.

Of major importance to any symposium on cancer chemotherapy is the observation that effective chemotherapy can be blocked by the presence of active or passive immunization against transplanted tumors.[1,2] This paradoxical evidence that immunologic enhancement can interfere with effective chemotherapy indicates that drug action may be directed not only to the tumor but to the host as well. Chemotherapy of cancer might work through suppression of tumor enhancing circulating antibody which could permit the active participation of cellular immune responses which could be primary factors in the control of tumor growth. Alternatively, the action of chemotherapy could mediate the lethal action of lymphocyte or macrophage "killer" cells that are programmed for lethal cytotoxic activity. Because of this, cancer chemotherapy should be directed at developing techniques for the enhancement of the host-versus-graft rejection phenomenon as the controlling factor in the treatment of malignancy. It is the purpose of this review to present the rationale for this viewpoint. In effect, we are seeking in cancer therapy the opposite of what those in transplantation immunity need. In addition, any success in the area of improving host-tumor rejection through cellular immune responses might also be of importance to our understanding of blastocyst implantation and fetal survival which could have added usefulness in population control.

Tumor Antigens

That immunologic mechanisms are involved in tumor induction and growth is well established. The presence of tumor specific antigens and the role of cellular immunity have been shown repeatedly since the first demonstration of tumor specific transplantation antigens (TSTA) in autochthonous tumors by Foley,[3] and numerous reviews have been written on the subject.[4-7] The application of this mechanism to clinical medicine has been particularly reinforced by the work of Gold and Freedman et al.,[8,9] who found carcinoembryonic antigens related to gastrointestinal malignancy in a majority of such cancer patients. The carcinoembryonic antigens or related "T" antigens have now been found to be present in metastatic cancer independent of gastrointestinal origin.[10,11] Tumor-specific antigens have been found for sarcomas,[12,13] renal cancer, melanoma,[14] Burkitt lymphoma, head and neck epithelioma,[15] and rhabdomyoma.[16]

Most recently, Hellstrom et al.,[17,18] using an in vitro colony inhibition technique, have shown that lymphocytes from children with neuroblastoma and Wilms' tumor can cross react to specifically inhibit in vitro neuroblastoma cells. The lymphocytes of mothers of children with this disease also possess cytocidal activity against these neuroblastoma cells in the absence of serum from the patient with neuroblastoma.[17,18] This clinical laboratory investigation was based on similar findings in rabbits with Shope papilloma virus-induced tumors that demonstrated that aggressive tumor growth correlated with inhibition by serum of cellular immune response.[18]

From the Medical College of Virginia, Health Sciences Center, Richmond, Virginia.

BCG and Immunologic Adjuvants

In a related area, the importance of cellular immune response is seen in the extensive studies with bacille Calmette-Guérin (BCG) or related bacterial products as adjuvants in the treatment of cancer. Bacille Calmette-Guérin, an attenuated form of tuberculosis infection, has been used on a large scale as an immunologic prophylactic approach for the control of tuberculosis since World War II. The use of BCG as an effective agent in the control of tumor growth was first observed by Halpern and Biozzi and others,[19,20] who demonstrated increased resistance of rats and mice to the growth of the T-8 and Ehrlich ascites tumors on the basis of its reticuloendothelial and immunologic enhancing action.[21,22]

In addition to its effects against transplanted and virus-induced tumors, BCG shows enhancement of host resistance against viruses and bacteria,[23,24] and recently has been shown to increase interferon production associated with viral infection and immunologic response.[25]

In other studies, antitumor results were reported by Old and Clarke[26] against S180 and Ca 755 which were related to reticuloendothelial stimulation and immunologic response.[27] This action of BCG was equally apparent in splenectomized animals,[28] and splenectomy, paradoxically, itself had antitumor effects. BCG adjuvant action as an antitumor agent required direct contact with the tumor cells in a guinea pig system used by Rapp.[29]

Apart from effects against transplanted and methylcholanthrene-induced tumors, BCG delays the appearance of tumors and prolongs survival of mice and hamsters inoculated with leukemia transplants and polyoma virus.[30,31]

Mathé[32] and Lamensans et al.[33] have shown inhibition of L1210 leukemia after intravenous and intraperitoneal injection of BCG. Enhanced tuberculosis resistance in studies of rabbits correlates with a decrease in the appearance of spontaneous uterine cancer.[34] Recent epidemiologic data in BCG-treated children support the fact that vaccination with BCG can decrease the incidence of leukemia and childhood solid tumors.[35]

Most recently, Mathé et al.[36–38a,b] have given BCG inoculation to patients with acute lymphocytic leukemia and have shown prolongation of the unmaintained remission period for 29 months to 5 years.[38a,b]

Similar results following BCG-induced return to tuberculin positivity have been reported by Sokal and Aungst[39] in regard to restoring chemotherapy response and enhancing survival in advanced (stage IV) Hodgkin's disease. Most recently, responses have been reported for melanoma after local intratumoral injection of BCG.[40]

Of clinical importance, immunologic and antitumor effects in animal systems have been obtained by Weiss et al.[41,42] using a methanol extract of tuberculosis which behaves like BCG; this biological agent is now under investigation. It possesses advantages over BCG in that it is a uniform preparation and does not require viable organisms for effectiveness.

Not only have BCG and related extracts of tubercle bacilli been shown to impede tumor growth; other agents include *Corynebacterium parvum*, which is under clinical test against advanced tumors and leukemia,[38a,b,40 43] and the synthetic polyanions, pyran copolymer[44] and the synthetic polynucleotide, polyinosine-cytosine Poly rI:rC.[45,46]

The clinical antitumor reaction of Poly rI:rC may relate to interferon induction but their behavior in man and laboratory animals can resemble that seen for bacterial endotoxins with fever and/or related hemorrhagic necrosis of tumors. However, Poly rI:rC and related synthetic and natural oligonucleotides as well as bacterial endo, toxins and synthetic polyanions increase immunologic responsiveness.[46] Recently-Mathé has indicated its usefulness in preventing relapse in pediatric leukemia.[38b]

The failure of tumors to evoke significant regression on the basis of tumor antigenicity may be due to anergy or failure of cellular immunity in the patient with advanced cancer.[47] This defect in immunologic response has been most notable in Hodgkin's disease[39] and lung cancer.[47] Attempts to reverse this have been made with BCG inoculation and, as mentioned previously, Sokal and Aungst[39] have found that 7 of 8 stage IV patients with Hodgkin's disease who failed to develop tuberculin positivity to BCG were dead within a year, whereas, of 24 patients with similar disease who developed tuberculin reactions, only one died. The 23 other patients were alive at the time of this writing, with a 30-month median survival rate that is still increasing. However, Mathé et al.[36,37] report negative effects on other solid tumors in relation to tuberculin reaction in 51 patients but give no details. Israël et al.[48] were able to produce positive reactivity in 50 per cent of tuberculin-negative patients with lung cancer after BCG inoculation, but the conversion did not result in significant improvement in survival. In the studies of Sokal and Aungst[39] and Israël et al.,[48] chemotherapy was administered concomitantly. The success of these agents as adjuvants may relate to the size of the tumor inoculum, as Mathé and others believe that the presence of tumor populations above 10^5 are not effectively controlled with immunotherapy. Similar implications are present in the work of Martin et al.,[49] where the reticuloendothelial system (RES) stimulator zymosan can make the difference in an adjuvant animal tumor system after surgery.

In regard to our laboratory studies with the synthetic polyanion, pyran copolymer, we have found that it is ineffective in pretreatment of syngeneic tumors but its action is effective on pretreatment when histocompatibility is not complete.[50] This action could be reversed by chemotherapy, e.g., methotrexate, and we are faced with a paradox in that chemotherapy, like splenectomy,[28] can impede or enhance the appropriate immune response, with similar paradoxical results, as is seen in the action of enhancing antibody.[1,2]

The importance of the successful use of immunologic adjuvants lies in their application as surgical adjuvants in the absence of observable tumor[51] and ascertaining the appropriate dosage and timing in conjunction with chemotherapy. Logically, the key to clinical success will depend on our ability to distinguish through in vitro methodology the relation of immunologic enhancement to the tumorcidal activity of the cellular immune or delayed hypersensitivity response. In this regard, it is of interest that Siegal[52] has found shark IgM capable of nonspecific inhibition of transplanted tumors in rodents. The nonspecific tumor-inhibiting capacity of IgM protein is of tremendous theoretical importance and is similar to what has been seen for the nonspecific antitumor activity of interferon.[53]

In another area, the study of blocking or enhancing antibody or of glycoprotein tumor antigens that interfere with tumor rejection is in its infancy. However, the concept of adjuvant enhancement of endogenous immune response is paralleled by the attempts to directly heighten the antigenicity of the tumor through coupling to haptens or with varied approaches to purification of tumor antigen. This chapter will not enter into a consideration of these approaches.

Skin Reactivity

Most recently it has been shown in mice that intracutaneous injection of living tumor cells can result in regression of implants elsewhere,[29,40,54] with the implication that the skin as an area for the production of immunologic response may be different from other areas of the body. This is supported by the work of Klein,[55] who showed that the quinone mustard (Trenimon) or dichloronitrobenzene (DCNB) sensitization of the skin of cancer patients resulted in slough of basal cell tumors and senile keratosis when the antigen was applied to the tumor in an ointment base. This allergic response of cutaneous tumors was much greater than that seen in normal skin, and one can transmit this pattern of response with the transfer of lymphocytes sensitized to DCNB. Unfortunately, this is not seen for visceral disease or metastatic cancer to the skin and, in this regard, it is of interest that pulmonary and cutaneous melanomas respond to chemotherapy (i.e., imidazole carboxamide or BCNU-vincristine) while visceral melanomas do not. More recently, the pattern of cutaneous allergic response to DCNB has been related to operative curability,[56] as has been seen for tuberculin or DCNB response in Hodgkin's disease or lung cancer.[39,47] The operative prognosis is poor if bowel or head and neck cancer patients do not sensitize adequately to DCNB regardless of clinical staging. We have confirmed this in head and neck cancer patients and this anergy is associated with limited prognosis and relatively poor response to chemotherapy.

Leukocyte Transfusions

One clinical approach that may bypass the above problems and enhance specific or nonspecific resistance to tumor growth is the use of leukocyte transfusions for the control of tumor growth.

This approach has been made in a number of early clinical studies.[57–63] The number of such efforts has increased in the past year to the point where utilization of leukocytes directed toward cancer immunotherapy was a substantial part of the Immunology, Clinical Trials Section of the recent Tenth International Cancer Congress in Houston, Texas.

In favor of this approach, recent advances in the technology of leukocyte separation via differential centrifugation will soon make leukapheresis available in most major hospital and research centers. This will provide large numbers of lymphocytes or monocytes (macrophages) for extended clinical trial as possible adjuncts in the treatment of malignancy.[64–67]

In the past, many clinical investigations of this type were restricted by the limited availability of leukocyte transfusions. For this and other reasons, many early studies primarily involved leukemics, with cellular therapy directed to the formation of radiation or chemotherapy induced chimeras. However, pioneering clinical programs, as reported by Nadler and Moore[63] and others[60,61,68] have involved cross-transplantation of tumors followed by intravenous administration of "sensitized" leukocytes (lymphocytes) obtained by venous drainage or thoracic duct cannulation at the height of host-graft rejection. More recently, these approaches have involved tissue culture technique with exposure of cultured autochthonous or isogeneic lymphocytes to the tumor or with lymphocytes returned to the recipient after lymphoblastic transformation following phytohemagglutinin exposure.[69–71] For example, in the case of McKhann and Aust,[68] thoracic duct cells from the cannulated patient are repeatedly exposed to growing tumor cells in tissue culture, and lymphocytes are reinfused until the thoracic duct cannula is plugged or the cells in the tissue culture fail. Similar techniques have been used by Aust et al.[69] Using another technique, a Peruvian group[72] utilizes lymphocytes or related macrophages obtained from transplanted tumors and neighboring tissue at the peak of regression and inflammatory reaction after rejection of the tumor in a volunteer recipient. These sensitized allogeneic cells are then given to the tumor host.

In other studies, Symes et al.[73] and Woodruff et al.[74,75] have explored the use of allogeneic spleen cells for the treatment of cancer with questionable antitumor effect. Peripheral blood lymphocytes and spleen cells are undoubtedly different in terms of their capability for such immunotherapeutic experiments. These factors have been reviewed recently[76,77] and may relate to lymphoblastic activation or macrophage lymphocyte inter-reaction. A lymphocyte activating factor is under clinical and laboratory study at the Sloan-Kettering Research Institute in New York.[78]

Eschbach et al.[79] have reported a cross-circulation study done between an acute myelocytic 15-year-old girl and a uremic 19-year-old boy. This was performed on a daily basis for two hour periods over four and a half months. No major toxic reactions were reported, and hematologic remission did occur in the leukemic girl. Both patients benefited from the study, with no apparent residual toxicity in the surviving uremic participant.

In relation to leukocyte transfusions, there is suggestive evidence of potential benefit in patients with melanoma and breast cancer, who constitute the majority of cases reported. In all these studies, there is little information on the localization and fate of the infused cells, and the in vitro antitumor effectiveness of these cells has not been reported. The number of cases in any series is small as related to uniformity of technique and patient selection so that one has to await a larger more detailed clinical experience.

Laboratory Observations

In regard to other theoretical considerations in support of the utilization of lymphocyte transfusions to patients with advanced cancer, observations have been made regarding a defect in lymphocytes in tumor-bearing animals. For example, apart from defects in skin testing, Schrek and Rabinowitz[80] and Holm and Perlman[81,82] clearly demonstrated the impaired phytohemagglutinin activity in lymphocytes in patients with Hodgkin's disease or chronic lymphocytic leukemia. In addition, as discussed previously, there is recent evidence that immune reactivity of patients with advanced cancer is impaired.[39,47,56] Cancer autotransplants are inhibited when their leukocytes are administered simultaneously[83] and histologic and tissue culture evidence of lymphocyte penetration of tumors is associated with host response and improved prognosis.[84,85]

In regard to allogeneic inhibition, it has been shown that the confrontation of tumor cells with incompatible cell types (allogeneic cells) leads to growth inhibition and tumor destruction via nonimmunological mechanisms.[76,86–91] Similar phenomena have been observed as possible mechanisms for the inhibition of ovulation by intrauterine devices. These developments might provide us with an opportunity to clinically approach the control of tumor growth in man without the need for prior sensitization of the "aggressor" donor cells, which is not always seen. There may be variable factors relating to qualitative or quantitative differences in the cells used.[92,93]

Although granulocytes can also produce in vitro plaques as a result of their lethal action or through alteration of the ability of cells to adhere to glass, phytohemagglutinin-stimulated lymphocytes are said to possess a more potent cytotoxicity than that seen for granulocytes.[94,95]

In support of the role of lymphocytes as potentially possessing clinical usefulness, as discussed previously, Mathé's group[36–38a,b] has been successful in inducing complete remission with leukocyte transfusions in patients who have acute leukemia. In this case, remissions are associated with graft-versus-host reactions, and the therapeutic index of this approach is subject to question. Mathé's group has also injected xenogeneic lymphoid cells from immunized rabbit spleens into pleural and peritoneal effusions of cancer patients with occasional "good" results.[37] However, toxicity without benefit was seen on utilization of efferent lymph node sheep lymphocytes following human tumor implantation for clinical antitumor effect.[96]

Cellular destruction produced by "aggressor" cells can be induced by using sensitized lymphocytes and macrophages.[97–128] In regard to the action of "aggressor" cells,[114–131] contact between "aggressor lymphoid cells" and the target is a factor. Cellular immunity is not always necessary because contact between the target cell and non-immune lymphocytes can cause destruction if they are sensitized by the presence of phytohemagglutinin (PHA)[122–126] or xenogeneic antibodies.[123] In this regard, a soluble toxic factor seems to be produced when "aggressor" and "target" cells are in contact.[114,132] This is associated with an enlargement of lymphocytes and the shut-down of protein synthesis in the target cells.

A critical number of lymphocytes also is necessary for nonspecific cytopathic effects. Target cell destruction is dependent on cell type since monolayers of peritoneal macrophages treated with spleen cells from normal or immunized animals show clear-cut destruction only when immunized cells are used.[133]

In support of the use of transfused lymphocytes for the development of enhanced cellular immune response, skin grafts are rejected in accelerated fashion after transfusion of cells from mixed splenic or blood cultures or from multiple transfusions. Only relatively few sensitized cells necessarily participate in rejection phenomena.[127,134,135] In this regard, the observation of Granger and Kolb[114] and others[136,137] has led to the development of techniques for determining tissue compatibility in that blastic transformation of mixed lymphocyte populations has been used as a predicting factor in regard to host-graft rejection as the pattern of blastic response correlates with the appearance of the host-graft rejection.[136,137] Where destruction of cells occurs, blastic transformation has been seen.[138] This blastic change, demonstrating a degree of incompatibility, is what one may need in regard to tumor rejection on the part of the host.

A strong rationale for the use of nonsensitized allogeneic lymphocytes is provided by the work of Hellstrom and Moller and their coworkers.[87,88,90,91,123,140] These observations have shown inhibition of the growth of parental tumors in F_1 hybrids independent of immune reactivity against the tumor graft which related to histocompatibility antigens from extracts of allogeneic cells.[87,88,113,136] These observations and those of others[86–91,136,137,139,140] suggest that available cells with histocompatibility antigens, which represent allogeneic differences between cell lines, may be all that is necessary for this pattern of inhibition or destruction. The reaction does not necessarily require intact cells as extracts of allogeneic lymphocytes in vitro cause chromosomal abnormalities in fibroblasts and embryonic cells.[141,142] In addition, destructive effects on tumor cells have been seen for allogeneic DNA[143]; Alexander and others[144] and Pilch et al.[145] have shown that RNA extracted from immunized cells can transfer cellular-mediated tumor rejection.

The limited success of previous clinical studies using leukocyte or lymphocyte transfusions could relate to the quality or quantity of "aggressor" lymphocytes administered. In relation to lethal effects produced by "aggressor" cells, another factor in addition to numbers and surface contact is the age of the cells used.[114,146,147] However, the survival capacity of lymphocytes is such that stored cells or cadaver blood could be a clinical source of cells.[146]

The possible antitumor benefits of lymphocyte infusion also include a consideration of autologous lymphocytes obtained from the same tumor-bearing host. It follows that if tumor antigenicity exists, then the lymphocytes of the tumor-bearing host should have been sensitized in vivo by patients with cancer.[39,47,48,148–150] Consequently, attempts have been made to increase the specific immunologic responsiveness of lymphocytes in the patient bearing tumor by activation with various adjuvants that would augment an otherwise ineffective immunologic antitumor attack on the tumor. Apart from BCG and related compounds, one approach for lymphocyte activation used by several investigators is phytohemagglutinin or other mitogenic agents added in vitro prior to reinfusions. As indicated, the need for PHA to enhance the cytotoxic action of "aggressor" cells has been observed,[122–126,132,134,135] and pretreatment of lymphocytes and/or macrophages by PHA or related agents may be required. On this basis, a clinical trial has been undertaken by Frenster and Rogoway[70,71] in which buffy coat leukocytes are exposed to PHA, appropriately washed, and then reinfused.

Clinical Studies of Leukocyte (Lymphocyte) Infusions

The successful transfer of lymphocytes from allogeneic human donors to patients with cancer (with the hope of producing therapeutic benefit) was reported by Nadler and Moore.[63] However, in these studies the source of the lymphocytes in each instance was the buffy coat of a second patient with the same histologic form of cancer as the recipient. Most recently, Moore's group has reported on those of allogeneic cultured lymphocytes.[151] Some definite responses were obtained in both these studies despite the fact that the actual quantity of lymphocytes that could be transferred under these circumstances was limited. Somewhat similar studies were carried out by Krementz et al.[60,61] Israël et al.[58,59] have reported 70 infusions of pooled allogeneic lymphocytes in 25 patients with advanced cancer. In this group, the general condition of 14 patients definitely improved after this form of immunotherapy, and there were definite objective signs of improvement in 9 of these patients. Mathé and his coworkers[36] have also employed allogeneic leukocytes for cancer therapy in man, but in their studies the leukocyte infusions have been combined with cancer chemotherapeutic agents, thereby allowing the development of graft versus host reactions. This combination makes analysis of results difficult although complete remissions of acute leukemia have been obtained. Both Israël and Mathé report control of malignant effusions by intrapleural or intraabdominal leukocyte administration.

The most critical concern as relates to clinical toxicity or leukocyte transfusions is the graft-versus-host reaction, the "secondary syndrome." As is well known, this phenomenon is dependent on the ability of circulating lymphoblasts to colonize the host to produce secondary disease. The consequences of secondary, graft-versus-host disease have been reviewed elsewhere,[7] and one might expect that we might find the greatest likelihood of this phenomenon to occur in immunosuppressed patients. We feel this danger is minimal and has not been seen in 24 patients treated with lymphocytes in our study but will always remain a calculated risk in any program particularly if cells are given to patients with immune depression and leukopenia from intensive chemotherapy.

In regard to clinical trials, at this time it is important to obtain appropriate matching as regards ABO incompatibility, for no leukocyte separation system is currently available that does not have its quota of contaminating red blood cells. However, new techniques are being devised for more effective separation of red blood cells. Our group[152] has given allogeneic lymphocytes to 24 recipients, who have received from one to 15 infusions of 10^{9-10}/cc lymphocytes with each transfusion from single or multiple donors over a three-week period. Up to 100 cc of lymphocytes (10^{9-10} cells) are given in a one hour infusion; fever and chills of a minor nature were observed in 3 patients. No graft-versus-host reactions have been seen, but careful selection is made to avoid treating patients who are immunodepressed.

Of the 24 patients treated, 17 have completed therapy receiving 9 units of lymphocytes from single donors over a 3 week period. Of 8 patients with melanoma in the study, 2 have shown objective response, 1 with a dramatic disappearance of all cutaneous, pulmonary and liver disease 6 weeks after his last infusion. One patient with gastric carcinoma showed transient objective and subjective improvement, as has one with osteogenic sarcoma.

In any program of lymphocyte infusion, the problem of selecting donors and a source of lymphocytes remains unanswered. Allogeneic lymphocytes obtained from peripheral blood or thoracic duct migrate to the small bowel lamina propria after brief residence in liver or lungs and there is some question as to their ability to react or activate host lymphocytes.[152–154] In relation to this, more recently it has been found that one can enhance immunologic reactivity in immunodepressed rodents by reacting donor peripheral blood lymphocytes with Poly rI:rC and recipient marrow cells.[155] Based on this, should lymphocyte infusions be given into the marrow space? What of the use of splenic or peritoneal macrophages to enhance lymphocyte antigenic response? Until more is known about human lymphocyte distribution and localization, there is no answer, but it is encouraging that sensitized lymphocytes are reported to localize in nodes adjacent to the presence of antigen.[154] In this regard, as discussed previously, the lymphocytes or macrophage "aggressor" cell-killing capacity reflects on its ability to home in and make contact with the tumor cell surface.

Rationale of Lymphocyte Infusion

Conceptually, the rationale of lymphocyte infusion can include several approaches: specific and nonspecific. There is no clear-cut evidence as to which concept is better, and therefore techniques that have been or will be used reflect one's point of view.

If one believes in the specific effects of lymphocytes or monocytes, then the ideal cells to obtain may be from healthy recipient volunteers who are rejecting a tumor graft. For this conceptual approach, the technique of grafting has varied from study to study, and ranges from utilizing untreated tumor to freeze-thawed, ultrasonicated and radiated cells and cell fractions with or without adjuvants to enhance their reactivity. Moore's group has eliminated the volunteer tumor graft recipient by using in vitro lymphocyte cultures.[151] In addition, one can use cured cancer or leukemia patients in remission (e.g., long- or short-term survivors of melanoma or bowel cancer where clinical TSTA antigens have been demonstrated or can be implied). Furthermore, one might logically use donors with benign or self-limited disease on the assumption that there are patterns of intrinsic host resistance that are immunologically related to the benign nature of the process (e.g., bladder papilloma, superficial melanoma, bowel polyps). In support of this approach, recent work has attempted to prognosticate the aggressiveness of malignancy by means of the number of lymphocytes infiltrating or reacting to the disease.[80,81] Alternatively, based on the in vitro work of the Hellstroms, one might anticipate success using the lymphocytes of mothers whose children have had neuroblastoma or Wilms' tumor for administration to children with this disease. Again, based on the work of the Hellstroms and the empiricism of Nadler, Moore and others,[17,18,60,61,63,76] it might be appropriate to use lymphocytes from patients with arrested or regressing disease produced by chemotherapy or radiation.

Although we have made attempts to obtain donors cured of their cancer (e.g. bowel cancer) we have clinical misgivings in using lymphocytes from any cancer patient cured or arrested because of our fear of coincident activation of their disease with removal of lymphocytes, despite the fact that our methodology does not significantly change the total count or differential of the donor. Our group is still attempting this despite a shortage of such donors and the obvious medicolegal implications.

In contrast to the above problems, if one believes in the nonspecific effect of lymphocytes, then the assumption is that allogeneic interaction will produce blastic transformation of recipient and donor cells that could lead to enhanced immune reactivity of the host against his own tumor. The contribution of donor lymphocytes could work against the tumor by also providing stimulatory oligonucleotides[45,46,156] or lymphocyte- or macrophage-produced transforming factors[77] that could stimulate host-tumor rejection. Alternatively, graft-versus-host reaction could be factors contributing to response. In our own group study, although we give ABO compatible cells and type the lymphocytes used, we do not select for compatible lymphocyte donors since we are seeking allogeneic stimulating effects rather than risking the questionable benefit of a lymphocyte graft.

Another alternative in relation to enhancing the immunologic response of transfused cells is to prime the donor with BCG, pertussis or related reticuloendothelial phagocytic-stimulating compounds. These could theoretically increase the availability of immunologically active cells.

In regard to the number of donor cells to be given, lymphocytes may transfer antigenic information via macrophages through specific or nonspecific antigen RNA transfer, and hence not many sensitized cells may be necessary.[144,145] However, either concept requires unknown volumes of leukocytes from single or multiple donors.

In our intramural cooperative program,[152] we have been using the Latham leukapheresis apparatus,[67] a differential centrifuge that permits us to conveniently salvage 10^{9-10} lymphocytes, i.e., 80 per cent of the leukocytes provided by single donors processed by the machine in a 2-hour period. Alternatively, the continuous flow centrifuge blood separator (American Instrument Company—AMINCO),[65] which is now commercially available, may extract 10^{10} leukocytes per donor but has not yet been adapted specifically for lymphocyte salvage. Although the cost of this machine ranges from $12,500 to $25,000, with the ancillary rotors and equipment, the true cost of initial investment is between $25,000 and $50,000, but their value to blood banking operations for platelet retrieval and washing or packing red blood cells makes them potentially self-sustaining in any major blood bank program. They will soon be available to most large medical centers. However, regardless of the number of lymphocytes or macrophages obtainable for programs for the cellular control of tumor growth, we are still handicapped by the problems of enhancing antibody or blocking antibody that may make cellular efforts useless. Unless chemotherapeutic or plasmaphoretic techniques could be developed to remove enhancing antibody, only a small number of patients with advanced cancer might be expected to respond. To offset this, in relation to our efforts, we are attempting to achieve improved specificity in the selection of lymphocyte donors. Attempts at this institution are being made to grow tumor cells in vitro and measure the killing capacity of a panel of lymphocyte donors.[156] If this program matures, we can then be more selective in choosing our donors. The hope of all lymphocyte transfusional programs is the development of enhanced antitumor selectivity of donors regardless of the specific or nonspecific action of the lymphocytes used.

References

1. Ferrer, J. F. and Mihich, E.: Prevention of therapeutically induced regression of sarcoma 180 by immunologic enhancement. Cancer Res. 28:245, 1968.
2. Mihich, G.: Modification of tumor regression by immunologic means. Cancer Res. 29:2345, 1969.
3. Foley, E. J.: Attempts to induce immunity against mammary adenocarcinomas in inbred mice. Cancer Res. 13:578, 1953.
4. Green, H. N., Anthony, H. M., Baldwin, R. W. and Westrop, J. W.: An immunological approach to cancer. London: Butterworths, 1967.
5. Zilber, L. A. and Abelev, G. I.: The Virology and Immunology of Cancer. Oxford: Pergamon, 1968.
6. Pinsky, C. M., Mitchell, S., Oettgen, H. F. and Schwartz, M. K.: Immune reactions to L-asparaginase in man. Proc. Amer. Ass. Cancer Res. 11:63, 1970 (abstract).
7. Klein, G. and Oettgen, H. F.: Immunological factors involved in the growth of primary tumors in human and animal hosts. Cancer Res. 29: 1741, 1969.
8. Gold, P. and Freedman, S. O.: Demonstration of tumor specific antigens in human colonic carcinomata by immunological tolerance and absorption techniques. J. Exp. Med. 121:439, 1965.
9. Gold, P.: Colon Cancer. Symposium, Immune Reactions to Cancer in Man. Cancer Res., 1971 (in press).
10. Hansen, H. J., Lance, K. P. and Krupey, J.: Demonstration of an ion-sensitive antigenic site on carcinoembryonic antigen using zirconyl phosphate gel. Clin. Res. 19:143, 1971.
11. Tal, C. and Halperin, M.: The presence of serologically distinct protein in serum of cancer pathology and in pregnant women. Israel J. Med. Sci. 5:708, 1970.
12. Eilber, F. R. and Morton, D. L.: Immunologic studies of human sarcomas. Proc. Amer. Ass. Cancer Res. 11:23, 1970 (abstract).
13. Hirshaut, Y.: Sarcomas. Symposium Immune Reactions to Cancer in Man. Cancer Res., 1971 (in press).
14. Alexander, P.: Melanoma. Symposium Immune Reactions to Cancer in Man. Cancer Res., 1971 (in press).
15. Henle, W.: Burkitt's lymphoma. Symposium Immune Reactions to Cancer in Man. Cancer Res., 1971 (in press).
16. Sinkovics, J. G., Shirato, E., Cabiness, J. R. and Martin, R.: Clinical tissue culture and immunological studies. Abstr. Tenth Int. Cancer Congress, 1970, p. 204.
17. Hellström, I. E., Hellström, K. E., Pierce, G. E. and Bill, A. H.: Demonstration of cell bound and humoral immunity against neuroblastoma cells. Proc. Nat. Acad. Sci. 60:1231, 1968.
18. Hellström, K. E. and Hellström, I. E.: Immunologic defenses against cancer. Hosp. Pract. 1:45, 1970.
19. Halpern, B. N., Biozzi, G., Stiffel, C. and Mouton, D.: Effet de la stimulation du système réticulo-endothélial par l'inoculation du bacille de Calmette-Guérin sur le développement de l'épithélioma atypique T-8 de Guérin chez le Rat. C. R. Soc. Biol. 153:919, 1959.
20. Biozzi, G., Stiffel, C., Halpern, B. N. and Mouton, D.: Effet de l'inoculation du

bacille de Calmette-Guérin sur le développement de la tumeur ascitique d'Ehrlich chez la Souris. C. R. Soc. Biol. 153:987, 1959.
21. Biozzi, G., Stiffel, C., Halpern, B. N. and Mouton, D.: Étude de la function phagocytaire dur sur au cours du developpement de tumeurs malignes. Ann. Inst. Pasteur 94:681, 1958.
22. Balner, H., Old, L. J. and Clarke, D. A.: Accelerated rejection of male skin isografts by female C57Bl mice infected with BCG. Proc. Soc. Exp. Biol. Med. 109:58, 1962.
23. Halpern, B. N.: Role du système reticulo-endothélial dans l'immunité antibacterienne et antitumorale. Colloques Int. Centre Nat. de la Recherche Scientifique 115:319, 1963.
24. Dubos, R. J. and Schaedler, R. W.: Effects of cellular constituents of mycobacteria on the resistance of mice to heterologous infections. I. Protective effects. J. Exp. Med. 105:703, 1957.
25. Stinebring, W. R. and Absher, M.: Production of interferon following an immune response. Ann. N.Y. Acad. Sci. 173:714, 1970.
26. Old, L. J. and Clarke, D. A.: Effect of bacillus Calmette-Guérin (BCG) infection on transplanted tumors in the mouse. Nature 184:291, 1959.
27. Old, L. J., Benacerraf, B., Clarke, D. A., Carswell, G. A. and Stockert, E.: The role of the reticuloendothelial system in the host reaction to neoplasia. Cancer Res. 21:1281, 1961.
28. Old, L. J., Clarke, D. A., Benacerraf, B. and Stockert, E.: Effect of prior splenectomy on the growth of sarcoma 180 in normal and bacillus Calmette-Guérin infected mice. Experientia 18:335, 1962.
29. Rapp, H. J.: Immunotherapy of guinea pig hepatoma. J. Nat. Cancer Inst., 1971 (in press).
30. LeMonde, P. and Clode, M.: Effect of BCG infection on leukemia and polyoma in mice and hamsters. Proc. Soc. Exp. Biol. Med. 111:739, 1962.
31. LeMonde, P. and Clode, M.: Influence of BCG infection on polyoma in hamsters and mice. Cancer Res. 26:585, 1966.
32. Mathé, G.: Immunothérapie active de la leucémie L1210 appliquée après la greffe tumorale. Rev. Franc. Etud. Clin. Biol. 13:881, 1968.
33. Lamensans, A., Mollier, M. F. and Laurent, M.: Action du BCG sur l'activité catalasique hepatique chez la Souris. Rev. Franc. Etud. Clin. Biol. 13:871, 1968.
34. Lurie, M. B.: Resistance to Tuberculosis: Experimental Studies in Native and Acquired Defensive Mechanisms. Cambridge: Harvard University Press, 1964.
35. Davignon, L. P., LeMonde, P., Robillard, A. and Frappier, G.: BCG vaccination and leukemia mortality. Lancet 2:638, 1970.
36. Mathé, G., Schwarzenberg, L., Amiel, J. L., Schneider, M., Cattan, A. and Schlumberger, J. R.: Approches immunologiques du traitement des cancers chez l'homme. Bull. Cancer 54:33, 1967.
37. Mathé, G., Amiel, J. L., Schwarzenberg, L., Schneider, M., Cattan, A. and Schlumberger, J. R.: The role of immunology in the treatment of leukemias and hepatosarcomas. Cancer Res. 27:2542, 1967.
38a. Mathé, G., Amiel, J. L., Schwarzenberg, L., Schneider, M., Cattan, A., et al.: Demonstration de l'efficacité de l'immunothérapie active dans la leucémie aigue lymphoblastique humaine. Rev. Franc. Etud. Clin. Biol. 13:454, 1968.
38b. Mathé, G.: Personal communication, 1970.
39. Sokal, J. E. and Aungst, C. W.: Response to BCG vaccination and survival in advanced Hodgkin's disease. Cancer 24:128, 1969.
40. Morton, D. L.: Immunologic aspects of melanoma and sarcoma. Presented at 7th Ann. Meeting of Reticuloendothelial Soc., 1970.
41. Weiss, D. W., Bonhag, R. S. and Leslie, P.: Studies on the heterologous immunogenicity of a methanol-insoluble fraction of attenuated tubercle bacilli (BCG). J. Exp. Med. 124:1039, 1966.
42. Weiss, D. W., Bonhag, R. S. and DeOme, K. B.: Protective activity of fractions of tubercle bacilli against isologous tumours in mice. Nature 190:889, 1961.
43. Mathé, G.: Les réactions immunologiques (spontanées ou à visées thérapeutiques) et l'evolution des cancers (revue générale). Europ. J. Cancer 1:1, 1965.
44. Regelson, W.: Anionic polyelectrolytes as antimitotic agents. Advances Chemother. 3:303, 1968.
45. Levy, H. B.: Interferon and interferon inducers in the treatment of neoplastic diseases. (Ch. 6 in this volume.)
46. Plescia, O. J. and Braun, W. (Eds.): Nucleic Acids in Immunology. New York: Springer Verlag, 1968.
47. Krant, M. J., Manskopf, G., Brandrup, C. S. and Madoff, M. A.: Immunologic alterations in bronchogenic cancer. Cancer 21:623, 1968.

48. Israël, L., Mawas, C., Bouvrain, A., Mannon, P. and Sors, Ch.: Étude de l'hypersensibilité retardée à la tuberculine chez 130 cancéreux adultes: Effets du BCG. Path. Biol. 15:597, 1967.
49. Martin, D. S., Hayworth, P. E. and Fugmann, R. A.: Enhanced cures of spontaneous murine mammary tumors with surgery: Combination chemotherapy and immunotherapy. Cancer Res. 30:709, 1970.
50. Wampler, G. and Regelson, W.: Immunoenhancing agents used in combination with chemotherapeutic drugs in three murine tumor systems. Abstr. 7th Ann. Meeting of Reticuloendothelial Soc., 1970, p. 25.
51. Regelson, W.: Chemotherapy of gastrointestinal neoplasms. (Ch. 13 in this volume.)
52. Siegal, M.: Personal communication, 1970.
53. Gresser, I., Boye-Brouty, D., Thomas, M. T. and Macieira-Coelho, A.: Interferon and cell division. I. Inhibition of the multiplication of mouse leukemia L1210 cells in vitro by interferon preparations. Proc. Nat. Acad. Sci. U.S.A. 66:1052, 1970.
54. Stewart, T. H. M. and Tolnai, G.: The regression of an inflammatory skin lesion by the induction of a delayed hypersensitivity reaction. Cancer 24:117, 1969.
55. Klein, E.: Hypersensitivity reactions at tumor sites. Cancer Res. 29:2351, 1969.
56. Eilber, F. R. and Morton, D. L.: Impaired immunologic reactivity and recurrence following cancer surgery. Cancer 25:362, 1970.
57. Andrews, G. A., Congdon, C. C., Edwards, C. L., Gengozian, N., Nelson, B. and Vodopick, H.: Preliminary trials of clinical immunotherapy. Cancer Res. 27:2542, 1967.
58. Israël, L., Mannoni, P., Delobel, J., Mawas, C., Gross, B., et al.: Notes sur les résultats des intradermo-réactions de lymphocytes viables, homologues et hétérologues chez des receveurs cancéreux et des témoins. Path. Biol. 15:593, 1967.
59. Israël, L., Mannoni, P., Mawas, C., Gineste, J. Gross, B. and Sors, C.: 70 perfusions de, lymphocytes homologues dans 25 cas de cancers avancés. Path. Biol. 15:603, 1967.
60. Krementz, E. T. and Samuels, M. S.: Tumor cross transplantation and cross transfusion in the treatment of abnormal malignant disease. Bull. Tulane Univ. Med. Faculty 26:263, 1967.
61. Krementz, E. T., Samuels, M., Wallace, J. H. and Benes, E. N.: Clinical Experiences in the Immunotherapy of Cancer. Abstr. Tenth Int. Cancer Cong., 1970, p. 203.
62. Amos, D. B.: Formal discussion of Marc A. Lappé and R. T. Prehn's paper, Immunologic surveillance at the macroscopic level: Nonselective elimination of premalignant skin papillomas. Cancer Res. 29:2379, 1969.
63. Nadler, S. H. and Moore, G. E.: Clinical immunologic study of malignant disease: Response to tumor transplants and transfer of leukocytes. Ann. Surg. 164:482, 1965.
64. Freireich, E. J., Judson, G. and Levin, R. H.: Separation and collection of leukocytes. Cancer Res. 25:1516, 1965.
65. American Instrument Company, Silver Spring, Maryland. Continuous-flow centrifuge blood cell separator. Transfusion 8:3, 1968.
66. Tullis, J. L., Eberle, W. G., II, Baudanza, P. and Tinch, R.: Platelet-pheresis: Description of a new technique. Transfusion 8:3, 1968.
67. Abbott Laboratories, North Chicago, Illinois. Latham blood processor.
68. McKhann, C. F. and Aust, J.: Immunotherapy of human tumors. Abstr. Tenth Int. Cancer Cong., 1970, p. 202.
69. Aust, J. C., Jagarlamoody, S. and McKhann, C. F.: Immunization of lymphocytes in vitro for immunotherapy of malignant disease. Surg. Forum 21:118, 1969.
70. Frenster, J. H. and Rogoway, W. M.: Clinical use of activated autologous lymphocytes for human cancer immunotherapy. Abstr. Tenth Int. Cancer Cong., 1970, p. 203.
71. Frenster, J. H. and Rogoway, W. M.: In vitro activation and re-infusion of autologous human lymphocytes. Lancet 2:979, 1968.
72. Miro-Quesada, O.: Personal communication, 1970.
73. Symes, M. O., Ridell, A. G., Immelman, E. J. and Tarblanche, J.: Immunologically competent cells in the treatment of malignant disease. Lancet 1:1054, 1968.
74. Woodruff, M. F. A. and Symes, M. O.: The use of immunologically competent cells in the treatment of cancer: Experiments with a transplantable mouse tumor. Brit. J. Cancer 16:707, 1962.
75. Woodruff, M. F. A. and Nolan, B.: Preliminary observations on treatment of advanced cancer by injection of allogeneic spleen cells. Lancet 2:426, 1963.
76. Hellström, K. E. and Hellström, I.: Cellular

immunity against tumor antigens. Advances Cancer Res. 12:167, 1969.

77. Lawrence, S. H.: Transfer factor and cellular immune deficiency disease. New Eng. J. Med. 283:411, 1970.
78. Oettgen, H. F.: Personal communication, 1970.
79. Eschbach, J. W., Jr., Epstein, R. B., Burnell, J. M. and Thomas, E. D.: Physiologic observations in human cross circulation. New Eng. J. Med. 273:997, 1965.
80. Schrek, R. and Rabinowitz, Y.: Effects of phytohemagglutinins on rats and normal and leukemic human blood cells. Proc. Soc. Exp. Biol. 113:191, 1963.
81. Holm, G. and Perlmann, P.: Impaired phytohemagglutinin-involved cytotoxicity in vitro of lymphocytes from patients with Hodgkin's disease or chronic lymphatic leukemia. Clin. Exp. Immunol. 2:351, 1967.
82. Holm, G. and Perlmann, P.: Phytohaemagglutinin-induced cytotoxic action of unsensitized immunologically competent cells on allogeneic and xenogeneic tissue culture cells. Nature 207:818, 1965.
83. Southham, C. B., Brunschwig, A., Levin, A. G. and Dixon, Q.: Effect of leukocytes on transplantability of human cancer. Cancer 19:1743, 1966.
84. Stewart, T. H. M.: The presence of delayed hypersensitivity reactions in patients toward cellular extracts of their malignant tumors. I. The role of tissue antigen, nonspecific reactions of nuclear material, and bacterial antigen as a cause for this phenomenon. II. A correlation between the histologic picture of lymphocyte infiltration of the tumor stroma, the presence of such a reaction, and a discussion of the significance of this phenomenon. Cancer 23:1368, 1380, 1969.
85. Richters, A., Sherwin, R. and Richters, V.: The quantitation of lymphocyte interactions with neoplastic and non-neoplastic human lung cells in an autologous in vitro system. Proc. Amer. Ass. Cancer Res. 10:72, 1969.
86. Hellström, K. E.: Differential behaviour of transplanted mouse lymphoma lines in genetically compatible homozygous and F_1 hybrid mice. Nature 199:614, 1963.
87. Hellström, K. E. and Hellström, I. E.: Syngeneic preference and allogeneic inhibition. *In* Palm, J. (Ed.): Isoantigens and Cell Interaction. Philadelphia: Wistar Institute Press, 1965, pp. 79–93.
88. Hellström, K. E., Hellström, I. E. and Bergheden, C.: Studies on allogeneic inhibition. III. Inhibition of mouse tumor cell colony formation in vitro by contact with lymphoid cells containing foreign H-2 antigen. Int. J. Cancer 2:286, 1967.
89. Hellström, K. E. and Hellström, I. E.: Allogeneic inhibition and its possible relation to cell-bound immunity in vitro. *In* Mihich, E. (Ed.): Immunity, Cancer and Chemotherapy. New York: Academic Press, 1967, p. 51.
90. Moller, E.: Cytotoxicity by non-immune allogeneic lymphoid cells. J. Exp. Med. 126:395, 1967.
91. Moller, G. and Moller, E.: Inhibition of tumor growth by confrontation with incompatible cells. Cancer 20:871, 1967.
92. Chernyakhovskaya, I. Y., Kadaggidze, Z. G., and Svet-Moldavsky, G. J.: Effect of syngeneic and allogeneic lymphocytes on L-cells and mouse embryo fibroblasts *in vitro*. Nature 214:1229, 1967.
93. Phillips, M. E.: Studies on the cytolytic effect of sensitized lymphoid cells and immune sera *in vivo* and *in vitro*. Int. Arch. Allergy 32:249, 1967.
94. Lundgren, G., Moller, G. and Zukoski, C. H.: Effects of human granulocytes and lymphocytes on human fibroblasts in vitro. Acta Path. Microbiol. Scand. 72:453, 1968.
95. Holm, G., Perimann, P. and Werner, B.: Phytohaemagglutinin-induced cytotoxic action of normal lymphoid cells on cells in tissue culture. Nature 203:841, 1964.
96. Mathé, G. and Alexander, P.: Personal communication, 1968.
97. Warnatz, H., Scheiffarth, F. and Schmidt, G.: Immunological studies of the influence of isologous lymphocytes on the growth of the Ehrlich ascites tumor. Int. Arch. Allergy 30:238, 1966.
98. Woodruff, M. F. A.: Immunological aspects of cancer. Lancet 2:265, 1964.
99. Foley, E. J.: Attempts to induce immunity against mammary adenocarcinomas in inbred mice. Cander Res. 13:578, 1953.
100. Old, L. J. and Boyse, E. A.: Immunology of experimental tumors. Ann. Rev. Med. 15:167, 1964.
101. Rosenau, W. and Moon, H. D.: Lysis of homologous cells by sensitized lymphocytes in tissue culture. J. Nat. Cancer Inst. 27: 471, 1961.
102. Rosenau, W. and Morton, D. L.: Tumor-specific inhibition of growth of methylcholanthrene-induced sarcomas *in vivo* and *in vitro* by sentized isologous lymphod cells. J. Nat. Cancer Inst. 36:825, 1966.

103. Alexander, P.: Immunotherapy of leukemia: The use of different classes of immune lymphocytes. Cancer Res. 27: 2521, 1967.
104. Hatler, B. G., Jr., Tusji, K., Amos, B. and Shingleton, W. W.: Cytotoxic effect of immune thoracic duct lymphocyte in a tumor setting. Surg. Forum 18:221, 1967.
105. Mathé, G.: Immunothérapie adoptive locale de la tumeur BP 8 sous forme ascitique chez la Souris. Rev. Franc. Etud. Clin. Biol. 11:1027, 1966.
106. Svet-Moldavsky, G. J. and Kadaghidze, Z. G.: Anti-tumor effect of activated lymphocytes. Lancet 2:641, 1968.
107. Hashimoto, Y., Sudo, H. and Ishidate, M.: Inhibiting effect of carcinostatic agents on antitumor activity of sensitized lymphoid cells. Gann 58:31, 1967.
108. Kakulas, B. A.: Destruction of differentiated muscle cultures by sensitized lymphoid cells. J. Path. Bact. 91:495, 1966.
109. Coulson, A. S., Gurner, B. W. and Coombs, R. R. A.: Macrophage-like properties of some guinea-pig transformed cells. Int Arch. Allergy 32:264, 1967.
110. Toolan, H. W.: Conditioning of the host. J. Nat. Cancer Inst. 14:745, 1953.
111. Rebuck, J. W., Monto, R. W., Monaghan, E. A. and Riddle, J. M.: Potentialities of the lymphocyte, with an additional reference to its dysfunction in Hodgkin's disease. Ann. N.Y. Acad. Sci. 73:8, 1958.
112. Berman, L.: Lymphocytes and macrophages in vitro: Their activities in relation to functions of small lymphocytes. Lab. Invest. 15:1084, 1966.
113. Sura, S. N., Chernyakhovskaya, I. Y., Kadaghidze, Z. G., Fuks, B. B. and Svet-Moldavsky, G. J.: Cytochemical study of interaction between lymphocytes and target cells in tissue culture. Exp. Cell Res. 48: 656, 1967.
114. Granger, G. A. and Kolb, W. P.: Lymphocytes in vitro cytotoxicity: Mechanism of immune and non-immune small lymphocytes mediated target on cell destruction. J. Immun. 101:111, 1968.
115. Govaerts, A. L. J.: Cellular antibodies in kidney homotransplantation. J. Immun. 85:516, 1960.
116. Koprowski, H. and Fernandes, M. V.: Autosensitization reaction in vitro. J. Exp. Med. 116:467, 1962.
117. Rosenau, W. and Moon, H. D.: Lysis of homologous cells by sensitized lymphocytes in tissue culture. J. Nat. Cancer Inst. 27:471, 1961.
118. Taylor, H. E. and Culling, C.: Cytopathic effect in vitro of sensitized homologous and heterologous spleen cells or fibroblasts. Lab. Invest. 12:884, 1963.
119. Wilson, D. B.: The reaction of immunologically activated lymphoid cells against homologous target tissue cells in vitro. J. Cell. Comp. Physiol. 62:273, 1963.
120. Granger, G. A. and Weiser, R. S.: Homograft target cells: Specific destruction in vitro by contact interaction with immune macrophages. Science 145:1427, 1964.
121. Granger, G. A. and Weiser, R. S.: Homograft target cells: Contact destruction in vitro by immune macrophages. Science 151:97, 1966.
122. MacKaness, G. B.: Cell-mediated immunity to infection. Hosp. Pract. 5:73, 1970.
123. Moller, F.: Contact-induced cytotoxicity by lymphoid cells containing foreign isoantigens. Science 147:873, 1965.
124. MacLennan, I.C.M. and Loewi, G.: The effect of peripheral lymphocytes from patients with inflammatory joint disease on human target cells in vitro. Clin. Exp. Immunol. 3:385, 1968.
125. Holm, G. and Perlmann, P.: Quantitative studies on phytohemagglutinin-induced cytotoxicity by normal human lymphocytes against homologous cells in tissue culture. Immunology 12:525, 1967.
126. Holm, G. and Perlmann, P.: Cytotoxic potential of stimulated human lymphocytes. J. Exp. Med. 125:721, 1967.
127. Wilson, D. B.: Quantitative studies on the behavior of sensitized lymphocytes in vitro. I. Relationship of the degree of destruction of homologous target cells to the number of lymphocytes and to the time of contact in culture and consideration of the effects of isoimmune serum. J. Exp. Med. 122:143, 1965.
128. Weiss, L.: Interaction of sensitized lymphoid cells and homologous target cells in tissue culture and in grafts: An electron microscope and immunofluorescence study. J. Immun. 101:1346, 1968.
129. Old, L. J., Boyse, E. A., Bennett, B. and Lilly, F.: Peritoneal cells as an immune population in transplantation studies. *In* Amos, D. and Koprowski, H. (Eds.): Cell Bound Antibodies. Philadelphia: Wistar Institute Press, 1963, pp. 89–99.
130. Old, L. J., Boyse, E. A., Clarke, D. A. and

Carswell, E. A.: Antigenic properties of chemically induced tumors. Ann. N.Y. Acad. Sci. 101:80, 1962.

131. Bennet, B., Old, L. and Boyse, E.: The phagocytosis of tumor cells in vitro. Transplantation 2:183, 1964.

132. Rigas, D. A. and Osgood, E. E.: Purification and properties of the phytohemagglutinin of phaseolus vulgaris. J. Biol. Chem. 212:607, 1955.

133. Stuart, A. E.: The effect of immunological lymphoid cells on tissue culture preparation of macrophages. J. Path. Bact. 93:673, 1967.

134. Najarian, J. S.: The role of the lymphocyte in homograft rejection. *In* Yoffey, J. M. (Ed.): The Lymphocyte in Immunology and Haemopoiesis. London: Edward Arnold, 1967, p. 266.

135. Burke, J. F.: Induced immunologic response to tumors. Cancer Res. 29:2363, 1969.

136. Evans, R.: Cultivation and in vitro characterization of mouse phagocytic cells. J. Reticuloendothel. Soc. 8:571, 1970.

137. Wolstenholme, G. E. W. and O'Connor, C. M. (Eds.): Cellular Aspects of Immunity. Boston: Little, Brown, 1959.

138. Sharp, J. A.: Adhesion of lymphocytes to large motile cells in cultures of rabbit thymus. Nature 209:828, 1966.

139. Nouza, K.: The theory, practice and treatment of graft versus host reactions. Rev. Franc. Etud. Clin. Biol. 13:747, 1968.

140. Moller, G. and Moller, E.: Growth inhibition by interaction between allogeneic cells: A model for the elimination of incompatible cells. Ann. Med. Exp. Fenn. 44:181, 1966.

141. Fialkow, P. J.: Chromosomal breakage induced by extracts of human allogeneic lymphocytes. Science 155:1676, 1967.

142. Fialkow, P. J. and Gartler, S. M.: Hyperploidy effect of lymphocyte extract on fibroblasts *in vitro*. Nature 211:713, 1966.

143. Glick, J. L.: Induction of an allogeneic-like inhibition by means of DNA obtained from untreated cells. *In* Plescia, J. and Braun, W. (Eds.): Nucleic Acids in Immunology. New York: Springer Verlag, 1968, pp. 414–428.

144. Alexander, P., Delorme, E. J. and Hall, J. G.: The effect of lymphoid cells from the lymph of specifically immunized sheep on the growth of primary sarcomata in rats. Lancet 1:1186, 1966.

145. Pilch, Y. H., Ramming, K. P. and Deckers, P. S.: Transfer of tumor immunity with RNA. Presented at NCI Cancer Immunology Conf., 1970 (in press, 1971).

146. McCullough, J., Benson, S. J., Tunis, E. J. and Quie, P. G.: Effect of blood bank storage on leukocyte function. Lancet 2:1333, 1969.

147. Moorhead, J. F., Connolly, J. J. and McFarland, W.: Factors affecting the reactivity of human lymphocytes in vitro. I. Cell number, duration of culture and surface area. J. Immun. 99:413, 1967.

148. Miller, D. G.: Patterns of immunologic deficiency in lymphomas and leukemias. Ann. Intern. Med. 57:703, 1962.

149. Robinson, E.: Immunology and PHA in cancer. Lancet 2:753, 1966.

150. Robinson, E.: PHA in cancer. Lancet 1: 213, 1967.

151. Moore, G. E. and Gerner, R. E.: Cytotherapy of cancer. Abstr. Tenth Int. Cancer Cong., 1970, p. 200.

152. Regelson, W. (Chairman), Wampler, G., Hossaini, A., Lawrence, W., Moon, J., et al. (Leukapheresis Task Force), Medical College of Virginia, Virginia Commonwealth University, Richmond, Virginia, 1970.

153. Hall, J. G. and Smith, M. E.: Homing of lymph-borne immunoblasts to the gut. Nature 226:262, 1970.

154. Griscelli, C., Vassalli, P. and McCluskey, R. T.: The distribution of large division lymph node cells in syngeneic recipient rats after intravenous injection. J. Exp. Med. 130:1427, 1969.

155. Moses, E. and Shearer, G.: Conversion of genetic low responders to a synthetic polypeptide into high responders by polynucleotides. Miles Symposium, Biological Effects of Polynucleotides (in press, 1971).

156. Escobar, M.: Work in progress, 1971.

The Effects of Chemotherapy on Hemostasis

By Isadore Brodsky, M.D. and James F. Conroy, D.O.

A PROPER UNDERSTANDING OF THROMBOPOIESIS and blood coagulation is increasingly important in understanding the pathogenesis and treatment of cancer. Neoplastic disease is a common cause of secondary thrombocytosis and a hypercoagulable state.[1-3] Studies indicate that fibrin deposition is important for the growth of primary tumors and their metastatic spread.[4-7] Fibrin is deposited, particularly at the periphery, and this provides an important latticework for tumor growth. Human cancer cells contain an agent that some have referred to as a cancer coagulative factor that induces fibrin formation and is thought to resemble certain thromboplastins. The action of this factor can be blocked by coumadin cogeners. The formation of an enveloping microthrombus around embolic tumor cells is also considered a decisive part of the mechanism of endothelial adherence and penetration.[4,6] It has been noted that clumped tumor cells are essential in establishing tumor metastases.[8] These considerations have recently led to investigations utilizing anticoagulants for treatment of neoplasia in both experimental animals and humans.[6,9,10]

An exaggeration of this hypercoagulable state may be responsible for the increasing frequency with which the phenomenon of disseminated intravascular coagulation (DIC) is being noted in clinical oncology.[3] In the animal the prototype of DIC is the generalized Shwartzman reaction. Rabbits made granulopenic with nitrogen mustard are protected from the generalized Shwartzman reaction when challenged by endotoxin. Thus, there is evidence that granulocytes are necessary for intravascular clot formation, perhaps by releasing a substance with thromboplastic activity. In contrast, thrombocytopenia associated with neoplastic disease is of clinical significance, has prognostic value, and may indeed precede the onset of clinical disease, as in the preleukemic state. Thrombocytopenia is a common preleukemic manifestation in the viral-induced and spontaneous murine leukemias.[11,12]

Current chemotherapeutic measures significantly affect hemostasis in regard to thrombocytopenia due to marrow suppression. Recent observations also indicate that other significant coagulopathies may be a direct result of chemotherapy. For example, the bleeding diathesis associated with mithramycin therapy is well documented but its mechanism is poorly defined.[13] To our knowledge, the first documented instance of DIC resulting directly from chemotherapy was reported from our institution.[3] A patient with acute granulocytic leukemia developed acute intravascular coagulation following a precipitous fall in the white blood cell count induced by combination chemotherapy with vincristine, methotrexate, 6-mercaptopurine and prednisone (VAMP). We believed that destruction of white blood cells resulted in release of a thromboplastic material. This patient was successfully treated with heparin therapy and subsequently entered complete hematologic remission. A summary of the events in this case is presented in Table 1.

Treatment with *Escherichia coli* L-asparaginase is frequently associated with the

---

From the Division of Hematology and Medical Oncology, Department of Medicine, Hahnemann Medical College and Hospital, Philadelphia, Pennsylvania.

Supported by grant No. CA-08024 from the National Institutes of Health.

TABLE 1.—*Effect of Chemotherapy and Heparin Therapy on Coagulation Profile in a Patient with Acute Myelomonocytic Leukemia*

Days of Chemo-therapy	*WBC × $10^3/mm^3$*	*Thrombin time in seconds at incubation of 10 min.*	*Platelet count × $10^3/mm^3$*	*Fibrinogen (mg/100 ml)*	*ELT (hr.)*	*Pro. time %*	*PTT (sec.)*	*C.T. (min.)*
0*	192	3.2	277		5–6	100	53.4	6
3†	128	16.5	122	45	5–6	57	69.3	11
4	8.4	10.0	106	45	5–6	52	114.8	
6	3.7	4.8	191	165	5–6	100	62.9	5
9‡	3.8	3.2	164		5–6	100	54.8	8
Normal Range		3.9–6.0	150–450	150–300	4.5–6.0	70–100	60–70	6–12

* Chemotherapy begun.
† Heparin begun.
‡ Heparin discontinued.
Abbreviations: ELT = euglobulin lysis time; PTT = partial thromboplastin time; Pro. time = one-stage prothrombin time; C.T. = Lee-White clotting time.

development of hypofibrinogenemia.[14] This complication will develop in approximately 80 to 90 per cent of patients treated with this drug. The main factors to be considered in the pathogenesis of this condition are (1) DIC, primarily associated with a fall in the white blood cell count during therapy, and (2) a possible decrease in the synthesis of fibrinogen during therapy.

We have recently concluded an intensive investigation of the coagulation mechanism

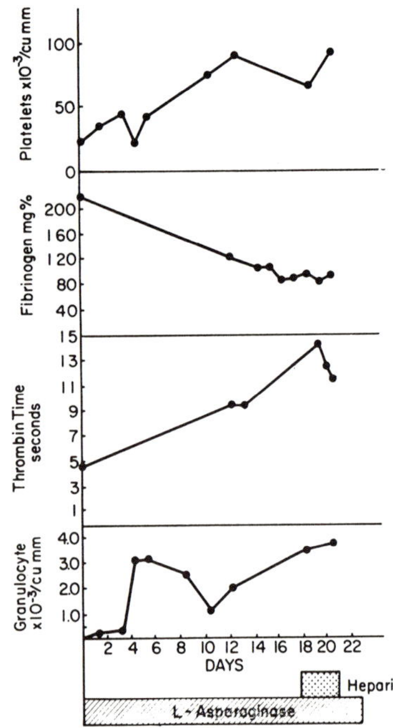

FIG. 1.—(Case 1: acute lymphoblastic leukemia.) Effects of L-asparaginase and subsequent heparin therapy on selected hematologic and coagulation parameters. Only the thrombin time obtained after 10 minutes' incubation is presented. Figures 1 through 7 from Brodsky et al.,[16] by courtesy of the British Journal of Haematology.

and, in particular, fibrinogen anabolism and catabolism, in six patients with hematologic or solid tumor neoplasms treated with L-asparaginase. A cohort method utilizing ^{75}Se-selenomethionine was employed to label the fibrinogen.[15] In four patients the study was performed during a period of L-asparaginase-induced hypofibrinogenemia, and in two patients fibrinogen was labeled 48 hours prior to the start of L-asparaginase therapy.[16]

The first patient treated was a 14-year-old girl with acute lymphoblastic leukemia who had become resistant to standard chemotherapeutic drugs (Fig. 1). Immediately prior to the start of L-asparaginase the platelet count was 35,000, the fibrinogen level was 220 mg%, the thrombin time was normal, and the white blood cell count was sharply decreased with blasts in the peripheral blood. With treatment (10,000 units of L-asparaginase daily) a sharp decrease occurred in the fibrinogen level from 220 to 80 mg% associated with a rise in the thrombin time. The platelet count rose, as did the white blood cell count. Split products of fibrinogen were not demonstrated. On the eighteenth day of therapy, heparin was started in a dose of 20,000 units per day. This was continued for 3 days and no significant change in the underlying coagulation mechanism was noted. Eventually a complete objective remission of the underlying leukemia was attained.

A second patient presented with a hypernephroma, with metastases to the lung and the adrenal glands (Fig. 2). Prior to the start of L-asparaginase administration, the platelet count was normal but the fibrinogen level was markedly elevated at 1000 mg%. The thrombin time and the white blood cell count were well within normal limits. During L-asparaginase therapy the fibrinogen level fell to approximately 400 mg%. It is important to note that, although the fibrinogen level decreased, it was still within normal limits. The thrombin time became prolonged, but again there were

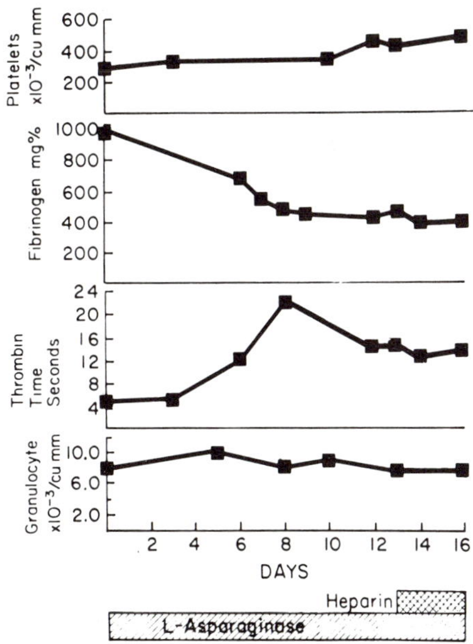

FIG. 2.—(Case 2: hypernephroma.) Effect of L-asparaginase and subsequent heparin therapy on selected hematologic and coagulation parameters. Only the thrombin time obtained after 10 minutes' incubation is presented.[16]

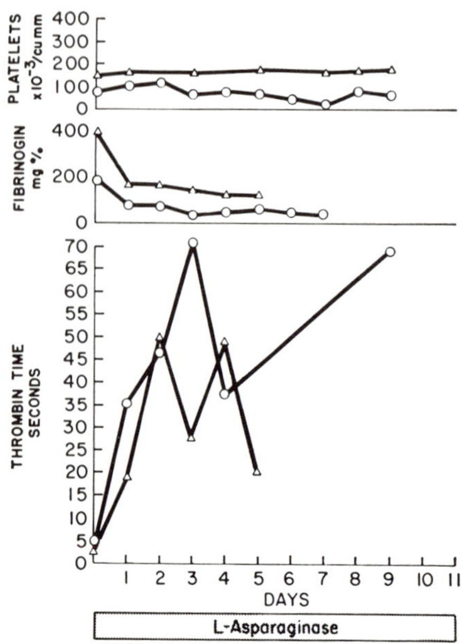

FIG. 3.—(Case 3 △—△ and Case 4 ○—○: lymphosarcoma.) Effect of L-asparaginase therapy on the platelet count, fibrinogen level, and thrombin time obtained after 10 minutes' incubation.[16]

no demonstrable split products, and heparin therapy had no effect on the underlying coagulation disorder.

The next two patients had lymphosarcoma. In one the fibrinogen level prior to therapy was 400 mg%, and in the other 200 mg% (Fig. 3). Significant hypofibrinogenemia developed, and again this was associated with a prolongation in the thrombin

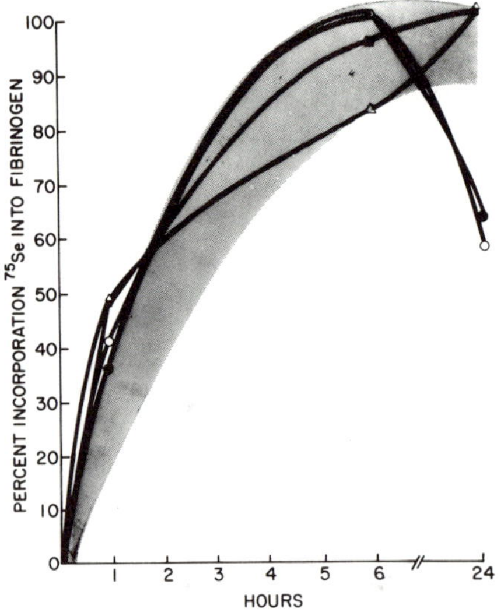

FIG. 4.—Anabolic phase of fibrinogen metabolism in Case 1 ●—●, Case 2 ■—■, Case 3 △—△, Case 4 ○—○. Stippled area: control range.[16]

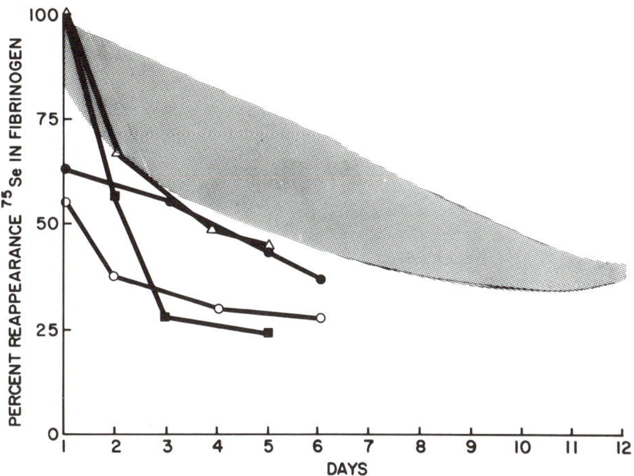

FIG. 5.—Catabolic phase of fibrinogen metabolism during L-asparaginase therapy in Cases 1 to 4. Stippled area: control range.[16]

time. The platelet count remained stable; split products were not demonstrable. In none of the four cases were we able to document primary fibrinolysis as measured by the euglobulin clot lysis time.[16]

The anabolic and catabolic phases of fibrinogen survival were determined in all four patients during the period of maximum hypofibrinogenemia (Fig. 4). The controls shown for comparison were obtained in ten subjects with normal coagulation. In the normal controls, during the anabolic phase, incorporation of radioactivity into fibrinogen reached its peak 6 hours after intravenous administration of selenomethionine. The radioactivity reached a plateau, and the catabolic phase started 24 hours later. In essence, the anabolic curves (that is, the synthesis of fibrinogen) in the patients treated with L-asparaginase were well within normal limits.

The catabolic phase of fibrinogen survival is presented in Figure 5. In the control group the normal fibrinogen survival was approximately 7.8 ± 2.8 days.[15] This is represented by the stippled area. In the patients treated with L-asparaginase overall fibrinogen survival ranged from 1.5 to 4 days. The fibrinogen survival represented the time in days from the 50 per cent point on the anabolic curve to the 50 per cent point on the catabolic curve. The shortest survival, one and a half days, was noted in one patient with lymphosarcoma whose fibrinogen level prior to treatment had been 200 mg % and had then fallen to 50. The next shortest survival, approximately 2 days, was noted in the patient with hypernephroma, whose fibrinogen survival fell from a level of 960 to 400 mg %.

In a second experiment, the effect of L-asparaginase on fibrinogen labeled with selenomethionine, before the start of enzyme therapy, was determined. Two patients with Hodgkin's disease were studied. On day zero 250 μc of selenomethionine was injected (Fig. 6). At this time both patients presented with hyperfibrinogenemia, the values being 600 and 800 mg %. Their thrombin times were normal. One patient had thrombocytosis and the other a normal platelet count. The anabolic phase of fibrinogen synthesis was determined and observations in the catabolic phase started. Two days later L-asparaginase in a dose of 10,000 units per day was begun. A constant fall in fibrinogen level in both patients occurred. The platelet counts remained almost constant and actually showed a slight rise.

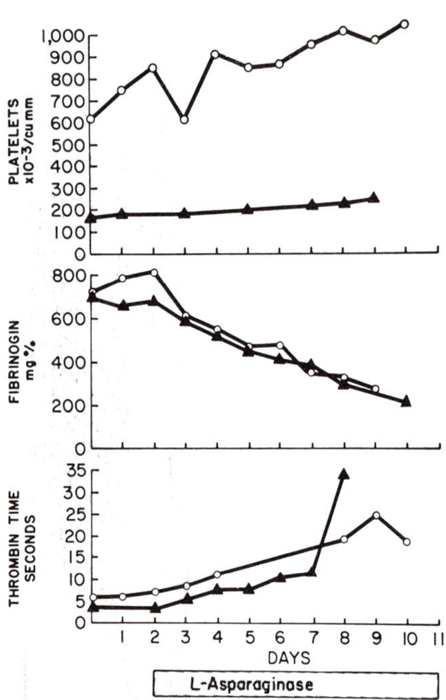

FIG. 6.—(Case 5 ○—○ and Case 6 ▲—▲: Hodgkin's disease.) Effect of L-asparaginase therapy on the platelet count, fibrinogen level, and thrombin time obtained after 10 minutes' incubation. ^{75}Se-selenomethionine was administered 2 days before start of L-asparaginase.[16]

The anabolic curves of fibrinogen synthesis in these two cases were normal and the catabolic curves were well within normal limits (Fig. 7).

On the basis of the above data one cannot support the contention that the hypofibrinogenemia in these cases was due to DIC. The factors opposing this particular concept are (1) the absence of any significant thrombocytopenia during L-asparaginase therapy (in fact, in some of the cases the platelet count actually rose); (2) split products of fibrinogen, a common occurrence in DIC, were not elevated and there was no evidence for primary fibrinolysis; and (3) in two patients short courses of heparin therapy had no effect on the abnormal coagulation parameters.

The final possibility, and the explanation that we favor, is that L-asparaginase can interfere with asparagine metabolism, leading to the synthesis of an abnormal fibrinogen with a decreased survival. Asparagine is a crucial amino acid in the process of fibrin polymerization.[7]

Initially the development of L-asparaginase therapy carried with it the hope that this form of treatment would be specific for the neoplastic cell. It is now quite apparent that L-asparaginase can also cause significant abnormalities in normal cells. Its effect on fibrinogen is highly constant. Of course, one might raise the question as to whether the induction of hypofibrinogenemia may have some significance in inducing a therapeutic effect. The question is obviously hypothetical but should be raised in view of experimental and clinical evidence that a significantly less potent agent, in terms of the coagulation mechanism, such as warfarin, can significantly influence the course of metastatic disease.[6,9,10]

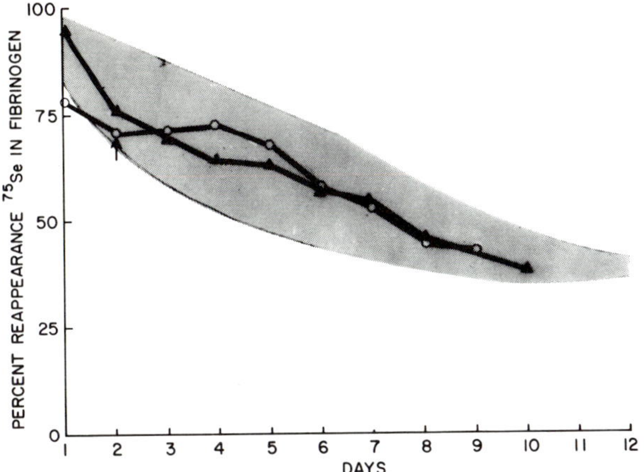

FIG. 7.—Catabolic phase of fibrinogen metabolism in Cases 5 and 6. ↑ indicates start of L-asparaginase therapy. Stippled area: control range.[16]

Laki[7] also speculated in 1968 that involvement of the clot in the growth of a tumor would be suggested if it were found that L-asparaginase reacted with the asparagine residues of fibrinogen. The demonstrated dysfibrinogenemia following L-asparaginase therapy adds strong support to Laki's hypothesis.[16]

A current problem in coagulation vis-à-vis chemotherapy revolves around a new agent, mithramycin. This drug has demonstrated antitumor effects on testicular and cerebral neoplasms. Its application and effective dosage are severely hampered by production of a severe bleeding diathesis. Hemorrhage of varying degrees has been reported in 59 per cent of patients. Hemorrhage was present in nearly all patients who died from drug toxicity. Vascular damage has been noted both in vivo and in vitro and has been considered an important factor in initiating the bleeding.[13] Thrombocytopenia did occur but was seldom of a degree to explain the bleeding diathesis. Altered platelet function has been observed.[13] Depression of factors II, V, VIII, and X has been regularly reported, as has an increase in fibrinolytic activity. Hepatic dysfunction is a regular occurrence with mithramycin. It would not be unreasonable to hypothesize drug-induced production of an abnormal clotting factor or fibrinogen such as is demonstrated with L-asparaginase.

Actinomycin D is known to inhibit the effect of vitamin K in inducing prothrombin synthesis and is also known to block DNA-dependent RNA synthesis.[17] In the absence of vitamin K, a regulatory gene has been postulated to repress the activity of the operon concerned with the elaboration of the vitamin K-dependent clotting proteins such as prothrombin. By combining with the repressor molecule, vitamin K may act to derepress the operator gene. The operator can then allow the structural genes to elaborate messenger RNA, which will serve as template for the synthesis of the vitamin K-dependent clotting proteins.

From a pharmacologic standpoint, with the development of newer chemotherapeutic agents and, in particular, specific enzymes such as L-asparaginase to treat malignancy, more emphasis will have to be placed on the effects of these drugs on the coagulation mechanism.

References

1. Levin, J. and Conley, C. L.: Thrombocytosis associated with malignant disease. Arch. Intern. Med. 114:497, 1964.
2. Davis, R. P., Theologides, A. and Kennedy, B. J.: Comparative studies of blood coagulation and platelet aggregation in patients with cancer and nonmalignant disease. Ann. Intern. Med. 71:67, 1969.
3. Leavey, R. A., Kahn, S. B. and Brodsky, I.: Disseminated intravascular coagulation—a complication of chemotherapy in acute myelomonocytic leukemia. Cancer 26:142, 1970.
4. Wood, S., Jr.: Pathogenesis of metastasis formation observed *in vivo* in the rabbit ear chamber. Arch. Path. 66:550, 1958.
5. Agostino, D., Cliffton, E. and Girolami, A.: Effect of prolonged coumadin treatment on production of pulmonary metastases in the rat. Cancer 19:284, 1966.
6. Ryan, J. J., Ketcham, A. S. and Wexler, H.: Warfarin treatment of mice bearing autochthonous tumors: effect on spontaneous metastases. Science 162:1493, 1968.
7. Laki, K. and Yancey, S. T.: Fibrinogen and the tumor problem. *In* Laki, K. (Ed.): Fibrinogen. New York: Marcel Dekker, 1968, p. 359.
8. Brodsky, I., Barin, M., Kahn, S. B., Lewis, G. and Tellem, M.: Metastatic malignant melanoma from mother to fetus. Cancer 18:1048, 1965.
9. Michaels, L.: Cancer incidence and mortality in patients having anticoagulant therapy. Lancet 2:832, 1964.
10. Ryan, J. J., Ketcham, A. S. and Wexler, H.: Reduced incidence of spontaneous metastases with long-term coumadin therapy. Ann. Surg. 168:163, 1968.
11. Brodsky, I., Kahn, S. B., Ross, E. M., Petkov, G. and Braverman, S. D.: Prelymphoid leukemia phase of Rauscher virus infection. J. Nat. Cancer Inst. 38:779, 1967.
12. Brodsky, I.: Thrombocytopenia, a prelymphoid leukaemic sign in AKR mice. Nature 223:198, 1969.
13. Monto, R. W., Talley, R. W., Caldwell, M. J., Levin, W. C. and Guest, M. M.: Observations on the mechanism of hemorrhagic toxicity in mithramycin therapy. Cancer Res. 29:697, 1969.
14. Bettigole, R. E., Himelstein, E. S., Oettgen, H. F. and Clifford, G. O.: Hypofibrinogenemia due to L-asparaginase: Studies of fibrinogen survival using autologous ^{131}I fibrinogen. Blood 35:195, 1970.
15. Brodsky, I., Siegel, N. H., Kahn, S. B., Ross, E. M. and Petkov, G.: Simultaneous fibrinogen and platelet survival with (^{75}Se) selenomethionine in man. Brit. J. Haem. 18:347, 1970.
16. Brodsky, I., Kahn, S. B., Vash, G., Ross, E. M. and Petkov, G.: Fibrinogen survival with (^{75}Se) selenomethionine during L-asparaginase therapy. Brit. J. Haem. 20: 477, 1971.
17. Olson, R. E.: Vitamin K-induced prothrombin formation antagonism by actinomycin-D. Science 145:926, 1964.

Biochemical Factors Predicting Response to Chemotherapeutic Agents

By THOMAS C. HALL, M.D.

THE PREDICTION OF RESPONSE TO ANTITUMOR AGENTS is an important subject, and will become increasingly so in the future. There are a number of reasons for this:

1. There are forms of leukemia in which it is difficult to induce remissions and which are rapid in course, such as acute myeloblastic leukemia, blastic crises of chronic myelocytic leukemia, and the drug resistant phases of acute lymphoblastic leukemia. In these patients one usually has time to choose only one drug regimen for trial; if one fails the patient is dead before a second regimen can be tried. Therefore, preselection of drugs on the basis of known drug sensitivity for inclusion in a clinical regimen becomes vital.

2. Drug combinations are increasingly being used to enhance their cytocidal effects and prolong remission. The composition of such combinations is usually decided empirically. If one could identify ineffective drugs and so *exclude* them, the unnecessary toxicity would be lessened. If one could identify potentially effective drugs and include them, effectiveness should increase.

3. The methods used most effectively to predict drug effectiveness, such as DNA inhibition, can often be used to determine more appropriate dosages, intervals and rates of administration. For example, our studies of the duration of daunomycin inhibition of DNA synthesis for leukemic cells suggest that the inhibition lasts 48 or more hours. Hence it seems unnecessary to give the drug more often than twice weekly, and the massive suppression of normal marrow proliferation induced by the daily schedules used up until now may not be necessary or desirable.

4. Clinical drug trials are very expensive; for example, $1,000 per case is a common figure. For a 100-patient trial, one-tenth of a million dollars is a low cost figure. In the instance of 5-fluorouracil (5-FU), it has been estimated that 0.5 million dollars, with much patient morbidity, was used to show that 5-fluorouracil was ineffective in acute leukemia. Using a simple in vitro phosphorylation method, 5-FU can, at one-hundredth the cost, be predicted to be ineffective in human leukemia, in a few months, with no patient morbidity.

The evaluation of attempts to predict drug responsiveness in human leukemia has been in the direction of increasing simplicity and precision, and decreasing cost. Such attempts can be based upon study of characteristics of (1) the host, (2) the drug, (3) the tumor cell, and (4) the dynamic interaction of the first three in controlled circumstances.

Examination of the *host* characteristics, such as normal marrow reactions as exemplified by platelet, granulocyte and hemoglobin estimates, are of some help statistically to describe patients who are poor risks for chemotherapy in general, but they are of little value in selecting specific drugs for individual patients.[1]

From the Division of Oncology and the Departments of Medicine and Pharmacology, University of Rochester Medical Center, Rochester, New York.

Supported in part by grants CA-11198 and PH69-39 from the U.S. Public Health Service.

Knowledge of the mode of *action of a drug* is also helpful, but only in a general way, i.e., anti-DNA metabolites are not very effective in the treatment of chronic lymphocytic leukemia, in which there is little DNA replication, and alkylating agents which are generally cytotoxic do not distinguish well between the rapidly dividing blast cells in normal marrow and those of acute leukemia.

Examination of the particular cell-drug relationship using the cells of a specific patient gets closer to the ideal. The parameter of cell function to be examined is important, and should be chosen because of the therapeutic possibilities. However, most initial efforts in this area had fundamental conceptual defects. Study of the effects of an anti-cell division drug such as methotrexate upon such vegetative functions of the cell as carbohydrate metabolism is not very helpful, as has been found by those who used impairment of glycolysis or respiration as possible predictive indices for drug sensitivity.[2] For this reason, the simple in vitro dye reduction tests were not successful.[3]

Effects upon cell growth in tissue culture are not likely to succeed when so little is known about human tumor tissue cultures that less than 5 per cent of patients' cells have established viable in vitro lines. Even in short-term 1- or 2-day cultures, one usually cannot set up the conditions for DNA synthesis to occur, and one examines the effects of drugs upon surviving but not dividing cells.

It is not helpful to look for short-term inhibition of uridine incorporation into RNA as a selective predicting system for DNA antimetabolites such as are commonly used in antileukemia therapy.[4]

It will usually be of little value to add drug to an in vitro system containing tumor cells and expect to observe a drug effect.[5] The reasons for this are multiple:

1. Some drugs need to be activated by organs of the host which are absent from the culture, i.e., the liver for cyclophosphamide. Such drugs will show much less effect in cultures than in vivo.[6]

2. The host may catabolize or eliminate the drug rapidly, i.e., renal excretions of methotrexate, or hepatic deamination of cytarabine. Such drug metabolism results in vivo in constantly shifting concentrations of drug in cells and fluids outside the cell, and these are difficult to reproduce in cell culture. As a result, depending upon the in vitro experimental design, the drug may be present in higher than physiologic concentrations for longer than therapeutic periods, and all the cells in culture show a common effect. Such studies can give hints as to probable mode of action, but hardly can be used for selective prediction.[7]

3. Ionic factors and pool sizes of other DNA substrates cannot be estimated with any precision in an in vivo system. Therefore, a model for effects of drug on cells similar to the actual in vivo therapeutic situation is virtually impossible in vitro.

4. The target tumor tissue and normal host tissue have almost never been looked at simultaneously in vitro. Such a method should suggest whether the differential effect desired in vivo was being achieved in vivo. A selective toxicity to the tumor should be preceded by greater uptake into tumor cells as compared with marrow or gastrointestinal mucosa, and followed by greater inhibition of DNA synthesis in the tumor than in the stem cells of marrow or intestinal crypts.

Our work in this area has been based upon the examination of three aspects of the drug-cell interaction. I wish to acknowledge the cooperation of my colleagues, David Kessel, Ph.D., DeWayne Roberts, Ph.D., Aly Nahas, Ph.D. and Bruce Hacker, Ph.D. in these areas.

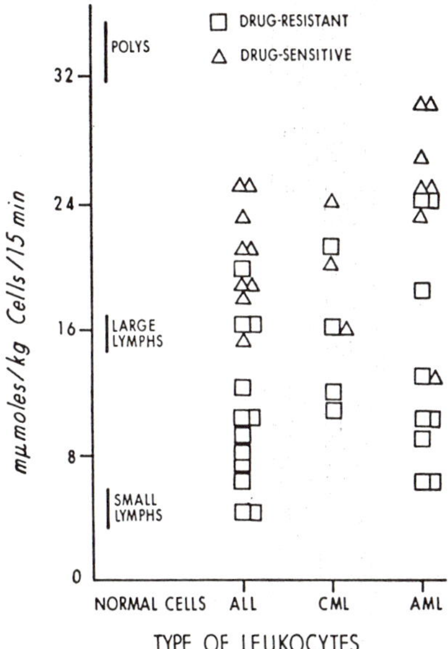

FIG. 1.—Uptake and retention of tritiated methotrexate by human white cells of several types. Incubation for 15 minutes in modified Eagle's medium at 10 mM/ml.

The first laboratory technique we use is the examination of the uptake and retention of labeled drugs by the malignant cell in vitro. These processes are usually performed as part of the vegetative functions of nondividing cells, and can therefore be examined during short periods, up to an hour, after removal of cells from the body. We have used the blast cells of leukemic peripheral blood and marrow, as well as the free-floating cells of malignant effusions in such studies.

Figure 1 shows that the uptake of tritiated methotrexate by human leukemic cells in vitro correlates very well with general and specific predictions of drug responsiveness.

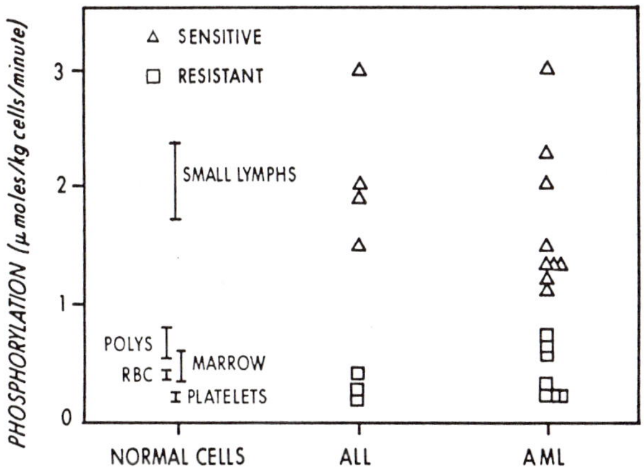

FIG. 2.—Uptake and phosphorylation of tritiated cytosine arabinoside by human white cells of various types. Conditions of incubation as in Figure 1.

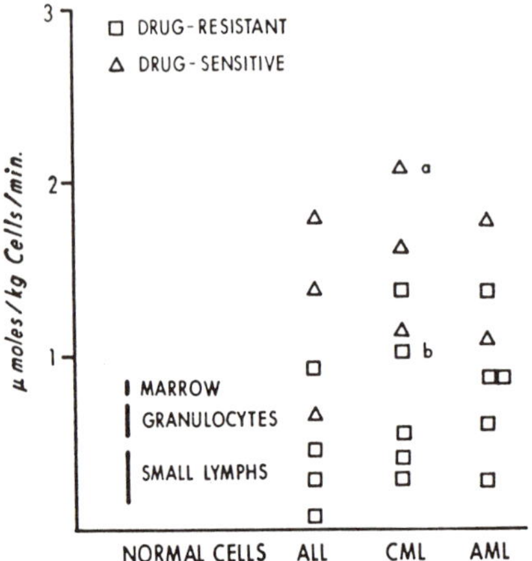

FIG. 3.—Conversion of 6-mercaptopurine to non-diffusable products by human leukocytes. Preparations a and b were from the same patient before and after development of drug resistance.

The low uptake by human leukemia, as compared to mouse ascites leukemia, correlates well with the *generally* higher sensitivity of mouse leukemias. The low uptake in all human small lymphocytes correlates well with the unresponsiveness of chronic lymphocytic leukemia to methotrexate (MTX). In most instances, high uptake by malignant cells is correlated with drug responsiveness, and low uptake is almost invariably correlated with drug resistance either innate, as in acute myeloblastic leukemia (AML), or acquired, as in acute lymphoblastic leukemia, after relapse occurring during treatment with methotrexate.

A similar situation exists with regard to cytarabine (Fig. 2). The retention of cytarabine's active phosphorylated derivative, by cells after incubation for 15 minutes in vitro, is high in the cells of patients who were later shown to be sensitive to the drug and low in those who were resistant.

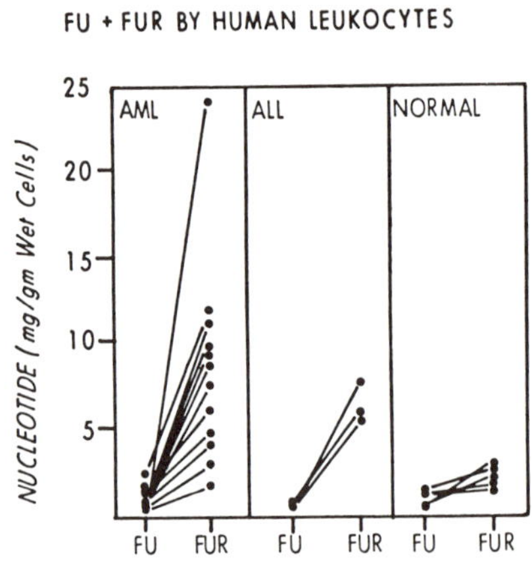

FIG. 4.—Uptake and phosphorylation of radioactive FU and FUR by human white cells. The lines connect different aliquots from single specimens incubated simultaneously but separately with each isotope. In most leukemic cells FUR is phosphorylated while FU is not, in contrast to normal cells.

Figure 3 shows that in patients who were resistant to 6-mercaptopurine (6-MP), there was low phosphorylation of the drug, whereas in sensitive patients, the drug was well taken up and retained. Note that there is some overlap, and in these cases one would like an additional test of whether the drug taken up to an intermediate extent would be effective therapeutically. These data have been obtained on whole cells. Winter and Davidson were unable to make such correlations using broken cells, nor were we able to do so. This requirement for whole human cells is in contrast to the situation for mouse leukemias, in which both intact and broken-cell phosphorylation correlates well with drug responsiveness.

The data in Figure 4 clearly show that 5-fluorouracil is not well phosphorylated by normal human cells and that the difference between leukemic cell uptake and normal cells is too low to permit selective drug toxicity to the leukemic blasts as opposed to normal marrow. The drug almost certainly will be extremely toxic to normal cells at the time when an antileukemic effect would be seen, or before. These data could have helped to prevent a clinical trial of 5-FU in leukemia at great cost in federal dollars and patient morbidity. It also indicates that another drug, 5-fluorouridine, which has almost never been tried in man, might have an antileukemic effect.

The second parameter which we have studied is the inhibition in neoplastic cells of target enzymes of antitumor drugs. Dihydrofolate reductase is the target enzyme for methotrexate. If the drug is to be effective, it must inhibit this enzyme for a substantial portion of the DNA synthesis time of target cells. Figure 5 shows the results seen

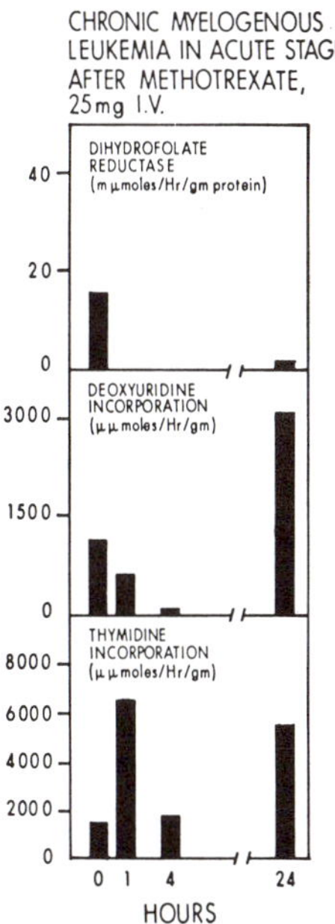

FIG. 5.—Changes observed in isolated leukemic blast cells after methotrexate 25 mg was given intravenously as a single pulse dose. A prompt decrease in the target enzyme dihydrofolate reductase (dHFR) is accompanied by inhibition of deoxyuridine incorporation into DNA, a reaction dependent upon dHFR. However, a compensatory increase of thymidine incorporation into DNA suggests that the dHFR block will not be effective in causing cessation of growth of the leukemic blasts.

when a "pulse" dose of methotrexate was given intravenously in the usual therapeutic range of 0.5 mg per kg. Cells were examined before drug administration and at intervals thereafter. In this patient, resistance to the drug was predicted by the lack of prolonged and substantial inhibition of the target enzyme. After a trial with methotrexate, clinical resistance to the drug was observed. Thymidylate synthetase, the target enzyme for drugs of the FU family, can also be measured. The specificity of the method for a single biochemical effect can be seen in that no change occurs in thymidylate synthetase, whereas the closely related enzyme falls and rises.

Figure 5 also demonstrates the third parameter which we have measured, namely, inhibition of DNA synthesis in the target cells, from the normal endogenous substrate deoxyuridine (UdR), or via the salvage pathway through thymidine (TdR), which is shown as percentage of inhibition relative to the initial untreated levels found at time zero.

By this technique, we avoid the objections cited above to adding the drug to cells in vitro. We give the usual clinical dose, and the patient's circulatory and catabolic processes establish clinical drug levels, rates of disappearance, pool sizes and cofactor concentrations which are the actual ones formed clinically during therapy.

This patient had a brief period of inhibition of DNA synthesis from UdR, but it was not maintained; there was an increase in DNA synthesis from TdR which biochemically would be expected to cause drug resistance and which may have been

TABLE 1.—*Acute Lymphoblastic Leukemia*

Patient	*Test drugs*	*Uptake and retention*	*Enzyme and inhibition*	*DNA block*		*Clinical response*
				UdR	*TdR*	
H.C.	6 MP	+				MTX + 6 MP
	MTX	±				→ Remission
S.M.	MTX	±				MTX → 0
S.P.	6 MP	0				6 MP → 0
	MTX	+				MTX → Remission
C.R.	MTX	+				MTX → Remission
W.R.	6 MP	+				6 MP + Pred. → Remission
J.C.	MTX		+		+	MTX → Remission
M.C.	MTX			+	+	MTX → Remission
D.M.	MTX	+	+	+	±	MTX → Remission
E.A.	MTX			+		MTX → 0
R.A.	MTX		±	+	+	MTX → Remission
	Cytarabine			+	±	Cytarabine → 0
G.A.	MTX	+				MTX → 0
J.R.	Cytarabine	+				Cytarabine → Remission
M.S.	Cytarabine	+				Cytarabine → 0
W.E.	MTX	+				MTX → 0
P.L.	6 MP	±				6 MP, VCR + Pred. → 0
						MTX + 6 MP, VCR + Pred. → 0
M.H.	Cyclophosphamide				+	Cyclophosphamide → Remission

Abbreviations: UdR = deoxyuridine; TdR = Thymidine; 6 MP = 6-mercaptopurine; MTX = methotrexate; VCR = Vincristine; Pred. = Prednisone; + = result in vitro suggesting drug effect in vivo; ± = result in vitro permissive of; 0 = no clinical benefit.

Usefulness of in vitro biochemical systems for predicting outcome of clinical treatment of acute lymphoblastic (lymphocytic) leukemia. Not all tests could be done on each patient. However, in vitro significant uptake of drug, or substantial inhibition of biosynthesis of DNA predicts for responsiveness in vivo.

mediated by drug-associated increases in thymidine kinase. Clinical resistance was found after prolonged drug administration.

A summary of our attempts to predict responses in 14 patients with acute lymphocytic leukemia is shown in Table 1. Because most of these patients were children, it was

TABLE 2.—*Patients with Acute Myeloblastic Leukemia Responding to Chemotherapy*

Patient	*Uptake and retention* Drug	Result	*DNA inhibition* Drug	UdR	TdR	*Prediction*	*Clinical treatment* Regimen	Response
EdTa	MTX	+	VAMP	+	+	+	VAMP	Complete
	6 MP	+						
J.C.	CA	+	CA	+	+	+	CA	Complete
R.W.	MTX	+	CA	+	+	+	MTX+CA	Toxic
	CA	±						
MiSm	CA	+	CA	+	±	±	CA	Partial
AnKa	(a) MTX	+	VAMP			±		Partial
	6 MP	0		±	±	±	VAMP	
	(b) CA	+	CA+VAMP	+	±		CA+VAMP	Partial
	(c) Daunomycin		Dauno	+	+	+	Dau+CA+VAMP	Complete
S.T.	MTX	+				+		
	CA	±					VAMP	Complete
	6 MP	±						
R.S.	MTX	±				±	VAMP	Partial
	CA	±						
	6 MP	0						
KeFo	MTX	±				±	CA+	
	6 MP	0					6 MP+	Complete
	CA	±					VCR	
	Dauno		Dauno	+	+	+	Dauno	Complete
KiMi	6 MP	+				+	CA+6 MP+	
	CA	+					VCR	Partial
FlLa	CA	0				0	CYT, CA, VCR	None
	MTX	±				±	MTX, CA, CYT	Partial
EsSt	MTX	+				+		
	CA	±				±		
			Pred	0	0	0	Pred, CA, MTX,	
			VCR	0	0	0	VCR	Partial
PeHa	CA	+	CA	0	0	0	CA+CYT	
			CYT	±	±	±		Complete
Gl0b	CA	±				±	CA	Complete
RoPe	6 MP	+				+	6 MP+MTX	Partial
	MTX	+						
	CA	+				+	CA	Complete
VaJo	CA	0				0		
	6 MP					0	6 MP+CA	Complete
JaFa			CYT		±	+	CYT	WBC Fall
(Blast Crisis)	6 MP	+				+	CYT+6 MP	Partial
	CA	–				–	CYT+6 MP+CA	No Change

In vitro analysis of drug uptake and retention, and inhibition of DNA synthesis in a group of patients with acute myelogenous leukemia who responded to subsequent clinical drug regimens. Positive uptakes and inhibition are usually associated with good clinical responses when the same drugs are given clinically later. Except for patient VaJo, remissions occurred only in patients who showed significant drug uptake.

Additional abbreviations: CA = Cytarabine; CYT = Cytoxan (cyclophosphamide).

TABLE 3.—*Patients with Acute Myeloblastic Leukemia Who Did Not Respond to Chemotherapy*

Patient	*Uptake and retention*		*DNA inhibition*			*Predic-*	*Clinical Treatment*	
	Drug	*Result*	*Drug*	*UdR*	*TdR*	*tion*	*Regimen*	*Response*
R.D.	CA	0	CA	0	0	0	CA	0
R.W.	6 MP	0	6 MP	0	0	0	6 MP	0
D.J.	CA	0					CA	0
A.W.	MTX	+					VAMP	0
	6 MP	0					VAMP+CA	0
	CA	0						
R.D.	MTX	+	MTX	+	0	0	VAMP	0
	6 MP	0	6 MP	±	0	0		
G.P.	CA	0	CA	±	±	±	CA	0
MaWe	6 MP	−				−	6 MP	0
Gl0b	6 MP	−				−	6 MP	0
C.W.	MTX	+				+	MTX	0
J.H.	CA	+	CA	±	±	±	CA, MTX+VCR	Poor Partial
	MTX	±	MTX	0	0	0		Partial
			VCR	0	0	0		
			CYT	+	+	±		
M.Mc	CA	±				±		
			VCR	±	±	±	CA+VCR	Poor Partial
ElDi	MTX	+	MTX	+	−	±	6 MP+177X	0
			+					
	6 MP	−	6 MP					
OsRe			Cytoxan	+	+PB	0	Cytoxan	0
				0	0B7			
ChWi	MTX	+				±	MTX	0
EsSt	6 MP	−				−	6 MP	0
MiGa	6 MP	−	CYT	0	0	0	6 MP+CYT	0
MaHa	6 MP	−				−	6 MP+CA	0
(blastic crisis)	CA	−				−		
LoCo	6 MP	−				−	6 MP	0
(blastic crisis)								
LiaBi	6 MP	−					6 MP	0
(blastic crisis)								

Studies similar to those in Table 2, on patients who later failed on clinical treatment with the drugs studied. A positive or ± prediction was only taken to before a state in which the leukemic cell could respond, not necessity to respond. However, in all patients except G.P., ElDi, and ChWi there was a 1:1 relationship between prediction and response.

not always possible to obtain enough blood on bone marrow to measure uptake of multiple drugs. In addition, it was not always possible to perform DNA studies before and after treatment.

However, we attempted to predict, using the available information, both successes and failures of treatment with the drugs the pediatricians planned to use. In 12 of the 14 cases, our predictions and the actual clinical results correlated well. In two cases, there was lack of correlation. We believe that when we can also do all our tests on each of these patients, our ability to predict with accuracy should approach 100 per cent.

Table 2 shows the comparable situation for acute myeloblastic leukemia, with data on all patients who had drug-induced complete or partial remissions. Again, the uncertainties of clinical practice are such that usually one does not get all the cells one needs to predict with confidence. However, for the most part, we could predict which type of response the patient would have. Of 19 drug trials, we predicted failure of response only twice, in patients G10b and VaJo, and in each instance only drug uptake data were available.

Predictions for drug resistance may be actually more useful in AML than in ALL, since one may wish to omit a toxic drug, such as daunorubicin, from a combination if pulse-dose studies show poor DNA inhibition. In acute lymphoblastic leukemias, drug sensitivity is so common that one is much less often forced into the use of very toxic multiple drug combinations.

Patients with AML who did not respond to treatment are listed in Table 3; we were able to identify the drugs which were subsequently shown to be ineffective in all but one of 19 trials. We have examined 38 patients with AML who were subsequently treated with drugs tested; in all but three predictive capacity was shown.

References

1. Eckhardt, S.: Criteria for the application of clinical chemotherapy. *In* Sellei, C., Eckhardt, S. and Németh, L. (Eds.): Chemotherapy of Neoplastic Disease. Budapest: Hungarian Acad. of Science, 1970, pp. 47–120.
2. Bickis, I. J., Henderson, W. D. and Quastel, J. H.: In vitro estimation of individual tumor sensitivity to anticancer agents. Cancer 19:103, 1966.
3. DiPaolo, J. A. and Dowd, J. E.: In vitro assessment of chemotherapeutic activity in cancer. N.Y. J. Med. 62:2127, 1962.
4. Cline, M. J. and Rosenbaum, E.: Prediction of in vivo cytotoxicity of chemotherapeutic agents by their in vitro effect on leukocytes from patients with acute leukemia. Cancer Res. 28:2516, 1965.
5. Foley, G. E. and Eagle, H.: The cytotoxicity of antitumor agents for normal human and animal cells in the first tissue culture passage. Cancer Res. 18:1012, 1958.
6. Brock, N.: Einige aktuelle Probleme der Tumortherapie mit Cyclophosphamide. Anglo-Germ. Med. Rev. 2:460, 1964.
7. Creasey, W. A., Papac, R. J., Markiw, M., Calabresi, P. and Welch, A. D.: Biochemical and pharmacological studies with 1-β-D-arabinofuranosylcytosine in man. Biochem. Pharm. 15:1417, 1966.

The Alteration of Biologic Activity by Modifying Dose Schedules of Cancer Chemotherapeutic Agents

By Edward Miller, M.D.

IN A PREVIOUS REPORT WE REVIEWED RESULTS of 10 years of clinical investigation relating to the alteration of biologic activity by changes in the dosages of cancer chemotherapeutic agents.[1] This report, although it contains some new material, is a review of the attempts to achieve more effective cancer therapy by manipulation of the dosages of chemotherapeutic agents. The antimetabolites are best suited for such attempts, because they are specific in their actions with regard to the metabolic stage of the cell cycle. Since most investigators have used 5-fluorouracil (FU), 5-fluoro-2′-deoxyuridine (FUDR), and methotrexate (MTX), this discussion will be limited to these compounds.

FU and FUDR

We have reported the changes in the metabolic pathways of FU and FUDR in man, when they are administered by continuous infusion.[2–4]

Since the activity of FU is decreased by continuous infusion, it has been demonstrated clinically that this method of administration of FU possesses no advantages over administration by intravenous injection.[2] However, modification of the dosage by injection of a single daily dose has been successful.[5–7] In these studies, the individual dose was reduced, and the doses were spaced at greater intervals. This method resulted in a marked reduction in toxicity, while maintaining approximately the same therapeutic efficacy. Additional attempts at modifying the dose schedule of FU—by short infusions (1–8 hours),[8] by weekly injections,[9] and by multiple daily doses[10]—have not shown any clinical advantages over the modified injection schedules cited above.

In contrast, we have demonstrated the increased activity of FUDR when it is

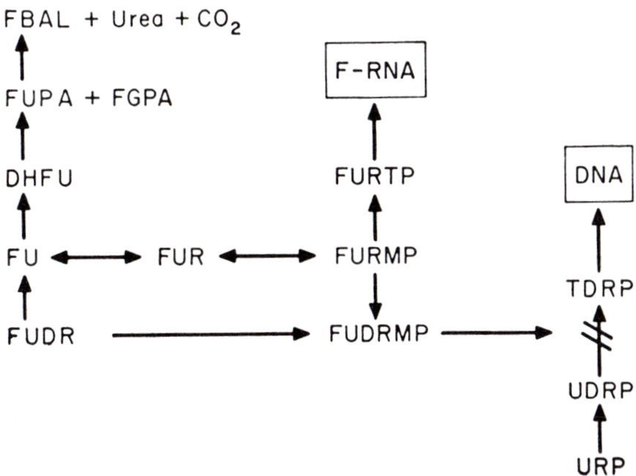

Fig. 1.—Metabolism of FU and FUDR.

From Hoffmann-La Roche Inc., Nutley, New Jersey.

continuously infused.[4] The amount administered by infusion (0.5–1.0 mg/kg/day) is approximately $\frac{1}{30}$ to $\frac{1}{40}$ that of the single daily dose (30 mg/kg/day). This dosage has reached its optimal use in regional arterial infusion.[11,12]

Reference to the metabolism of FU and FUDR (Fig. 1) provides a partial explanation for the clinical phenomena noted above. Three hours after intravenous injection of 15 mg/kg of FU in man, none of the drug can be detected in the blood.[13] Most of the FU is catabolized in the liver and excreted as innocuous breakdown products. Approximately 80 per cent is excreted as CO_2 in the lungs, and about 15 per cent as urea and α-fluoro-β-alanine in the urine.[14,15] Hence, only a fraction of the dose is anabolized to 5-fluoro-2′-deoxyuridine monophosphate (FUDRMP), the "lethal nucleotide." By blocking the enzyme thymidylate synthetase, FUDRMP inhibits DNA synthesis, thereby producing an antineoplastic effect in malignant cells and toxicity in normal cells.[16,17]

When FUDR is administered by intravenous injection, it is rapidly cleaved to FU and follows the same metabolic route.[14] When molar equivalents of FU and FUDR are given by injection, the toxic and therapeutic effects have been observed clinically to be the same.[18,19] However, the continuous infusion of FUDR apparently results in the direct anabolic conversion to FUDRMP.[4]

The results from clinical investigation of dosages of FU and FUDR indicate that the activity of these compounds depends upon the amount of drug anabolized to the nucleotide FUDRMP per unit of time. Our initial report demonstrated that the total amount of FU administered means nothing if anabolism does not occur.[2] In that study, patients received total doses of FU as high as 540 mg/kg over a period of 5 weeks, with no sign of either response or toxicity. It is apparent that anabolism occurs only after a certain threshold has been exceeded. Beyond this threshold, the liver is unable to catabolize all of the FU. This is evident also in the studies using intravenous injections.

To maintain response, that rate of anabolism of FU must be maintained which will destroy more tumor cells than are being replaced.

Methotrexate

At the previous symposium in 1965, we presented our preliminary results with the continuous infusion of methotrexate (MTX) in 30 patients with a wide spectrum of malignancies.[1] A subsequent published report described the results in a series of 161 patients with solid tumors.[20] The dose schedule was either (a) 5 mg/day by continuous infusion, or (b) 1.25 mg four times daily orally. The intent of both schedules was to maintain a constant low level of MTX in the tissues. Of 148 patients who received an adequate trial, there was a response (i.e., tumor regression of at least 50 per cent associated with clinical benefit for at least 2 months) in 52 (35 per cent). The duration of response ranged from 2 to 15 months, the average being 4.4 months. This compares favorably with earlier studies of MTX in solid tumors, when the compound was given orally or intravenously in large single daily doses.[21–23]

However, Condit and his colleagues have said: "To compare different dose schedules of the same drug, a tumor should be employed which responds with regularity to the drug being used. In man, with the folic acid antagonists, we have acute leukemia in children and choriocarcinoma in women."[23]

One woman with choriocarcinoma (Fig. 2) and one woman with chorioadenoma (Fig. 3) were treated with MTX in oral doses of 1.25 mg four times daily. Each

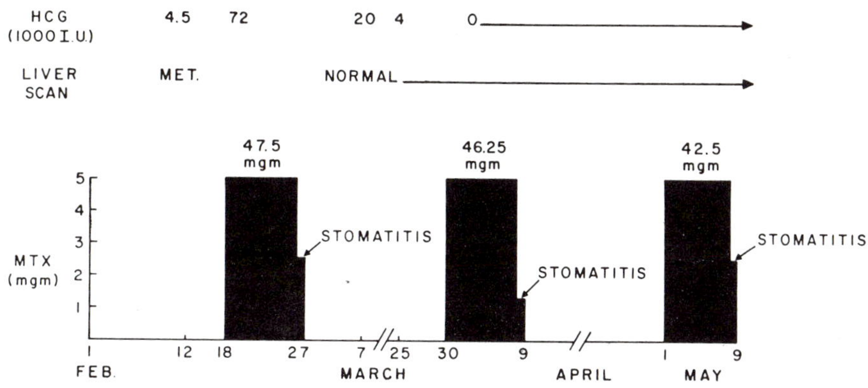

FIG. 2.—Treatment information: 23-year-old female patient with choriocarcinoma with metastases.

patient received three courses of MTX, although all signs of disease were gone after the first course. Both patients remain free of disease 3 and 2 years respectively, with no further therapy. Not only was there complete response in both patients, but the only sign of toxicity for all six courses was moderate stomatitis.

These two cases tend to confirm our conclusion made after our initial study—namely, that the sustained presence of MTX in the tissues is more significant than a high concentration in the blood.[24] This is compatible with assay studies, which have shown that after a single dose of MTX, orally or intravenously, most of the intact drug is rapidly excreted in the urine.[25,26]

The biologic effects of MTX are due to its inhibition of the enzyme folic acid reductase,[27] which cuts off the supply of tetrahydrofolic acid, a coenzyme in methylation reactions essential for DNA synthesis.[28]

The daily administration of 5 mg of MTX, by either continuous infusion or multiple oral doses, produces activity of MTX equivalent to that produced by larger single daily doses given for longer periods of time. There is also a suggestion that toxicity may be lessened without sacrificing efficacy.

DISCUSSION

In seeking optimal dosages for antimetabolites, we mean those which will produce

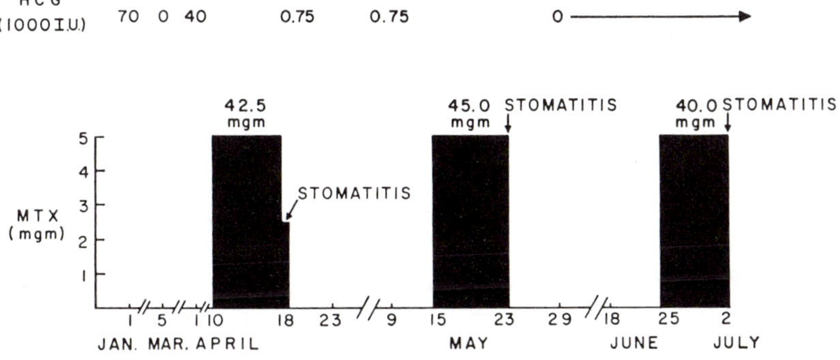

FIG. 3.—Treatment information: 17-year-old female patient with chorioadenoma.

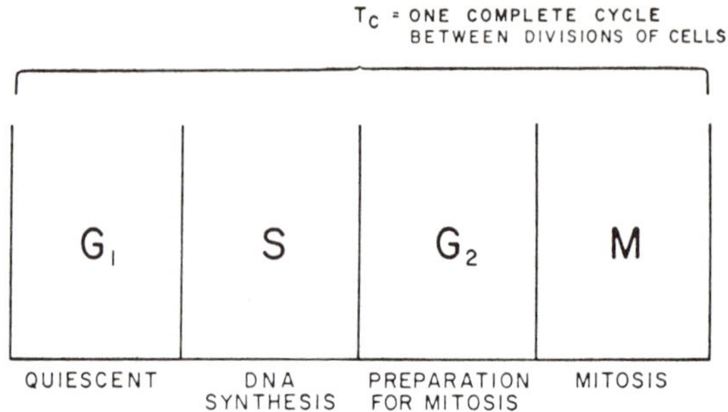

FIG. 4.—Generation time (Tc) of a cell. Adapted from Merkle et al., [29] with permission.

the greatest efficacy with the least toxicity. In addition to the changes in metabolism, there are other factors which will affect the efficiency of an antimetabolite.

Figure 4 is a schematic representation of the generation time (T_c) of a cell.[29] Since FU, FUDR, and MTX inhibit DNA synthesis, it is obvious that only those cells in S phase (i.e., proliferating cells) will be sensitive to the action of these agents. Therefore, it is essential to establish the T_c and the duration of the S phase, not only for the specific tumor under attack, but also for the normal proliferating tissues of the body. The gastrointestinal mucosa in man, for example, has a T_c of at least one day with an S phase of approximately 9 to 14 hours.[30] These cells are among the most rapidly proliferating in the body. Hence, the antimetabolites cause high percentages of toxicity in the gastrointestinal tract.

But the duration of S phases is not enough information. The number of cells in S phase at a given time is also of significance. If there are more normal cells than tumor cells in S, at the time of a single dose, the result will be toxic effects with little or no antitumor effect. This may account for some of the nonresponders encountered clinically.

Another point to consider is the entry of the agent (or its active form) into the cells in S phase. This, of course, is the heart of the matter. For if there were great differences between tumor and normal cell permeability, there would be no problem in cancer chemotherapy. However, we know there are slight differences, or we would not achieve any success at all. By giving just enough antimetabolite to enter all sensitive tumor cells, but *not* enough to enter all the sensitive normal cells, an optimal effect can be obtained. The infusion of low doses of FUDR and MTX may be successful through this mechanism. This may also explain why high single doses of FU produce severe toxicity although the response rate is unchanged. With all the sensitive tumor cells covered, the excess drug then satures the sensitive normal cells.

Many others factors are to be considered in cancer chemotherapy, but they are not within the scope of this chapter. The modification of dosages is only a part of this complex area of medicine. However, we feel it can be rewarding from the viewpoint of the clinician and his patient. Some cancers which were considered totally resistant to certain agents have been shown to yield. In tumors already known to be sensitive, better and longer responses have been possible in many instances.

The cure of cancer is, of course, the ultimate goal. This will be possible when agents are found with sufficiently high therapeutic margins (or possibly with other modalities). In the meantime, we believe that the control of a cancer is also a valid goal. By control, we mean the destruction of cancer cells at a rate faster than they can be replaced. In some cases, this may be clinically as effective as a cure. In many cases, it will greatly improve the quality of survival time in a grateful patient.

References

1. Miller, E. and Sullivan, R. D.: The alteration of biologic activity of cancer chemotherapy agents by prolonged infusion. *In* Brodsky, I. and Kahn, S. B. (Eds.): Cancer Chemotherapy. New York: Grune & Stratton, 1967.
2. Sullivan, R. D., Young, C. W., Miller, E., Glatstein, N., Clarkson, B. and Burchenal, J. H.: Clinical effects of the continuous administration of fluorinated pyrimidines (5-fluorouracil and 5-fluoro-2′-deoxyuridine). Cancer Chemother. Rep. 8:77, 1960.
3. Miller, E., Sullivan, R. D., Young, C. W. and Burchenal, J. H.: Clinical effects of continuous infusion of anti-metabolites: Prevention of toxicity of 5-fluoro-2′-deoxyuridine by thymidine. Proc. Amer. Ass. Cancer Res. 3:251, 1961.
4. Sullivan, R. D. and Miller, E.: The clinical effects of prolonged intravenous infusion of 5-fluoro-2′-deoxyuridine. Cancer Res. 25: 1025, 1965.
5. Cudmore, J. T. P. and Groesbeck, H. P.: Comparison of high-dosage and low-dosage maintenance therapy with 5-fluorouracil in solid tumors. Cancer 17:230, 1964.
6. Williams, H. M.: Clinical evaluations of various dose schedules of 5-fluorouracil. Clin. Res. 12:289, 1964.
7. Ansfield, F. J.: A less toxic fluorouracil dosage schedule. J.A.M.A. 190:686, 1964.
8. Hall, T. C., Cavins, J. A., Khung, C. L., Griffiths, C. T., Dederick, M. M. and Yount, W. J.: Time and vehicle studies of a safe and effective method for administration of 5-fluorouracil. Cancer 19:1008, 1966.
9. Mackman, S., Ramirez, G. and Ansfield, F. J.: Results of 5-fluorouracil (NSC-19893) given by the multiple daily dose method in disseminated breast cancer. Cancer Chemother. Rep. 51:483, 1967.
10. Jacobs, E. M., Bateman, J. R., Luce, J. K., Wood, D. A. and the Western Cooperative Cancer Chemotherapy Group: Treatment of cancer with weekly intravenous 5-fluorouracil. Proc. Amer. Ass. Cancer Res. 8:34, 1967.
11. Sullivan, R. D., Watkins, E., Jr., Rodriguez, F. R., Miller, E. and Norcross, J. W.: Continuous arterial infusion chemotherapy of human liver cancer using 5-fluoro-2′-deoxyuridine: Autodetoxification studies and clinical effects. Proc. Amer. Ass. Cancer Res. 4:66, 1963.
12. Sullivan, R. D.: Continuous arterial infusion cancer chemotherapy. Surg. Clin. N. Amer. 42:365, 1962.
13. Clarkson, B., O'Connor, A., Winston, L. and Hutchison, D.: The physiologic disposition of 5-fluorouracil and 5-fluoro-2′-deoxyuridine in man. Clin. Pharmacol. Ther. 5:581, 1964.
14. Chaudhuri, N. K., Mukherjee, K. L. and Heidelberger, C.: Studies on fluorinated pyrimidines. VII. The degradative pathway. Biochem. Pharmacol. 1:328, 1958.
15. Mukherjee, K. L., Boohar, J., Wentland, D., Ansfield, F. J. and Heidelberger, C.: Studies on fluorinated pyrimidines. XVI. Metabolism of 5-fluorouracil-2-C^{14} and 5-fluoro-2′-deoxyuridine-2-C^{14} in cancer patients. Cancer Res. 23:49, 1963.
16. Cohen, S. S., Flaks, J. G., Barner, H. D., Loeb, M. R. and Lictenstein, J.: The mode of action of 5-fluorouracil and its derivatives. Proc. Nat. Acad. Sci. U.S.A. 44: 1004, 1958.
17. Harbers, E., Chaudhuri, N. K. and Heidelberger, C.: Studies on fluorinated pyrimidines. VIII. Further biochemical and metabolic investigations. J. Biol. Chem. 234: 1255, 1959.
18. Young, C. W., Ellison, R. R., Sullivan, R. D., Levick, S. N., Kaufman, R., et al.: The clinical evaluation of 5-fluorouracil and 5-fluoro-2′-deoxyuridine in solid tumors in adults. Cancer Chemother. Rep. 6:17, 1960.
19. Ellison, R. R.: Clinical applications of the fluorinated pyrimidines. Med. Clin. N. Amer. 45:677, 1961.
20. Sullivan, R. D., Miller, E., Zurek, W. Z., Oberfield, R. A. and Ojima, Y.: Re-evaluation of methotrexate as an anticancer drug. Surg. Gynec. Obstet. 125:819, 1967.
21. Burchenal, J. H., Karnofsky, D. A., Kingsley-Pillers, E. M., Southam, C. M., Myers, W. P. L., et al.: The effects of the folic acid antagonists and 2,6-diaminopurine on neoplastic disease, with special reference to acute leukemia. Cancer 4:549, 1951.
22. Schoenbach, E. B., Colsky, J. and Greenspan, E. M.: Observations on the effects of

the folic acid antagonists, aminopterin and amethopterin, in patients with advanced neoplasms. Cancer 5:1201, 1952.
23. Condit, P. T., Shnider, B. I. and Owens, A. H., Jr.: Studies on the folic acid vitamins. VII. The effects of large doses of amethopterin in patients with cancer. Cancer Res. 22:706, 1962.
24. Methotrexate in the treatment of cancer (a symposium). Brit. Med. J. 2:954, 1961.
25. Liguori, V. R., Giglio, J. J., Miller, E. and Sullivan, R. D.: Effects of different dose schedules of amethopterin on serum and tissue concentrations and urinary excretion patterns. Clin. Pharmacol. Ther. 3:34, 1962.
26. Freeman, M. V.: The fluorometric measurement of the absorption, distribution and excretion of single doses of 4-amino-10-methylpteroylglutamic acid (amethopterin) in man. J. Pharmacol. Exp. Ther. 122:154, 1958.
27. Werkheiser, W. C.: Specific binding of 4-amino folic acid analogues by folic acid reductase. J. Biol. Chem. 236:888, 1961.
28. Delmonte, L. and Jukes, T. H.: Folic acid antagonists in cancer chemotherapy. Pharmacol. Rev. 14:91, 1962.
29. Merkle, T. C., Stuart, R. N. and Gofman, J. W.: The calculation of treatment schedules for cancer chemotherapy. Lawrence Radiation Laboratory, University of California, Livermore, California, 1965.
30. Lipkin, M., Sherlock, P. and Bell, B.: Cell proliferation kinetics in the gastrointestinal tract of man. II. Cell renewal in stomach, ileum, colon, and rectum. Gastroenterology 45:721, 1963.

II. CHEMOTHERAPY OF SOLID TUMORS

Chemotherapy and Hormonal Therapy of Carcinoma of the Breast

By IRWIN H. KRAKOFF, M.D.

AT THE HAHNEMANN SYMPOSIUM on Cancer Chemotherapy in November 1965, I was privileged to present a paper[1] bearing the same title as this one. It would be exciting to be able to state that developments in the therapy of breast cancer have occurred at such a pace that the older paper is completely outmoded. Unfortunately, however, that has not been the case—with minor exceptions and additions the review in 1965 is still applicable.

The focus of this discussion is on the management of recurrent or metastatic breast cancer. It is recognized that in the primary therapy of carcinoma of the breast there are controversies regarding the type of surgery to be employed and whether or not to use radiation therapy preoperatively or immediately postoperatively (Fig. 1). These controversies are outside the realm of this particular discussion, but it should be noted that at this late date these questions still exist. Although plans are being developed for a nationwide cooperative study comparing radical and simple mastectomy, no such attempt has been made until now. Several recent articles in popular women's magazines[2] may have lent additional heat to the controversy.

The menopause is considered a dividing line in determining the management of patients with recurrent breast cancer since the hormonal status and, therefore, the therapy of premenopausal women, differ from those of postmenopausal women.

RADICAL MASTECTOMY

Conservative local management	More extensive local management	Systemic procedures
Radiation therapy	Extended radical mastectomy	Adjuvant chemotherapy
Simple mastectomy + radiation therapy (McWhirter)	Pre and/or postop radiation therapy	Castration (premenopausal patient)
	Simple mastectomy, remaining breast	Prophylactic hormone or chemotherapy

FIG. 1.—Sequence of therapy in early breast cancer.

From the Medical Oncology Service, Department of Medicine, Memorial Hospital for Cancer and Allied Diseases, and the Division of Chemotherapy Research, Sloan-Kettering Institute for Cancer Research, New York, New York.

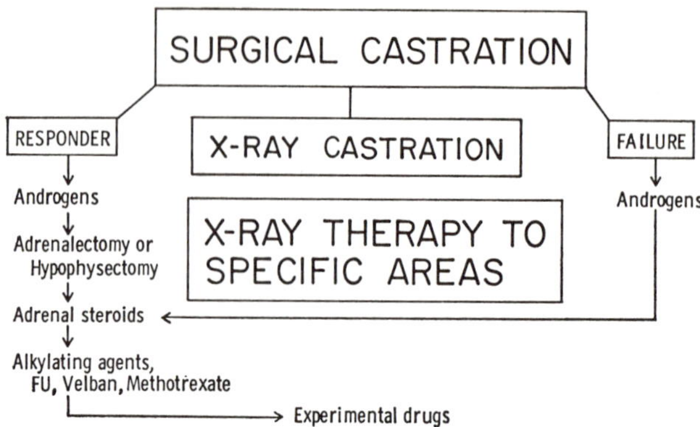

FIG. 2.—Sequence of therapy in recurrent breast cancer in premenopausal women.

PREMENOPAUSAL PATIENTS

Since there is some residual ovarian function after the cessation of menses, women who are less than one year postmenopausal are considered for purposes of therapy to be premenopausal. As shown in Figure 2, surgical castration should be the initial approach to the management of recurrent breast cancer in the premenopausal group. It can be anticipated that improvement will occur in 30 or 40 per cent of premenopausal women so treated. X-ray castration is sometimes considered as an alternative to surgical removal of the ovaries, but this is generally less satisfactory, since the effects of surgical castration are more quickly apparent and variations in dose can raise some question as to the completeness of castration by X-ray. Therefore, the preferred approach in most centers is surgical removal of the ovaries.

An additional question that must be considered is the value of prophylactic castration at the time of radical mastectomy versus therapeutic castration done when there is evidence of recurrent disease. Although it has been shown that prophylactic castration results in delay of recurrence, this was not reflected in a difference of survival time. In a study by Kennedy and his coworkers,[3] and in our own experience[4] (Figs. 3 and 4), the period from onset of disease to death was similar in two groups: one castrated prophylactically and the other therapeutically at the time of recurrence. Since it is difficult to predict which patients will enjoy a surgical cure and which will develop recurrent disease, it is apparent that if prophylactic castration is performed, a large number of patients will be included for whom this procedure would not have been necessary. In addition, as shown in Figure 2, the response to castration is an important guide in determining further therapy for these patients, and the performance

INTERVAL FROM MASTECTOMY TO FIRST RECURRENCE (MONTHS)

	Number of Patients	Mean	Median	Mode
Prophylactic	201	36.3	22.0	18.0
Non-prophylactic	323	31.8	21.0	12.0

FIG. 3.—Influence of "prophylactic" castration on time of recurrence of breast cancer. Prophylactic castration appears to delay slightly the recurrence of disease.

SURVIVAL FROM FIRST RECURRENCE (MOS.)

	Number patients	Mean	Median	Mode
Prophylactic	186*	19.8	13.0	9.0
Non-prophylactic	323	25.0	17.0	11.0

* 15 Patients still living.

FIG. 4.—Influence of "prophylactic" castration on survival time in patients who develop recurrent breast cancer. Although recurrence appears to be delayed somewhat, there is no influence on overall survival.

of prophylactic castration deprives one of this guide. On these bases, it is considered that therapeutic surgical castration is preferable to prophylactic castration in the premenopausal group.

If a response occurs to surgical castration, no further therapy should be employed until there is evidence of further recurrence of the disease. If minor solitary lesions appear, these can be satisfactorily treated with X-ray therapy. When more generalized reactivation of the disease occurs, the institution of androgen therapy may provide another period of improvement. If that fails, or if there is improvement and subsequent relapse, two additional surgical procedures can be considered. Since the adrenal glands are a source of estrogen, bilateral adrenalectomy can result in improvement in about 30 per cent of those patients who had previously responded to castration. Similarly, hypophysectomy can result in suppression of adrenal function and the removal of growth hormone. This procedure, too, can result in improvement in about 30 per cent of those who have responded to castration.[4] In those patients who have failed to respond to castration, the response rate to hypophysectomy or adrenalectomy is less than 10 per cent.[5,6] The response rate and survival times of patients who have had adrenalectomy are similar to those of patients who have had hypophysectomy. The choice of procedure depends primarily on the availability of a skilled surgeon to perform either procedure. There appears to be no advantage to the sequential use of these operations.

In patients who fail to respond to any of these procedures or who relapse after an initial response, the use of adrenal cortical steroids may provide brief periods of improvement. Finally, the use of nonhormonal chemotherapeutic agents (discussed in detail below) can be considered for patients when other forms of therapy have been exhausted.

Postmenopausal Patients

As shown in Figure 5, the initial choice of therapy in this group of patients, i.e., those women who are more than 5 years postmenopausal, should be estrogens. It can be anticipated that approximately one-third of postmenopausal patients will respond to estrogen therapy. In those who fail to respond or in those who respond and then relapse, androgen therapy may provide some additional benefit. In those who respond to estrogen or androgen and subsequently relapse, hypophysectomy or adrenalectomy should be considered, since approximately half of that group can be expected to show an additional response to one of these ablative procedures. Of those who have failed to respond to hormonal therapy, the response rate to hypophysectomy or adrenalectomy is less, i.e., about 25 per cent.

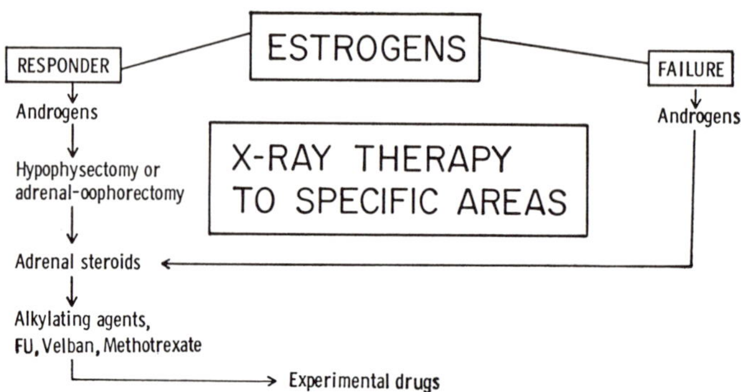

FIG. 5.—Sequence of therapy in recurrent breast cancer in postmenopausal women.

As with the premenopausal group, adrenal cortical steroids may produce brief improvement in those patients who have failed to respond to hormonal therapy or who have relapsed afterward, and nonhormonal chemotherapeutic agents can produce further periods of response.

A third group of hormonal agents, the progestins, are known to produce some responses in recurrent and metastatic breast cancer. Their precise role in its management has not yet been thoroughly defined and is still under investigation.

The value of response to endocrine therapy can be measured in terms of symptomatic improvement and also in increased length of survival (Fig. 6).[7]

NONHORMONAL CHEMOTHERAPY

Table 1 enumerates specific agents used in breast cancer. Nonhormonal agents should be reserved for those patients who have failed to respond to hormonal measures or who have responded, have relapsed, and are no longer responsive. For patients in these categories, three classes of compounds may be useful: the polyfunctional alkylating agents, the fluorinated pyrimidines and the plant alkaloid vinblastine. A large number of polyfunctional alkylating agents can be used in the treatment of recurrent or metastatic breast cancer (as well as in other tumors). These appear to have similar biologic activities and to produce similar degrees of tumor regression.

ENDOCRINE RESPONSE VS SURVIVAL TIME

Evaluation therapy	Number of cases	Percentage patients deceased (12 month intervals)					
		0-12	13-24	25-36	37-48	49-60	≥61
Beneficial response	158	7.0	27.2	24.0	16.5	10.1	**15.2**
Failure	685	44.4	32.0	11.8	5.9	2.0	**3.9**

FIG. 6.—Influence of endocrine therapy on survival time in recurrent breast cancer.

TABLE 1.—*Specific Agents Used in Breast Cancer*

Agents	*Principal route of administration*	*Usual dose*	*Acute toxic signs*	*Major late toxic manifestations*
Steroid Hormones				
Androgens			None	Fluid retention, masculinization
Testosterone propionate	I.M.	50–100 mg 3 times weekly		
Fluoxymesterone (Halotestin)	Oral	10–20 mg/day		
Estrogens				
Diethylstilbestrol;	Oral	1–5 mg 3 times daily	Occasional nausea and vomiting	Fluid retention, feminization, uterine bleeding
ethynylestradiol (Estinyl)	Oral	0.1–1.0 mg 3 times daily		
Progestins				
Hydroxyprogesterone caproate (Delalutin);	I.M.	1 gm 2 times weekly	None	
6-methylhydroxyprogesterone (Provera)	Oral I.M.	100–200 mg/day 200–600 mg twice a week	None	
Adrenal Cortical Compounds				
Cortisone acetate;	Oral	50–300 mg/day		
hydrocortisone acetate	Oral	50–200 mg/day	None	Fluid retention, hypertension, diabetes, increased susceptibility to infection
Prednisone (Meticorten)	Oral	20–100 mg/day		
Polyfunctional Alkylating Agents				
Methylbis (β-chloroethyl) amine (HN2, Mustargen)	I.V.	0.4 mg/kg in single or divided doses	Nausea and vomiting	Therapeutic doses moderately depress peripheral blood cell count; excessive doses cause severe bone marrow depression, with leukopenia, thrombocytopenia, and bleeding. Maximum toxicity may occur two or three weeks after last dose. Dosage, therefore, must be carefully controlled. Alopecia and hemorrhagic cystitis occur occasionally with cyclophosphamide
Chlorambucil (Leukeran)	Oral	0.1–0.2 mg/kg/day 6–12 mg/day	None	

TABLE 1.—*Specific Agents Used in Breast Cancer* (*contd.*)

Agents	*Principal route of administration*	*Usual dose*	*Acute toxic signs*	*Major late toxic manifestations*
Polyfunctional Alkylating Agents				
Cyclophosphamide (Endoxan, Cytoxan)	I.V.	3.5–5.0 mg/kg per day for 10 days (40–60 mg/kg) (Total dose)	Nausea and vomiting	Bone-marrow depression, hemorrhagic cystitis, alopecia
	Oral	50–300 mg/day		
Triethylenethio phosphoramide (thio-TEPA)	I.V.	0.2 mg/kg daily for 4-5 days	None	
Antimetabolites				
5-Fluorouracil (5-FU)	I.V.	12 mg/kg daily for 5 days; smaller dose 1 or 2 times a week for maintenance	None	Stomatitis, gastrointestinal injury, bone-marrow depression
4-Amino-N^{10}-methylpteroylglutamic acid (methotrexate)	Oral	2.5–5.0 mg/day	None	Oral and digestive tract ulcerations; bone-marrow depression, with leukopenia, thrombocytopenia and bleeding
Miscellaneous Drugs				
Vinblastine (Velban)	I.V.	0.1–0.15 mg/kg/week	Nausea and vomiting	Alopecia, muscular weakness, areflexia, bone-marrow depression
Vincristine (Oncovin)	I.V.	0.015–0.05 mg/kg/week	None	Areflexia, peripheral neuritis, paralytic ileus, mild bone-marrow depression
o,p′-DDD	Oral	2–10 gm/day	Nausea and vomiting	Skin eruptions, diarrhea, mental depression, muscle tremors
Quinacrine (Atabrine)	Intracavitary	100–200 mg/day × 5	Local pain, fever	

The choice of an alkylating agent depends on factors related to route and rate of administration rather than to any specificity for carcinoma of the breast. Nitrogen mustard is a rapidly acting compound which can be given intravenously. Thio-TEPA can also be given intravenously and provides the advantage that, when given in divided doses, it does not cause nausea and vomiting such as occur uniformly with nitrogen mustard. Cyclophosphamide may be given either intravenously or orally. Any of these compounds can produce regressions in about one-fourth of patients with soft tissue disease, and in a smaller number of patients with osseous metastases. These regressions, unfortunately, are usually brief, but in occasional patients maintenance therapy with an oral alkylating agent may result in prolonged periods of benefit.

5-Fluorouracil and 5-fluoro-2′-deoxy-β-uridine have been used in breast cancer, as in other types of tumors. It appears that about 15 per cent of patients with breast cancer treated with these agents can experience responses. Although in one study[10] it was reported that fluorodeoxyuridine produced favorable responses more frequently than fluorouracil, this has not been the general experience. In most centers, these two compounds are considered similar in their effect on breast cancer as well as on other tumors. Vinblastine, an alkaloid derived from the periwinkle, has also been shown to produce responses in some patients.[11] With this compound, too, the duration of response is usually brief.

As in other neoplastic diseases, an effort has been made in breast cancer to use multiple anticancer agents with differing mechanisms of action and with differing toxicity in order to improve therapeutic responses. Cooper[8] has recently reported the results of one such combination regimen which, he states, has produced extraordinary results. This program utilizes a combination of vincristine, cyclophosphamide, prednisone, 5-fluorouracil and methotrexate. Other groups are presently studying the effects of other three-, four- and five-drug combinations. Either nitrogen mustard or thio-TEPA may be given intrapleurally in patients with intractable pleural effusions due to metastatic disease. This can prevent recurrence of pleural effusions in approximately 70 per cent of the patients treated.[9]

Some consideration should be given to the so-called adjuvant use of chemotherapeutic agents at the time of surgery. Studies have been in progress for several years to determine whether the administration of cytotoxic drugs, at and immediately after surgery would result in an increased surgical cure rate or in delay in recurrence. Each of these drugs is capable of producing significant bone marrow depression, with depletion of leukocytes and platelets, depression of immune responses, and gastrointestinal toxicity and their indiscriminate use is therefore not recommended.

A nationwide adjuvant chemotherapy study utilizing thio-TEPA has recently been reviewed.[12] There appeared to be no increase in either cure rate or survival time in postmenopausal women. In premenopausal patients, there was some delay in recurrence time and a slight increase in 5-year survival.

There inevitably will be patients who have exhausted the usefulness of hormonal measures, and who have failed to respond or have exhausted their responsiveness to the conventional nonhormonal chemotherapeutic agents. For these patients, it is appropriate to consider the use of an experimental agent under investigation at that time. Several centers throughout the country are engaged in the evaluation of these experimental drugs and, for patients with evaluable disease, transfer to such a center may provide them with an opportunity to participate in such a program.

References

1. Krakoff, I. H.: Chemotherapy and hormonal therapy of carcinoma of the breast. *In* Brodsky, I. and Kahn, S. B. (Eds.): Cancer Chemotherapy: Basic and Clinical Applications. New York: Grune & Stratton, 1967, pp. 77–83.
2. Maynard, F.: Breast cancer: is there an alternative to surgery? Woman's Day, November 1970, p. 6.
3. Kennedy, B. J., Mielke, P. W., Jr. and Fortuny, I. E.: Therapeutic castration versus prophylactic castration in breast cancer. Surg. Gynec. Obstet. 118:524, 1964.
4. Kaufman, R. J.: Personal communication.
5. Pearson, O. H. and Ray, B. S.: Hypophysectomy in the treatment of metastatic mammary cancer. Amer. J. Surg. 99:544, 1960.
6. MacDonald, I.: Endocrine ablation in disseminated mammary carcinoma. Surg. Gynec. Obstet. 115:215, 1962.
7. Escher, G. C. and Kaufman, R. J.: Advanced breast cancer: factors influencing survival. Acta Un. Int. Cancr. 19:1039, 1963.
8. Cooper, R. G.: Combination chemotherapy in hormone-resistant breast cancer. Proc. Amer. Ass. Cancer Res. 10:15, 1969.
9. Weisberger, A. S.: Direct instillation of nitrogen mustard in the management of malignant effusions. Ann. N.Y. Acad. Sci. 68:1091, 1958.
10. Ansfield, F. J. and Curreri, A. R.: Further clinical comparison between 5-fluorouracil and 5-fluorodeoxyuridine. Cancer Chemother. Rep. 32:101, 1963.
11. Frei, E.: *In* Clinical Staff Conference: Breast Cancer. Combined Clinical Staff Conference at the National Institutes of Health. Ann. Intern. Med. 63:321, 1965.
12. Fisher, B., Ravdin, R. G., Ausman, R. K., Slack, N., Moore, G. E. and Noer, R. J.: Surgical adjuvant chemotherapy in breast cancer. Ann. Surg. 168:337, 1968.

Chemotherapy of Gastrointestinal Neoplasms

By William Regelson, M.D.

TWO OBSERVATIONS OF IMMEDIATE CLINICAL INTEREST have recommended themselves to me since our review[1] for the previous symposium, and those of others.[2–6] One is the implied success of 5-fluorouracil (5-FU) as adjuvant chemotherapy in operable or inoperable cancer of the bowel at the time of primary surgery when given in the absence of clinical disease.[7–13] Results in this early patient population indicate that 5-FU delays local recurrence and prolongs 5- and 8-year[14] survival. 5-FU is more valuable as an adjuvant than as a palliative (its usual use) in patients with advanced cancer. The other observation relates to the work of Moertel et al.[6] and others,[15] suggesting that in patients with advanced cancer, the combination of 5-FU with supervoltage radiotherapy significantly prolongs survival of patients with inoperable gastrointestinal cancer. Similar results appear to be developing in the statistical appraisal of the Veterans Administration Surgical Adjuvant Cancer Chemotherapy Study.[13] These observations, although preliminary in character, represent practical clinical possibilities as relates to technique and concept available to all.

Elsewhere the situation in regard to new chemotherapy has not been particularly promising beyond the important observation that 5-FU can be effectively administered by mouth as induction or maintenance treatment.[16–18]

In relation to other drugs, bis-dichloro-nitrosourea (BCNU) has value, and mitomycin C is still undergoing tests clinically[6,19–21] but may be ineffective in patients who have not responded to 5-FU.[19] Streptozotocin is extremely promising for pancreatic carcinoma[22,23] and carcinoid, and bleomycin for esophageal and gastric carcinoma presents new hope.[24,25]

The best of the new drugs may be camptothecin sodium, which is still in limited supply[26] and undergoing phase II evaluation,[27] and 1-(2-chloroethyl)-3-cyclohexyl-1-nitrosourea (CCNU) an orally active cogener of the nitrosourea alkylating agent BCNU.[25,27] In other areas, combination chemotherapy has not yet clearly defined itself as better than 5-fluorouracil alone although the concept of combination chemotherapy has proved its value in leukemia, lymphoma and melanoma. Lerner has reported that weekly maintenance of 5-FU (10 mg/kg per week) with hydroxyurea (80 mg/kg per week) may be more effective than either drug alone in prolonging survival of patients with metastatic bowel carcinoma to the liver.[28]

For these reasons adjuvant chemotherapy with 5-fluorouracil, and/or alkylating agents and radiotherapy, remains our best hope to change patterns of survival in gastrointestinal cancer from the dismal mortality rate, 67 to 98 per cent within 5 years. Perhaps the combination of chemotherapy with techniques for earlier diagnosis and/or immunotherapy which is now becoming feasible, thanks to the work of Gold[29] and others who have demonstrated tumor-specific antigens, might provide new possibilities for the future.

From the Medical College of Virginia, Health Sciences Center, Richmond, Virginia.

Adjuvant Chemotherapy

The concept of adjuvant chemotherapy with 5-fluorouracil represents the most outstanding approach to the treatment of gastrointestinal malignancy. This means the use of 5-fluorouracil in treating patients after surgery in the absence of evident disease. This is based on the observations of Curreri's group,[9–11] who, employing a "second look" operative procedure, gave 5-fluorouracil for a minimum of four courses postoperatively to the point of toxicity in patients with Duke's B and C carcinoma (lymph node involvement) of the bowel following curative resection. In this population, on second look, there were 25 of 29 patients who had no evident disease at the end of a year, with 3 patients having recurrence, one at 57 months from his "negative" second look. From past experience, one would have expected that at the end of a year 40 to 50 per cent of patients in this "second look" population would have evidence of active disease. What is more impressive, Mackman et al.[10] investigated a group of 23 patients who were thought to be curable prior to surgery, but were found to have adjacent structures involved. Tumor was resected and in this population, following multiple courses of 5-fluorouracil, 14 of 23 patients were free of tumor (3 false negatives) and 3 of 9 patients had local disease that was successfully resectable. Of 6 patients with palliative resection, 2 had no disease at second look (1 false negative), but the surviving patient was apparently free of disease 7 years later despite biopsy-proved metastases to liver, omentum, and pelvic peritoneum.

This work, although impressive in itself, is further supported by work done by Rousselot et al.[7,8,14] In their study, 5-fluorouracil was instilled intraluminally for a half-hour after a two-tape procedure localizing 5-FU to the involved segment of the bowel. After a half-hour of intraluminal regional administration of 5-FU (30 mg/kg), resection was done and the patient was given two intravenous doses of 5-FU (10 mg/kg once a day for 2 days). For Duke's C or Stage III carcinoma, there is a 5-year projected survival of 64 per cent, as compared to an in-house survival of 27 per cent and national survival averages in the range of 32 per cent. A recent 8-year report on this population by this group indicates an 8-year survival of 57 per cent.[14] This program is now being conducted as a cooperative study in the New York City area[12] utilizing a randomization technique for ongoing comparison with untreated controls.

Unfortunately, a cooperative study designed by Curreri to test these observations in a major national program did not receive support. However, we have conducted such a study in cooperation with the University of Virginia and have 37 patients in a randomized study utilizing the Rousselot intraluminal approach combined with the multiple courses of 5-FU used by Curreri[9] and Mackman and Curreri.[10,11] In our study, 5-fluorouracil is given intraluminally and intravenously as in Rousselot's program, but, in addition, 1 month later 5-fluorouracil is given orally, 12 mg/kg once a day for 4 days, then 6 mg/kg every other day for seven doses or to the point of toxicity every other month for 1 year. The rationale for the use of oral 5-FU will be discussed later.

In regard to past experience with adjuvant chemotherapy conducted by the Veterans Administration for colorectal and gastric carcinoma, thio-TEPA was the drug of choice, with only a single course at the time of surgery.[30–33]

In another cooperative study on colorectal cancer by the Clinical Drug Evaluation Program, there was no improvement in combined 2- or 3-year survival statistics, but follow-up data indicated that female patients who received the initial high dose showed a significant decrease in recurrent colorectal disease at 5 years.[33] In men, there were negative results with HN2 (Mustargen) and thio-TEPA (TSPA) given similarly for gastric and colorectal cancer on both high- and low-dosage regimens. Why the sex difference, with women being favored, has still not been established.

In TSPA and HN2 for gastric cancer there was no difference in terms of 30-day, 30-month or 45-month survival rates. Similar negative experiences have been seen for a single trial of 2′-deoxy-5-fluorouridine (FUDR).[34] However, in a group in whom tumor tissue was left behind, 3-year survival at both high (0.8 mg/kg) and low (0.6 mg/kg) dosages of TSPA was 20 per cent compared to 6 per cent for the controls.[33] This was felt to be of borderline significance but may be pertinent to the results of recent adjuvant studies with 5-fluorouracil.[7–14] The action of thio-TEPA as an adjuvant is controversial, as is seen in completely opposite reports of responses in carcinoma of the breast.[35,36]

As reported in our earlier review,[1] increased survival for patients with gastric cancer has also been reported by the Viennese group[37] with cyclophosphamide (Cytoxan) or mitomycin similar to that reported in patients with bronchogenic cancer. In the Viennese study, the group showing increased survival showed the greater toxicity, as evidenced by leukopenia. Similar survival relations to leukopenic doses have been made by Moertel and Reitemeier,[6] but toxicity need not necessarily accompany therapeutic effectiveness with 5-fluorouracil.[1]

In contrast with the earlier Veterans Administration studies,[30–34] a more recent randomized program involving 5-fluorouracil in repeated courses[13,38] has been undertaken. In this new study, treatment is started between the fourteenth and the thirtieth day postoperatively with 5-fluorouracil, 12 mg/kg daily for 5 days, for maximum single doses of 1.0 gm. The 5-FU is given at 6- to 8-week intervals until the nineteenth postoperative month. The development of this ongoing study was based on an earlier program beginning in 1965 that divided patients into good and poor risk categories. In that study, survival of treated patients at 18 months indicated the likelihood that 5-FU exerted a clinically significant protective action in preventing recurrence and is consistent with the experience of others[7–14] which should lead to a definitive answer as to the value of adjuvant chemotherapy.

Adjuvant therapy utilizing chemotherapy and immunotherapy is theoretically successful where tumor population is minimal.[39,40] This provides justification for the use of immunologic adjuvants such as bacillus Calmette-Guérin (BCG), *Corynebacterium parvum* or related stimuli to cellular immune response.[41]

Of interest in relation to immunologic response are the prolonged survivals reported for electrocoagulation procedures in both operable and inoperable carcinoma of the bowel.[42,43] The value of immunologic enhancement and electrocoagulation as techniques to stimulate immune resistance remains to be ascertained.

Oral 5-Fluorouracil

As mentioned previously, we have an extensive program utilizing oral 5-FU. In this regard, oral 5-fluorouracil has been demonstrated to be effective utilizing ^{14}C tagged material in a study by the Arthur D. Little group under contract to the Cancer Chemotherapy National Service Center. On the basis of tagged material, some 50 per cent of drug is absorbed by mouth. This has been reported by earlier workers,[44–46] confirmed in dogs and rats,[47,48] and subsequently by Khung et al.,[16] as well as by us[17,18] in some 200 patients. This has recently been confirmed by Lahiri et al.[49] and

Irwin et al.[50] The latter group believes that oral 5-FU may be more effective against hepatic implants than the parenteral drug.

In oral administration of 5-FU* we utilize the Hoffmann-LaRoche ampules, 12 mg/kg of the drug in juice at breakfast. This is given by the standard loading technique once a day for 4 days and then every other day to toxicity, or, in a modified program, giving the drug once a day for 6 days, 1 week off, and then twice a week indefinitely or to relapse. When they are given 5-FU orally, approximately 20 per cent of patients have some mild nausea, which can be handled by readjusting the dosage downward. Oral ulceration or diarrhea is rarely seen. Primary toxicity is manifested by depression of the blood cell count, which can be controlled initially by counts once a week and then every other week. As is true for most standard chemotherapy, the dosage is halved if the leukocyte count is 5000–3000 per cubic millimeter, and stopped if the count is less than 3000 per cubic millimeter. Administering 5-FU orally is more convenient. It is our impression, confirmed by the experience of Khung et al.[16] and others,[49,50] that our response rate with the oral method is essentially the same as with the intravenous route, and we feel that the pattern of response is similar to that seen with prolonged intravenous infusions. It is important to emphasize that some patients who fail to respond, or who relapse, while being given 5-FU orally will respond when the drug is given by the standard intravenous push. We believe that 5-fluorouracil given either intravenously or orally selects for a 15 to 20 per cent responding population, and responses can be seen without toxicity, as described by others.[1] The convenience of the oral route will undoubtedly make for greater use of 5-FU, with less hazard to patients. Given orally, 5-FU is ideal for surgical adjuvant programs. I do not mean to denigrate the proved effectiveness of parenteral 5-FU, but I know of many patients who are not given maintenance therapy or repeated loading doses because of the inconvenience and greater toxicity of parenteral 5-FU. Renewed comparative study of parenteral versus oral 5-FU is in order with particular regard to its place in prolonged adjuvant chemotherapy.

Parenteral 5-FU

Although Moertel et al.[51] found FUDR more effective than 5-FU, the former has only recently become available, and the difference between the two agents is controversial in regard to response rates.[1] What is important is that the response to these related drugs seems to be the same in cancer of the colon as in rectal cancer.[52]

In regard to intravenous 5-FU, more investigators are finding the weekly maintenance programs as valuable as the loading dose technique.[52–55] A comparative study by Ramirez et al.[55] in both colorectal and breast cancer appears to adequately settle the issue as to the appropriate value of weekly administration of 5-FU.

Radiation Synergy

As discussed in our previous review,[1] the action of chemotherapeutic agents with radiation may provide additive or synergistic effects. The most effective agent in this regard has been reported to be 5-FU[1,6] with clinical results in cancer of the stomach, colon, pancreas and liver. Previous results represented only small population samples, but in a randomized, double-blind study Moertel et al.[6,56] have shown, in 183 patients

* 5-FU as a dissolvable tablet has been made available by the Calgon Company and will undergo clinical study.

TABLE 1.—*Prolonged Survival with Combination Therapy*

No. of patients	*Carcinoma*	*Time treated with 5-FU (months)*	*Time treated with placebo (months)*
50	Stomach	13.5	5.8
68	Pancreas	11.4	6.8
65	Large Bowel	22.5	16.8

with inoperable localized gastrointestinal carcinoma, that survival of these patients can be prolonged when 5-FU is combined with radiation therapy (3500–4000 rads were delivered by cobalt-60 teletherapy or 6 MV linear accelerator and combined with 5-FU, 15 mg/kg per day for 3 days, or placebo). These results are promising because they show no major toxicity in the responding group (Table 1).

The results of the recent preoperative VA study with FUDR have shown, on recent reanalysis, suggestive improvement in survival.[38]

Further results of mitomycin C or AB 132 in this regard are academic, as these compounds are not clinically available. However, recent data for AB 132 indicate surprisingly enhanced 5-year survival in carcinoma of the lung which may be applicable for AB 132 in view of AB 132's gastrointestinal antitumor activity and laboratory evidence of synergizing effects with radiation.[57,58]

I believe that for localized inoperable carcinoma of the bowel, adjuvant 5-FU and radiation therapy may be appropriately used, but radiation dosage should be adjusted to a concept of palliation rather than cure.

New Agents

In relation to cancer chemotherapy of gastrointestinal neoplasms, no new agents of major consequence have been reported, with the exception of bleomycin for esophageal or gastric carcinoma with or without concomitant radiation therapy.[24,25] Bleomycin has minimal marrow depressant activity but produces characteristic skin lesions and pulmonary fibrosis. Let us hope its true place in gastrointestinal neoplasia will be more rapidly ascertained than that of mitomycin C, which, although it shows activity against gastric and bowel cancer, remains unavailable because of toxicity despite reported response rates not unlike those seen with 5-FU.[1,6,19–21] The problem of late toxicity is the drawback of mitomycin, delaying its commercial availability and, as mentioned earlier, it appears to be ineffective when given after failure of 5-FU treatment.[19] Similar late toxicity, despite a significant level of response, has been reported by Moertel et al.[6,59] for bis-dichloro-nitrosourea (BCNU), which is available from the Cancer Chemotherapy National Service Center. A better cogener of BCNU, CCNU, is absorbable by mouth and is showing activity against bowel cancer.[27]

Although methotrexate in large intermittent dosage, with or without citrovorum factor "save," has been reported to produce responses in gastrointestinal cancer[1] in a major study of the Eastern Oncology Cooperative Study Group (EOCSG), it has not proved itself valuable in the treatment of gastrointestinal cancer at oral doses of 0.25 mg/kg or 0.6 mg/kg twice weekly. However, reports of response, as presented in my earlier review,[1] keep appearing.[6,60]

The role of heparin as an agent in preventing metastases has been explored as an adjuvant in Germany; its rationale in clinical therapy deserves serious consideration.[1]

Combination chemotherapy represents a hope in future programs,[1] although no combinations have yet proved to be better than 5-FU alone. Cytoxan plus 5-FU is well tolerated in bowel cancer[61] and has been combined with methotrexate and vincristine to successfully treat breast cancer. In this regard, Costanzi and Coltman[62] have seen significant response in two pancreatic cancers with the above combination. Moertel's group is having success with the combined use of 5-FU and BCNU in this disease.[27] The rationale for the simultaneous use of multiple drugs to hit various phases of the mitotic cycle and to avoid resistance is self-evident, but to my knowledge no optimal program has yet established itself.

Secreting Tumors

Streptozotocin, an antibiotic derived from *Streptomyces achromogenes*, shows activity against the L1210 animal tumor system.[22] This drug has been found to be diabetogenic in experimental animals, producing selective toxicity for pancreatic beta cells. For this reason, it is now in study for its effects on pancreatic carcinoma and has had successful clinical trial in 16 of 23 islet cell tumors.[30] Safely tolerated therapeutic dosage remains to be determined but appears to be in the range of 1 gram per square meter per week for 2 weeks escalated to effective dosage. In regard to islet cell tumors, responses have also been seen for tubericidin.[25] For palliation in secreting tumors, the use of diazoxide as an antagonist to insulin hypoglycemia is well established.[63]

Other special bowel tumors of secretory character such as carcinoid respond to Cytoxan and 5-FU[1] and mitomycin C, and the side effects can be mitigated by diets low in niacin and tryptophan or by administration of alpha-methyldopa, methysergide, or cyproheptadine, as reported previously.[1] Moertel[27] and others[25] have reported responses of carcinoid to streptozotocin. Cinanserin (Squibb), a drug which is available for laboratory experimentation but which has been withdrawn from clinical use, is an extremely potent antiserotonin agent which should be tried if possible. Camptothecin[27] is under clinical trial, and phase II studies will be of interest.[26]

References

1. Regelson, W.: Chemotherapy of gastrointestinal cancer. *In* Brodsky, I. and Kahn, S. B. (Eds.): Cancer Chemotherapy. New York: Grune & Stratton, Inc., 1967, pp. 84–107.
2. Regelson, W.: Perspectives and prospects in the chemotherapy of gastrointestinal cancer. Med. Coll. Va. Quart. 3 (2): 119, 1967.
3. Sherlock, P., Ehrlich, A. N., Pavon, E. E. and Paglia, M. A.: Treatment of gastrointestinal cancer: Current status and recent progress. Gastroenterology 53:630, 1967.
4. Oberfield, R. A. and Sullivan, R. D.: New concepts in chemotherapy of advanced gastrointestinal cancer. Lahey Clin. Found. Bull. 16:197, 1967.
5. Moertel, C. G. and Reitemeier, R. J.: Chemotherapy of gastrointestinal cancer. Surg. Clin. N. Amer. 47:929, 1967.
6. Moertel, C. G. and Reitemeier, R. J.: Advanced Gastrointestinal Cancer: Clinical Management and Chemotherapy. New York: Harper & Row, 1969.
7. Rousselot, C. M., Cole, D. R., Grossi, C. F., Conte, A. J. and Gonzalez, R. M.: Intraluminal chemotherapy (HN2 or 5-FU) adjuvant to operations for cancer of the colon and rectum. II. Follow-up report of 97 cases. Cancer 20:829, 1967.
8. Rousselot, C. M., Cole, D. R., Grossi, C. E., Conte, A. J., Gonzalez, E. M. and Pasternack, B. S.: A five year progress report on the effectiveness of intraluminal chemotherapy (5-fluorouracil) adjuvant to surgery for colon rectal cancer. Amer. J. Surg. 115: 140, 1968.

9. Curreri, A. R. and Mackman, S.: Reoperation in carcinoma of the colon following resection and adjuvant chemotherapy. Surg. Gynec. Obstet. 123:274, 1966.
10. Mackman, S., Curreri, A. R., and Ansfield, F. J.: Second look operation for colon carcinoma after fluorouracil therapy. Arch. Surg. 100:527, 1970.
11. Mackman, S. and Curreri, A. R.: The second look operation for carcinoma of the colon after administration of 5-fluorouracil. Amer. J. Surg. 115:227, 1968.
12. Grossi, C. F.: Personal communication (St. Vincent's Hospital, New York), 1970.
13. Keehan, R. J.: Veterans Administration Surgical Adjuvant Cancer Chemotherapy Study: Progress Report No. 32, 1970.
14. Rousselot, L. M., Cole, D. R., Grossi, C. E., Conte, A. J., Gonzalez, E. M. and Pasternack, B. S.: Adjuvant chemotherapy of 5-fluorouracil in surgery for colo-rectal cancer: Eight year progress report (in press, 1971).
15. Henderson, I. W. D., Lipowska, B. and Lougheed, S. E.: Clinical evaluation of combined radiation and chemotherapy in gastrointestinal malignancies. Amer. J. Roentgen. 102:545, 1968.
16. Khung, C. L., Hall, T. C., Piro, A. J. and Dederick, M. M.: A clinical trial of oral 5-fluorouracil. Clin. Pharmacol. Ther. 7:527, 1966.
17. Regelson, W.: Work in progress, 1971.
18. Regelson, W., Lawrence, W., Jr. and Horsely, S., III.: Work in progress, 1971.
19. Ansfield, F. J.: Clinical study of mitomycin C (NSC 26980) in colorectal cancer. Cancer Chemother. Rep. 53:287, 1969.
20. Jones, R. J., Jr., Moore, G. E., Olson, K. B., Colsky, J. and McKenzie, D.: Phase II studies of the effect of mitomycin C in treatment of human cancer. Abstr. X Int. Cancer Cong., 1970, p. 476.
21. Moertel, C. G., Reitemeier, R. J. and Hahn, R. G.: Mitomycin C therapy in advanced gastrointestinal cancer. J.A.M.A. 204: 1045, 1968.
22. National Cancer Institute, Program Analysis Branch, Chemotherapy: Chemotherapy Fact Sheet, streptozotocin (NSC 85998), 1969.
23. Taylor, S. and Moertel, C. G.: Personal communication (St. Luke's and Presbyterian Hospital, Chicago, Illinois and Mayo Clinic, Rochester, Minnesota), 1970.
24. Wada, T.: Chemotherapy for esophageal cancer by bleomycin. Abstr. X Int. Cancer Cong., 1970, p. 492.
25. Carter, S.: Program Analysis Branch, Chemotherapy, National Cancer Institute. Personal communication, 1970.
26. Gottlieb, J. A., Guarino, A. M. and Block, J. B.: Initial pharmacological studies and clinical evaluation of comptothecin sodium. Abstr. X Int. Cancer Cong., 1970, p. 399.
27. Moertel, C. G.: Personal communication (Mayo Clinic, Rochester, Minnesota), 1970.
28. Lerner, Harvey J.: Personal communication (University of Pennsylvania Hospital, Philadelphia, Pennsylvania), 1971.
29. Gold, P.: Colon Cancer. Symposium on immune reactions to cancer in man. Cancer Res. (in press, 1971).
30. Sharp, G. S. and Benefiel, W. W.: 5-Fluorouracil in the treatment of inoperable carcinoma of the colon. Cancer Chemother. Rep. 44:27, 1965.
31. Dwight, R. W.: Adjuvant chemotherapy in cancer of the large bowel: An interim report of the Veterans Administration Surgical Adjuvant Cancer Chemotherapy study. Trans. New Eng. Surg. Soc. 63:109, 1962.
32. Dwight, R. W., Higgens, G. A. and Keehn, R. J.: Factors influencing survival after resection in cancer of the colon and rectum. Am. J. Surg. 117:512, 1969.
33. University of California, Los Angeles, California Statistical Unit: 17th Report on Colo-Rectal Clinical Trials. Adjuvant Cancer Chemotherapy Studies, 1957–1965.
34. Serlin, O., Wolkoff, J. S., Amadeo, J. M and Keehn, R. J.: Use of 5-fluorodeoxyuridine (FUDR) as an adjuvant to the surgical management of carcinoma of the stomach. Cancer 24:223, 1969.
35. Donegan, W. L.: Prolonged surgical adjuvant chemotherapy with thio-TEPA for mammary carcinoma: A progress report. Abstr. X Int. Cancer Cong., 1970, p. 500.
36. Mrazek, R. G. and McDonald, G. O.: Surgery and adjuvant chemotherapy in the treatment for breast carcinoma. Abstr. X Int. Cancer Cong., 1970, p. 501.
37. Karrer, K.: The importance of dose schedule in adjuvant chemotherapy. Abstr. X Int. Cancer Cong., 1970, p. 500.
38. Keehn, R. J. and Higgins, G. (Veterans Administration, Surgical Adjuvant Cancer Chemotherapy Study Group, National Research Council): Personal communication, 1970.
39. Mathé, G., Schwarzenberg, L., Amiel, J. L., Schneider, M., Cattan, A. and Schlumberger, J. R.: The role of immunology in the treat-

ment of leukemias and hematosarcomas. Cancer Res. 27:2542, 1967.

40. Klein, G. and Oettgen, H. F.: Immunologic factors involved in the growth of primary tumors in human or animal hosts. Cancer Res. 29:1741, 1969.
41. Regelson, W.: Immunological factors and chemotherapy. (Ch. 8, this volume.)
42. Strauss, A. A., Appel, M., Saphir, O. and Rabinovitz, A. J.: Immunologic resistance to carcinoma produced by electrocoagulation. Surg. Gynec. Obstet. 121:989, 1965.
43. Madden, J. L. and Kandalaft, S.: Electrocoagulation: A primary and preferred method of treatment for cancer of the rectum. Ann. Surg. 166:413, 1967.
44. Kennedy, B. J. and Theologides, A.: The role of 5-fluorouracil in malignant disease. Ann. Intern. Med. 55:719, 1961.
45. Khung, C. L.: The use of 5-fluorouracil orally in patients with advanced cancer. Proc. Amer. Ass. Cancer Res. 6:45, 1965.
46. Ellison, R. R.: Experience with fluorinated pyrimidine in adenocarcinoma of the lower intestinal tract. N.Y. J. Med. 61:2364, 1962.
47. Cole, D. R., Rousselot, L. M., Slattery, J. and Conte, A. J.: Absorption patterns of intraluminal injected 5-fluorouracil in the isolated right colon of the dog. Surgery 55:252, 1964.
48. Cole, D. R., Grossi, C. E., Conte, A. J. and Rousselot, L. M.: Adjuvant intraluminal chemotherapy with 5-fluorouracil in simulated colon cancer in the rat. Chemotherapia 11:158, 1966.
49. Lahiri, S. R., Boileau, G. and Hall, T. C.: 5-Fluorouracil (5-FU) by mouth in metastatic colo-rectal carcinoma. Proc. Amer. Soc. Clin. Oncol. 1971.
50. Irwin, L. E. and Pugh, R. P., Jr.: 5-Fluorouracil given once weekly: Comparison of intravenous and oral administration. Proc. Amer. Soc. Clin. Oncol. 1971.
51. Moertel, C. G., Reitemeier, R. J. and Hahn, R. H.: Comparative response to carcinoma of the rectum and carcinoma of the colon to fluorinated pyrimidine therapy. Cancer Chemother. Rep. 53:283, 1969.
52. Jacobs, E. M., Reeves, W. J., Jr., Wood, D. A., Pugh, R., Braunwald, J. and Bateman, J. R.: Treatment of cancer with weekly intravenous 5-fluorouracil: Study by the Western Cooperative Cancer Chemotherapy Group (WCCCG), Abstr. X Int. Cancer Cong., 1970, p. 480.
53. Nadler, S. H. and Moore, G. E.: A clinical study of fluorouracil. Surg. Gynec. Obstet. 127:1210, 1968.
54. Hart, G. D., Maxwell, S. B. and Soots, M. C.: Systemic 5-fluorouracil for palliation of gastrointestinal cancer. Appl. Ther. 10:670, 1968.
55. Ramirez, G., Korbitz, B. C., Davis, H. L., Jr., and Ansfield, F. J.: Comparative study of monthly courses versus weekly doses of 5-fluorouracil (NSC 19893). Cancer Chemother. Rep. 53:243, 1969.
56. Moertel, C. G., Childs, D. S., Reitemeier, R. J., Colby, M. Y. and Holbrook, M. A.: Combined 5-fluorouracil and supervoltage radiation therapy of advanced gastrointestinal carcinoma: A controlled evaluation. Proc. Amer. Ass. Cancer Res. 6:46, 1965.
57. Ambrus, J.: Personal communication (Roswell Park Memorial Institute, Buffalo, New York), 1970.
58. Regelson, W. and Pierucci, O.: The effect of radiation on splenomegaly induced by the Friend leukemia virus and its modification by ethyl-N-bis(2,2-dimethyl-ethylamidinophosphoro)-carbamate (AB 132), actinomycin D, and AET. Radiat. Res. 22:368, 1964.
59. Moertel, C. G., Reitemeier, R. J. and Hahn, R. G.: Therapy of advanced gastrointestinal cancer with 1-3-bis-(2-chlorethyl)-1-nitrosourea (BCNU). Clin. Pharmacol. Ther. 9:652, 1968.
60. Ward, W. W., Jr. and Mullins, F.: Methotrexate therapy of advanced gastrointestinal malignancy. J. Indiana Med. Ass. 62:355, 1969.
61. Mullen, J. M., Rosenbaum, E., Colombo, O., Barros, C., Louge, E. L. and Brea, M. M.: Cyclophosphamide plus 5-fluorouracil in slow intravenous infusion: Clinical subacute toxicity study. Abstr. X Int. Cancer Cong., 1970, p. 480.
62. Costanzi, J. J. and Coltman, C. A., Jr.: Combination chemotherapy using cyclophosphamide, vincristine, methotrexate and 5-fluorouracil in solid tumors. Cancer 23: 589, 1969.
63. Hunt, P. S.: Adult hypoglycemia associated with neoplasia: A report of three cases, with a note on the use of diazoxide. Aust. New Zeal. J. Surg. 35:295, 1966.

Chemotherapy and Hormonal Therapy in Neoplasms of the Ovary and Uterus

By G. Lennard Gold, M.D. and Mahmoodullah Baig, M.D.

MANY ADVANCES IN ONCOLOGY since the previous Hahnemann symposium on cancer chemotherapy are applicable to the topic of this chapter. Malignant tumors of the female genital tract can be considered representative of a number of organ sites of tumor growth, for lessons learned here may be applied elsewhere in research and clinical practice. A team approach is necessary for maximal effort and best patient care. The surgeon, the radiotherapist and the internist-oncologist must pool their varied funds of knowledge to continue the advances already established. Although the gynecologist knows the anatomy and clinical aspects of genital tumors, the far-reaching effects of neoplastic cells, newer theories and the toxic manifestations of recently developed drugs require the collaboration of other disciplines.

Ovarian Carcinoma

Primary carcinoma of the ovary represents about 5 per cent of all cancers in women,[1] and the probability of a woman's developing ovarian cancer during her life is about 0.9 per cent. Unfortunately, no complaints specifically indicate the presence of an ovarian tumor in its earliest stages. In many cases, these tumors have spread beyond the pelvis at the time of diagnosis, and this accounts for the poor prognosis. Approximately 10 per cent of patients live 3 years after the onset of chemotherapy.

The 5-year survival rate reported by various authors is 20 to 40 per cent.[2–5] The combination of surgery, irradiation and chemotherapy has yielded most of the encouraging experiences in the management of disseminated ovarian cancer. Alkylating agents in systemic chemotherapy of ovarian carcinoma were first used in 1952 by Rundles and Barton,[6] who demonstrated the favorable effects of triethylene melamine (TEM). Seligman et al.[7] observed short-term palliation after intravenous administration of hemisulfur mustard. Recently, the oral administration of substituted mustards has gained favor because of its convenience and negligible gastrointestinal toxicity. Ovarian cancer is responsive to thio-TEPA,[8,9] chlorambucil,[10] phenylalanine mustard,[11] and cyclophosphamide.[12] Other chemotherapeutic drugs, e.g., antimetabolites, antibiotics and alkaloids, are inferior to alkylating agents. An objective response to alkylating agents may be anticipated in 40 to 50 per cent of patients with palpable or measurable tumor. Although no one agent has demonstrated clinical superiority over the others, infrequently does an alkylating agent succeed after another fails.

Increased survival time has been reported with the combination of various alkylating agents and radiation either concurrently or sequentially.[13–16] Hreshchyshyn and Graham,[17] employing thio-TEPA in the initial treatment and chlorambucil for maintenance therapy, reported a good response in 17 per cent (22 of 130). They defined *good*

From the Division of Oncology, Department of Medicine, Georgetown University School of Medicine, Washington, D. C.

Supported in part by grant CA-08119 from the National Cancer Institute, National Institutes of Health.

response as more than 25 per cent measurable regression or more than 50 per cent palpable regression of the tumor, lasting more than 3 months and associated with symptomatic improvement, with ascites or pleural effusion suppressed completely in 26 per cent (13 of 50) or partially in 38 per cent (19 of 50). An increased median survival time (MST) was noted by Hreshchyshyn when thio-TEPA was given after irradiation (X-ray alone: MST = 4 months; X-ray and thio-TEPA: MST = 13.5 months), and the MST of 13.5 months was observed if the two agents were administered concurrently.

Kottmeier,[18] in a randomized study of 219 cases of inoperable ovarian carcinoma, noted that, on the average, patients who received combined therapy (radiation therapy plus a course of thio-TEPA intravenously) lived longer than those who were treated with radiation therapy alone.

Decker et al.[12] reported that of patients with recurrent, progressive ovarian cancer treated with cyclophosphamide alone (65 patients) or with radiation added (39 patients), about 36.5 per cent seemed to respond favorably; that is, there were objective remissions in 22 and arrest of progression of the tumor in 16 for at least 12 months. Masterson and Nelson[19] reported on a larger series of patients treated with chlorambucil and found a 50 per cent response rate.

Rutledge[20] treated 338 patients with advanced ovarian cancer with phenylalanine mustard. He defined objective response as a 50 per cent decrease in the size of the tumor mass and control of serous effusions. About 50 per cent of the patients in his series experienced objective response.

At the Mount Sinai Hospital (New York), Greenspan and Fieber[21] reported on a group of patients treated with a combination of methotrexate and thio-TEPA. They found that 21 of 30 patients responded favorably, as shown by objective regression in tumor size. This was probably the beginning of combination chemotherapy, for this report was published in the early 1960's.

Smith and Rutledge[22] treated 47 patients with serous, mucinous, and undifferentiated adenocarcinoma with combination chemotherapy. The combination consisted of actinomycin D, 5-fluorouracil and cyclophosphamide. This regimen was found to be effective in 38 per cent of the patients with serous or undifferentiated adenocarcinoma. The dose of actinomycin D was 500 gamma per day for 5 days; 5-fluorouracil was given in a dose of 6 to 8 mg/kg in 500 ml of 5% dextrose and water as an intravenous drip, for 1 to 2 hours daily for 5 days; the cyclophosphamide dose was 5 to 7 mg/kg, given as a direct intravenous push, daily for 5 days. These 5-day courses were repeated every 4 weeks, if the patient had recovered from hematologic and gastrointestinal toxicity. Their criterion for complete response was the disappearance of malignancy for 3 months or longer; a partial response was defined as a decrease in tumor size for 3 months or longer.

The differences in the percentages of patients showing objective responses in various published series are related to many factors, among them the time a remission must last to be considered response, the relation of drug administration to radiation therapy, and variations in type and grading of the tumor material.

Chemotherapy is not curative, but it has proved extremely useful for advanced ovarian carcinoma. Cooperative studies and the careful collaboration of the radiation therapist, the surgeon and the chemotherapist, combined with the continued search for new diagnostic techniques, is required to improve the outlook for patients with ovarian neoplasms.

Carcinoma of the Cervix

Epidermoid carcinoma of the cervix is still an enigma for the cancer chemotherapist. When vincristine first appeared on the scene, a few investigators suggested that satisfactory tumor regression could be produced in a minority of patients treated. We have had the opportunity to treat a number of patients with easily measurable metastatic cervical carcinoma but no favorable responses were noted. We suggest that other approaches may reap benefits that have eluded the chemotherapist. The epidemiologists have noted correlations between early age of first coitus, multiple sexual partners, uncircumcised male partners, and an increased incidence of cervical cancer. A venereally transmitted virus has been suggested and a high incidence of antibodies to herpesvirus Type 2 has been found in the serum of patients with invasive carcinoma.[23] Other workers have found an increased incidence of in situ carcinomas in women with genital herpes.[24] The association with herpesvirus Type 2 and epidermoid cervical carcinoma may also point the way to a new therapeutic approach, an immunologic one.

Continued and widespread use of the Papanicolaou smear technique should increase the number of cures of early lesions by surgery and X-ray therapy, thereby obviating the use of drugs.

Despite the high incidence of epidermoid carcinoma of the cervix, the experience of a number of authors bears out the belief that this lesion is one of the most resistant encountered. Alkylating agents, antimetabolites, and actinomycin D have proved unsatisfactory.[25] However, Papavasiliou et al.[26] reported that a combination of methotrexate and cyclophosphamide produced complete remissions in 3 of 23 patients, and partial remissions in 7 of 23 patients treated.[26] The Eastern Clinical Drug Evaluation Program (ECDEP)[27] reported on the treatment with 5-fluorouracil of 15 patients with cervical carcinoma, with 5 of the 15 patients responding, and on a similar percentage of responders in several references.[27] Again, the ECDEP[28] reported that 7 of 26 patients responded to chlorambucil and 4 of 18 patients responded to mitomycin C.[29] Although these results are interesting, they seem to be at variance with those of other investigative groups.

Endometrial Carcinoma

The incidence of endometrial carcinoma is related to age; about 75 per cent of the patients are postmenopausal at the time of diagnosis.[30] It is well known that in addition to age, the triad of obesity, hypertension and diabetes frequently is associated with endometrial cancer.[31] According to McKay, 50 per cent of such patients are obese, over 50 per cent have hypertension, 10 per cent have clinical diabetes, and approximately 50 per cent have abnormal glucose tolerance curves.[32]

In endometrial carcinoma, the size of the uterus, absence of cervical involvement, and type of histologic differentiation are factors which bear a direct relation to patient survival.[33] Up to 80 per cent of patients may survive more than 5 years when the uterus is not enlarged and the tumor is well differentiated. However, when the cancer is no longer confined to the uterus, the 5-year cure rate decreases to about 20 per cent.[34]

In 1961, Kelly and Baker[35] commenced clinical trials with progesterone (in oil) and 17-α-hydroxyprogesterone caproate in the therapy of far-advanced endometrial carcinoma. They reported objective regression lasting from 9 months to 4.5 years in 6 of

20 patients, and subsequently reported objective remissions in 32 per cent of their patients.[36]

Anderson[37] observed remissions in 8 of 20 patients (40 per cent) with advanced endometrial cancer treated with medroxyprogesterone. Smith et al.[38] treated 42 patients with this agent and obtained a significant response in 17 of 42 for 3 to 42 months (the average being 16.3 months) and a favorable clinical response in 19 of 42 patients.

Frick[39] reported objective remissions in 4 of 22 cases with disseminated endometrial carcinoma treated with 17-α-hydroxyprogesterone caproate. Mussey and Malkasian[40] reported their results in 20 patients treated with 17-α-hydroxyprogesterone caproate. Objective improvement occurred in 5 and an equivocal response was obtained in 4 more patients.

Kennedy[41] noted an objective improvement in 10 of 41 patients (24.4 per cent) who received 17-α-hydroxyprogesterone caproate and in 9 of 34 patients (26.5 per cent) who received dihydroxyprogesterone acetophenide. The mean duration of improvement was more than 35 months and more than 18.5 months, respectively. Similar objective responses have been reported by other investigators.[42–44]

Objective responses are more often seen in slowly growing, well-differentiated tumors. The clinical extent of the neoplasm seems to influence the response rate. Pulmonary and bony metastases respond well to progestational agents, while pelvic, abdominal and lymph node metastases respond poorly.

The dosage of 17-α-hydroxyprogesterone caproate is 500 mg administered intramuscularly 3 times a week; the dosage of medroxyprogesterone is about 150 mg injected intramuscularly 3 times a week.

If adequate therapy is administered, 30 to 55 per cent of patients will show objective remission.[44] Progestational agents are exceptionally free of toxic reactions when compared to other anticancer drugs. Therefore, there are no contraindications to progestational therapy in patients with disseminated endometrial carcinoma.

Chemotherapy with other antitumor drugs is of questionable value for patients who fail to respond or who are no longer responsive to progestational therapy. In a few patients, brief remissions with alkylating agents have been reported,[45] and Kennedy[41] has observed short-term objective improvement in 2 of 6 patients treated with hydroxyurea.

References

1. Ratzkowski, E. and Hochman, A.: Survival of patients with primary cancer of the ovary: An analysis of 146 cases. Cancer 16: 1578, 1963.
2. Stone, M. L., Weingold, A. B., Sall, S. and Sonnenblick, B.: Factors affecting survival of patients with ovarian carcinoma. Surg. Gynec. Obstet. 116:351, 1963.
3. Cutler, S. J., Ederer, F. G., Griswold, M. H. and Greenberg, R. A.: Survival of patients with uterine cancer, Connecticut, 1935–54. J. Nat. Cancer Inst. 24:519, 1960.
4. Kent, S. W. and McKay, D. G.: Primary cancer of the ovary: An analysis of 349 cases. Amer. J. Obstet. Gynec. 80:430, 1960.
5. Munnell, E. W.: The changing prognosis and treatment in carcinoma of the ovary: A report of 235 patients with primary ovarian carcinoma, 1952–1961. Amer. J. Obstet. Gynec. 100:790, 1968.
6. Rundles, R. W. and Barton, W. B.: Triethylene melamine in the treatment of neoplastic disease. Blood 7:483, 1952.
7. Seligman, A. M., Rutenburg, A. M., Persky, L. and Friedman, O. M.: Effect of 2-chloro-2′-hydroxydiethyl sulfide (hemisulfur mustard) on carcinomatosis with ascites. Cancer 5:354, 1952.

8. Bateman, J. C. and Winship, T.: Palliation of ovarian carcinoma with phosphoramide drugs. Surg. Gynec. Obstet. 102:347, 1956.
9. Hreshchyshyn, M. M.: A critical review of chemotherapy in the treatment of ovarian carcinoma. Clin. Obstet. Gynec. 4:885, 1961.
10. Masterson, J. G., Calame, R. J. and Nelson, J.: A clinical study on the use of chlorambucil in the treatment of cancer of the ovary. Amer. J. Obstet. Gynec. 79:1002, 1960.
11. Burns, B. C., Jr., Rutledge, F. and Gallagher, H. S.: Phenylalanine mustard in the palliative management of carcinoma of the ovary. Obstet. Gyn. 22:30, 1963.
12. Decker, D. G., Mussey, E., Malkasian, G. D., Jr. et al.: Cyclophosphamide in the treatment of ovarian cancer. Clin. Obstet. Gynec. 11:382, 1968.
13. Burns, B. C., Jr., Underwood, P. B., Jr. and Rutledge, F. N.: A review of carcinoma of the ovary at The University of Texas M. D. Anderson Hospital and Tumor Institute at Houston. *In* Cancer of the Uterus and Ovary. Chicago: Year Book Medical Publishers, 1969, p. 123.
14. Decker, D. G., Mussey, E., Malkasian, G. D., Jr. et al.: Adjuvant therapy for advanced ovarian malignancy. Amer. J. Obstet. Gynec. 97:171, 1967.
15. Lebherz, T. B., Huston, J. W., Austin, J. A. et al.: Sustained palliation in ovarian carcinoma. Obstet. Gynec. 25:475, 1965.
16. Long, R. T., Johnson, R. E. and Sala, J. M.: Variations in survival among patients with carcinoma of the ovary: Analysis of 253 cases according to histologic type, anatomical stage and method of treatment. Cancer 20:1195, 1967.
17. Hreshchyshyn, M. M. and Graham, J. B.: Chemotherapy of ovarian cancer. Int. Surg. 47:398, 1967.
18. Kottmeier, H. L.: Treatment of ovarian cancer with thioTEPA. Clin. Obstet. Gynec. 11:428, 1968.
19. Masterson, J. G. and Nelson, J. H., Jr.: The role of chemotherapy in the treatment of gynecologic malignancy. Amer. J. Obstet. Gynec. 93:1102, 1965.
20. Rutledge, F.: Chemotherapy of ovarian cancer with melphalan. Clin. Obstet. Gynec. 11:354, 1968.
21. Greenspan, E. M. and Fieber, M.: Combination chemotherapy of advanced ovarian carcinoma with the antimetabolite, methotrexate, and the alkylating agent, thioTEPA. J. Mount Sinai Hosp. N.Y. 29:48, 1962.
22. Smith, J. P. and Rutledge, F.: Chemotherapy with treatment of cancer of the ovary. Amer. J. Obstet. Gynec. 107: 691, 1970.
23. Rawls, W. E., Tompkins, W. A. and Figueroa, M. E. et al.: Herpesvirus Type 2: Association with carcinoma of the cervix. Science 161:1255, 1968.
24. Naib, Z. M.: Exfoliative cytology of viral cervico-vaginitis. Acta Cytol. 10:126, 1966.
25. Hreshchyshyn, M. M.: Experiences with chemotherapy in gynecologic cancer. New York J. Med. 64:2431, 1964.
26. Papavasiliou, C., Angelakis, P. G. and Papakyriakides, L.: Treatment of cervical carcinoma by methotrexate (NSC-740) combined with cyclophosphamide (NSC-26271). Cancer Chemother. Rep. (Part I) 53:255, 1969.
27. Moore, G. E., Bross, I. D., Ausman, R. et al.: Effects of 5-fluorouracil (NSC-19893) in 389 patients with cancer. Eastern Clinical Drug Evaluation Program. Cancer Chemother. Rep. 52:641, 1968.
28. Moore, G. E., Bross, I. D., Ausman, R. et al.: Effects of chlorambucil (NSC-3088) in 374 patients with advanced cancer. Eastern Clinical Drug Evaluation Program. Cancer Chemother. Rep. 52:661, 1968.
29. Moore, G. E., Bross, I. D., Ausman, R. et al.: Effects of mitomycin C (NSC-26980) in 346 patients with advanced cancer. Eastern Clinical Drug Evaluation Program. Cancer Chemother. Rep. 52:675, 1968.
30. Geisler, H. E. and Gibbs, C. P.: Invasive carcinoma of the endometrium: A 5 to 16 year follow-up of 183 patients. Amer. J. Obstet. Gynec. 102:516, 1968.
31. Cohen, C. J.: Treatment problems in endometrial cancer. Clin. Obstet. Gynec. 10:625, 1967.
32. McKay, D. G.: A review of the status of endometrial cancer. Cancer Res. 25:1182, 1965.
33. Breen, J. L.: Gynecologic oncology in the aged. Clin. Obstet. Gynec. 10:498, 1967.
34. Anderson, J. E., Meltzer, H. D., Scarborough, J. E. et al.: Adenocarcinoma of the endometrium. Cancer 18:955, 1965.
35. Kelley, R. M. and Baker, W. H.: Progestational agents in the treatment of carcinoma of the endometrium. New Eng. J. Med. 264:216, 1961.
36. Kelley, R. M. and Baker, W. H.: The role of progesterone in human endometrial cancer. Cancer Res. 25:1190, 1965.

37. Anderson, D. G.: Management of advanced endometrial adenocarcinoma with medroxyprogesterone acetate. Amer. J. Obstet. Gynec. 92:87, 1965.
38. Smith, J. P., Rutledge, F. and Soffar, S. W.: Progestins in the treatment of patients with endometrial adenocarcinoma. Amer. J. Obstet. Gynec. 94:977, 1966.
39. Frick, H. C., 2d: Progestational drugs in the management of endometrial cancer. Metabolism 14 (Suppl.):348, 1965.
40. Mussey, E. and Malkasian, G. D., Jr.: Progestogen treatment of recurrent carcinoma of the endometrium. Amer. J. Obstet. Gynec. 94:78, 1966.
41. Kennedy, B. J.: Progestogens in the treatment of carcinoma of the endometrium. Surg. Gynec. Obstet. 127:103, 1968.
42. Kistner, R. W., Griffiths, C. T. and Craig, J. M.: Use of progestational agents in the management of endometrial cancer. Cancer 18:1563, 1965.
43. Talley, R. W.: Medroxyprogesterone acetate (NSC-26386) in metastatic adenocarcinoma of the endometrium and cervix. Cancer Chemother. Rep. 46:27, 1965.
44. Kistner, R. W. and Griffiths, C. T.: Use of progestational agents in the management of metastatic carcinoma of the endometrium. Clin. Obstet. Gynec. 11:439, 1968.
45. Hreshchyshyn, M. M. and Holland, J. F.: Chemotherapy in patients with gynecologic cancer. Amer. J. Obstet. Gynec. 83:468, 1962.

Hematologic Neoplasms During Pregnancy

By Robert L. Capizzi, M.D.

THE LAST TWO DECADES have witnessed rapid advances in cancer chemotherapy. The use of specific, tailor-made drugs which affect vital cellular processes have not only prolonged the useful lives of cancer patients but have also led to a greater understanding of basic molecular mechanisms. This development, however, has not been without its perils, for on occasion therapy may produce problems in addition to those of the basic disease. Considerations of drug toxicity always enter our minds when we treat a patient who has cancer, but with the pregnant cancer patient we must also consider the consequences of our therapy on the fetus, both the immediate effects, namely, abortions, prematurity and malformations, and the delayed effects, mutagenesis and carcinogenesis.

Since the therapy of these diseases and the sequelae of such therapy are covered elsewhere in this volume, this chapter will deal only with the effects of pregnancy on the course of leukemia and lymphoma, and vice versa, as well as the effects of the diseases and their therapy on the fetus.

Incidence of Neoplasms During Pregnancy

The better control of other complications of pregnancy has resulted in a relative increase in the incidence of cancer during pregnancy. The published records of one hospital show that during the 1950s cancer had accounted for more deaths in obstetric patients than any other condition.[1] In the Memorial and James Ewing Hospital series, breast, lymphoma, gynecologic and bone neoplasms were the most common types of cancer in pregnancy.[2]

Contrary to some reports,[3,4] the coincidence of hematologic malignancies and pregnancy is probably not rare when this incidence is adjusted for age and sex. The incidence of acute leukemia in the general population was summarized by Tivey,[5] who found that acute leukemia may account for 50 to 500 of 100,000 hospital admissions. However, these figures are only an estimate of order of magnitude and include both sexes and all ages. In their review, Yahia et al.[6] reported that the annual death rate from acute leukemia in the entire female population is 2 per 100,000. They estimate that the death rate for females in the age group 15 to 45 is 1 per 100,000. This series also reported 2 pregnant patients with acute leukemia among 75,000 deliveries. Harris's report included one pregnant patient with acute leukemia occurring among 40,000 births, stillbirths and abortions at the Toronto General Hospital.[7] Similar data were reported from the Swedish Cancer Registry.[8] It might be concluded, then, that acute leukemia in the childbearing age group is a rare disease, but when one considers the statistics relating to age and sex, its concurrence with pregnancy is probably not as rare as was thought to be. Similar comments can be made for chronic granulocytic leukemia.

Since the occurrence of Hodgkin's disease is predominantly in the child-bearing age group,[9] its concurrence with pregnancy is not rare. The natural incidence of Hodg-

---

From the Molecular Biology Branch, Experimental Medicine Department, Medical Research Laboratory, Edgewood Arsenal, Maryland.

kin's disease for females in the age group 15 to 44 years has been reported as approximately 1.3 in 100,000.[10] This is to be contrasted with the reported incidence of Hodgkin's disease in pregnancy of approximately 1 in 6,000.[11,12] Hennessy and Rottino found 35 cases at one hospital over an 18-year period; however, they made no mention of the total number of deliveries.[13]

Since lymphosarcoma[9] and multiple myeloma[14] occur mostly in older persons, the data on their association with pregnancy are sparse. As of 1968 there were only 3 case reports in the world's literature concerning pregnancy in patients with multiple myeloma.[14–16]

Effect of Pregnancy on Course of Disease

Consideration of the vast anatomical and hormonal changes which occur during pregnancy presents a very important question: What effect will the pregnancy have when superimposed on a malignant process? The consensus is that pregnancy exerts no deleterious effect on the course of the acute and chronic leukemias[3,17–24] and Hodgkin's disease[13,25–29] except insofar as early gestation might present an obstacle to vigorous therapy.[23] This assertion is supported by the following data. Comparison of a number of pregnant patients who had acute or chronic leukemia or Hodgkin's disease with a corresponding nonpregnant group reveals similar data as to age at onset, natural history, cell type and morphology, and, most important, survival time. Furthermore, therapeutic abortions have not influenced the survival time in any of these diseases.

The average age at onset of acute leukemia in pregnancy does not differ significantly from that in the general population. In 126 patients reported in the American and Swedish literature, the average age at onset was 28 years.[6,8,30] For the population at large (both male and female), the median age for the onset of acute granulocytic

TABLE 1.—*Comparison of Leukemic Cell Type in Pregnant and Nonpregnant Women*

Period (Ref. and year)	*CGL*	*CLL*	*ALL*	*AGL*	*AML*	*Unclassified or Blast Cell*	*Erythro*	*Mixed*	*Total and %*
Pregnant									
Up to 1943	41	3	9	17	2	3	0	0	75
(30–1943)	54.7	4.0	12.0	22.7	2.7	4.0	0	0	%
Up to 1958	89	4	16	37	7	0	0	0	153
(21–1958)	58.2	2.6	10.4	24.1	4.6				%
1957–1963	22	0	8	28	6	4	2	1	69
(4–1964)	31.9		11.5	40.0	8.6	5.8	2.9	1.4	%
Average of 1958 and 1964 Reports	45	1.3	10.8	35.8					%
Nonpregnant									
1962	46	8	12	36					102
(33-1962)	45	7.8	11.8	35.2					%

Abbreviations for types of leukemia: *CGL* = chronic granulocytic; *ALL* = acute lymphocytic; *AML* = acute monocytic; *CLL* = chronic lymphocytic; *AGL* = acute granulocytic; *Erythro* = erythromyelogenous.

leukemia is 29 years, and the average age for 1,000 cases of acute leukemia of all diagnostic types in both sexes is 26.8 years.[5] In Sheehy's review of 89 cases of chronic granulocytic leukemia associated with pregnancy, the median survival time was 2.5 years.[21] This compares favorably with the median survival time of 2.6 years for 2,000 nonpregnant patients reported by Tivey.[5]

Consistent with the natural history of these diseases,[5,31] most diagnoses of chronic leukemia[21] and Hodgkin's disease[27] were made before the onset of pregnancy, whereas most diagnoses of acute leukemia were made during pregnancy.[6,30,32]

A comparison of leukemic cell types affecting pregnant and nonpregnant patients is shown in Table 1. The reviews of pregnant leukemic patients which appeared in 1943[30] and 1958[21] compare favorably with regard to diagnostic categories. However, the series reported in 1964[4] showed a decrease in the incidence of chronic granulocytic leukemia and an increase in acute granulocytic leukemia. In comparison, the figures for 102 nonpregnant females between the ages of 15 and 45[33] were intermediate between the earlier[21] and later reports[4] for pregnant patients. However, if one averages the figures for the 1958 and 1964 reports,[21,4] the diagnostic breakdown compares very favorably with those for the nonpregnant group.[33] This would indicate that the diagnostic types affecting pregnant and nonpregnant patients do not differ. These changes in the relative proportions of each cell type are also consistent with the epidemiologic studies of Court-Brown and Doll.[34]

The effect of pregnancy on the course of Hodgkin's disease has been well documented by Barry et al.[27] Eighty-four of 347 females with Hodgkin's disease in the age group 18–40 became pregnant during the course of their disease one or more times, for a total of 112 pregnancies. The most common tissue diagnosis in both groups was Hodgkin's granuloma, and the median survival time for the pregnant group was 90 months compared to 52 months for the nonpregnant group. Of 54 10-year survivors, 22 were of the pregnant group and 28 of the nonpregnant group, and the survival of 16 patients who underwent therapeutic abortion was approximately equal to those who went to term.[27] In the series reported by Hennessy and Rottino,[13] the 5- to 15-year survival in Hodgkin's disease was no different whether or not the woman had undergone a pregnancy during the course of her disease; the survival rate was 42 per cent (5-year) and 39 per cent (15-year).

Similarly, lack of effect of pregnancy on the course of melanoma,[35–37] cancer of the cervix,[37,38] sarcoma of the soft somatic tissues,[39] thyroid cancer,[37,40] gastro-intestinal cancer,[37,41] and breast cancer[42–46] has been reported.

Effect of Disease on Pregnancy

Fertility in the patient with leukemia and lymphoma is a relative problem and is more a manifestation of the patient's constitutional status than of actual disease. Consequently, there are reports in the literature of multiple births and pregnancies occurring in the patient with leukemia or lymphoma.[8,13,17,21,26,27,47]

Although pregnancy has not affected the course of the leukemias, these diseases have had a distinct effect on the course of gestation. In general, antineoplastic drug and irradiation therapy, along with improved supportive therapy with whole blood, blood products and antibiotics, has significantly lessened morbidity and prolonged survival.[33,48–50] The effects of therapy on maternal and fetal survival in acute and chronic leukemia are shown in Tables 2 and 3.

Despite the fact that hemorrhage and infection account for most of the morbidity

TABLE 2.—*Effect of Acute Leukemia on Pregnancy*

Therapy	*Before 1943*[30] *Supportive*	*1943 to 1956*[6] *Steroids or antimetabolites*	*1954 to 1964*[32] *Steroids and/or antimetabolites*
No. of patients	34	30	59
% Maternal survival to delivery	70	80	93
% Fetal survival	41	62	64

and mortality in acute leukemia,[33] these were not serious problems at the time of delivery, abortion or cesarean section.[7,30] However, parturient patients with decreased fibrinogen levels[6,23] and increased fibrinolytic activity have been reported.[6] Fibrinogen levels should, therefore, be monitored in the pregnant patient with acute leukemia, especially the promyelocytic variety.

The presence of Hodgkin's disease has not exerted a significant effect on the course of 430 pregnancies occurring in 342 women.[13,26–28] The reported incidence of spontaneous abortions for patients with Hodgkin's disease[12,28] is approximately the same as that reported for all pregnancies (7–8 per cent vs. 10 per cent).[51]

The question of transmission of disease from mother to fetus must also be considered. Although congenital leukemia has been reported to occur in infants born of hematologically normal mothers,[33] there has not been a report of congenital leukemia present at birth in a child of a mother with leukemia. The closest possibility to inherited leukemia is in the case report by Cramblett et al.[52] The diagnosis of acute lymphoblastic leukemia was made in the mother 8 days post partum, but she had had symptoms, petechiae and bleeding, at 7 months of pregnancy. The blood of the infant at 1 week of age was normal, but at 9 months of age the child had the full manifestations of acute lymphoblastic leukemia and died 3 months later.[52] The long-term follow-up of children born of leukemic or lymphomatous mothers has also failed to reveal disease transmission to the offspring.[32,53] Several reviews of the world's literature, one from 1866 to 1950, revealed only 9[54]; another, from 1862 to 1963, revealed 24 instances of transmission of maternal malignant disease to the products of conception.[55] In most instances the metastases were confined to the placenta, but the fetus had proved involvement in 8 cases; the most common diseases were melanoma and Hodgkin's disease.[55]

Although studies in animals have shown that the fetus is more tolerant to the transplantation of living homologous normal[56] or neoplastic cells[57] than at any other time in life, direct experimental evidence does prove the placenta to be an effective barrier to the transmission of malignant disease from mother to fetus. Reported attempts

TABLE 3.—*Effect of Chronic Leukemia on Pregnancy*

Therapy	*1943—Erf*[19] *Blood, Fowler's solution, brewer's yeast*	*1958—Sheehy*[21] *Blood, antimetabolites, irradiation to spleen, alkylating agents*
No. of patients	66	89
% Maternal survival to delivery	65	96.5
% Fetal survival		83.8

to transmit leukemia to fetal mice by injecting pregnant females with leukemic cells were unsuccessful. The offspring of these leukemic mothers, whether in utero, in the neonatal period, or at age 3 months, were found to be free of leukemia despite advanced leukemic infiltration of the mother's uterus before, at, or shortly after parturition. When tested by direct inoculation, these offspring showed no immunity to leukemia.[58]

Human maternal hematopoietic cells, both normal[59] and neoplastic,[60] have been shown to cross the placental barrier. In the case reported by Rigby et al., quinacrine-labeled leukemic cells were detected by ultraviolet fluorescence in the peripheral blood of the child at birth. However, leukemia did not develop in the child.[60] The fact that some cells do get through, yet do not produce disease is probably due to a genetic variability imparting host resistance, since mice have been shown to vary in their susceptibility to leukemic virus.[61]

Therapeutic Abortion

In considering therapy for the pregnant leukemic or lymphomatous patient, the question of therapeutic abortion arises. The consensus is that on the basis of the diseases themselves, therapeutic abortion is not indicated.[3,12,13,26–28,62–66] Studies of one disease, breast cancer, in which it might be thought that termination of pregnancy would benefit the patient, have also proved to the contrary.[42–46] Myles[28] gives the following indications for interruption of pregnancy in Hodgkin's disease: "(1) Where the Hodgkin's disease is localized to the inguinal or abdominal region and adequate deep X-ray therapy cannot be applied without the risk of producing an abnormal fetus, and (2) where deep X-rays have been administered to the abdominal region at a time when, unknowingly, a very early pregnancy was present." Also to be considered are the unwitting administration of a very large dose of an antimetabolite or alkylating agent either alone or in combination very early in the course of the pregnancy, as might be the case in certain experimental protocols, and the psychological effects of a continued pregnancy in a dying mother. It is perhaps best stated by Boronow[55] that "one's philosophy regarding termination of pregnancy in the presence of extra-pelvic malignancy will follow precisely his attitude toward abortion in the presence of any chronic debilitating and potentially lethal illness."

Fetal Hazards from Therapy

The increase in fetal survival has lagged behind the increase in maternal survival,

Table 4.—*Fetal Hazards due to Therapy*

1. Death in utero
2. Premature birth
3. Teratogenesis
   a. Anatomical
   b. Behavioral
4. Specific organ suppression
5. Long-term effects
   a. Retarded physical and/or mental growth and development
   b. Sterility
   c. Mutation
   d. Cancer
   e. Teratogenic in subsequent generations

largely because of the added hazard associated with chemotherapy to the viability and integrity of the fetus. Some fetal hazards arising from therapy of the mother are shown in Table 4. There is a uniqueness in the fetal response to drugs. Drug effect on the fetus may be influenced by the stage of gestation, the dose and duration of therapy,[67] sex, species and strain.[68,69] Individual genetic factors are not to be minimized, for an entire spectrum of effects, ranging from fetal resorptions to apparent normalcy, can be seen within one litter. Furthermore, the dose which produces fetal effects may not have perceptible effects on the mother.[70-72]

Death in utero can be manifested as fetal resorptions, abortions, or stillbirths with or without malformations. Delayed growth and development in utero and prematurity constitute added risks to the neonate. Those that survive the lethal effects of the drugs may have various structural malformations which may or may not affect long-term viability. These and other considerations in teratogenesis have been reviewed in greater detail.[68,69,73-80]

An area which has not received much attention is human behavioral teratology. Werboff and Gottleib have shown that the administration of various drugs to pregnant animals affected the learning potential, emotionality, sexual activity, and resistance to audiogenic seizures in the offspring without producing any gross or histologic alterations.[81] Similarly, normal litter mates of animals with hydrocephalus did not learn a maze as well as untreated controls and in addition had electroencephalographic changes.[77] A similar relation might be sought for in human behavioral problems.

Treatment of the mother with large doses of steroids or cytotoxic drugs during the last trimester of pregnancy has produced suppression of the adrenal glands[6] and bone marrow[82] in the neonate.

Long-term effects of drug exposure in utero include retarded physical and/or mental growth and development, sterility, and premature aging.[79,83] Subtle point mutations may occur in the developing fetus, so that altered coding for certain proteins may later be manifested as disease. Most drugs useful in the treatment of leukemia or lymphoma are carcinogenic in one species or another,[78,83-86] and in view of the time lag for carcinogenesis,[87] exposure in utero might be responsible for some neoplastic process appearing later in life,[78] as has been shown to occur in mice.[88,89] Finally, a source of concern for future generations stems from studies of the effect of deep X-ray on mice and on the fruit fly, *Drosophila melanogaster*. Evidence of deformity was shown to be delayed ordinarily until the third and subsequent generations. In humans, deformity due to irradiation appears to be carried as a recessive trait and although the fetus actually irradiated may be normal, deformity may appear in a second or third generation.[90] The increasing incidence of leukemia[34] and of Hodgkin's disease[10,31] might be significant in this regard.

Therapy

It is difficult to adequately assess the fetal effects of maternal chemotherapy from the literature. The reasons for this are that most of the data exist as case reports and the number of patients treated with a single drug is small, and that the regimens are varied and most patients have been treated with a combination of drugs either in a simultaneous, sequential or overlap-sequential fashion, which makes it difficult to isolate the effects of one drug or to assess drug-drug interaction. This is compounded by the fact that the organism which is the target of our concern—the fetus—is a very rapidly changing biologic system, and its susceptibility or resistance to various agents, including drugs and irradiation, changes markedly with its stage of development. Also, it is well known that drugs in combination, either multiple antineoplastic drugs or other drugs used for entirely different purposes, may alter the activity of anticancer drugs in a positive or negative fashion.

Unfortunately, most case reports do not note the use of drugs (e.g. sedatives, tranquilizers, antibiotics) that can be given in conjunction with antineoplastic agents. The following studies indicate the importance of such documentation. Gibson and Becker have shown that phenobarbital, a drug which induces liver drug-metabolizing enzymes, decreased the teratogenicity of cyclophosphamide, whereas SKF-525A, a drug which inhibits this enzyme system, enhanced its teratogenicity. This, incidentally, also suggests that the teratogenic effect of cyclophosphamide might be due to some mechanism other than alkylation.[91] Similarly, the teratogenic potential of 5-fluorouracil can be enhanced by the natural pyrimidines uracil and thymine.[92]

Radiation

The effect of radiation on the fetus depends upon the age of the embryo as well as the dose delivered to it.[93–98] The fetus is most sensitive in early gestation, when major organ formation is taking place,[99] and exposures as small as 5 R have produced an increased number of anomalies in animals.[97] Dekaban tabulated the periods of relative sensitivity to direct irradiation and found that the human fetus is most sensitive between 3 and 11 weeks of pregnancy; death or any number of malformations might ensue depending on the exposure. Beyond 20 to 25 weeks of gestation, the only effects of irradiation are those which might be observed following heavy ionizing irradiation given at any time during postnatal life; these include epilation and bone marrow depression.[100] Court-Brown and Abbatt[101] have stated that there is no threshold below which the danger of carcinogenesis would not exist, and therefore children exposed to radiation effects in utero may have late carcinogenic effects. However, the study of Wells and Steer[102] found no correlation between diagnostic X-ray examination of the abdomens of mothers during pregnancy and the development of leukemia in childhood. The incidence of leukemia and lymphoma in various irradiated populations, whether these people were irradiated for diagnostic, therapeutic, occupational or military purposes, has been very well reviewed by Latourette.[103]

When X-ray therapy is directed to areas outside the abdomen and inguinal region, shielding the abdomen with lead above, below and on the sides will eliminate exposure for externally scattered irradiation.[104,105] However, internal scatter of irradiation, an inverse function of voltage, must also be considered. Becker and Hyman[105] measured the amount of internal scatter in a phantom when 1000 R was administered via a 15 × 15 cm portal to the mid-chest and the fetal dose was estimated at 20 cm from the inferior margin of the treated area. With a 250 kv source, the fetal dose was 9.0 R; with a cobalt 60 source, 2.9 R; and with a 22.5 MV source, less than 0.1 R.

Radiation therapy was administered to 30 patients during the course of 31 pregnancies; 28 had Hodgkin's disease,[7,12,19,26,62,64–66,106–118] one had acute lymphoblastic leukemia,[17] and the other had chronic myelocytic leukemia.[19] Therapy was directed to extra-abdominal sites in 28 instances.[7,12,19,25,62,64,65,106–112,114–118] It was given as whole-body or "spray" in 3.[17,26,113] Twenty-two normal (on gross examination) children were born; the mothers of 9 had undergone irradiation either at the time of conception or during the first trimester. Two fetuses died with their mothers during gestation; they had no gross malformations. Two patients had hysterotomies in the fifth month and their fetuses were not reported to have congenital malformations.[19,107] There were five deaths in the neonatal period or early infancy. One mother had received 50 R of whole-body irradiation in the eighth month of pregnancy. Her baby was born prematurely (weight 1280 gm) and died 6 hours after birth. Postmortem examination revealed no anatomical malformations.[17] Another mother with chronic granulocytic leukemia received irradiation therapy directed to the spleen and long bones during the course of two pregnancies. In the first instance treatment was given during the eighth month of gestation. At term a hydrocephalic baby was born which had intermittent unexplained fevers until its death at age 2. This same patient became pregnant again and received an unspecified amount of irradiation to her spleen and long bones. Malignant hyperpyrexia developed in her second child 5 days after birth, and the child died on the tenth day. Fever in this case rose as high as 110°F. Postmortem examination of the child was inconclusive but toxoplasmosis was suspected.[19] Although in these two instances the X-ray beams were not aimed directly at the fetus, internal scatter could have affected their thermal regulatory centers. Two other neonatal deaths occurred on the fourth day of life. One newborn whose mother received a total of 9900 R to the chest throughout pregnancy died with pulmonary atelectasis.[62] The other, whose mother received 900 R to the chest in the fourth month of pregnancy, died with acute yellow atrophy of the liver, pneumonia and pulmonary edema.[7] Neither report listed congenital anomalies.

Ten patients were treated with a combination of irradiation and drugs. Nine of these patients had the irradiation directed to an abdominal site[29,82,119–121]; however, in only one case could the X-rays have affected the fetus directly. This was in a patient with multiple myeloma who received a total of 1500 R (which may have been started at the time of conception) over a 2-month period to the lower lumbar spine. A normal baby was born at term.[14] In most cases irradiation was combined with single drug therapy including triethylene melamine, steroids, busulfan, vinblastine, 6-mercaptopurine and urethane. There were 4 premature births; two were from mothers treated with 6-mercaptopurine in addition to irradiation of the spleen[29,119] and two were from mothers treated with busulfan, 6-mercaptopurine and irradiation to the spleen.[29,119] Three of the children survived. In the one neonatal death, the mother received 125 mg of 6-mercaptopurine during the first, eighth, and ninth months of gestation and 4–6 mg of busulfan from the second to eighth month inclusive, with splenic irradiation during the second month. The 6-mercaptopurine and busulfan were not administered concomitantly. The mother had a difficult labor necessitating cesarean section. The infant's birth weight was 1077 gm; it had multiple congenital anomalies and died at 10 weeks of age.[119]

Steroids

Administration of adrenal corticosteroids to pregnant animals is associated with a very high incidence of cleft palate in the offspring. The importance of genetics in the explanation for this defect is shown by a study in which the anomaly could be produced in almost 100 per cent of certain strains of mice, whereas others are immune.[122,123]

A summary of studies in humans follows. Steroids were administered to a total of 363 pregnant women, mostly for non-neoplastic diseases.[6,23,82,124–136] The timing of therapy during gestation was unspecified in most cases; 351 women received steroids only. The fetal problems were as follows: 1 abortion,[124] 9 stillbirths,[6,124] 16 premature births,[23,124] 6 cleft palates,[6,124–126] masculinization of 1 female,[126] and hypoadrenalism in 2 infants; 1 of the infants died[6] and the other was effectively treated with adrenal replacement therapy.[129] The death of 1 other premature infant in this review[131] could also have been due to unrecognized hypoadrenalism because of gland suppression by exogenous steroids, since the mother had received exogenous steroids throughout pregnancy. The need and value of steroids in these infants should be kept in mind, especially since the deterioration of the infant, once established, is rapid and relentless. This clinical observation is supported by experimental data which show that cortisol passes from the maternal to the fetal circulation via the placenta in relatively constant ratios[137] and that the developing fetus biosynthesizes essentially no cortisol.[138]

Folate Antagonists

Administration of one of the folate antagonists aminopterin or methotrexate to animals produces a high percentage of abortions and fetal malformations. Thiersch et al.[139,140] reported that the timing of antifolate administration is important and that the fetus had definite periods of drug sensitivity; the fetus in early gestation is more sensitive than later in pregnancy. Furthermore, nonlethal doses may produce malformations in a viable fetus.[141] However, the fetal response to drugs is unique, and varies to such a degree that a given fetus can survive its litter mates and evidence no harm.[80]

The effect of aminopterin on the human fetus has been determined largely from its use as a therapeutic or criminal abortifacient. Its effectiveness in this regard is marked, but only if given early in the first trimester. Of 36 patients who took the drug in the first trimester,[7,142–146] 26 aborted spontaneously within a matter of weeks.[7,142,145] Of 6 who aborted later or who had surgical evacuation of the uterus, 4 had malformed fetuses[142,145] and 2 were normal on gross examination.[145] Four patients went to term and delivered 3 babies with multiple congenital anomalies; 2 of them lived.[143,144,146] One patient was treated during the first trimester with methotrexate, actinomycin D and chlorambucil, with the diagnosis of recurrent choriocarcinoma. She went to term and delivered normal twins.[147] Five patients received methotrexate or aminopterin during the second or third trimester along with steroids, 6-mercaptopurine, vincristine or demecolcin. One patient had a spontaneous abortion; 4 went to term and delivered normal infants.[23,73,130,135,148]

Busulfan

Ten patients were treated with busulfan during the first trimester; 8 conceived while on therapy.[24,149–156] There were 2 premature births[150,155]; 8 went to term and delivered normal babies.[24,148,151–154,156] Two patients treated during the second and third trimester delivered normal term infants.[157,158] These observations are supported by experiments in animals which show that busulfan is the least active of all alkylating agents with regard to teratogenesis.[70]

6-Mercaptopurine

The fetal effects of 6-mercaptopurine in pregnancy are somewhat more difficult to interpret because most of the patients were treated with a combination of drugs, as mentioned earlier. However, one does get the impression that 6-mercaptopurine especially when administered during the first trimester, is associated with an increased rate of prematurity: 5 of 7 for those treated during the first trimester[23,119,130–132,134] and only 3 of 12 for those treated during the second or third trimester.[23,33,73,130,133,135,136,148,159]

Other Drugs

Other antineoplastic drugs which have been given to pregnant patients include chlorambucil,[160] cyclophosphamide,[161] triethylene melamine,[25,162,163] mechlorethamine,[27,162,164,165] vinblastine,[120,121,166,167] urethane,[14,16,18,168,169] and procarbazine.[170] However, their number is too small to allow anything but an anecdotal review. The aborted fetus of a mother treated with chlorambucil was found to have an absent kidney.[160] In animals this drug has been associated with a high number of genitourinary abnormalities.[171] One patient treated with cyclophosphamide delivered a baby with multiple congenital anomalies.[161]

Finally, a topic tangential to the above is the effect of chemotherapy or irradiation on the parental gamete prior to fertilization. There are sufficient animal studies to show that fetal effects, from resorptions to malformations or sterility of a viable fetus, may occur if conception takes place within a critical period after drug therapy. Data supporting this have been derived largely through the dominant lethal test, which is used to detect chemical mutagens.[172–176] Irradiation[176] and the alkylating agents triethylene melamine, thio-TEPA and TEPA[173] have produced positive results in animal systems, and effects on both the male[173–176] and female[172] gametes have been observed. Such studies provide the physician with better information so that he may counsel his patients who are on therapy and who may desire to have children. The increasing use of antineoplastic agents for non-neoplastic diseases emphasizes the need for such information.

Recommendations

I should like to make the following suggestions for the management of the pregnant patient with leukemia or lymphoma:

Where there is a chance for a cure, such as in the early stages of Hodgkin's disease, therapy should be as aggressive as it would be in a nonpregnant patient. The only indication for therapeutic abortion might be when the pregnant uterus is in the direct line of radiation therapy. Extra-abdominal and splenic irradiation can be safely used, with proper fetal shielding and the use of high speed equipment, so as to minimize internal scatter. The inclusion of pregnant women in multiple drug experimental protocols would be unjustifiable.

Where therapy is strictly palliative, the goal is to preserve the life of an already doomed mother so as to allow the vaginal delivery of an unaltered, viable infant. This would include adequate supportive care with blood, blood products, and antibiotic therapy as indicated, and the use of other drugs directed at the basic disease process. Indications for cesarean section should be for obstetric reasons or to deliver a viable infant from a dying mother. Chemotherapy during pregnancy should be restricted to one drug whenever feasible. This would lessen the risk to the fetus and allow better pharmacologic documentation.

Antimetabolites, especially the folate antagonists, should be avoided in the first trimester, if possible, since they pose an increased risk of abortion, prematurity and malformation. The agent 6-mercaptopurine in the smallest dose possible is probably safer than methotrexate.

Steroids may be associated with an increased incidence of prematurity, masculinization of the female and cleft palate. If administered for a prolonged period of time, especially during the last trimester, one should be alert for signs of hypoadrenalism in the newborn.

Busulfan, probably the safest alkylating agent with regard to the fetus, has been used throughout pregnancy without significant untoward effect.

Other drugs useful in the treatment of leukemia and lymphoma have not been administered to sufficient numbers of patients during pregnancy to allow adequate comment. However, if one can extrapolate from animal experiments to man, it would be safe to say that any anticancer agent administered to a pregnant patient in sufficient dosage and at the crucial time in gestation will harm the fetus.[177]

A strong plea should be made for the painstaking documentation and reporting of all drugs, especially anticancer drugs, used during pregnancy, for both their immediate and long-term effects on the fetus; this would increase our knowledge of therapeutics, human pharmacology and teratology.

REFERENCES

1. D'Espo, D. A.: Twenty-five years of obstetrics. Bull. Sloane Hosp. Women 5:1, 1959.
2. Barber, H. R. K. and Brunschwig, A.: Gynecologic cancer complicating pregnancy. Amer. J. Obstet. Gynec. 85:156, 1963.
3. Dameshek, W. and Gunz, F.: Clinical Features. *In* Leukemia, ed. 2. New York: Grune & Stratton, Inc., 1964.
4. Maloney, W. C.: Management of leukemia in pregnancy. Ann. N.Y. Acad. Sci. 144: 857, 1964.
5. Tivey, H.: The natural history of untreated acute leukemia. Ann. N.Y. Acad. Sci. 60:322, 1954.
6. Yahia, C., Hyman, G. A. and Phillips, L. L.: Acute leukemia and pregnancy. Obstet. Gynec. Survey 13:1, 1958.
7. Harris, L. J.: Leukemia and pregnancy. Canad. Med. Ass. J. 68:234, 1953.
8. Ask-Upmark, E.: Leukemia and pregnancy. Acta Med. Scand. 170:635, 1961.
9. Razis, D. V., Diamond, H. D. and Craver, L. F.: Familial Hodgkin's disease: Its significance and implications. Ann. Intern. Med. 51:933, 1959.
10. Cole, P., MacMahon, B. and Aisenberg, A.: Mortality from Hodgkin's disease in the United States. Lancet 2:1371, 1968.
11. Palacios-Costa, N., Chauanne, F. C. and Zebel-Fernandez, O.: An. d. ateno, Buenos Aires, 127, 1945. Cited by Kasdon, S. C.: Pregnancy and Hodgkin's disease with a report of three cases. Amer. J. Obstet. Gynec. 57:282, 1949.
12. Stewart, H. C., Jr. and Monto, R. W.: Hodgkin's disease and pregnancy. Amer. J. Obstet. Gynec. 63:570, 1952.
13. Hennessy, J. P. and Rottino, A.: Hodgkin's disease in pregnancy. Amer. J. Obtset. Gynec. 87:851, 1963.
14. Kosova, L. A. and Schwartz, S. O.: Multiple myeloma and normal pregnancy: Report of a case. Blood 28:102, 1966.
15. Giordano, C.: Mieloma múltiplo gravidez (primeira observaçao da casuística mundial). Matern. Infanc. 24:158, 1965.
16. Rosner, F., Soong, B. C., Krim, M. and Miller, S. P.: Normal pregnancy in a patient with multiple myeloma. Obstet. Gynec. 811:820, 1968.
17. Grier. R, M. and Richter,H. A.: Pregnancy with leucaemia. Amer. J. Obstet. Gynec. 37:412, 1939.
18. Gillim, D. L.: Leukemia and pregnancy. Amer. J. Obstet. Gynec. 70:1047, 1955.
19. Erf, L. A.: Leukemia and lymphosarcoma complicated by pregnancy: Cellular changes produced in guinea pigs by extracts of "leukemic" placenta. Amer. J. Clin. Path. 17:268, 1947.
20. Slentz, W. A.: Leukemia and pregnancy: Report of 4 cases and review of the literature. Ann. Intern. Med. 35:59, 1951.
21. Sheehy, T. W.: An evaluation of the effect of pregnancy on chronic granulocytic leukemia. Amer. J. Obstet. Gynec. 75:788, 1958.
22. Auer, J.: Acute myelogenous leucemia in pregnancy. Amer. J. Obstet. Gynec. 63:445, 1952.
23. Frenkel, E. P. and Myers, M. C.: Acute

leukemia and pregnancy. Ann. Intern. Med. 53:656, 1960.
24. Williams, D. W.: Busulfan in early pregnancy. Obstet. Gynec. 27:738, 1966.
25. Smith, R. B., Sheehy, T. W. and Rothberg, H.: Hodgkin's disease and pregnancy. Arch. Intern. Med. 102:777, 1958.
26. Bichel, J.: Hodgkin's disease and pregnancy. Acta Radiol. 33:427, 1950.
27. Barry, R. M., Diamond, H. D. and Craver, L. F.: Influence of pregnancy on the course of Hodgkin's disease. Amer. J. Obstet. Gynec. 84:445, 1962.
28. Myles, T. J. M.: Hodgkin's disease and pregnancy. J. Obstet. Gynaec. Brit. Emp. 62:884, 1955.
29. Lee, R. A., Johnson, C. F. and Halon, D. G.: Leukemia during pregnancy. Amer. J. Obstet. Gynec. 84:455, 1962.
30. McGoldrick, J. L. and Lapp, W. A.: Leucemia and pregnancy: Case report and review of the literature. Amer. J. Obstet. Gynec. 46:711, 1943.
31. Shimkin, M. B., Mettier, S. R. and Bierman, H. R.: Myelocytic leukemia: An analysis of incidence, distribution and fatality. Ann. Intern. Med. 35:194, 1951.
32. Hoover, B. A. and Schumacher, H. R.: Acute leukemia in pregnancy. Amer. J. Obstet. Gynec. 96:316, 1966.
33. Boggs, D. R., Wintrobe, M. M. and Cartwright, G. E.: The acute leukemias. Analysis of 322 cases and a review of the literature. Medicine. 41:163, 1962.
34. Court-Brown, W. M. and Doll, R.: Adult leukaemia: Trends in mortality in relation to aetiology. Brit. Med. J. 2:1063, 1959.
35. George, P. A., Fortner, J. G. and Pack, G. T.: Melanoma with pregnancy. A report of 115 cases. Cancer 13:854, 1960.
36. White, L. P., Linden, G., Breslow, L. and Harzfeld, L.: Studies on melanoma: The effect of pregnancy on survival in human melanoma. J.A.M.A. 117:235, 1961.
37. Phelan, J. T.: Cancer and pregnancy. New York J. Med. 68:3011, 1968.
38. Kinch, R. A. H.: Factors affecting the prognosis of cancer of the cervix in pregnancy. Amer. J. Obstet. Gynec. 82:45, 1961.
39. Cantin, J. and McNeer, G. P.: The effect of pregnancy on the clinical course of sarcoma of the soft somatic tissues. Surg. Gynec. Obstet. 125:28, 1967.
40. Breese, M. W.: Cancer of the thyroid in women of childbearing age. Amer. J. Obstet. Gynec. 86:616, 1963.
41. O'Leary, J. A. and Bepko, F. J., Jr.: Rectal carcinoma and pregnancy. Amer. J. Obstet. Gynec. 84:459, 1962.
42. White, T. T.: Prognosis of breast cancer for pregnant and nursing women: Analyses of 1,413 cases. Surg. Gynec. Obstet. 100:661, 1955.
43. Holleb, A. I. and Farrow, J. H.: The relation of carcinoma of the breast and pregnancy in 283 patients. Surg. Gynec. Obstet. 115:65, 1962.
44. Harrington, S. W.: Carcinoma of breast: Results of surgical treatment when the carcinoma occurred in the course of pregnancy or lactation or when pregnancy occurred subsequent to operation. Ann. Surg. 106:690, 1937.
45. Randall, L. M.: Clinical problems: Carcinoma of the breast and pregnancy. Amer. J. Obstet. Gynec. 78:1353, 1959.
46. White, T. T. and White, W. C.: Breast cancer and pregnancy: Report of 49 cases followed 5 years. Ann. Surg. 144:384, 1956.
47. Miles, F. T. and Wheeler, D.: Myelogenous leukemia and pregnancy: A report of 2 cases. Canad. Med. Ass. J. 52:407, 1945.
48. Mangalik, A., Boggs, D. R., Wintrobe, M. M. and Cartwright, G. E.: The influence of chemotherapy on survival in acute leukemia III. A comparison of patients treated during 1958–1964 with those treated in 2 sequentially preceding periods. Blood 27: 490, 1966.
49. Freireich, E. J., Gehan, E. A., Sulman, D., Boggs, D. R. and Frei, E.: The effect of chemotherapy on acute leukemia in the human. J. Chronic Dis. 14:593, 1961.
50. Kiczak, J., Lapis, J. and Majewska, M.: Odległe wyniki leczenia myleranem przewlekłych białaczek szpikowych. Pol. Arch. Med. Wewnet. 36:607, 1966.
51. Eastman, N. J. and Hellman, L. M. (Eds.): Williams' Obstetrics, 12th ed. New York: Appleton-Century-Crofts, 1961.
52. Cramblett, H. G., Friedman, J. L. and Najjar, S.: Leukemia in an infant born of a mother with leukemia. New Eng. J. Med. 259:727, 1958.
53. Diamandopoulos, G. T. and Hertig, A. T.: Transmission of leukemia and allied diseases from mother to fetus. Obstet. Gynec. 21:150, 1963.
54. Bender, S.: Placental metastases in malignant disease complicated by pregnancy. Brit. Med. J. 1:980, 1950.

55. Boronow, R. C.: Extrapelvic malignancy and pregnancy. Obstet. Gynec. Survey 19:1, 1964.
56. Billingham, R. E., Brent, L. and Medawar, P. B.: The antigenic stimulus in transplantation immunity. Nature 178:514, 1956.
57. Koprowski, H.: Immunological tolerance in tumor transplantation. Fed. Proc. 16: 592, 1957.
58. Burchenal, J. H.: Experimental studies on the relation of pregnancy to leukemia. Amer. J. Cancer. 39:309, 1940.
59. Macris, N. T., Hellman, L. M. and Watson, R. J.: The transmission of transfused sickle-trait cells from mother to fetus. Amer. J. Obstet. Gynec. 76:1214, 1958.
60. Rigby, P. G., Hanson, T. A. and Smith, R. S.: Passage of leukemic cells across the placenta. New Eng. J. Med. 271:124, 1964.
61. Gross, L.: Viral etiology of leukemia and lymphoma. Blood 25:377, 1965.
62. Kasdon, S. C.: Pregnancy and Hodgkin's disease. Amer. J. Obstet. Gynec. 57:282, 1949.
63. Klawans, A. H.: Pregnancy complicated by Hodgkin's disease. Amer. J. Obstet. Gynec. 43:895, 1942.
64. Kushner, J. I.: Pregnancy complicating Hodgkin's disease. Amer. J. Obstet. Gynec. 42:526, 1941.
65. Nagel, M.: Lymphogranulomatose maligne et grossesse: Trois nouvelles observations. Bruxelles Med. 32:1659, 1952.
66. Tenenblatt, W. and Horton, C. E.: Hodgkin's disease and pregnancy: Review of the literature and report of a case. West. J. Surg. Obstet. Gynec. 59:120, 1951.
67. Ingalls, T. H., Curley, F. J. and Prindle, R. A.: Experimental production of congenital anomalies. New Eng. J. Med. 247:758, 1952.
68. Karnofsky, D. A.: Drugs as teratogens in animals and man. Ann. Rev. Pharmacol. 5:447, 1965.
69. Cahen, R. L.: Experimental and clinical chemoteratogenesis. Advances Pharmacol. 4:263, 1966.
70. Murphy, M. L., Del Moro, A. and Lacon, C.: The comparative effect of five polyfunctional alkylating agents on the rat fetus, with additional notes on the chick embryo. Ann. N.Y. Acad. Sci. 68:762, 1958.
71. Chaube, S., Kury, G. and Murphy, M. L.: Teratogenic effects of cyclophosphamide (NSC-26271) in the rat. Cancer Chemother. Rep. 51:363, 1967.
72. Gibson, J. E. and Becker, B. A.: The teratogenicity of cyclophosphamide in mice. Cancer Res. 28:475, 1968.
73. Sokal, J. E. and Lessman, E. M.: Effect of cancer chemotherapeutic agents on the human fetus. J.A.M.A. 172:1765, 1960.
74. Kalter, H.: Teratology and pharmacogenetics. Ann. N.Y. Acad. Sci. 151:997, 1968.
75. Committee on Teratology. Commission on Drug Safety: Final Report. Chicago, 1963.
76. Commission on Drug Safety: Report of Conference on prenatal effects of drugs. Chicago, 1963.
77. Commission on Drug Safety: Workshop in Teratology, University of Florida College of Medicine, Gainesville, Florida, 1964.
78. DiPaolo, J. A. and Kotin, P.: Teratogenesis-oncogenesis: A study of possible relationships. Arch. Path. 81:3, 1966.
79. Karnofsky, D. A.: Late effects of immunosuppressive anticancer drugs. Fed. Proc. 26:925, 1967.
80. DiPaolo, J. A.: Teratogenic agents: Mammalian test systems and chemicals. Ann. N.Y. Acad. Sci. 163:801, 1969.
81. Werboff, J. and Gottleib, J. S.: Drugs in pregnancy: Behavioral teratology. Obstet. Gynec. Survey 18:420, 1963.
82. Bierman, H. R., Aggeler, P. M., Thelander, H., Kelly, K. H. and Cordes, F. L.: Leukemia and pregnancy: A problem in transmission in man. J.A.M.A. 161:220, 1956.
83. Conklin, J. W., Upton, A. C. and Christenberry, K. W.: Further observations on late somatic effects of radiomimetic chemicals and X-rays in mice. Cancer Res. 25:20, 1965.
84. Kelly, M. G., O'Gara, R. W., Gadekar, K., Yancey, S. T. and Oliverio, V. T.: Carcinogenic activity of a new antitumor agent, N - isopropyl - α-(2 - methyl - hydrazino) - p - toluamide, hydrochloride (NSC-77213). Cancer Chemother. Rep. 39:77, 1964.
85. Krakoff, I. N. and Karnofsky, D. A.: Growth-inhibiting drugs: Their anticancer, anti-immune and teratogenic effects. *In* Di Palma, J. R. (Ed.): Drill's Pharmacology in Medicine. New York: McGraw-Hill, 1965, p. 1231.
86. Shimkin, M. B.: Biological tests of carcinogenic activity. Arch. Environ. Health 16: 522, 1968.
87. Videbaek, A.: Chlornaphazin (Erysan) may induce cancer of the urinary bladder. Acta Med. Scand. 176:45, 1964.
88. Druckrey, H., Preussmann, R. and Ivan-

kovic, S.: N-nitroso compounds in organotropic and transplacental carcinogenesis. Ann. N.Y. Acad. Sci. 163:676, 1969.

89. Rice, J. M.: Transplacental carcinogenesis in mice by 1-ethyl-1-nitrosourea. Ann. N.Y. Acad. Sci. 163: 813, 1969.

90. Giles, A. M.: Pregnancy following pelvic irradiation. J. Obstet. Gynaec. Brit. Emp. 56:1041, 1949.

91. Gibson, J. E. and Becker, B. A.: Effect of phenobarbital and SKF-525-A on the teratogenicity of cyclophosphamide in mice. Teratology 1:393, 1968.

92. Wilson, J. G., Jordan, R. L. and Schumacher, H.: Potentiation of the teratogenic effects of 5-fluorouracil by natural pyrimidines. I. Biological aspects. Teratology 2:91, 1969.

93. Russell, L. B.: Effects of low doses of X-rays on embryonic development in the mouse. Proc. Soc. Exp. Biol. Med. 95:174, 1957.

94. Roland, M. and Weinburg, A.: Radiation effects on the unborn embryo immediately after conception. Amer. J. Obstet. Gynec. 72:1167, 1951.

95. Murphy, D. P.: Outcome of 625 pregnancies in women subjected to pelvic radium or roentgen irradiation. Amer. J. Obstet. Gynec. 18:179, 1929.

96. Hammer-Jacobsen, E.: Congenital malformations induced by radiation. Strahlentherapie 116:152, 1961.

97. Rugh, R.: Low levels of X-irradiation and the early mammalian embryo. Amer. J. Roentgen, 87:559, 1962.

98. Edwards, J. H.: Congenital malformation of the central nervous system in Scotland. Brit. J. Prev. Soc. Med. 12:115, 1958.

99. Hazards of radiation. Editorial. Brit. Med. J. 2:716, 1962.

100. Dekaban, A.: Abnormalities in children exposed to X-irradiation during various stages of gestation: Tentaive timetable of radiation injury to the human fetus. Part I. J. Nucl. Med. 9:471, 1968.

101. Court-Brown, W. M., and Abbatt, J. D.: Incidence of leukemia in ankylosing spondylitis treated with X-rays. Lancet 1:1283, 1955.

102. Wells, J. S. and Steer, C.: Relationship of leukemia in children to abdominal irradiation of mothers during pregnancy. Amer. J. Obstet. Gynec. 81:1059, 1961.

103. Latourette, H. B.: Induction of lymphoma and leukemia by diagnostic and therapeutic irradiations. Radiol. Clin. N. Amer. 6:57, 1968.

104. Kaplan, G., Collica, C. and Rubenfeld, S.: Gonadal exposure incident to roentgen therapy. Radiology 76:887, 1961.

105. Becker, M. H. and Hyman, G. A.: Management of Hodgkin's disease coexistent with pregnancy. Radiology 85:725, 1965.

106. Paviot, J., Levrat, M. and Jarricot, H.: Observation anatomoclinique d'un cas de granulome malin: Grossesse intercurrente; stenose des grosses bronches. Lyon Med. 150:437, 1932.

107. McDonald, I.: Hodgkin's disease in pregnancy. J. Obstet. Gynec. Brit. Comm. 63:931, 1956.

108. Hartweg, H. and Braun, H.: Lymphogranulomatose und Schwangerschaft. Strahlentherapie 94:213, 1954.

109. Summers, J. E. and Reid, W. C.: Hodgkin's disease complicated by pregnancy. J.A.M.A. 137:787, 1948.

110. Dyes, O.: Lymphogranulomatose und Schwangerschaftsunterbrechung. Munchen. Med. Wschr. 86:605, 1939.

111. Mertens, W.: Lymphogranulomatose und Schwangerschaft. Strahlentherapie 94:213, 1954.

112. Hartvigsen, B.: Hodgkin's disease and pregnancy. Acta Radiol. 44:317, 1955.

113. Portmann, U. V. and Mulvey, B. E.: Hodgkin's disease and pregnancy: Report of 4 cases. Cleveland Clin. Quart. 17:149, 1950.

114. McSwain, B. and Haber, A.: Hodgkin's disease complicated by pregnancy. Southern Med. J. 44:105, 1951.

115. Adair, F. L. (Ed.): Obstetrics and Gynecology. Vol. 2. Philadelphia: Lea and Febiger, 1940.

116. Olmsted, G. S.: Hodgkin's disease and pregnancy: The outcome of 625 pregnancies in women subjected to pelvic radium or roentgen irradiation. Amer. J. Obstet. Gynec. 18:179, 1929.

117. Brougher, J. C.: Pregnancy in Hodgkin's disease. West. J. Surgery Obstet. Gynecol. 57:430, 1949.

118. Bastenie, S. F. and Snoeck, J.: Un cas de granulomatose maligne décelé et soigné au cours d'une grossesse, reste sans récidive pendant trois ans. Bruxelles Med. 16:290, 1935.

119. Diamond, L., Anderson, M. M. and McCreadie, S. R.: Transplacental transmission of busulfan (Myleran) in a mother with leukemia. Pediatrics 25:85, 1960.

120. Rosenzweig, A. I., Crews, Q. E., Jr. and Hopwood, H. G.: Vinblastine sulfate in

Hodgkin's disease in pregnancy. Ann. Intern. Med. 61:108, 1964.

121. Lacher, M. J.: Use of vinblastine sulfate to treat Hodgkin's disease during pregnancy. Ann. Intern. Med. 61:113, 1964.

122. Fraser, F. C. and Fainstat, T. D.: Production of congenital defects in the offspring of pregnant mice treated with cortisone. Pediatrics 8:527, 1951.

123. Fraser, F. C., Kalter, H., Walker, B. E. and Fainstat, T. D.: The experimental production of cleft palate with cortisone and other hormones. J. Cell. Comp. Physiol. 43 (Suppl.):237, 1954.

124. Bongiovanni, A. M. and McPadden, A. J.: Steroids during pregnancy and possible fetal consequences. Fertil. Steril. 2:181, 1960.

125. Popert, A. J.: Pregnancy and adrenal cortical hormones. Brit. Med. J. 1:967, 1962.

126. Cohlan, S. Q.: Teratogenic agents and congenital malformations. J. Pediat. 63: 650, 1963.

127. Sato, H.: Effect of adrenocorticoids during pregnancy. Lancet 2:1235, 1963.

128. Board, J. A., Lee, H. M., Draper, D. A. and Hume, D. M.: Pregnancy following kidney homotransplantation from a nontwin: Report of a case with concurrent administration of azathioprine and prednisone. Obstet. Gynec. 29:318, 1967.

129. Morgan, J. E. and Reyes, C. T.: The association of acute lymphatic leukemia and pregnancy. Obstet. Gynec. 8:642, 1956.

130. Rothberg, H., Conrad, M. E. and Cowley, R. G.: Acute granulocytic leukemia in pregnancy: Report of 4 cases with apparent acceleration by prednisone in one. Amer. J. Med. Sci. 237:194, 1959.

131. Merskey, C. and Rigal, W.: Pregnancy in acute leukemia treated with 6-mercaptopurine. Lancet 2:1268, 1956.

132. Ravenna, P. and Stein, P. J.: Acute monocytic leukemia in pregnancy: Report of a case treated with 6-mercaptopurine in the first trimester. Amer. J. Obstet. Gynec. 85:545, 1963.

133. Shumacher, H. R.: The use of 6-mercaptopurine in late pregnancy. Amer. J. Obstet. Gynec. 74:1361, 1957.

134. Sinykin, M. B. and Kaplan, H.: Leukemia and pregnancy: A case report. Amer. J. Obstet. Gynec. 83:220, 1962.

135. Coopland, A. T., Friesen, W. J. and Galbraith, P. A.: Acute leukemia in pregnancy. Amer. J. Obstet. Gynec. 105:1288, 1969.

136. Loyd, H. O.: Acute leukemia complicated by pregnancy. J.A.M.A. 178:1140, 1961.

137. Midgeon, C. J., Prystowsky, H., Grumbach, M. M. and Byron, M. C.: Placental passage of 17-hydroxycorticosteroids: Comparison of the levels in maternal and fetal plasma and effect of ACTH and hydrocortisone administration. J. Clin. Invest. 35:488, 1956.

138. Gardner, L. I.: Newer knowledge of adrenocortical disturbances. Pediat. Clin. N. Amer. 4:889, 1957.

139. Thiersch, J. B., and Philips, F. S.: Effect of 4-amino-pteroylglutamic acid (aminopterin) on early pregnancy. Proc. Soc. Exp. Biol. Med. 74:204, 1950.

140. Thiersch, J. B.: The effect of 6-mercaptopurine on the rat fetus and reproduction of the rat. Ann. N.Y. Acad. Sci. 60:220, 1955.

141. Murphy, M. L. and Karnofsky, D. A.: Effect of azaserine and other growth inhibiting agents on fetal development of the rat. Cancer 9:955, 1965.

142. Thiersch, J. B.: Therapeutic abortion with a folic acid antagonist, 4-aminopteroylglutamic acid (4-amino PGA) administered by the oral route. Amer. J. Obstet. Gynec. 63:1298, 1952.

143. Meltzer, H.: Congenital anomalies due to attempted abortion with 4-aminopteroylglutamic acid. J.A.M.A. 161:1253, 1956.

144. Warkany, J., Beadury, P. H. and Hornstein, S.: Attempted abortion with aminopterin (4-amino-pteroylglutamic acid). Amer. J. Dis. Child. 97:274, 1959.

145. Goetsch, C.: An evaluation of aminopterin as an abortifacient. Amer. J. Obstet. Gynec. 83:1474, 1962.

146. Shaw, E. B. and Steinbach, H. L.: Aminopterin-induced fetal malformation: Survival of infant after attempted abortion. Amer. J. Dis. Child. 115:477, 1968.

147. Li, M. C.: Management of choriocarcinoma and related tumors of uterus and testes. Med. Clin. N. Amer. 45:661, 1961.

148. Hill, J. M. and Loeb, E.: Cited by Sokal, J. E. and Lessmann, E. M.: Effects of cancer chemotherapeutic agents on the human fetus. J.A.M.A. 172:1765, 1960.

149. Ruiz-Reyes, G. and Tamayo-Perez, R.: Leukemia and pregnancy: Observation of a case treated with busulfan (Myleran). Blood 18:764, 1961.

150. White, L. G.: Busulfan in pregnancy. J.A.M.A. 179:973, 1962.

151. Sherman, J. L. and Locke, R. V.: Use of busulfan in myelogenous leukemia during pregnancy. New Eng. J. Med. 259:288, 1958.
152. Neu, L. T.: Leukemia complicating pregnancy. Missouri Med. 59:220, 1962.
153. Dennis, L. H. and Stein, S.: Busulfan in pregnancy: Report of a case. J.A.M.A. 192:715, 1965.
154. Smalley, R. V. and Wall, R. L.: Two cases of busulfan toxicity. Ann. Intern. Med. 64:154, 1966.
155. Izumi, H. M.: Myleran in pregnancy: Report of a case. J.A.M.A. 161:969, 1956.
156. Uhl, N., Eberle, P. and Quellhorst, E.: Busulfan treatment in pregnancy: A case report with chromosome studies. German Med. Monthly. 14:383, 1969.
157. Earll, J. M. and May, R. L.: Busulfan therapy of myelocytic leukemia during pregnancy. Amer. J. Obstet. Gynec. 92: 580, 1965.
158. Korbitz, B. C. and Reiquam, C. W.: Busulfan in chronic granulocytic leukemia: A spectrum of clinical considerations. Clin. Med. 76:16, 1969.
159. Sandberg, A. A., cited by Sokal, J. E., and Lessmann, E. M.: Effect of cancer chemotherapeutic agents on the human fetus. J.A.M.A. 172:1765, 1960.
160. Shotton, D. and Monie, L. W.: Possible teratogenic effect of chlorambucil on a human fetus. J.A.M.A. 186:74, 1963.
161. Greenberg, L. H. and Tanake, K. R.: Congenital anomalies probably induced by cyclophosphamide. J.A.M.A. 188:423, 1964.
162. Boland, J.: Reticuloses: Clinical experience with nitrogen mustard in Hodgkin's disease. Brit. J. Radiol. 24:513, 1951.
163. Wright, J. C.: The effect of triethylene melamine and of triethylene phosphoramide in human neoplastic diseases. Acta Un. Int. Canc. 11:220, 1955.
164. Zoet, A. G.: Pregnancy complicating Hodgkin's disease. Northwest Med. 49: 373, 1950.
165. Deuschle, K. W. and Wiggins, W. S.: The use of nitrogen mustard in the management of two pregnant lymphoma patients. Blood 8:576, 1953.
166. Armstrong, J. G., Dyke, R. W., Fouts, P. J. and Jansen, C. J.: Delivery of a normal infant during the course of oral vinblastine sulfate therapy for Hodgkin's disease. Ann. Intern. Med. 61:106, 1964.
167. Nordlund, J. J., DeVita, V. T. and Carbone, P. P.: Severe vinblastine-induced leukopenia during late pregnancy with delivery of a normal infant. Ann. Intern. Med. 69: 581, 1968.
168. Imber, I. and Meharg, J. G.: Leukemia and pregnancy treated with urethane. Amer. J. Obstet. Gynec. 69:438, 1955.
169. Creskoff, H. J., Fitz-Hugh, T. and Frost, J. W.: Urethane therapy in leukemia. Blood 3:896, 1948.
170. Wells, J. H., Marshall, J. R. and Carbone, P. P.: Procarbazine therapy for Hodgkin's disease in early pregnancy. J.A.M.A. 205: 935, 1968.
171. Monie, I. W.: Chlorambucil-induced abnormalities of urogenital system of rat fetuses. Anat. Rec. 139:145, 1961.
172. Generoso, W. M.: Chemical induction of dominant lethals in female mice. Genetics 60:181, 1968.
173. Epstein, S. S. and Shafner, H.: Chemical mutagens in the human environment. Nature 219:385, 1968.
174. Cattanach, B. M., Pollard, C. E. and Isaacson, J. H.: Ethyl methanesulfonate-induced chromosome breakage in the mouse. Mutat. Res. 6:297, 1968.
175. Moutschen, J.: Mutagenesis with methyl methanesulfonate in the mouse. Mutat. Res. 8:581, 1969.
176. Schroder, J. H.: Dominant lethal mutation after irradiation of mouse spermatogonia with 600 R of X-rays. Intern. J. Radiat. Biol. 16:377, 1970.
177. Karnofsky, D. A.: Mechanisms of action of certain growth-inhibiting drugs. *In* Wilson, J. G. and MacKany, J. (Eds.): Teratology, Principles and Techniques. Chicago: University of Chicago Press, 1965.

Topical 5-Fluorouracil Chemotherapy for Premalignant and Malignant Epidermal Neoplasms

By EDMUND KLEIN, M.D., HALINA MILGROM, M.D., HOWARD L. STOLL, M.D., FREDERICK HELM, M.D., MARY J. WALKER, M.S., AND OLE A. HOLTERMANN, M.D., PH.D.

THE PURPOSE OF THIS CHAPTER is to review the background and current status of local chemotherapy. This approach, pursued for the past decade, has resulted in new methods of therapy for superficially located neoplasms.[1-3] The superficial location of tumors in the skin and subcutaneous tissues permits considerably more investigative flexibility than is afforded by deep-seated tumors. Cutaneous tumors have therefore been used as model systems in animals and in man for exploring the interactions among tumor, host and exogenous factors. Local administration of tumor agents permits manipulation of superficial tumors and adjacent tissues without major adverse changes in the overall status of the host and his defense mechanisms. Cutaneous tumor models therefore made it possible to study the effects of immunologic factors upon the course of tumors and to develop immunotherapeutic approaches to malignant disease.[4-6]

In the course of these studies, it became apparent that locally administered antitumor agents could profoundly affect the course of superficially located tumors. The effects of locally administered antitumor agents were shown to result in palliation of cutaneous metastases of disseminated tumors.[1-3] Local chemotherapy was subsequently found to result in control of premalignant and malignant epidermal lesions. These observations formed the basis of topical chemotherapy with 5-fluorouracil (5-FU)[7] for premalignant and malignant lesions of the skin which has recently come into widespread use.

Initial studies on mice with carcinogen-induced and transplanted tumors indicated the safety and effectiveness of a number of antitumor agents administered to superficially located neoplasms. Local administration of antitumor agents resulted in regressions of malignant lesions in the skin and subcutaneous tissues. The incidence of methylcholanthrene-induced papillomas and squamous cell carcinomas was also reduced by concurrent local applications of chemical carcinogens and cytostatic agents, thus suggesting the possibility of prophylaxis by local chemotherapy.

Bone marrow depression and other signs of systemic toxicity were not encountered in several species during topical administration of antitumor agents to tumors or normal depilated skin comprising up to 30 per cent of the body surface. Studies on local administration of ^{14}C-labeled 5-FU revealed minimal or nondetectable levels of radioactive carbon in the blood tissues.

To assess further the potential hazards of applying anticancer drugs directly to

---

From the Department of Dermatology, Roswell Park Memorial Institute, Buffalo, New York.

Supported in part by the Albert and Mary Lasker Foundation, New York, New York; grant No. 5-G03-RM-00013-03A1 from the Regional Medical Program of Western New York; grant No. CA-08678 from the National Cancer Institute and grant No. AI 09479-01 from the National Institute of Allergy and Infectious Diseases, National Institutes of Health; grant No. T-429 from the American Cancer Society, New York, New York; grant No. G-64-RP-15 from the United Health Foundation of Western New York; and the Arcade Community Chest, Arcade, New York.

tumors, initial clinical studies were carried out on cutaneous lesions in patients with advanced disseminated malignant disease[2,3] prior to investigation of the less serious primary cutaneous neoplasms.[8,9]

Various categories of antimitotic agents were investigated in our initial studies. These agents included several types of antimetabolites (folic acid antagonists, substituted purines and pyrimidines, and other analogues); alkylating agents (nitrogen mustard and derivatives, aziridyl compounds); antibiotics (actinomycin D, mitomyocin C, Mithramycin, and derivatives); alkaloids (e.g. vinblastine, vincristine); and a number of other agents (e.g. derivatives of steroid hormones). Approximately 30 different agents with antimitotic activities and, when possible, congeners without cytostatic action were included in these studies.

Tumors studied initially included several types of adenocarcinoma, malignant melanoma, cutaneous lymphomas, metastatic squamous cell carcinoma, and several types of sarcoma which had metastasized to the skin.[3] Various modes of administration and dosages were explored in patients with multiple, clinically equivalent tumors[9] to provide the basis of subsequent, more definitive studies whose protocols specified double-blind placebo-controlled investigations.[8,10]

It was clear from the initial studies that locally administered antitumor agents markedly altered the course of neoplasms. In appropriate conditions, complete regressions of malignant lesions were induced.[3,11] Systemic toxic effects were not encountered, even when the antitumor agents were administered locally at concentrations several orders of magnitude above the maximal levels which could be attained in tumors or surrounding tissues by systemic administration.[12] Local side effects were relatively minor and temporary and were limited to irritation of the skin and subcutaneous tissues, which underwent rapid recovery.[7]

Tumor destruction occurred with minimal or no effects on surrounding tissues.[12] If local chemotherapy was continued after the tumor had begun to disappear, normal granulation tissue started to form and re-epithelialization of the site previously occupied by tumor occurred.[7] These observations indicated that in certain situations antitumor agents will eradicate malignant cells without preventing the reduplication of non-neoplastic cells.

It was therefore apparent that selective antitumor effects could be readily induced in a large variety of malignant tumors by a number of different biochemical agents.[3] The selectivity of their action may be due to differences in their effects on malignant and nonmalignant cells. Alternatively, defense mechanisms of the host may be able to exert their effects, if the integrity of the tumor cell is compromised by chemotherapeutic agents, while similar damage to the normal cell is repaired or circumvented. A further possibility is that chemical agents produce changes in the tumor cells that result in expression of antigenic characteristics, thus leading to an effective and selective antitumor reaction mediated by immune mechanisms of the host.[4,6]

In view of the selective induction of regressions in lesions treated with local chemotherapy, and the lack of systemic toxicity, this approach was extended to a group of approximately 100 patients with various types of disseminated malignant disease. Regressions including complete tumor eradication were observed in 46 patients. Marked effects were noted in cutaneous metastases of adenocarcinoma, primary and metastatic squamous cell carcinoma, and in Kaposi's hemorrhagic sarcoma; 50 to 70 per cent of 140 lesions treated showed partial to complete regressions. The response rate was particularly satisfactory in 15 patients with Kaposi's hemorrhagic sarcoma; 14 patients showed significant responses including 6 patients with more than 90 per cent of tumors undergoing complete involution as a result of vinblastine or vincristine administered locally or in combination with systemic chemotherapy.[13] Less marked although significant effects were noted in cutaneous lesions of lymphomas, sarcomas, melanomas and miscellaneous other tumors, with a response rate of approximately 30 per cent of more than 100 lesions treated in 44 patients. These findings are consistent with our previous observations.[3]

Highly satisfactory results of local and, in particular, topical chemotherapy were subsequently obtained in patients with extensive premalignant and primary malignant epidermal tumors.[2,11,14–17] Several cytostatic agents investigated in exploratory studies were selected for more intensive investigation. These agents, 5-fluorouracil (5-FU), 5-mercaptouracil (5-MU), dimethylurethimine (AB 132), nitrogen mustard (NH), and actinomycin D (Ac-D), were submitted to double-blind placebo-controlled studies; of these agents 5-FU showed statistically highly significant effects ($p > 0.001$) resulting in tumor eradication in a group of 32 patients.[8] Topical 5-fluorouracil was therefore investigated further in order to delineate the types of cutaneous neoplasms for which it was effective,[18] to evaluate various modes of administration,[10] and to develop optimal methods for treatment.[19,20] As a result of these studies,[7,15,17] which have extended over the past ten years, topical 5-FU was found to be highly effective in the management of premalignant keratoses and extensive multiple superficial epidermal carcinomas (basal cell carcinomas, squamous cell carcinomas). In appropriate circumstances 5-year cure rates were more than 90 per cent in several thousand premalignant lesions treated in more than 150 patients and more than 80 per cent in over 1,000 superficial basal cell carcinomas treated in a group of 50 patients.[7] The response rate in nodular or infiltrative lesions of basal cell carcinoma and squamous cell carcinoma was approximately 60 per cent of 120 lesions in 86 patients.[7,19,20] The results in patients with nodular lesions are considerably less satisfactory than those obtained by surgery or radiation therapy, which approximate a cure rate of 98 per cent. Recent studies indicate that modification of the methods using topical 5-FU can result in considerably higher cure rates[21] than those obtained in initial trials.

The effect of topical 5-FU on epidermal neoplasms is selective. Inflammatory reactions are limited predominantly to the sites of lesions, usually with minimal and readily reversible effects on the normal skin or other tissues. The deeper lying epidermal appendages such as the hair roots and glands are usually spared and regenerate. As the neoplastic cells undergo involution, they are being largely replaced by connective tissue in the dermis and normal epithelium in the surface epidermis. As a rule, therefore, healing proceeds without scarring and with restoration of normal skin color and texture.

Exposure to the sun is a major and frequently primary factor in most patients with premalignant and malignant epidermal lesions, which occur usually as multiple neoplasms either concurrently or sequentially or both in the sun-exposed areas. It was, therefore, of significance to find that topical 5-FU resulted in inflammatory reactions in clinically undiagnosed lesions which then underwent involution. Neoplastic epidermal lesions are thereby detected at considerably earlier stages than would otherwise be possible, and are prevented from progressing into clinically more significant problems.

Topical 5-FU Therapy in Superficial Premalignant and Primary Malignant Epidermal Lesions

The procedures for topical chemotherapy described below have been developed for the management of premalignant keratoses (solar, X-ray–induced), and for superficial basal cell carcinomas (e.g. multiple basal cell nevoid syndrome, late radiation dermatitis) and squamous cell carcinomas in situ. These methods are less satisfactory for patients with arsenical dermatitis and associated premalignant and malignant lesions, or infiltrative lesions of basal cell carcinomas or squamous cell carcinomas. Modifications of presently used procedures of topical chemotherapy are under investigation for the management of arsenical dermatitis and infiltrative lesions, but have not yet been adequately evaluated.

Topical 5-FU therapy is indicated primarily for the management of extensive multiple actinic keratoses, multiple extensive superficial basal cell carcinomas and syndromes characterized by large numbers of squamous cell carcinomas in situ. Premalignant keratoses include those caused by sunlight, or other sources of ultraviolet light, and precancerous lesions arising in late radiation dermatitis undergoing malignant degeneration. Malignant epidermal lesions suitable for topical 5-FU include particularly multiple superficial basal cell carcinomas and squamous cell carcinomas, which are not adequately managed by surgery or radiation therapy because of persistent tumor formation involving extensive areas of the body surface. Several syndromes, such as the multiple basal cell nevoid syndromes, xeroderma pigmentosum, late radiation dermatitis and severely sun-damaged skin, have therefore been markedly benefited by topical 5-FU therapy.

The concentration of topical 5-FU indicated for the majority of keratoses and malignant epidermal lesions ranges from 1 per cent to 20 per cent, although further changes in both directions are indicated at times. The average concentration found to be satisfactory for the majority of lesions is 5 per cent 5-FU in a cream base.[20] The use of 5-FU solutions in propylene glycol has also been explored[12] but was found to be less satisfactory in our hands for reasons stated below. The lower range of 5-FU concentrations (1 per cent, 2 per cent) is primarily indicated for the management of lesions associated with late X-ray dermatitis and for patients with atrophic or severely sun-damaged skin. The lower concentrations of 5-FU may also be used when it is desired to avoid a brisk inflammatory reaction. In the latter case, administration of low concentrations of topical 5-FU requires at least 6 to 10 weeks and results in lower cure rates. Residual lesions are then treated with higher concentrations of topical 5-FU, but since these are much fewer than initially, they can be treated individually, and the overall reaction to 5-FU is milder. Areas undergoing treatment may be washed in the usual manner. At the height of the reaction, the use of soap may result in discomfort and can be replaced by water compresses. The use of water-soluble cosmetic agents may be helpful to cover sites at which reactions are occurring without interfering with treatment, although administration of these agents may result in or increase discomfort.

Topical 5-FU has virtually no serious systemic or local side effects. Since the presence of keratoses or multiple superficial epitheliomas usually indicates the likelihood of other clinically undetectable lesions, the application of the topical chemotherapeutic preparation should initially not be limited to the sites of clinically overt involvement but should be extended to the normal appearing skin of the area under treatment for the purpose of eradicating unrecognized early lesions. Except for the treatment of residual lesions following a recent course of topical chemotherapy, the 5-FU preparation should be applied to the general area involved, such as the entire forehead or the entire face including the apparently normal skin between the lesions. Application of the cream is carried out twice daily. A thin layer of 5-FU cream is gently applied to the premoistened area with a moistened finger, which may be protected by a rubber glove or fingercot. Discomfort, even at the height of the inflammatory reaction, is usually minor, but gentle administration facilitated by premoistening reduces irritation and results in minimal interference with the healing process.

The response to topically administered 5-FU consists of one or more of the following reactions in the sequence listed: erythema, edema, vesiculation, erosion, ulceration, exudation, necrosis, granulation tissue formation, re-epithelialization, and healing. The onset of healing is indicated by re-epithelialization, as a rule starting at the margin of the lesions where tumor involution usually reaches completion earlier, since the tumor as a rule has less substance at its periphery than at more central parts of the lesion. A course of topical 5-FU usually requires from 2 to 4 weeks. Administration of 5-FU is continued through the various stages of the inflammatory reaction including the period of necrosis and at least the onset of re-epithelialization. Exfoliative specimens or biopsies provide more definitive guidelines as to the presence of residual neoplastic cells. With some experience, the time at which 5-FU administration may be discontinued is readily recognized. A brisk reaction lasting for 3 to 7 days which usually begins to subside is an indication for discontinuing topical 5-FU administration. Alternatively, administration of 5-FU may be continued until healing has progressed far enough to indicate that residual tumor is not likely to be present, since viable neoplastic tissue will not be replaced by normal tissue. A relatively safe period for attaining eradication of keratoses and superficial epitheliomas is a 4-week course.

Application of 5-FU without a covering dressing is usually sufficient for premalignant keratoses and for superficial epitheliomas. To accelerate the reaction to topical 5-FU therapy and to render it more effective in lesions which appear to be resistant, frequently as a result of deeper infiltration, occlusion with a plastic dressing (e.g. a polyethylene sheet, transparent wrap, Telfa pads) is used.[20] The discomfort may be increased because occlusive treatment may intensify the inflammatory reaction induced by 5-FU.

Since the carcinogenic effects of ultraviolet radiation in sunlight or of X-rays in producing premalignant or malignant epidermal neoplasms are cumulative and onset of these lesions may follow variable periods of latency, new lesions may continue to develop in patients with extensive involvement after an initial course of topical 5-FU, although the incidence may be considerably reduced. Resistance to topical 5-FU has not been encountered after an initial course of therapy with this agent. Subsequent courses of 5-FU therapy are therefore indicated in patients with an otherwise appreciable incidence of new lesions, and should be repeated at intervals which will range from 6 months to 2 years as determined by the frequency of new lesions. In some patients with exceedingly frequent de novo development of keratoses or epitheliomas, an almost continuous maintenance regimen with topical 5-FU may be indicated.

Necrosis resulting from the inflammatory response to topical 5-FU is almost invariably superficial. Infection has not been demonstrated in lesions undergoing topical therapy since the antimitotic action of 5-FU results in inhibition of the growth of microorganisms. Attention to residual necrotic exudate after discontinuation of topical 5-FU therapy, however, is indicated. As a rule, specific therapy is not required. Local administration of antibiotic preparations, such as topical polymyxin, bacitracin, or other antimicrobial agents, is usually sufficient but rarely needed. Necrotic exudate following topical 5-FU therapy can usually be controlled by lukewarm tap water or saline compresses. Treatment of the associated discomfort with topical anti-inflammatory agents (e.g. corticosteroids) and mild analgesics (e.g. aspirin) is usually adequate but also rarely required.

The most frequently encountered side effects leading to appreciable necrotic exudate result from local nonspecific irritation of the skin, more frequently found in the flexural folds such as the nasolabial or infraorbital regions. These side effects are usually the result of inadvertent retention of 5-FU in the affected regions, which are thus exposed to the equivalent of occlusive administration of the antimitotic agent. Nonspecific irritations are usually treated adequately by preventing the topical 5-FU preparation from reaching the affected sites. This can more readily be accomplished with 5-FU cream preparations than solutions since the former can be more effectively confined to the sites of their application. In general, treatment of other areas does not require interruption. Nonspecific irritations during topical 5-FU therapy are usually readily reversible and improve within 24 to 48 hours after avoiding contact with 5-FU at the affected sites. If discomfort is more severe, compresses with lukewarm tap water or saline solution are helpful. Treatment of the associated discomfort with mild analgesics (e.g. aspirin) and topical corticosteroid preparations is usually adequate. Topical steroids should be applied four or more times per day confined to the affected areas, which should have been premoistened with tap water, and should be limited to a period of 48 to 72 hours. More protracted administration of topical steroids, particularly to areas involving mucocutaneous junctions such as the vermilion border, may result in delayed healing.

The patient should be warned prior to instituting topical 5-FU therapy that the appearance of the reaction, particularly if the face or other exposed areas are involved, may be unsightly. He should also be assured of the temporary nature and relative innocuousness of the inflammatory reaction to topical 5-FU and of the excellent cosmetic results. This can be readily accomplished by showing the patient a sequence of photographs of the status prior to treatment, during or at the height of the reaction, and the end result.

Less intensive management with topical 5-FU is employed for the treatment of actinic keratoses and basal cell epitheliomas associated with late radiation dermatitis. This regimen may also be used for the management of solar keratoses and superficial epitheliomas associated with conditions other than late radiation dermatitis if a brisk inflammatory reaction to 5-FU is to be avoided for cosmetic or other reasons. The course of treatment will be correspondingly protracted, and isolated residual lesions will require additional, more intensive treatment (which, however, may then be confined to the sites of involvement since the majority of lesions will already have been eradicated by a preceding course at lower concentrations of topical 5-FU). The overall reaction will be comparatively mild and in many instances limited to erythema, which can be readily covered by appropriate cosmetic preparations.

While less intensive management is elective for other patients, it is essential that initially low concentrations of topical 5-FU be used in patients with radiation dermatitis. Consequently, a low concentration of topical 5-FU (usually 1 per cent) should be employed initially and administration should be limited to a small area to evaluate the intensity of the response. The concentration of 5-FU and the frequency of application may then be increased (or decreased) as indicated by the intensity of the reaction. For some patients with late radiation dermatitis, application of 1 per cent 5-FU cream once every second or third day or even less frequently may be indicated and will prove satisfactory for the control of neoplastic lesions. Alternatively, the concentrations may have to be decreased to as low as 0.01 per cent to avoid an excessive reaction. Conversely, concentrations of 5-FU may have to be increased up to 20 per cent or higher and may have to be applied as often as 4 times a day for protracted periods in order to treat resistant lesions. It may further be desirable to sequentially treat relatively small areas in patients with radiation dermatitis at any one time to avoid the appreciable discomfort of a widespread intensive reaction. The procedures found adequate for the management of radiation dermatitis in the initial course frequently provide the basis for subsequent courses since these patients usually require repeated treatment. Some patients may require almost continual therapy with topical 5-FU for adequate control because even in moderately severe late radiation dermatitis the incidence of new lesions can be appreciable. Since neoplasia associated with radiation dermatitis may be serious, leading to highly invasive basal cell or squamous cell carcinomas, early or prophylactic treatment as made possible by topical chemotherapy is indicated.

Extensive and close monitoring of patients under topical 5-FU therapy has failed to reveal evidence of systemic toxicity. Bone marrow depression has not been documented even in patients in whom extensive areas of the body surface (up to 50 per cent) were treated concurrently for periods of 8 to 12 weeks.

Unless there are other unrelated indications, routine laboratory studies are usually not required. In rare instances allergic reactions to 5-FU have been encountered. These are of the immediate type and do not usually require treatment, except for discontinuation of 5-FU. Exposure to sun should be avoided during 5-FU therapy, since the intensity of the reaction is frequently increased. When exposure to sun cannot be adequately prevented, the use of a sunscreen agent should be instituted.

The methods of topical 5-FU therapy have been described as a prototype of topical chemotherapy because they have been proved to be effective and have become widely used clinical procedures. It should be pointed out that the management of individual problems by local chemotherapy may require considerable modification of the methodology described above. These modifications include the use of antitumor agents other than 5-FU, the combination of two or more chemical antitumor agents, and the concurrent use of ionizing radiation or of immunotherapy. Concentrations of antitumor agents may have to be adjusted to individual requirements, the mode of administration may have to be altered (e.g. intralesional injections), and the frequency and duration of administration may require variation as indicated by the behavior of the tumor under treatment. Discussion of the results obtained by local chemotherapy will be limited to the use of 5-FU in the common types of epidermal neoplasms, since this experience is based on more extensive data than are available for other antitumor agents. Unless otherwise stated, the results presented were obtained with the methods as described above and are based on a follow-up of 5 years or longer.

Premalignant Keratoses

By far the most common epidermal neoplasms are actinic keratoses, the vast majority of which are caused by exposure to the ultraviolet radiation of the sun. The lesions therefore predominate on sun-exposed areas such as the face, the arms and the back of the hands. They also occur on other areas of the body surface which have been exposed to the sun as a result of occupational or recreational activities. Solar keratoses are almost exclusively limited to the white race; their incidence is higher in fair individuals than in those with darker complexions. Sun-induced keratoses and frankly malignant epidermal lesions occur with an exceedingly high incidence in albinism or in depigmented areas (vitiligo scars) regardless of racial origin. Solar keratoses present as multiple lesions varying in size from less than a millimeter to several centimeters in diameter, with irregular outlines, vary in color from red to brownish and usually have a rough scaly surface which may be elevated above surrounding skin. The incidence of solar keratoses has been estimated to be from 5 million to 20 million people in the United States.

There has been considerable debate about the propensity of solar keratoses to be transformed into squamous cell carcinomas, as well as debate regarding metastatic dissemination. The issue is clouded by the de novo development of squamous cell carcinomas in the skin of patients who have had extensive exposure to sun, since ultraviolet radiation may result in the direct formation of squamous cell carcinoma without prior recognizable induction of solar keratoses. If conversion of solar keratoses to squamous cell carcinoma occurs, it is protracted and has been estimated to involve between 2 and 5 per cent of premalignant keratoses over periods of up to 20 years. Since early squamous cell carcinomas and solar keratoses resemble each other clinically and since the incidence of carcinomas in areas involved by solar keratoses is high, the nature of the origin of squamous cell carcinoma is largely of academic interest; treatment and removal of potentially as well as actually malignant lesions are indicated in any event.

A patient with extensive solar keratoses and multiple squamous cell carcinomas in situ is shown in Figure 1. It should be pointed out that the lesions suspected of being squamous cell carcinomas should be treated definitively and as rapidly as possible, which usually requires surgery or radiation therapy. In patients who have extensive involvement with multiple lesions, however, the clinical diagnosis of each squamous cell carcinoma may be complicated since numerous biopsies are required. Furthermore, since microscopic diagnosis of squamous cell carcinoma is dependent on adequate sampling, efforts should be made to obtain specimens from areas which have appreciable infiltration around or subjacent to suspicious lesions, particularly where marked exophytic components are present. It is frequently not practical to perform biopsy on every suspicious lesion when the number of tumors is large or extensive areas are confluently involved. Until the development of topical chemotherapy, it was therefore difficult or impossible to treat all involved areas.

In our experience with patients with extensive solar keratoses, we have found that topical 5-FU therapy resulted in unmasking clinically undiagnosable and therefore unsuspected lesions of squamous cell carcinoma. In general, the reaction at sites involved by squamous cell carcinoma is more intense than in keratoses. Biopsies or exfoliative cytology of areas which reacted with more severity than those involved by the majority of keratoses frequently revealed evidence of squamous cell carcinomas in situ. Since these lesions usually respond to topical 5-FU therapy, further management may not be required, except for careful periodic observation of the sites suspected or found to be involved by squamous cell carcinoma. Lack of recurrence over a 3- to 5-year period usually indicates lasting eradication. However, any solar keratosis may contain incipient squamous cell carcinoma which would be unrecognizable

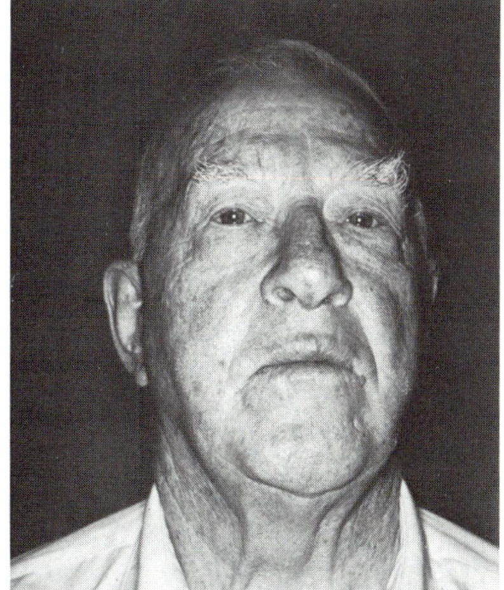

FIG. 1.—Multiple solar keratoses and squamous cell carcinomas in situ prior to therapy with topical 5-fluorouracil (5-FU).

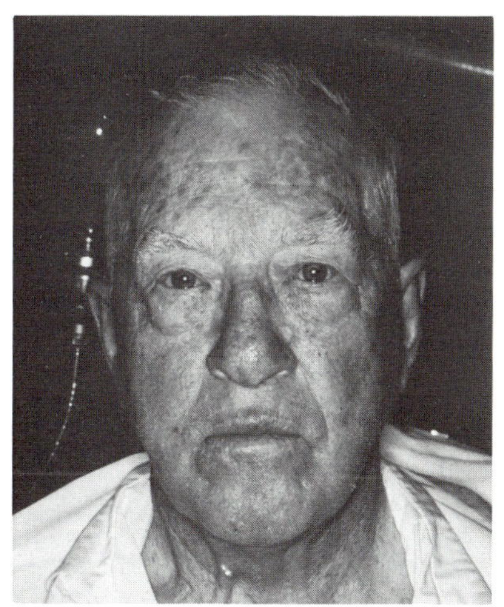

FIG. 2.—Onset of reaction after 7 days of topical applications of 5 per cent 5-FU cream twice daily to the forehead. Note the increase in the number of apparent lesions as compared to the pretreatment state.

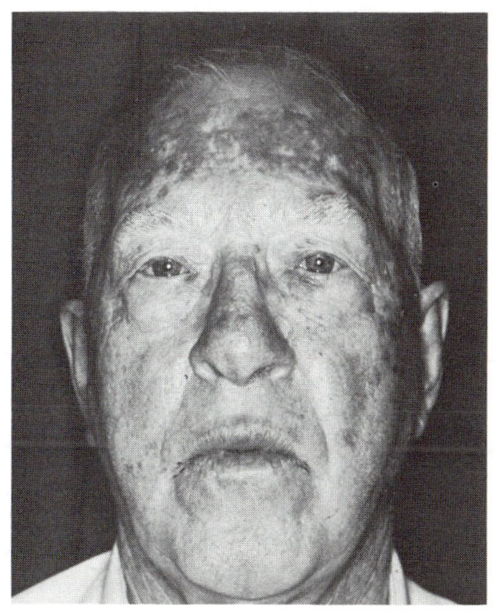

FIG. 3—Height of reaction occurs within 15 days of twice daily applications of 5 per cent 5-FU cream to the forehead. Large number of lesions have become apparent, resulting in confluent erosions. Sparing of the uninvolved skin is apparent by lack of reaction.

clinically or by the reaction to 5-FU. Therefore, biopsies should be done on lesions which fail to resolve after adequate topical 5-FU therapy and such lesions treated by the most effective method available for definitive management.

Treatment of solar keratoses is indicated as a therapeutic measure for the removal of these lesions and as a prophylactic measure for preventing the development or progression of incipient squamous cell carcinoma. The majority, if not all, of the lesions will usually undergo resolution, thus reducing the problems of management of extensive involvement to relatively few lesions. Biopsies should be done on residual lesions after a course of 5-FU which has resulted in clearing of most of these lesions, which should be followed carefully to determine whether they contain early squamous cell carcinoma or are resistant keratoses. If infiltrative squamous cell carcinoma is present, surgery or radiation therapy is indicated. Alternatively, if keratosis or squamous cell carcinoma in situ is present, administration of 5-FU may be repeated, preferably under occlusion or at a higher concentration and for a more protracted period than the initial course. More than 90 per cent of lesions which have failed to respond to the initial course will be adequately treated following a second, more

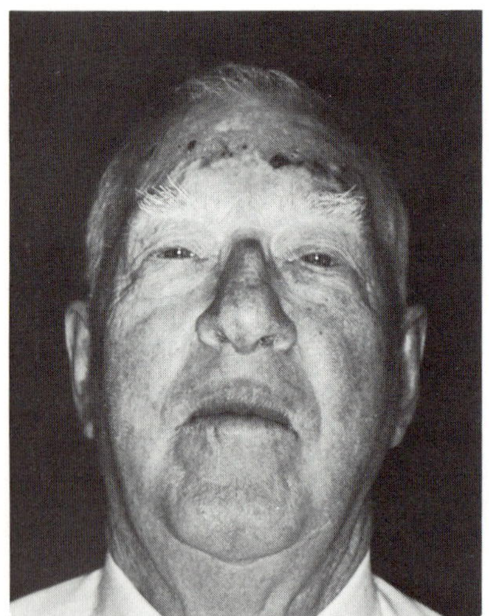

FIG. 4.—Healing has taken place over most of the previously involved areas despite continued administration of topical 5-FU cream. Areas still showing marked reaction are indicative of more intense involvement and represent sites at which actinic keratoses include squamous cell carcinomas in situ.

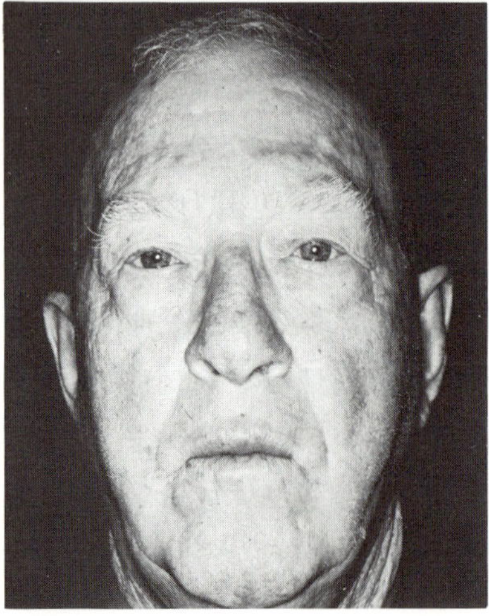

FIG. 5.—Complete healing takes place within 3 to 4 weeks of discontinuing topical 5-FU. Depigmented scars are largely due to procedures used prior to topical chemotherapy.

intensive course of topical 5-FU. In a group of approximately 200 patients with extensive solar keratoses followed for periods of 5 years or longer, 5 per cent 5-FU cream was found to result in resolution of at least 95 per cent of lesions treated. The number of lesions per patient varied from 5 clinically diagnosable areas to more than 1,000 lesions.

Onset of the reaction to topical 5-FU usually occurs within 5 to 10 days, although in second or subsequent courses it may occur earlier, although in some patients it may take up to 3 weeks before a reaction supervenes. The intensity of the reaction will be determined by the concentration of 5-FU and the frequency of application. Occlusion accelerates the onset of the reaction and increases the intensity as well as the effectiveness of the response. We have used occlusion to bring about rapid onset of the reaction and continued with subsequent open administration of the agent in order to decrease the time required for an adequate course of topical 5-FU therapy.

The various stages of the response are illustrated in Figures 2 to 5. Figure 2 shows the onset of the reaction which consists of erythema at sites involved by clinically recognizable lesions as well as in areas in which the presence of keratoses or other epidermal neoplasms could not be otherwise detected. Under continued administration of topical 5-FU the reaction then proceeds to erosion, ulceration and the formation of a necrotic exudate (Fig. 3). At this stage re-epithelialization commencing from the margin of the lesions may become apparent. This indicates that the tumor is undergoing resolution and is being replaced by normal granulation tissue and epidermis. Necrosis usually takes 2 to 3 weeks to become apparent. In most patients, topical 5-FU therapy may be terminated at this stage. However, the only definitive basis for concluding that therapy has been adequate is provided by histologic examination of biopsy specimens or exfoliative cytology. As a rule this is impractical and not indicated since the trauma of biopsies or the difficulty of evaluating cytologic specimens frequently exceeds more practical alternative management. If therapy is stopped at this stage and found not to have resulted in complete regression, most lesions will nevertheless have resolved. Residual lesions may be treated with a second course of topical 5-FU, the application of which is then limited to the sites showing continued involvement. Alternatively, topical 5-FU therapy may be continued for a week following the onset of necrosis, which usually prolongs the duration of healing, but almost invariably results in regression of more than 90 per cent of lesions.

Continued administration of topical 5-FU permits healing to proceed (Fig. 4), although it may delay recovery. Thus, where there is doubt, or for those patients with a previous history of large numbers of residual lesions, 5-FU therapy may be continued, preferably at a reduced concentration, until healing has proceeded almost to completion. It is a fairly simple matter to have the pharmacist cut the concentration of 5-FU in a coarse preparation by adding a compatible vanishing base in the appropriate proportions.

In the group of patients under observation for 5 years or longer, we found the most satisfactory results (in terms of 5-year cure rates) to follow a 4-week course of topical administration of 5 per cent 5-FU cream in a vanishing base, with applications of the preparation twice a day. Comparative studies in which the 5 per cent 5-FU cream was used on one-half of the face and then followed on the other half of the face by application of 5-FU propylene glycol at concentrations of 5 per cent, 2 per cent, and 1 per cent demonstrated the superiority of topical 5-FU cream over other types of preparations in several respects. The 5-year cure rate with the 5 per cent 5-FU cream exceeded 95 per cent, while the cure rates following use of the propylene glycol preparation amounted to 88 per cent for the 5 per cent 5-FU solution, 77 per cent for the 2 per cent 5-FU solution, and less than 75 per cent for the 1 per cent 5-FU solution.

Furthermore, the incidence of side effects such as nonspecific dermatitis involving the nasolabial and infraorbital folds was appreciably more common when the 5-FU solutions were used. The reasons for the more common incidence of side effects is inability to confine the solution to the sites of intended application with resulting accumulation of 5-FU in the flexor folds. For these reasons treatment with 5-FU solutions usually has to be discontinued or interrupted once side effects have occurred. Resumption of therapy with 5-FU solutions is frequently associated with repeated nonspecific dermatitis. On the other hand, 5-FU cream can be applied in such a manner that a minimum of the preparation will find its way into the flexor folds. The incidence of side reactions can thereby be minimized. When side effects do occur, therapy with 5-FU cream can be continued with appropriate precaution to prevent the cream from coming into contact with sites of nonspecific irritation. Thus, the incidence of side effects can be reduced, the management of side effects is facilitated, and interruption of therapy can be avoided with the use of the 5-FU cream preparation.

Basal Cell Carcinomas

Basal cell carcinomas are the most common skin cancers. They are also the most common cancers in the white race. Although most basal cell carcinomas occur on sun-exposed areas, approximately 30 per cent of these lesions are found in areas which are not exposed to the sun. Basal cell carcinomas are malignant lesions which are characterized primarily by local invasion; if metastases occur at all, they are extremely rare. Their clinical characteristics include a "pearly" border surrounding a lesion which varies in size, shape, color, degree of infiltrate, nodularity, erosion, and ulceration or exophytic tumor components. For purposes of this chapter, basal cell carcinomas are divided into the superficial type, with minimal invasion of the underlying dermis, and the nodular type, which extends into the dermis and may have advanced into the subcutaneous tissues.

Though clinical differentiation of basal cell carcinomas from other types of tumors such as squamous cell carcinomas and malignant melanoma can be made with a high degree of statistical accuracy, definitive diagnosis of any one lesion is possible only on the basis of biopsy. In the presence of multiple superficial lesions encountered in various skin cancer syndromes such as the multiple basal cell nevoid syndrome, late radiation dermatitis with malignant degeneration, arsenical dermatitis, xeroderma pigmentosum and extensive solar damage to the skin, it is not practical to perform a biopsy on every lesion. However, a number of biopsies have to be taken in order to determine the nature of the lesions. Infiltrating tumors should be treated definitively and as rapidly as possible; topical therapy with 5-FU is indicated particularly for patients with multiple lesions which involve extensive areas of the body surface. In these patients surgery or radiation therapy frequently is inadequate since the high incidence of new lesions and the extent of existing lesions make concurrent therapy of involved areas impractical. Nevertheless, it must be borne in mind that squamous cell carcinomas or malignant melanoma may develop in patients with multiple basal cell carcinomas and that therapy for these potentially metastasizing and rapidly invasive lesions is optimally accomplished by radiation therapy or surgery.

Topical 5-FU therapy was proved to be highly effective for patients with multiple superficial basal cell carcinomas, whereas it was found to be less satisfactory for patients with nodular basal cell carcinomas. The 5-year cure rate in a group of approximately 50 patients with multiple superficial basal cell carcinomas associated with the various syndromes enumerated above was 80 per cent or more following topical 5-FU therapy. The 5-year cure rates for nodular basal cell carcinomas employing the method described above using an occlusive regimen of 20 per cent 5-FU cream was 56 per cent in a group of approximately 100 patients. Recent data[21] indicate that more protracted courses of topical 5-FU may considerably increase the cure rate for nodular basal cell carcinomas. These approaches, however, are still in the investigative stages and should not be considered as a routine form of therapy.

The pattern of response of superficial basal cell carcinomas (Figs. 6–10) to topical 5-FU resembles closely that described for the treatment of solar keratoses. Figure 6 shows superficial basal cell carcinomas prior to therapy. The lesions are flat and minimally infiltrated, and have slight, if any, nodularity. The margins are irregular and may or may not be sharply demarcated from the surrounding uninvolved skin. The lesions may be covered by intact but neoplastic epidermis or may be ulcerated.

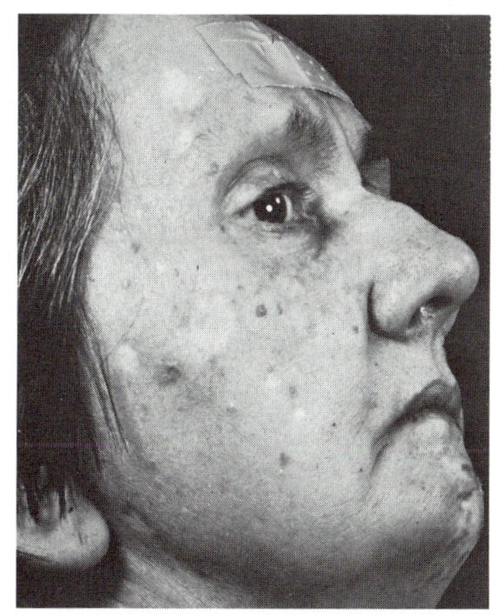

FIG. 6.—Patient with multiple superficial and nodular basal cell carcinomas prior to topical chemotherapy. Nodular basal cell carcinomas are present on the cheek, forehead (covered with tape) and chin. Those lesions present on the cheek, temple, nasolabial fold, chin, upper lip, nose and forehead are of the superficial type. Depigmented areas are atrophic scars from previous surgical and radiation procedures for the removal of basal cell carcinomas.

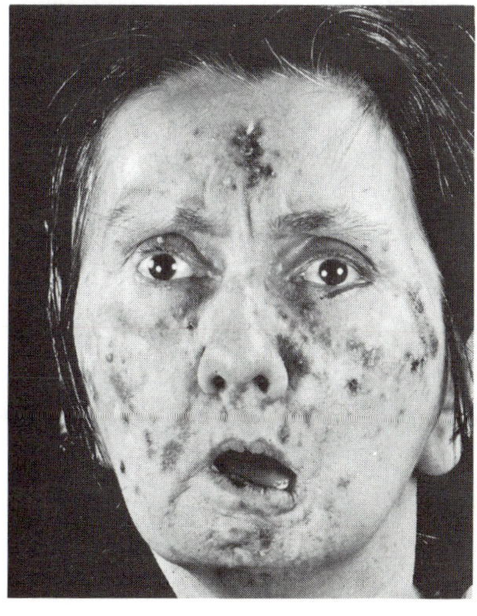

FIG. 7.—Two weeks following daily administration of 20 per cent 5-FU cream. The patient shows selective reaction at the sites of lesions. Nonspecific reaction is apparent around the left nasolabial fold. Skin not involved by basal cell carcinomas including sites of atrophic scars does not show reaction. The reaction is well tolerated by severely retarded patients who are otherwise difficult to manage.

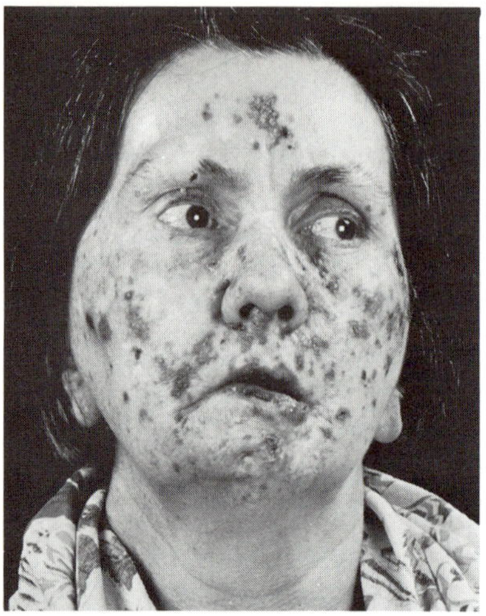

FIG. 8.—Reaction following 4 weeks of topical administration of 5-FU cream twice a day is shown. The reaction has subsided at a number of sites at which basal cell carcinomas have undergone involution. Nonspecific reaction around nasolabial folds has subsided except where carcinomas were present. Recovery of nonspecific reaction in the region of the nasolabial fold occurred within 48 hours of withholding direct administration of 5-FU cream to areas where side effects were apparent. Marginal re-epithelialization of lesions on both cheeks and upper lip indicates that tumor involution has occurred. Topical 5-FU therapy was continued for 5 more days.

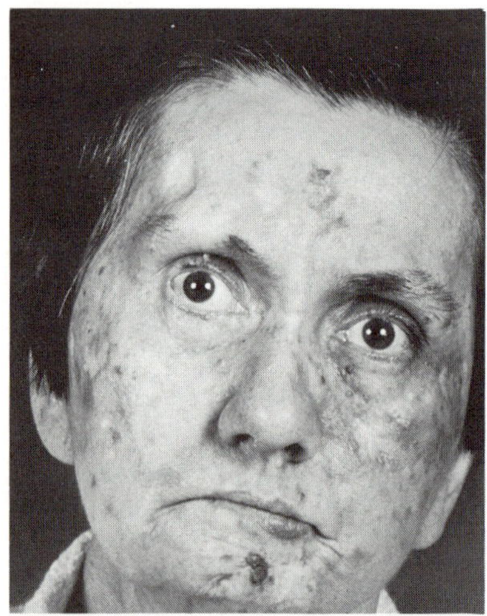

FIG. 9.—Ten days following discontinuation of topical 5-FU. The majority of lesions have progressed toward healing. Residual pigmentation frequently accompanied by erythema at sites of previous involvement fades spontaneously over the ensuing 3 to 6 weeks.

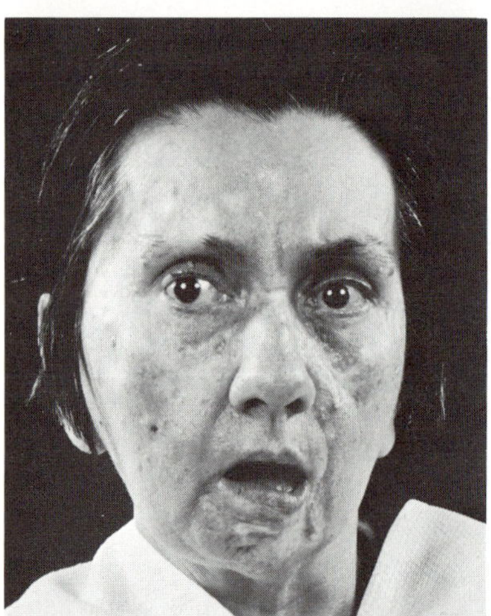

FIG. 10.—Three weeks after discontinuing topical 5-FU therapy, most lesions have disappeared and healed. Pigmentation has also disappeared. Residual nodular basal cell carcinoma on the right cheek is the only lesion which requires further treatment.

The size may vary considerably and the color may range from that of normal skin to various shades of red, brown or yellow. Figure 7 illustrates the onset of the response to topical 5-FU. As in actinic keratoses, the initial reaction to topical chemotherapy is erythema accompanied by varying degrees of edema limited to the sites involved by basal cell carcinoma lesions. The reaction may remain at that stage until the erythema gradually fades as neoplastic cells are being replaced by normal epidermis. Alternatively, the reaction will proceed to erosion and ulceration accompanied or followed by a necrotic exudate (Fig. 8). While topical administration of 5-FU is being continued and the tumor undergoes resolution, starting usually at the edges of the lesion, the neoplastic tissue is replaced by granulation tissue and normal epithelium (Fig. 9). In the absence of nodules within the lesions, therapy can usually be discontinued at that stage. In the presence of nodules, topical therapy should be continued until the nodules are no longer detectable and exfoliative cytologic specimens or biopsies fail to show residual neoplastic cells. It will be noted that as therapy is continued, re-epithelialization proceeds while the tumor undergoes resolution. Thus, healing may be impeded but is not prevented by topical 5-FU. Topical administration of this agent may therefore be continued until most or all of the lesions have undergone re-epithelialization. Since involvement of the underlying dermis by superficial basal cell carcinoma is minimal, healing after topical chemotherapy as a rule proceeds with minimal or no scar formation.

More than 95 per cent of residual superficial lesions respond to a subsequent 4-week course of 20 per cent 5-FU cream twice a day under occlusion. Erosions after administration of a 20 per cent 5-FU preparation are usually more marked than after the use of 5 per cent 5-FU and healing may be correspondingly delayed.

The results of topical 5-FU administration in nodular basal cell carcinomas are less satisfactory than in superficial lesions. Topical 5-FU therapy is not indicated for the routine management of solitary nodular basal cell carcinomas, since the results of surgery or radiation therapy show cure rates of approximately 98 per cent. In our experience a 4-week course of daily applications of 20 per cent 5-FU cream under occlusion results in cure rates of approximately 60 per cent. A second 4-week course following an interval of one month after termination of the first course of topical 5-FU raises the cure rate to approximately 70 per cent. An uninterrupted course of 8 to 10 weeks results in cure rates of approximately 80 per cent. Since surgery or radiation therapy requires considerably less time for treatment, these modalities are more desirable for the management of nodular basal cell carcinomas as far as both expediency and superior cure rates are concerned. The cosmetic results of effective topical 5-FU therapy for nodular basal cell carcinomas may be superior to those obtained by other modalities, but this consideration does not justify the selection of topical chemotherapy as the treatment method.

There may be occasions on which topical 5-FU therapy can offer advantages over surgery or radiation therapy or when it may be optimally used in conjunction with these methods. Consideration may be given to the use of topical chemotherapy in patients of advanced age in whom extensive surgical procedures or radiation therapy may not be indicated for a variety of reasons. The presence of multiple nodular basal cell carcinomas in close proximity to one another may justify an attempt to remove some of the lesions by topical chemotherapy to reduce the number of sites requiring surgery or plastic repair or the extent of the area which has to be irradiated. In this way surgical procedures may be simplified and the need for plastic repair may be reduced or eliminated. Similar considerations may pertain to sites at which radiation may result in functional impairment, such as carcinomas of the upper lip or the eyelids. It is essential that sites of infiltrative basal cell carcinoma treated with topical 5-FU be followed up at least every 3 months for 2 to 3 years and every 6 months thereafter to detect recurrences as early as possible.

Squamous Cell Carcinoma

Therapy of squamous cell carcinoma should be prompt and definitive; this can best be assured by surgery or radiation therapy. For multiple squamous cell carcinomas in situ, as in patients with extensive solar skin damage, arsenical dermatitis resulting in cutaneous malignant lesions or late radiation dermatitis undergoing malignant degeneration, topical chemotherapy may be indicated, when surgery or radiation therapy is not feasible because large areas are involved by multiple or extensive lesions. Topical chemotherapy in these patients should be limited to superficial lesions, whereas infiltrative tumors require surgical removal or radiation. Topical chemotherapy for multiple squamous cell carcinomas in situ is used in a manner similar to that described for solar keratoses and superficial basal cell carcinomas. Because of the potential seriousness of squamous cell carcinomas, we have preferred to use a 20 per cent 5-FU cream applied twice daily under occlusion, even when large areas were involved with multiple lesions such as the entire back or chest. For this purpose we used a plastic vest to provide occlusion. The reaction of multiple intraepidermal squamous cell carcinomas (Figs. 11–15) to topical 5-FU is analogous, but usually more intense than that of actinic keratoses or superficial basal cell carcinomas. The onset of the reaction (see Fig. 12) is marked by erythema which may be accompanied by a nonspecific reaction involving the hair follicles or the orifices of the sebaceous glands. The latter side effects are readily reversed following discontinuation of occlusive dressings. Administration of topical 5-FU, however, can be continued without occlusion while the side effects are subsiding (see Fig. 13). Thus, topical therapy is initiated under occlusion and then continued on an open basis. Satisfactory results are obtained in that 90 per cent or more of superficial squamous cell carcinomas (in situ) were found to undergo resolution in a group of 20 patients. Residual lesions which are relatively few as compared to the number initially present can then be readily treated surgically or by radiation therapy.

An ever-present danger of squamous cell carcinoma, whether treated by surgery, radiation therapy, or topical chemotherapy, is local extension or recurrence and metastatic spread. Despite a biopsy which indicates an in situ lesion, sampling may

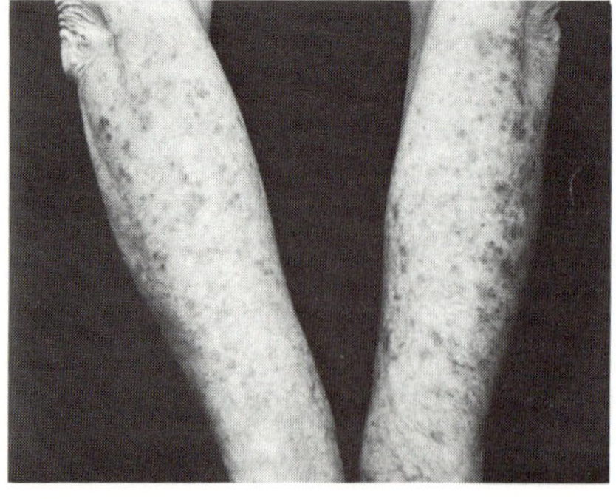

FIG. 11.—A patient with multiple squamous cell carcinomas and keratoses associated with arsenical dermatitis prior to topical 5-FU chemotherapy.

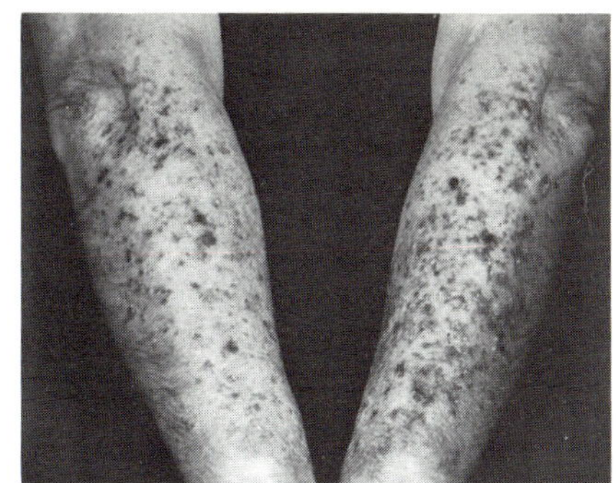

FIG. 12.—Intense reactions at sites involved by squamous cell carcinomas and arsenical keratoses are apparent after administration of 20 per cent 5-FU cream twice daily under occlusion for 5 days.

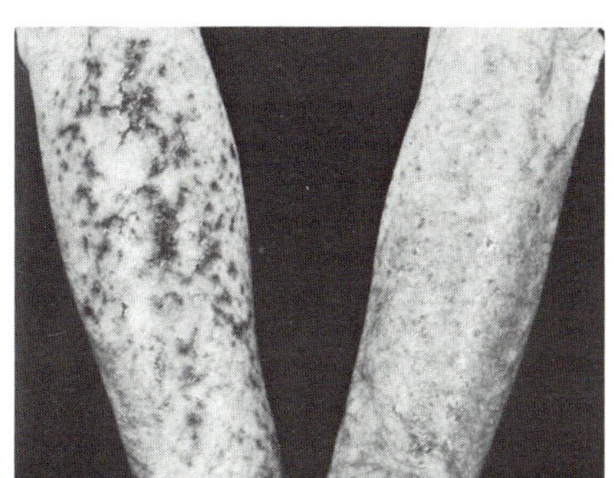

FIG. 13.—Reaction is considerably more marked on the right arm, where occlusion has been continued for 14 more days, although some areas are beginning to heal. The left arm has almost completely recovered despite continued open application of topical 5-FU.

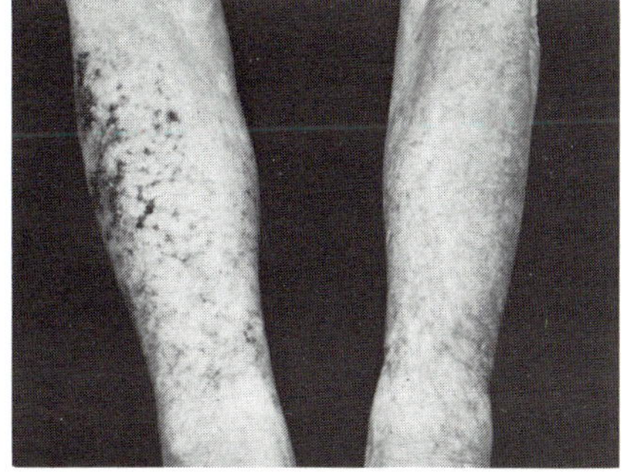

FIG. 14.—Ten days after discontinuation of occlusive dressings but continued topical (open) administration of 20 per cent 5-FU cream, the right arm is proceeding toward healing, while the left arm, to which open topical administration of 20 per cent 5-FU has been continued, has undergone complete recovery.

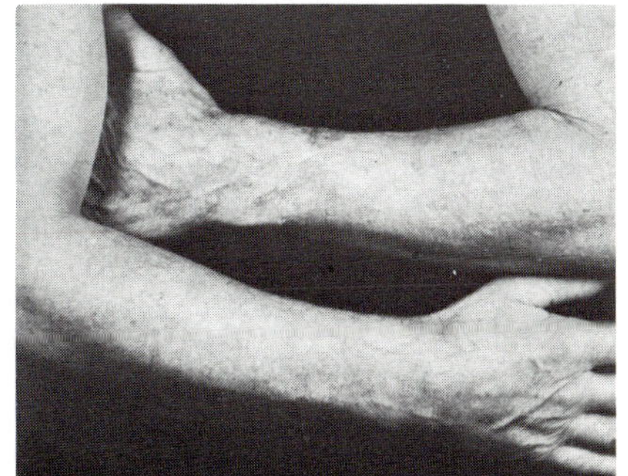

FIG. 15.—Complete recovery has taken place 4 weeks after discontinuing topical 5-FU.

not have been adequate and the tumor may have penetrated through the basement membrane. From the clinical appearance it is impossible to determine whether an inflammatory reaction is caused by the response to topical 5-FU or by an extension of the tumor. In any event, progression of tumor requires discontinuation of topical 5-FU therapy and excision of the tumor. This contingency resembles analogous observations after surgery or radiation therapy, when it is difficult to determine whether onset of an intense inflammatory reaction accompanied by extension of tumor is associated with the reaction to treatment or the natural course of the tumor.

More recently[12,21,22] topical chemotherapy has been used to manage squamous cell carcinomas when surgery or radiation therapy is not appropriate because of the large size of the lesions, advanced age, or poor operative risk of the patient, or, in the case of agitated patients, inability to confine radiation therapy to the site requiring treatment. Topical 5-FU therapy on these occasions has been useful as a palliative procedure and in several instances appears to have resulted in eradication of lesions that could not be managed by other modalities. Evaluation of the results of topical chemotherapy in large squamous cell carcinomas in those conditions has not proceeded far enough or long enough to consider topical chemotherapy only as a last resort, and even then primarily as an investigative approach. Treatment in those conditions requires protracted periods (up to several months), with intensive monitoring by means of frequently repeated biopsies to determine the nature of the response.

Discussion

The results of topical chemotherapy indicate that this modality provides the treatment of choice for extensive premalignant and multiple superficial malignant lesions of the skin that cannot be adequately managed by surgical procedures or radiation therapy. Although most of the results reported above were obtained with topical preparations of 5-FU, preliminary studies suggest that analogous results may be obtained with a number of other antimitotic agents, such as vinblastine, bleomycin, and 5-mercaptouracil, 2-deoxyuridine[12,13,23] and a number of other agents.[24–30] It therefore appears that further studies are indicated to explore other agents, either alone or in combination, or with radiation therapy.

Studies on multiple lesions involving extensive areas of the body surface further indicated that concurrent or sequential combinations of surgery and/or radiation therapy with topical chemotherapy can provide an effective approach to the management of otherwise intractable disease. Combined management, therefore, including reconstructive and plastic surgery,[21,22] chemosurgery,[31] chemotherapy and immunotherapy,[6] has been extensively used by us and others.

An important development arising from studies carried out in parallel with chemotherapy was the observation that delayed hypersensitivity reactions elicited by topical administration of cutaneous sensitizing agents resulted in selectively destructive effects on epidermal neoplasms and other tumors involving the skin.[4–6,30,32,33] It was found that combinations of topical chemotherapy with immunotherapy resulted in more rapid resolution of tumors and in eradication of epidermal neoplasms that could not be eliminated by topical chemotherapy or immunotherapy alone.[6] Thus, topical administration of cytostatic agents was found not to inhibit host defense mechanisms such as immunologic antitumor activity, and could be advantageously and possibly synergistically used in conjunction with stimulation of antitumor immunity.

The mechanisms by which topically applied antimitotic agents exert their selective antitumor effects on epidermal neoplasms are not fully understood. Inhibition of DNA synthesis by 5-FU through inhibition of thymidylate synthetase may be an important factor. The possibility of the incorporation of 5-FU derivatives (FUR) into RNA of tumor cells, and the resultant formation of fraudulent macromolecules which are incompatible with cellular integrity or which elicit an immune or other defense reaction on the part of the host, has not been excluded. The selective nature of the antitumor response, emphasized by the fact that tumors undergo involution while normal granulation tissue and epidermis grow, indicates that nonspecific inhibition of cellular reduplication cannot be the only factor. If this were so, both neoplastic and normal tissues should be affected in the same way. Therefore, a mechanism responsible for a selective action against tumor cells and not, at least to the same extent, against their normal counterparts must be present. Furthermore, a number of antimitotic agents that exert their inhibitory effects by different mechanisms produce the same degree of selectivity in their antitumor effects when administered locally to the tumor site. It therefore appears that factors common to the mechanisms of different chemical agents are operative in producing similar selective effects on superficially located malignant tumors. Further exploration of the mechanisms by which local chemotherapy produces selective antitumor effects may be of value in providing guidance for more effective chemotherapy by local as well as systemic management.

References

1. Klein, E.: Studies on local chemotherapy of neoplasms in the skin. Presented at the Stephen Rothman Research Meeting, Academy of Dermatology, Chicago, Ill., 1961.
2. Klein, E., Milgrom, H., Helm, F., Ambrus, J., Traenkle, H. L. and Stoll, H. L.: Tumors of the skin. I. Effects of local use of cytostatic agents. Skin 1:81, 1962.
3. Klein, E.: Tumors of the skin. VIII. Local chemotherapy of metastatic neoplasms. N.Y. J. Med. 68:877, 1968.
4. Klein, E.: Differential immunologic reaction in normal skin and epidermal neoplasms. Fed. Proc. 26:430, 1967.
5. Klein, E.: Tumors of the skin. X. Immunotherapy of cutaneous and mucosal neoplasms. N.Y. J. Med. 68:900, 1968.
6. Klein, E.: Hypersensitivity reactions at tumor sites. Cancer Res. 29:2351, 1969.
7. Klein, E., Stoll, H. L., Milgrom, H., Helm, F. and Walker, M. J.: Tumors of the skin. XII. Topical 5-fluorouracil for epidermal neoplasms. J. Surg. Oncol. 3:331, 1971.
8. Klein, E., Stoll, H. L., Milgrom, H., Case, R. W., Traenkle, H. L., et al.: Tumors of the skin. IV. Double-blind study on effects of local administration of anti-tumor agents in basal cell carcinoma. J. Invest. Derm. 44:351, 1965.
9. Klein, E., Stoll, H. L., Milgrom, H., Case, R. W., Traenkle, H. L., et al: Tumors of the skin. V. Local administration of antitumor agents to multiple superficial basal cell carcinomas. J. Invest. Derm. 45:489, 1965.
10. Stoll, H. L., Jr., Klein, E., and Case, R. W.: Tumors of the skin. VII. Effects of varying the concentration of locally administered 5-fluorouracil on basal cell carcinomas. J. Invest. Derm. 49:219, 1967.
11. Klein, E., Stoll, H. L., Miller, E., Milgrom, H., Helm,, F. et al.: Local administration of 5-fluorouracil. Proc. Amer. Ass. Cancer Res. (April) 1966, p. 37.
12. Klein, E.: Tumors of the skin. IX. Local cytostatic therapy of cutaneous and mucosal premalignant and malignant lesions. N.Y. J. Med. 68:886, 1968.
13. Burgess, G. H., McEvoy, B., Calamel, P., Ezdinli, E. and Klein, E.: Studies on the vincaleukoblastine alkaloids in Kaposi's hemorrhagic sarcoma. (In preparation.)
14. Klein, E., et al.: Local chemotherapy in cutaneous and mucosal neoplasia. Presented at Annual Meeting of American College of Physicians, 1967
15. Dillaha, C. J., Jansen, G. T., Honeycutt, W. M. and Bradford, A. C.: Selective cytotoxic effect of topical 5-fluorouracil. Arch. Derm. 88:247, 1963.

16. Goldman, L.: The response of skin cancer to topical therapy with 5-fluorouracil. Cancer Chemother. Rep. 28:49, 1963.
17. Dillaha, C. J., Jansen, T., Honeycutt, M. W. and Holt, G. A.: Further studies with topical 5-fluorouracil. Arch. Derm. 92:410, 1965.
18. Klein, E., Milgrom, H., Helm, F., Traenkle, H. L., Case, R. W., et al.: Local administration of anti-tumor agents. Proc. Amer. Ass. Cancer Res. 6:36, 1965.
19. Klein, E., Stoll, H. L., Milgrom, H., Traenkle, H. L., Graham, S. and Helm, F.: Tumors of the skin. VI. Study on effects of local administration of 5-fluorouracil in basal cell carcinomas. J. Invest. Derm. 47:22, 1966.
20. Stoll, H. L., Jr. and Klein, E.: Tumors of the skin. XI. Effect of occlusive dressing on the local administration of 5-fluorouracil to superficial basal cell carcinoma. J. Invest. Derm. 52:304, 1969.
21. Litwin, M. S., Ryan, R. F., Reed, R. J. and Krementz, E. T.: Topical chemotherapy of cutaneous malignancy of the head and neck. Southern Med. J. 62:556, 1969.
22. Klein, E., et al.: Unpublished data.
23. Schwartz, S. H., Bardos, T. J., Burgess, G. H. and Klein, E.: Cytostatic and immunologic activity of 5-mercaptouracil desoxyriboside in the management of multiple superficial basal cell epitheliomas. J. Med. 1:174, 1970.
24. Sullivan, M., Zall, L. and McCulloch, H.: Failure of podophyllin in the treatment of cutaneous carcinoma. Bull. Hopkins Hosp. 90:368, 1962.
25. Pillat, A.: Oertliche Chemotherapie der Karzinome am Aeusseren Auge durch Bayer E39. Arztliche Fortbildung 9:1, 1959.
26. Haserick, J. R., Richardson, J. H. and Grant, D. J.: Remission of lesions in mycosis fungoides following topical application of nitrogen mustard: A case report. Cleveland Clin. Quart. 26:144, 1959.
27. Van Scott, E. J., Shaw, R. K., Crounse, R. G. and Condit, P. T.: Effects of methotrexate on basal cell carcinoma. Arch. Derm. 82:762, 1960.
28. Siebeck, R.: Zur Indikation der Chemotherapie von Lidkarzinomen. Med. Mschr. 16:743, 1962.
29. Belisario, J.: Recent assessments in the aetiology and therapy of skin carcinomas. Indian J. Derm. 29:191, 1963.
30. Helm, F., Klein, E., Traenkle, H. L. and Rivera, E. P.: Studies on the local administration of 2,3,5-tri-ethylene-imino-1,4-benzoquinone (Trenimon) to epitheliomas. J. Invest. Derm. 45:152, 1965.
31. Mohs, F. E.: Chemosurgery in Cancer, Gangrene and Infections. Springfield, Ill.: Charles C Thomas, 1956.
32. Cavins, J. A.: Topical immunotherapy of multiple superficial skin tumors. Abstracts of Tenth International Cancer Congress, Houston, Texas, 1970, pp. 206–207.
33. Levin, A., Stjernsward, J., De Schryver, A. and Johansson, B.: Effect of delayed hypersensitivity reactions on human skin neoplasms. Abstracts of Tenth International Cancer Congress, Houston, Texas, 1970, pp. 207–208.

Chemotherapy of Endocrine Neoplasms

By JOHN R. DURANT, M.D.

I REVIEWED FEMALE CHORIOCARCINOMA and thyroid and adrenal cancer at the previous Hahnemann Symposium on Cancer Chemotherapy.[1] The purpose of this chapter is not to rehash that material but rather to highlight a few recent developments and the associated controversy. It is a measure of the progress of cancer research that five years ago I could rather confidently call one of the subjects of this paper the only cancer for which chemotherapy seemed to be curative. Other contributors to this symposium will probably now claim a number of other examples, including testicular cancer, acute leukemia, Burkitt's lymphoma, and Hodgkin's disease.

CHORIOCARCINOMA

Choriocarcinoma can now be cured in approximately 75 per cent of American women by the use of methotrexate and actinomycin D.[2,3] Adequate therapy has generally been guided by the use of an assay for chorionic gonadotrophin. This discussion of choriocarcinoma and its treatment will center on certain implications raised by these two facts. First, since choriocarcinoma usually develops from preexistent benign trophoblastic disease, it seems reasonable to attempt to prevent fatal disease in all women by treating early, that is, when there is either nonmetastatic but malignant disease or persistent benign disease. A few examples of the results of this approach will be discussed. Second, it is increasingly obvious that it is necessary for the therapist to understand the sensitivity of the various assays for human chorionic gonadotrophin (HCG) and the consequent possibilities.

In a number of studies now available for examination, women with nonmetastatic trophoblastic disease were treated with chemotherapy. The rationale for therapy is that in approximately 40 per cent of patients with elevations of HCG for more than 60 days, invasive malignant trophoblastic disease will develop. Since we cannot know which of these patients will have spontaneous remission, it seems reasonable to treat them all. Ross et al.[4] reported 44 such patients in 1967. Only three did not completely respond. Metastasis occurred in one patient and she died. The other two required hysterectomy to remove residual intrauterine foci of active disease. That such a program is not only successful in saving lives but may also preserve childbearing function was demonstrated by an examination of the subsequent obstetrical histories of these 44 women as well as 3 others with nonmetastatic disease and 11 with known choriocarcinoma confined to the uterus. In 21 patients 29 pregnancies occurred. Of these there were 22 live births, 2 as yet undelivered pregnancies, 3 early spontaneous abortions, and 1 stillborn. One child, born by cesarian hysterectomy, died after unsuccessful surgery for tetralogy of Fallot.[5] Brewer et al.[6] chose a somewhat different approach. Fifty-one patients with molar pregnancy were followed with serial titers for 60 days, with a follow-up of 2 to 4½ years. They found elevated titers at 60 days in 15 (29.4 per cent) of the women. In four women with elevated titers of

---

From the Cancer Research and Training Program, University of Alabama School of Medicine, Birmingham, Alabama.

500 IU or less, no treatment was given, and no serious consequences were noted. The other 11 women were all successfully treated with drugs and/or surgery.

Treatment in both the previously cited series was exactly the same as for newly diagnosed metastatic trophoblastic disease. Methotrexate and actinomycin D were given repeatedly until titers were normal and then for at least two more courses. The patients in the first series stayed in the hospital for an average of 58 days, during which they were so treated for 35 days.[5] Despite this disadvantage, this approach seems warranted in that it successfully prevents fatal disease in 40 per cent of these women, especially since reproductive function is usually preserved.

This rationale has been further extended by a group of Japanese investigators. They undertook prophylactic treatment of all patients with hydatidiform mole but did not wait 60 days. Shortly after the diagnosis was established, 107 patients received 10 mg of methotrexate daily by mouth for 7 days. Two additional groups of patients were followed up. There were 42 who received no therapy and 39 who received miscellaneous other chemotherapeutic agents not including actinomycin D. In none of the 107 patients treated with methotrexate did choriocarcinoma develop. In each of the other two groups choriocarcinoma developed in 3 patients; 4 of them died. Toxicity was tolerable. There were no deaths attributable to the drugs, and 23 patients experienced no toxicity.[7] This method could probably be carried out safely in most clinics on an outpatient basis, thus obviating the long hospitalization required for the more intensive therapy given to patients with persistent elevations of HCG. On the other hand, a great many patients would be treated with and exposed to a toxic drug which they probably do not need. The extent of such unnecessary treatment is indicated by the reported incidence of molar pregnancy in the United States of about 1 in 2,000.[8] Choriocarcinoma develops in less than 1 per cent of these women.[9] Thus, although an aggressive prophylactic approach may be justified in Asia, where malignant transformation may be frequent, such a program does not seem warranted in the United States. At the present time it seems feasible to follow up all cases of nonmetastatic trophoblastic disease with serial titers and to delay treatment for 60 days. Those with marginal elevations at that time may be safely followed up until the course of their disease is established.

Follow-up and treatment are necessarily interwoven with an understanding of the meaning of elevated chorionic gonadotrophin titers. Because this problem arises infrequently and is not always well understood, and because of its implications for therapy of this and, indeed, other malignant diseases, a brief discussion may be helpful. Ordinary pregnancy tests become positive at a level of approximately 500 International Units (IU).[10] Levels of 50 IU HCG are normally present in premenopausal women because of luteinizing hormone (LH), which cannot be distinguished from HCG by any of the methods known today.[11] Thus, there is a gap of 50 to 500 IU, perhaps resulting in a negative pregnancy test, but the woman may still be secreting HCG. That this small amount of HCG is important is illustrated by the fact that 25 per cent of 44 women with nonmetastatic trophoblastic disease had levels persistently in this range[4] and by the realization that to be sure a tumor is eradicated all HCG should be shut off.

Tests more sophisticated and sensitive than the usual pregnancy test are necessary for the proper diagnosis and treatment of trophoblastic disease. The most common method is the mouse uterine weight assay, which is ten times as sensitive as a pregnancy test and can detect 50 IU,[10] all of which may actually be LH. Other newer tests depend upon immunologic assays. The most commonly used method is based on inhibition of agglutination. In this system HCG-coated red blood cells or latex particles are suspended in an unknown body fluid which is being tested. To this suspension an anti-HCG antibody is added. If there is HCG in the suspension fluid, it will combine with the antibody, and the coated red cells or particles will remain in suspension. On the other hand, if there is no HCG in the suspension fluid, the antibody will combine with the HCG on the particle surface and cause agglutination. A test is positive when agglutination is inhibited because of the substance being tested for in the suspension medium. The amount of the substance in the test fluid is roughly proportional to the number of dilutions up to which the inhibition continues to occur.[12,13] Unfortunately, this simple method is probably not reliable enough for use in treatment of trophoblastic disease. More recently a very sensitive radioimmunoassay method has been devised. This test may ultimately be easier to perform than the mouse assay technique. It is estimated that the sensitivity of this procedure is so great that it can detect as little as 2×10^{-3} IU of HCG.[14,15] At present, for clinical purposes it is best to obtain a mouse uterine weight assay by sending specimens to one of the established trophoblastic disease centers.

The sensitivity of the radioimmunoassay has some interesting therapeutic implications. Oncologists have become increasingly concerned with testing for subclinical cancer so that they may decide whether to treat apparently normal patients with more chemotherapy or initiate it after some other form of therapy such as surgery or irradiation. Acute leukemia, for instance, is estimated to enter complete clinical remission when a total tumor cell load of approximately 10^9 cells remains.[16] Such a large number of cells weighs only about one gram and is about as likely to be found in a patient as is the proverbial needle in a haystack. For each tumor being treated there is a great need for a biologically detectable tag which will accurately quantify the amount of tumor possibly remaining. The fetal antigen of colon carcinoma reported by Gold and coworkers[17] may be an example of this type of substance, and HCG is clearly another. Simple mathematics will clarify the importance of accurate and sensitive tests for HCG in the therapy of choriocarcinoma. If the radioimmunoassay can detect as little as 2×10^{-3} IU and if estimates of 5×10^{-5} IU/cell/day are accurate,[18] then the radioimmunoassay can detect as few as 40 HCG-producing cells[19] ($2 \times 10^{-3}/5 \times 10^{-5}$). The ability to treat such a small tumor cell load and accurately determine the need for continued therapy is obviously important. Forty remaining cells will bring us to the brink of cure. Normal titers contain up to 50 IU, however. If such a titer is due to choriocarcinoma rather than background LH, a "normal" level will indicate a rather large tumor cell load. The number of these cells can be easily calculated from the equation $1:5 \times 10^{-5} = X:50$. Solving for X gives a value of 10^6. Thus, at the time a normal titer is reached in the course of treating a patient with trophoblastic disease, as few as no tumor cells and as many as 10^6 may be remaining. The logic of treating for several courses beyond a normal titer is clearly established.

It is theoretically possible to solve this problem mathematically. If one assumes that all viable tumor cells are secreting HCG, one can calculate the probable number of tumor cells present in any patient by knowing the total excretion in a 24-hour period. This information can be plotted on semilog paper over the course of time, and a plot of the regression of the tumor can be obtained. Theoretically, then, the problem of inability to distinguish between low titers all due to LH and those due to HCG could

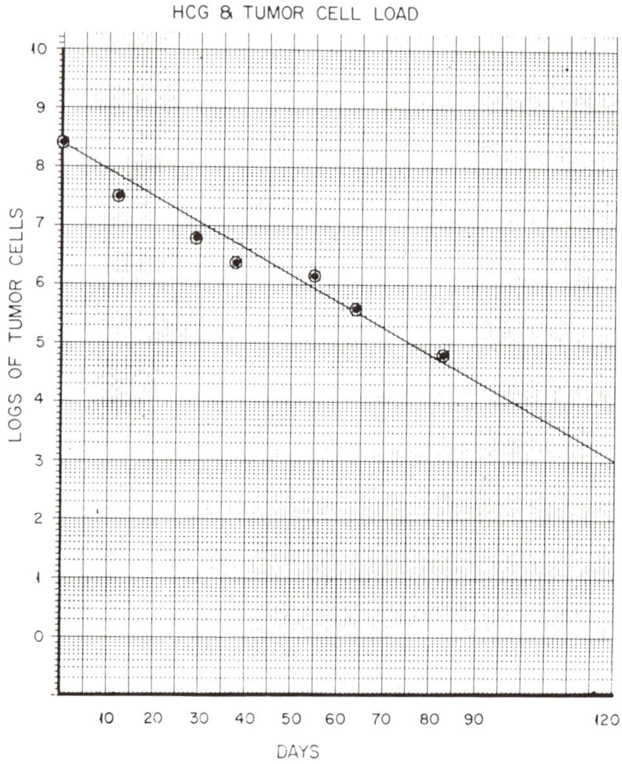

Fig. 1.—Smooth regression line obtained by converting 24-hour excretion of human chorionic gonadotropin (HCG) to the total number of tumor cells in a patient with choriocarcinoma. This indicates that therapy was equally effective at all points continuously. The entire curve could be shifted downward were some of the HCG actually luteinizing hormone (LH).

be overcome by plotting regression lines and treating for a long enough time to cause the regression line to cross the zero line at less than 5×10^{-5} IU/day. Bagshawe was able to construct smooth regression curves (Fig. 1) in about one-third of his patients, and treatment continued to the zero point resulted in a relapse rate of less than 4 per cent. On the other hand, when, for reasons unknown, an uneven curve was produced, the relapse rate was much higher, approximately 25 per cent. It is not clear what is responsible for the satisfactory translation of kinetic theory into practice in one group and not in the other, but the partial success is encouraging to oncologists who have become accustomed over the years to almost total failure.

Thyroid Cancer

The treatment of thyroid cancer has changed very little in the past five years. The patient who has a well-established diagnosis resulting from clinical signs and symptoms is generally subjected, if possible, to a total thyroidectomy. If this is not possible, as much tumor as possible is removed. The Pittmans at our institution have recently reviewed our approach to the problem of the patient with residual thyroid cancer following surgery.[20] It is my conviction that most such patients should receive a trial with thyroid hormone, even those with anaplastic carcinoma. In addition, if the patient has a well-differentiated carcinoma, investigation of the possibility of the use of ^{131}I is indicated. Exogenous thyroid administration is discontinued; the patient is given 20 mCi of ^{131}I, scanned and counted at 4, 6, and 24 hours later. If there is any indication of uptake, the patient is treated with ^{131}I, and administration of thyroid hormone is resumed the following day. Approximately one-half the patients treated in this fashion at the University of Alabama have responded. An example of the results of a somewhat different technique is the series from the Melbourne Cancer Institute from 1955 to 1965. Sixty-seven patients with known metastatic carcinoma from the thyroid and 31 with metastatic disease of unknown primary site were scanned only at 24 hours. Seventeen of the known thyroid cancers and 1 of the unknown primary cancers demonstrated uptake in the metastases. Fourteen patients were treated, 2 of whom had not had thyroidectomy and 4 of whom still had evidence of functional thyroid tissue in the neck. Of the 14, 7 manifested objective responses, 2 of which were complete. Of the 7 who failed to respond, 2 showed symptomatic improvement. All of the responding patients had well-differentiated forms of thyroid cancer.[21]

There is an increasing awareness of the value of supervoltage high dose external irradiation for some patients with thyroid carcinoma. Smedal et al.[22] found that about 15 per cent of all patients with thyroid cancer seen at the Lahey Clinic had well-differentiated but locally inoperable disease. They elected to treat this type of patient with external 2 MEV radiation therapy, administering 4,800 to 5,000 rads in 6 weeks. Their patients have had a mean survival of 9.5 years, and in only 5 of 32 patients was there failure to achieve local control. For anaplastic carcinoma, in which the natural history is such that local invasion rather than distant metastasis is the usual cause of death, a more hopeful approach with external radiation therapy is now possible. Rafla,[23] at the Manitoba Cancer Treatment and Research Foundation, reported on 38 patients over the course of 15 years. Eight of these had reticulum cell sarcoma and are excluded from this discussion. Of the remaining 30, 25 were able to be treated by aggressive, high dose radiation therapy, usually after as much surgical removal of the tumor as possible. Six of these patients (approximately 25 per cent) were alive without evidence of recurrence, including 2 treated with radiation therapy alone. One patient still had evidence of disease, but the remainder had died of their disease. These two reports clearly illustrate the value of external radiation therapy given to locally inoperable tumor of any histologic type.

Most of the interest in thyroid cancer, however, centers on the meaning of many recent studies reported concerning its prevalence and its usual biologic quiescence. These studies have frequently suggested to students of the disease that surgery modifies the course of few, if any, patients, that thyroid nodules should not be removed for fear of cancer, and that patients with established thyroid cancer are best not treated surgically. A review of some of this material is of interest.

The argument and counterargument run along these lines: A great deal of information indicates that a thyroid nodule is almost never malignant; that even if it is malignant, the natural history of the disease suggests that it is either so "benign" that nothing needs to be done or so malignant that nothing can be done. Perhaps so, but thyroid cancer does kill, some anaplastic carcinomas are cured, and well-differentiated lesions can undergo transition to anaplastic carcinoma. Thus, appropriate management of all thyroid cancer consists in surgical removal. The evidence supporting these opposite points of view is illustrated by a number of studies.

Sampson et al.[24] recently reviewed the prevalence of thyroid cancer at autopsy in one Japanese and six American studies and added their own data from the Japanese National Institute of Health/Atomic Bomb Casualty Commission Life Span Study in Hiroshima and Nagasaki. In the combined American series there were 3,267 autopsies in which thyroid cancer was sought as an incidental finding. Histologic evidence for this diagnosis was found in 67 patients. The prevalence varied from 1 per cent to 4 per cent with an overall average of a little more than 2 per cent. Yet, even in reports from cancer centers, thyroid cancer is responsible for only a very few deaths. At the Memorial Hospital in New York City only 50 patients in a series of 7,361 autopsies died either as a result of thyroid cancer or its treatment,[25] and at the M. D. Anderson Hospital up to 1966 there were only 105 deaths from this cause.[26] In general hospitals, the rate is even lower, with a group of Boston hospitals collectively noting a rate considerably less than 1 autopsy in 1,000.[27] The data from the Atomic Bomb Survey population are even more striking.[24] From the fixed population in this area 3,067 consecutive autopsies were available for study. Primary carcinoma of the thyroid was found in 536 cases. Of these, 525 were classified as papillary and 11 were other histologic types, mostly follicular. Of the 525 papillary carcinomas, 518 were occult (less than 1.5 cm in size and not detected during life). Of the 536 cases of thyroid cancer, there were 18 in which the disease was clinically evident. Of the 518 cases in which the cancer was not clinically apparent, there was only one case of a clinically inapparent thyroid cancer found to explain death from metastatic malignancy of unknown origin. Thus, of the 536 cases of thyroid cancer found in this population, 518 were clinically inapparent, and of this latter kind only one was clinically important.

Not only is occult primary disease clinically unimportant, but even its metastases seem to be of little consequence. One hundred twenty-eight patients with clinically inapparent thyroid cancer were studied carefully for cervical node metastases. Of these, 20 were found to contain one or more foci of nodal metastases. From this the authors calculated that at least 3 per cent of the Japanese population has clinically insignificant metastatic thyroid cancer.[28] Somewhat similar findings are reported by another Japanese group.[29] These data are further supported in the United States by Woolner et al., who found that the prognosis for thyroid cancer of the well differentiated type was benign whether or not lymph node dissection was done.[30] These studies, and many others like them, tend to encourage the belief that surgery is never indicated for thyroid cancer, apparently reducing the problem to absurdity.

Further contribution to the evidence suggesting the uselessness of looking for thyroid cancer comes from the Framingham study.[31] Of 5,127 people who were followed up for 15 years, 218 had nodules either at the beginning of the study or during it. Of the 199 nodules found initially, 45 were surgically examined and found to be benign. The remainder have all been followed up for 15 years, and none have any sign of cancer of the thyroid. During the course of the study, 67 new nodules were found. Thirteen of these were surgically removed and all found to be benign.

Thus, in this highly selected review, it appears that thyroid carcinoma cannot be detected with any reliability by biopsy of suspicious lesions, and that it is often present and metastasizes without affecting the patient's health, and only rarely causes death.

Despite the above, it is clear that cancer of the thyroid does kill some people, even those who have well-differentiated tumors. Perhaps the most important factor which should cause the physician to take a more careful look at the problem is the question of transition from well-differentiated to poorly differentiated cancer. In the Memorial

Hospital series, 50 patients died as a result of thyroid cancer or its treatment. Of these patients 4 of 10 with papillary thyroid cancer and 2 of 10 with follicular cancer underwent a transition to a more malignant, anaplastic variety.[25] At the M. D. Anderson Hospital, 27 of 554 thyroid cancers were classified as spindle or giant cell. Of these 27, 23 operative specimens were available for study; all these patients had well-differentiated tumor prominent in the cancer. Four were small biopsy specimens only and could not be used for real analysis.[26] Rafla[23] reported a long history of a thyroid mass in one patient that began to enlarge rather suddenly. Examination of the surgical specimen showed well-differentiated papillary carcinoma in one area with anaplastic carcinoma adjacent. Such experiences have led to the speculation that most, if not all, anaplastic carcinomas of the thyroid arise from previously untreated or poorly treated well-differentiated tumors.

Two recent cases at the University of Alabama (kindly provided by Dr. William A. Maddox) will illustrate this phenomenon and its rather characteristic clinical course.

Case #1.—About 2 years before admission, this 67-year-old white man first noted a mass about 2.5 cm in diameter in the upper part of the right side of his neck. It had increased in size slowly until about 2 months before admission, when it suddenly seemed to grow rapidly. Shortly thereafter hoarseness, sore throat, and dysphagia developed.

On physical examination there was a large 8 × 12 cm mass involving the thyroid gland, and a number of 1.5 to 3 cm nodes were noted bilaterally in the cervical and supraclavicular area. Indirect laryngoscopy revealed that the right vocal cord was paralyzed.

Biopsy of a right cervical node was interpreted as well-differentiated follicular carcinoma of the thyroid (Fig. 2). A chest X-ray film revealed probable bilateral pulmonary metastases.

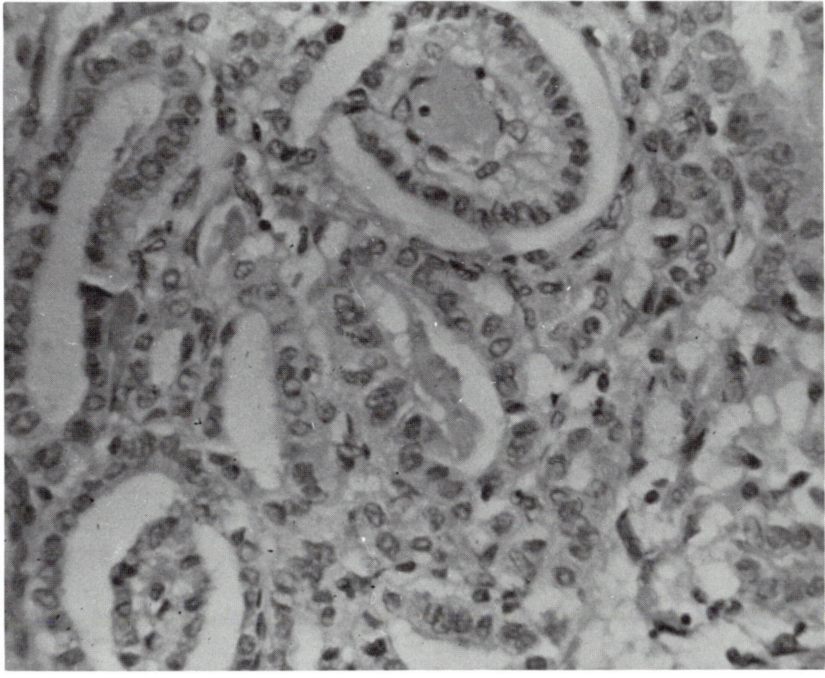

FIG. 2.—(Case # 1) Photomicrograph of well-differentiated follicular carcinoma of the thyroid. Hematoxylin and eosin (H&E), ×100. Figures 2 through 5 by courtesy of William A. Maddox, M.D.

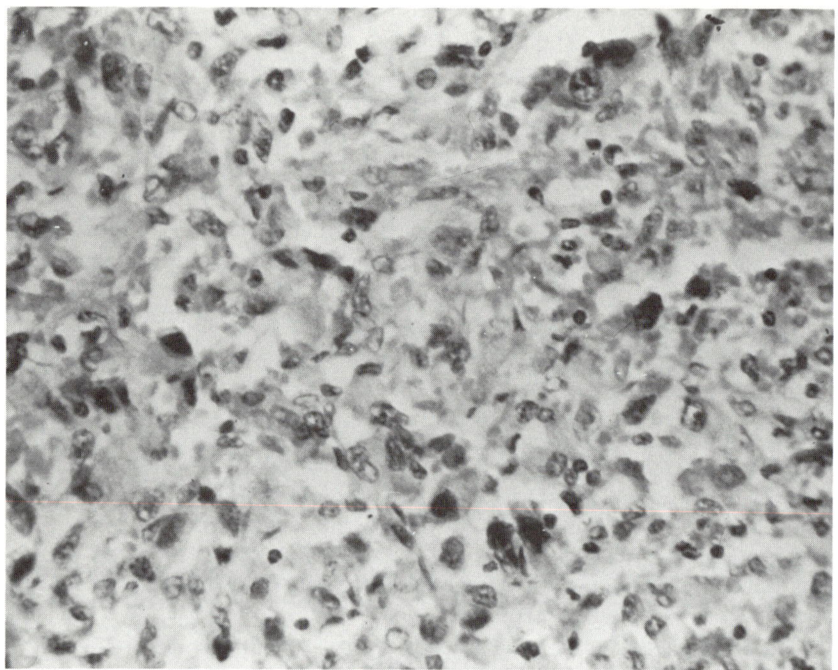

FIG. 3.—(Case # 1) Photomicrograph of anaplastic carcinoma of the thyroid. H&E, ×100.

He was taken to the operating room, where a subtotal thyroidectomy was carried out. Nineteen of 22 jugular nodes removed were positive for carcinoma. The operative specimen revealed a large cancer of the mixed, papillary-follicular type with areas of undifferentiated cancer (Fig. 3).

The postoperative course of the patient was stormy, and he died 8 days after operation. At autopsy there was extensive undifferentiated carcinoma with metastases in the lung, heart, adrenals, pancreas, bone marrow, kidney, and posterior pituitary.

Case #2.—A 75-year-old white woman manifested hoarseness at age 65. Her physician examined her, found partial paralysis of a vocal cord, and recommended an unknown type of exploratory operation on her neck which the patient refused. She noted no change at all in her status for 9½ years, when rather suddenly she noted increasing hoarseness and a mass in the right side of her neck. In addition, she reported a 20-lb. weight loss during the previous 6 months.

On examination, it was seen that the left lobe of the thyroid was not enlarged but was much firmer than normal. A 3-cm node was noted in the right jugular chain. On indirect laryngoscopy the left vocal cord was found to be completely paralyzed. The remainder of the examination was unremarkable.

At operation a tumor originating in the left lobe of the thyroid was found in juxtaposition to the cricoid cartilage entrapping the left recurrent laryngeal nerve. The tumor had adhered to the larynx, had invaded the esophagus, and was found in bilateral cervical and upper mediastinal lymph nodes. A modified right radical neck dissection, total thyroidectomy, partial left neck dissection, mediastinal dissection, and tracheostomy were done, with successful removal of all the known tumor. Pathologic examination revealed a mixed carcinoma with papillary (Fig. 4), follicular, and undifferentiated giant cell carcinoma (Fig. 5).

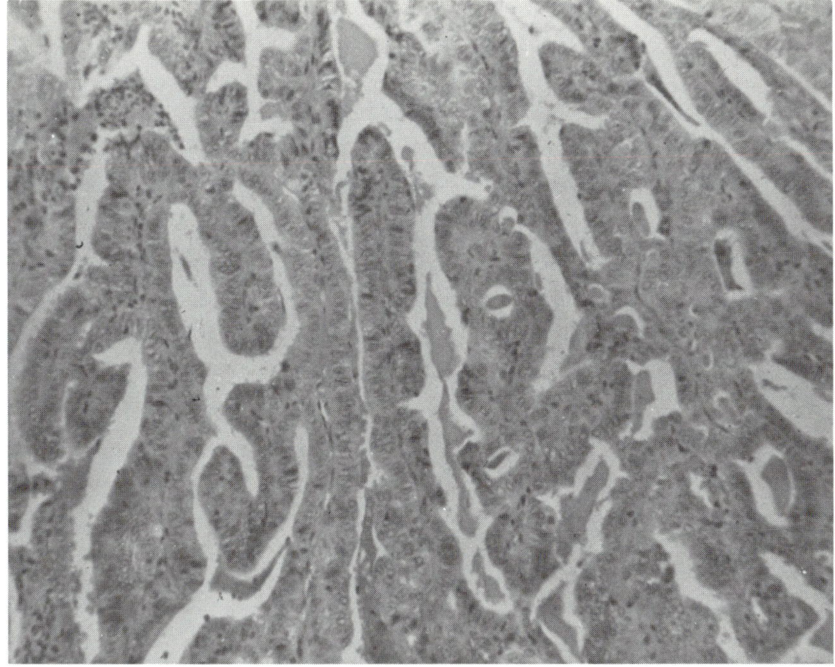

FIG. 4.—(Case # 2) Photomicrograph of papillary carcinoma of the thyroid. H&E, ×25.

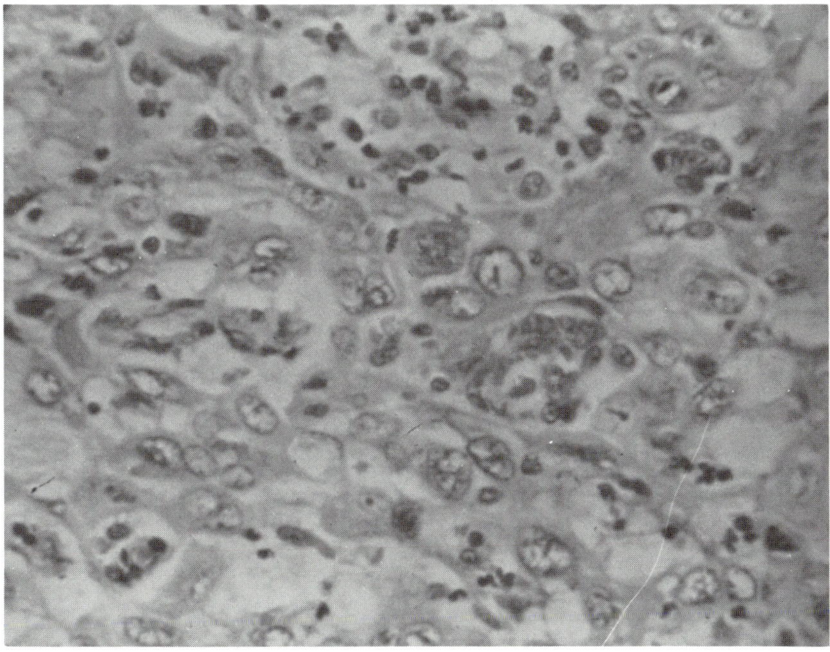

FIG. 5.—(Case # 2) Photomicrograph of giant-cell anaplastic carcinoma of the thyroid. H&E, ×400.

The patient made an uneventful postoperative recovery and 6 months later was without evidence of disease.

In both cases it seems likely that a well-differentiated carcinoma developed a number of years previously. Slow growth was noted at first, but then a rather sudden increase in symptoms and signs occurred, and the patients sought surgical attention. In both instances well-differentiated carcinomas were found in combination with more anaplastic forms.

The important question raised by these and similar cases is whether all well-differentiated tumors should be aggressively removed to prevent later fatal transition to an aggressive and much less treatable form.

At the University of Alabama we steer a middle course between benign neglect and aggressive surgery. It seems likely that clinically apparent carcinoma does kill patients, and the Pittmans have suggested the following strong indications for exploration of the neck for carcinoma of the thyroid[20]:

1. Children
2. Cold nodules
3. Pressure symptoms not otherwise explained
4. Stony hard thyroid mass
5. Recent appearance or growth
6. Hot nodules in children
7. Nodules associated with pheochromocytoma (because of the great association of medullary [solid] carcinoma of the thyroid with pheochromocytoma)
8. History of X-ray treatment, especially in childhood, of the neck
9. Psammoma bodies seen on roentgenograms of the neck

We contend that these indications will yield a higher frequency of thyroid cancers which are or will become clinically significant, and that therapy does influence the course of the disease.

Adrenal Carcinoma

Adrenal Cortex

The status of the chemotherapy of adrenal cortical carcinoma was well reviewed in 1966 by Hutter and Kayhoe[32]; they reported the results of treating 138 patients with mitotane (*o,p'*-DDD; Lysodren). The usual dose of *o,p'*-DDD for a patient was about 10 grams a day, given orally in divided doses. Toxicity was primarily gastrointestinal, cutaneous, or in the central nervous system. Only 28 per cent of the patients with abnormally high levels of steroid excretion failed to have at least a 30 per cent reduction or more of these levels. Such a response did not, however, indicate a good therapeutic response. Only 34 per cent of the patients treated had a decrease in measurable disease. All of these also had a decrease in abnormally high steroid levels. The mean duration of steroid response was 5 months and that of measurable disease 10 months. There was a suggestion from survival curves that survival was improved by treatment. The survival rate in those patients without abnormal steroid excretion appeared as good as in those with abnormal steroid excretion. A response in steroid levels, when achieved, usually occurred within 4 weeks and a decrease in measurable tumor within 6 weeks.

Survival is somewhat better than it used to be.[33] In the patients whose response to treatment was studied, the females had a 50 per cent survival of greater than 56 months and the males had a 50 per cent survival of 20 months. Further supporting an improved survival is the report from Memorial Hospital of 34 cases encountered from 1935 to 1967. None of these patients was cured, but 3 survived with disease more than 5 years. The 30 patients who died lived an average of 3 years from the onset of symptoms, with females living 0.9 years longer than males.[34]

Adrenal Medulla

This subject was reviewed at the previous symposium on cancer chemotherapy. Since that time, no specific agent has been found for the control of malignant pheochromocytoma. Nevertheless, some significant advances in the understanding of the biochemistry of the sympathetic nervous system have become widely known and may contribute considerably to symptomatic control for victims of malignant pheochromocytoma. The concept of alpha and beta receptors and the differing pharmacology of their blockade have suggested that the alpha blocker phenoxybenzamine, as well as the beta blocker propranolol, may help to control the inexorable symptomatic course of the patient with this malignancy.[35] Unfortunately, beta blockade may sometimes be contraindicated because of associated cardiac failure, and the patient may not respond to alpha blockade. This clinical circumstance may be successfully met by the use of alpha-methyl-tyrosine, which blocks the rate-limiting step in catecholamine synthesis by inhibiting the hydroxylation of tyrosine to dopa; it is more specific than alpha-methyldopa.[36] Jones et al.[37] have successfully relieved symptoms in two patients with malignant pheochromocytoma in this fashion. This drug will undoubtedly receive wider attention for this purpose.

INSULINOMA

Streptozotocin, a 1-methyl, nitrosourea-glucosamine antibiotic derived originally from *Streptomyces achromogenes*, has been used recently in the treatment of metastatic insulinoma.[38] Carter et al.[39] report that the Cancer Therapy Evaluation Branch of the National Cancer Institute has to date acquired data on 23 patients with metastatic insulinoma who were treated with streptozotocin. Of the 23 observed, 20 of the tumors were functional, with hypersecretion of insulin. Objective evidence of remission was noted in approximately 70 per cent of the patients.

The total intravenous dosages administered to this group of patients ranged from 1.5 to 40 gm and were most often given on a weekly schedule. Major adverse reactions included nephrotoxicity and gastrointestinal effects. Nephrotoxicity was the main dose-limiting side effect.[40] At present the recommended dosage of streptozotocin for insulinoma is 1 gram per square meter of body surface area per week, administered intravenously.[39]

REFERENCES

1. Durant, J. R.: Chemotherapy of endocrine tumors. *In* Brodsky, I. and Kahn, S. B. (Eds.): Cancer Chemotherapy: Basic and Clinical Applications. New York: Grune & Stratton, 1967, p. 119.
2. Lewis, J., Jr.: Chemotherapy for metastatic gestational trophoblastic neoplasms. Clin. Obstet. Gynec. 10:330, 1967.
3. Lewis, J., Ketcham, A. S. and Hertz, R.: Surgical intervention during chemotherapy of gestational trophoblastic neoplasms. Cancer 19:1517, 1966.
4. Ross, G. T., Hammond, C. B. and Odell, W. D.: Chemotherapy for nonmetastatic gestational trophoblastic neoplasms. Clin. Obstet. Gynec. 10:323, 1967.

5. Hammond, C. B., Hertz, R., Ross, G. T., Lipsett, M. B. and Odell, W. D.: Primary chemotherapy for nonmetastatic gestational trophoblastic neoplasms. Amer. J. Obstet. Gynec. 98:71, 1967.
6. Brewer, J. I., Torok, E. E., Webster, A. and Dolkart, R. E.: Hydatidiform mole: A follow-up regimen for identification of invasive mole and choriocarcinoma and for selection of patients for treatment. Amer. J. Obstet. Gynec. 101:557, 1968.
7. Koga, K. and Maeda, K.: Prophylactic chemotherapy with amethopterin for prevention of choriocarcinoma following removal of hydatidiform mole. Amer. J. Obstet. Gynec. 100:270, 1968.
8. Parsons, L. and Sommers, S.: Textbook of Gynecology. Philadelphia: W. B. Saunders, 1962.
9. MacGregor, C., Ontiveros, E., Vargas, E. and Valenquela, S. L.: Hydatidiform mole: Analysis of 145 patients. Obstet. Gynec. 33:343, 1969.
10. Taymor, M. L.: Bioassay and immunoassay of human chorionic gonadotropin (HCG). Clin. Obstet. Gynec. 10:303, 1967.
11. Marshall, J. R., Hammond, C. B., Ross, G. T., Jacobson, A., Rayford, P. and Odell, W. D.: Plasma and urinary chorionic gonadotropin during early human pregnancy. Obstet. Gynec. 32:760, 1968.
12. Mishell, D. R. and Davajan, V.: Quantitative immunologic assay of human chorionic gonadotropin in normal and abnormal pregnancies. Amer. J. Obstet. Gynec. 96:231, 1966.
13. Haskins, A. L.: Quantitative assay of human chorionic gonadotropin: A comparison of immunoassay and bioassay. Amer. J. Obstet. Gynec. 97:777, 1967.
14. Odell, W. D., Rayford, P. L. and Ross, G. T.: Simplified partially automated method for radioimmunoassay of human thyroid-stimulating, growth, luteinizing, and follicle-stimulating hormones. J. Lab. Clin. Med. 70:973, 1967.
15. Ross, G.: Estimates of doubling times in hormone-producing cells of normal and neoplastic trophoblast. *In* Lund, C. J. and Choate, J. W. (Eds.): Transcript of the Fourth Rochester Trophoblast Conference, 1967, p. 324.
16. Schabel, F. M., Jr.: Drug treatment of malignant tumors of man and animals: A rational approach to cancer chemotherapy. Southern Med. Bull. 57 (No. 1): 40, 1969.
17. Gold, P., Gold, M. and Freedmann, S. O.: Cellular location of carcinoembryonic antigens of the human digestive system. Cancer Res. 28:1331, 1968.
18. Bagshawe, K.: An analysis of tumor growth based on HCG production by trophoblastic tumors. *In* Lund, C. J. and Choate, J. W. (Eds.): Transcript of the Fourth Rochester Trophoblast Conference, 1967, p. 305.
19. Schabel, F. M., Jr.: Concept and practice of total tumor cell kill. Presented at Tenth Int. Cancer Cong., Cancer Therapy: Experimental Models and Clinical Trials, Houston, Texas, 1970.
20. Pittman, J. A. and Pittman, C. S.: Thyroid nodules and cancer. Mod. Treatm. 6:534, 1969.
21. Andrews, J. T. and Minty, C. C.: Investigation and treatment of metastatic thyroid carcinoma with radioiodine. Clin. Radiol. 20:237, 1969.
22. Smedal, M. I., Salzman, F. A. and Meissner, W. A.: The value of 2 MV roentgen-ray therapy in differentiated thyroid carcinoma. Amer. J. Roentgen. 99:352, 1967.
23. Rafla, S.: Anaplastic tumors of the thyroid. Cancer 23:668, 1969.
24. Sampson, R. J., Key, C. R., Buncher, C. R. and Iijima, S.: Thyroid carcinoma in Hiroshima and Nagasaki. J.A.M.A. 209: 65, 1969.
25. Silverberg, S. G., Hutter, R. V. P. and Foote, F. W.: Fatal carcinoma of the thyroid: Histology, metastases, and causes of death. Cancer 25:792, 1970.
26. Ibanez, M. L., Russell, W. O., Albores-Saavedra, J., Lampertico, P., White, E. C. and Clark, R. L.: Thyroid carcinoma: Biologic behavior and mortality. Cancer 19:1039, 1966.
27. Vanderlaan, W. P.: The occurrence of carcinoma of the thyroid gland in autopsy material. New Eng. J. Med. 237:221, 1947.
28. Sampson, R. J., Hisao, O., Key, C. R., Buncher, C. R. and Iijima, S.: Metastases from occult thyroid carcinoma: An autopsy study from Hiroshima and Nagasaki, Japan. Cancer 25:803, 1970.
29. Yagawa, K., Takahashi, S. and Murata, T.: Clinicopathological study of latent thyroid carcinoma. Abstr. Proc. of 25th Ann. Meeting, Jap. Cancer Ass., 1966, p. 106.
30. Woolner, L. B., Lemmon, M. L., Beahrs, O. H., Black, B. M. and Keating, F. R.: Occult papillary carcinoma of the thyroid gland: A study of 140 cases observed in a 30-year period. J. Clin. Endocr. 20:89, 1960.

31. Vander, J. B., Gadston, E. A. and Dawles, T. R.: The significance of non-toxic thyroid nodules: Final report of a fifteen-year study of the incidence of thyroid malignancy. Ann. Intern. Med. 69:537, 1968.
32. Hutter, A. M. and Kayhoe, D. E.: Adrenal cortical carcinoma: Results of treatment with o,p′-DDD in 138 patients. Amer. J. Med. 41:581, 1966.
33. Hutter, A. M. and Kayhoe, D. E.: Adrenal cortical carcinoma: Clinical features of 138 patients. Amer. J. Med. 41:572, 1966.
34. Huves, A. G., Hajdu, S. I., Brasfield, R. D. and Foote, F. W., Jr.: Adrenal cortical carcinoma: Clinicopathologic study of 34 cases. Cancer 25:354, 1970.
35. Boréus, L. O., Broberger, U., Nergårdh, A. and Zetterqvist, P.: Malignant pheochromocytoma in a child: Treatment with a combination of alpha- and beta-adren, ergic blockade. Acta Paediat. Scand. 57:36-1968.
36. α-Methyl-tyrosine and phaeochromocytoma (Annotations). Lancet 2:1130, 1968.
37. Jones, N. F., Walker, G., Ruthven, C. R. J. and Sandler, M.: α-Methyl-*p*-tyrosine in the management of phaeochromocytoma. Lancet 2:1105, 1968.
38. Schreibman, P. H., de Koliren, L. G. and Arky, R. A.: Metastatic insulinoma treated with streptozotocin. Ann. Intern. Med. 74:399, 1971.
39. Carter, S. K., Broder, L. and Friedman, M.: Streptozotocin and metastatic insulinoma. (Editorial Notes) Ann. Intern. Med. 74:445, 1971.
40. Sadoff, L.: The nephrotoxicity of streptozotocin. Cancer Chemother. Rep. 54:457, 1970.

Refinements in the Treatment of Children with Solid Tumors

By AUDREY E. EVANS, M.D.

TREATMENT OF CANCER IN CHILDHOOD was discussed at the previous symposium on the same subject. In particular, the advances made in the treatment of Wilms' tumor, neuroblastoma, and soft tissue sarcomas were noted and the regimens outlined.[1] Today it would be gratifying to report further advances, so that the results of treatment of all tumors would equal those reported at that time for children with Wilms' tumor. Alas, such spectacular advances have not occurred. The survival rate of children with Wilms' tumor is still unique in childhood cancer.

A plea was made at the earlier symposium for a combined approach to the child with cancer, using all three treatment modalities of surgery, radiation therapy, and chemotherapy for maximal effect. Careful follow-up and aggressive early retreatment of recurrence or metastasis was also stressed. During the present decade, we hope to see not only advances but refinements of treatment, allowing one to employ only those methods and agents which have proved to be valuable.

In the past 5 years, an attempt has been made to define not only the best treatment but also the extent of treatment, with the hope of doing the greatest good with the least harm. It is well known that the secondary effects of treatment can be damaging and, at times, even lethal in themselves. These considerations apply especially to children, whose tissues contain rapidly dividing and differentiating cells unlike the corresponding structures in adults. The late sequelae of radiation therapy given to children have been described by O'Malley and his colleagues,[2] Tefft and coworkers,[3] and Filler et al.[4] The unwanted side effects include radiation nephritis, hepatitis and secondary primary tumors arising from irradiated tissues. The ill effects of chemotherapy are not so well known. The production of leukopenia and possibly alteration in the immune response following vigorous treatment leave patients susceptible to infection by a variety of organisms. Death can be the result. In similar fashion, resistance of the host to the tumor might be decreased if such an interaction does, in fact, exist.

In children with neuroblastoma, Bill and Morgan have shown a correlation between good survival and an adequate total lymphocyte count, which suggests that cell-mediated immune responses may play a role in resistance of the host to the tumor.[5] The presence of tumor antibodies has been demonstrated for several neoplasms, but the part they play in the prevention of metastasis has yet to be defined.

In view of the foregoing and similar considerations, and because there are now available several agents and methods of treating cancer, it is important to define the role of each one in the management of the disease. The rapidly growing tissues of children are unusually susceptible to antimitotic agents, and treatment should be limited to those known to be beneficial. Perhaps the 1970s will take us past the age of

---

From the Department of Oncology, Children's Hospital of Philadelphia, Philadelphia, Pennsylvania.
Supported in part by U.S. Public Health Service Grant CA 11796 from the National Cancer Institute and grant RR 05506 from the Division of Research Facilities and Resources.

haphazard treatment when therapy was given in the belief that any treatment was better than none.

To illustrate some ways in which the effects of various treatment modalities are being tested, it might be helpful to discuss the current cooperative group studies being conducted in this country. The work of many pediatric groups was originally devoted to investigating the effect of chemotherapy in leukemia or metastatic cancer. More recently, the effects of regimens incorporating sharply defined methods of total combined care are being compared. Many study protocols specify details of the primary surgical management, radiation therapy, and the chemotherapy to be used. In addition, data regarding clinical evolution are obtained for analysis, in an attempt to better understand the natural history of the disease and its influence on prognosis. The investigation currently being conducted by the National Wilms' Tumor Study Group is a good example of such a protocol. One might ask, why is a study of this tumor necessary? It is already known that surgical removal, radiation therapy, and at least two chemotherapeutic agents are effective means of destroying the tumor. Surely, combining them all would lead to the best results.

Wilms' Tumor

The National Wilms' Tumor Study (NWTS) design has as its primary objective the refinement of treatment methods known to be of value. A previous study, conducted by Children's Cancer Study Group A (CCSGA) and reported by Wolff et al.,[6] showed that actinomycin D, given to children with Wilms' tumor at periodic intervals for 15 months after surgery, caused a significant decrease in recurrent or metastatic disease. Long-term follow-up of those children has shown that about 80 per cent of patients receiving "prophylactic" actinomycin D remained free of disease for 2 years or more, as compared with approximately 50 per cent of those who had received one course only. Wolff et al. pointed out, however, that the recurrence rate should not be confused with the survival rate. Earlier reports by Farber had shown that aggressive management could save patients with recurrent or metastatic disease, and this fact has been confirmed in the CCSGA study. Investigations by others suggest that the survival figures for the two groups originally reported by Wolff et al. are little different.[7] The difference between the recurrence rate and the survival rate represented the patients who survived after retreatment of their metastases.

This leads to an important series of questions. What are the relative risks entailed in giving chemotherapy to or withholding it from seemingly disease-free patients if a high proportion of them can still be salvaged when metastases develop? Is it better to ablate occult metastases in those who harbor them but, in so doing, expose a sizeable proportion of such patients unnecessarily to the dangers of chemotherapy? Or is it better to wait and treat vigorously with radiation and chemotherapy those children in whom metastases do develop, knowing success to be less than universal if such a policy is followed? The committee that designed the NWTS considered the question and decided that, on balance, prevention where possible was better than retreatment when necessary. It is conceded that this is a debatable point.

In the current NWTS, two specific questions are being asked:

1. Is postoperative radiation therapy necessary for the treatment of patients with well-encapsulated localized lesions, after what appears to be their total removal?

2. Which of the two chemotherapeutic agents, actinomycin D and vincristine,

known to be effective against Wilms' tumor, gives the better result, and can this result be improved by their use in combination?

Secondary objectives of the study are to determine what effect the state of disease at diagnosis has on the prognosis and to obtain epidemiologic information regarding the possible associated diseases in the patients and their families. The patients were grouped as follows:

Group I.—Tumor is limited to the kidney and is completely resected. The surface of the renal capsule is intact. The tumor is not ruptured before or during removal. There is no residual tumor apparent beyond the margins of resection.

Group II.—Tumor extends beyond the kidney but is completely resected. There is local extension of the tumor, i.e., penetration beyond the pseudocapsule into the perirenal soft tissues, or periaortic lymph node involvement. The renal vessels outside the kidney substance are infiltrated or contain tumor thrombi. There is no residual tumor apparent beyond the margins of resection.

Group III.—Residual nonhematogenous tumor confined to the abdomen. Any one or more of the following may occur: 1. The tumor has been ruptured or biopsy performed before or during surgery. 2. There are implants on the peritoneal surfaces. 3. There are involved lymph nodes beyond the abdominal periaortic chains. 4. The tumor is not completely resectable because of local infiltration into vital structures.

Group IV.—Hematogenous metastases. Deposits beyond Group III, e.g., lung, liver, bone and brain.

Group V.—Bilateral renal involvement either initially or subsequently. (Patients in this group with bilateral disease are not included in the study but information on them is compiled.)

It will be at least 4 more years before any definitive answers from this study will be forthcoming. In the meantime, I believe that conventional treatment of children with Wilms' tumor remains surgical removal of the primary lesion, postoperative irradiation therapy to the tumor bed, and actinomycin D given at the time of surgery and at three-month intervals for 12 to 18 months. In the presence of metastatic disease, radiation therapy in curative doses should be delivered to the tumor bed and all sites of disease, together with a combination of actinomycin D and vincristine. The survival rate of children with metastases, whether present at diagnosis or developing subsequently, has been reported by Farber to be as high as 50 per cent.[8] Thus, such children should be treated with the reasonable hope that they will be cured.

Neuroblastoma

The treatment of patients with neuroblastoma is also dependent upon the extent of disease at diagnosis. In an attempt to determine the influence of this factor on prognosis, an analysis was made of the physical findings on 100 patients entered in two CCSGA studies.[9] From the data obtained, a system of staging was devised:

Staging of Neuroblastoma

Stage I.—Tumors confined to the organ or structure of origin.

Stage II.—Tumors extending in continuity beyond the organ or structure of origin but not crossing the midline. Regional lymph nodes on the homolateral side may be involved.

Stage III.—Tumors extending in continuity beyond the midline. Regional lymph nodes may be involved bilaterally.

Stage IV.—Remote disease involving the skeleton, organs, soft tissue, and distant lymph node groups, etc. (see Stage IV-S).

Stage IV-S.—Patients who would otherwise be in Stage I or II, but who have remote disease confined to one or more of the following sites: liver, skin or bone marrow (without radiographic evidence of bone metastasis on complete skeletal survey).

Using the staging criteria, data on patients at the Children's Hospital of Philadelphia between 1947 and 1967 were analyzed in a similar fashion. Table 1 shows the 2-year survival figures derived from both the Children's Hospital and the CCSGA patients.[10]

As one would expect, the patients with localized disease do relatively well, whereas few of those with bone metastases survive. Table 1 also points up the well-known fact that the prognosis for younger children is much better than for those two years and older. What is not so well known is the excellent survival rate of patients with metastatic disease who fall into a special category, here called Stage IV-S. These patients, with disease spread to certain sites and without X-ray evidence of bone metastases, apparently do as well as those who have Stage I disease. This kind of analysis is valuable because it may serve as a guide to the type and amount of treatment that children with neuroblastoma should receive. For example, Stage I patients probably do not require any treatment other than surgery.

At present, there is no evidence that chemotherapy has altered the survival rate of patients with neuroblastoma by suppressing the growth of occult metastases, as actinomycin D (dactinomycin) has done for those with Wilms' tumor. Sutow reported the survival rates of patients with Wilms' tumor and neuroblastoma seen at 35 institutions in the United States.[11] Two years, 1957 and 1963, were selected for analysis. The former was chosen as a sample year when chemotherapy for patients with solid tumors was not used routinely. The latter year was selected because actinomycin D, vincristine and cyclophosphamide (Cytoxan) were in common use for the treatment of Wilms' tumor and neuroblastoma. The two test years were shown to be valid because a significant difference was detected in the survival rates for patients with Wilms' tumor. Little or no difference could be detected in the case of neuroblastoma. To be sure, the analysis was retrospective and encompassed many institutions without any attempt being made to evaluate the type of treatment individual patients had received.

Many investigators are currently engaged in attempting to define the role of chemotherapy in this disease. For example, members of the CCSGA are conducting a prospective investigation to determine the value of cyclophosphamide in the treatment of patients with localized neuroblastoma. All patients have as complete a removal of

TABLE 1.—*Two-Year Survival of 234 Children with Neuroblastoma*

Age (Yrs.)	*Stage* I	(%)	II	(%)	III	(%)	IV	(%)	IV-S	(%)	Total	(%)
<1	10/11	91	14/15	93	2/4	50	4/17	24	18/20	90	48/67	72
<2	4/5	80	5/8	63	3/7	43	0/26	0	1/1	100	13/47	28
>2	2/3	67	4/12	33	3/13	23	3/88	3	2/4	50	14/120	12
Total	16/19		23/35		8/24		7/131		21/25		75/234	
Survival (%)	84		66		33		5		84		32	

the primary tumor as possible, followed by postoperative radiation therapy if it is indicated. Thereafter, one-half of the patients receive intermittent courses of cyclophosphamide for one year. Until the value of chemotherapy has been defined, its use might well be limited to those patients two years of age or older with Stage II disease and all patients with Stage III and Stage IV tumors. It is difficult to decide its value in patients with Stage IV-S because several of the 25 patients enumerated in Table 1 survived without any chemotherapy. Perhaps those patients with evidence of disease in the bone marrow should be treated vigorously in the hope that small nests of cells can be prevented from growing and developing into symptomatic metastases. However, infants under one year of age, with lesions restricted to the liver or skin, or both, seem to survive with no additional treatment beyond removal of the primary tumor. It must be emphasized that current standard practice remains surgery, radiation therapy, and chemotherapy for all patients considered at risk. The foregoing analysis is an attempt to define the risks.

Several investigators have reported good responses in patients with metastatic neuroblastoma after treatment with cyclophosphamide and vincristine (singly or in combination) and, also, daunomycin.[12–14] The objective response rate is usually between 30 and 40 per cent, and a few long-term survivals of patients with bone metastases have occurred. This is not good enough, and the search for a better method goes on. For example, the current CCSGA study compares the effect of vincristine combined with cyclophosphamide versus a regimen using the same combination plus cytosine arabinoside.

Soft-Tissue Sarcomas

The treatment of rhabdomyosarcoma and allied soft-tissue sarcomas has traditionally rested upon complete surgical removal, including amputation when necessary. The need for such radical procedures has been questioned recently with regard to tumors arising in the orbit, and it has been suggested that radiation therapy alone in this situation might suffice. Similar considerations apply perhaps to other sites as well. Indeed, the role of radiation therapy is under active discussion revolving around two points:

1. Can radiation therapy be used as primary treatment, thus obviating radical surgery?
2. Should radiation therapy be given postoperatively to all patients, regardless of whether or not the surgical margins seem clear of tumor?

For example, with regard to the female pelvic structure, there is no hesitation in giving treatment when there is doubt regarding the adequacy of the excision, but excellent results have been obtained following complete removal alone. When the primary tumor is found to be localized at surgery, and microscopic examination of the surgical specimen shows a good margin of normal tissue surrounding the tumor, many radiation therapists believe that there is no indication for additional radiation. The dose normally delivered leads to considerable damage to normal structures and is too high a price to pay for radiation given for "prophylactic" purposes.

The perennial hope is that a better chemotherapeutic agent can be found that will obviate both radiation therapy and surgery. Even a less efficient agent, or combination of agents, would be of value if it would permit less radical surgical and radiotherapeutic procedures by cleaning up small foci of residual tumor cells. There have been some encouraging results along these lines. Recently, a study was designed by

CCSGA to determine whether actinomycin D and vincristine could suppress recurrent or metastatic disease in children with rhabdomyosarcoma. All patients had primary removal of the tumor, and most received postoperative irradiation. One group then continued without chemotherapy and the other received cyclic courses of actinomycin D and vincristine for one year. Preliminary results, using life table analysis, show a significant difference in the metastatic rate between those patients who received "prophylactic" chemotherapy and those who did not. Included in the group receiving chemotherapy were some patients with microscopic and, indeed, gross residual disease who have survived without recurrence or metastases. These preliminary data, derived from a small group of patients so far treated, suggest that "prophylactic" chemotherapy may be useful in patients with soft-tissue sarcomas, as it is in patients with Wilms' tumor, and, we hope, with equally good results. If this proves to be true, the basic approach to the treatment of soft-tissue sarcomas may change, and surgical and radiation therapy can be less radical.

Current Treatment for Other Tumors

The past 5 years have not produced major advances in the treatment of other tumors. Chemotherapy is being employed in a "prophylactic" manner for both osteogenic sarcoma and Ewing's tumor. I know of no agent which has a consistent effect on osteogenic sarcoma, but there are initial reports that chemotherapy may reduce the number of patients with Ewing's tumor in whom metastases develop. Hustu and Pinkel[15,16] have reported treatment of a small number of patients with vincristine and cyclophosphamide, leading to long-term survival in more than half. Some tumors of the central nervous system, such as medulloblastoma, are proving responsive to chemotherapy. There are reports of good effects after treatment with intrathecal methotrexate, intravenous vincristine and nitrosourea. Comparative studies are difficult to design and evaluate, but several are currently under way.

References

1. Evans, A. E.: Chemotherapy of solid tumors in children. *In* Brodsky, I. and Kahn, S. B. (Eds.): Cancer Chemotherapy. New York: Grune & Stratton, 1967, pp. 133–139.
2. O'Malley, B., D'Angio, G. J. and Vawter, G. F.: Late effects of roentgen therapy given in infancy. Amer. J. Roentgen. 89: 1067, 1963.
3. Tefft, M., Vawter, G. F. and Mitus, A.: Secondary primary neoplasms in children. Amer. J. Roentgen. 103:800, 1968.
4. Filler, R. M., Tefft, M., Vawter, G. F. and Mitus, A.: Hepatic lobectomy in childhood: Effects of x-ray and chemotherapy. (In press.)
5. Bill, A. H. and Morgan, A.: Evidence for immune reactions to neuroblastoma and future possibilities for investigation. J. Pediat. Surg. 5:111, 1970.
6. Wolff, J. A., Krivit, W., Newton, W. A., Jr. and D'Angio, G. J.: Single versus multiple dose dactinomycin therapy of Wilms' tumor. New Eng. J. Med. 279:290, 1968.
7. Wolff, J. A.: Personal communication.
8. Farber, S.: Chemotherapy in the treatment of leukemia and Wilms' tumor. J.A.M.A. 198:827, 1966.
9. Evans, A. E., D'Angio, G. J. and Randolph, J.: A proposed staging for children with neuroblastoma. Cancer 27:374, 1971.
10. Evans, A. E., D'Angio, G. J., Johnson, D. and Koop, C. E.: Observations on the management of children with neuroblastoma; Concepts derived from a new staging system. (In press.)
11. Sutow, W. W., Gehan, E. A., Heyn, R. M., Kung, F. H. et al.: Survival in Wilms' tumor and neuroblastoma. Pediatrics 4: 800, 1970.
12. James, D. H., Hustu, O., Wrenn, E. L. and Pinkel, D.: Combination chemotherapy of childhood neuroblastoma. J.A.M.A. 194: 123, 1965.

13. Evans, A. E., Heyn, R. M., Newton, W. A., Jr. and Leikin, S. L.: Vincristine sulphate and cyclophosphamide for children with metastatic neuroblastoma. J.A.M.A. 207: 1325, 1969.
14. Samuels, L., Newton, W. A., Jr. and Heyn, R. M.: Daunorubicin therapy in advanced neuroblastoma. Cancer 27:831, 1971.
15. Hustu, O. and Pinkel, D.: Treatment of Ewing's sarcoma with concurrent radiotherapy and chemotherapy. J. Pediat. 73:249, 1965.
16. Pinkel, D.: Personal communication.

Chemotherapy of Genitourinary Neoplasms

By Paul Gonick, M.D.

THE RESPONSE OF GENITOURINARY MALIGNANCY to chemotherapy varies from the high responsiveness of carcinomas of the prostate and testes, through the relative resistance of tumors of the genitourinary epithelium, to the almost uniform resistance of the adenocarcinomas of the renal parenchyma.

The material presented in this chapter will cover what is known of the chemotherapy of these three groups of tumors. It is recognized that dactinomycin and vincristine have improved survival of patients with Wilms' tumor of the kidney, and *o-p'*-DDD has been effective in treating patients with adrenal carcinoma. The therapy of these tumors is discussed in other chapters.

Carcinoma of the Prostate

The use of diethylstilbestrol in the treatment of carcinoma of the prostate marked the beginning of cancer chemotherapy, since this chemical was the first synthetic substance with anticancer activity.[1] Thirty years after Huggins' original paper, orchiectomy and estrogen therapy are still the main therapies for disseminated cancer of the prostate, and the use of these modalities has doubled or tripled survival in prostatic cancer patients.[2]

Several different dosages of diethylstilbestrol have been reported.[3] However, recent reports by the Veterans Administration Cooperative Research Group (VACRG) have shown up to 25 per cent increased mortality from cardiovascular diseases in a group of prostatic cancer patients treated with diethylstilbestrol (5 mg daily), when compared with a similar group of patients who were not treated with estrogen.[4] When a dosage of 5 mg per day of diethylstilbestrol was compared with a dosage of 1 mg per day in a subsequent study, the VACRG found similar antitumor effect but decreased cardiovascular toxicity at the latter dosage. Dosage of 0.2 mg per day of diethylstilbestrol was found to be ineffective.[5]

A new antiandrogen, cyproterone acetate, has been shown to be effective in treating a group of patients with prostatic cancer who had had no previous chemotherapy. Cyproterone has little or no estrogenic effect and is related to progestational hormones. Unfortunately, it does not appear to be any more effective than estrogens, and is of little value in treating the patient whose tumor no longer responds to estrogen.[6] The overall response rate to estrogens or orchiectomy is about 50 per cent, with remissions lasting 1 to 2 years.

Plan of Therapy

Stage I, or latent carcinoma (incidental finding at the time of prostatectomy). Therapy: Observation or, in rare cases, radical prostatectomy.

Stage II (nodule or induration without spread beyond the prostatic capsule). Therapy: Biopsy and either observation or radical prostatectomy, depending upon the age and condition of the patient.

From the Division of Urology, Department of Medicine, Hahnemann Medical College and Hospital, Philadelphia, Pennsylvania.

Stage III (local spread with a fixed prostate but no evidence of metastasis). Therapy: Biopsy and observation or radiation therapy, depending upon the age and condition of the patient.

Stage IV (lymph node or other organ metastases). Therapy: Biopsy and observation. Orchiectomy or diethylstilbestrol (1 mg per day orally) when the patient manifests symptoms of metastasis or the tumor rapidly increases in size.

Those patients whose symptoms are not relieved or whose malignancies progress rapidly usually do not respond to changes in the dosage of hormones.[4] However, a small number of patients may respond to the following maneuvers; these alternatives are offered for those who either fail after orchiectomy or estrogen therapy or relapse after remission:

1. Orchiectomy (despite previous administration of estrogens).
2. Switch to other estrogens (e.g., chlorotrianisene (Tace) or polyestradiol phosphate (Estradurin)).
3. Local external irradiation.
4. Diethylstilbestrol 4,4′-diphosphoric ester (Stilphostrol), 0.5 gm per day, by slow intravenous drip for 5 days.
5. Prednisone, 5 to 30 mg per day.
6. ^{32}P, with or without stimulation by androgens.[7]
7. Alkylating agents, followed by resumption with diethylstilbestrol, 1 mg per day.[8]
8. Adrenalectomy or hypophysectomy. Once the tumor is resistant to hormones, adrenalectomy or hypophysectomy rarely induces a response. Furthermore, these procedures require that the patient be in good medical condition and capable of following advice concerning hormone replacement. Thus, their use in the debilitated and elderly patient with carcinoma of the prostate is greatly limited.
9. Androgens: On rare occasions, estrogen-resistant prostatic cancer has responded to testosterone propionate, 100 mg intramuscularly, 3 times a week.[9]

The efficacy of conjugated estrogenic hormones (Premarin) and medroxyprogesterone acetate (Provera), with or without diethylstilbestrol, is presently being investigated by the VACRG. Immunotherapy with malignant prostatic cells grown in tissue culture or with frozen thawed tumor extracts may play a role in future therapy.

Cancer of the Testes

Chemotherapy of certain testicular cancers has yielded disease-free intervals of 2 years in 30 per cent of patients with metastatic disease. The concept of maintenance chemotherapy and prophylactic chemotherapy has gained support in the last five years.

The histologic and cellular types in testicular neoplasms are important in choosing the most effective form of chemotherapy. It is, therefore, imperative to examine multiple sections of the original tumor and to obtain a biopsy of metastatic deposits.

Seminoma

Seminomas are radiosensitive, and radiation therapy can usually control metastases. However, when the course of radiation is completed, or if there is widespread metastasis, a course with an alkylating agent such as chlorambucil (Leukeran), 6 to 10 mg per day to total dosage of 3 to 5 mg/kg or until toxicity is shown, or cyclophosphamide (Cytoxan), 150 to 300 mg per day to a total dosage of 50 mg/kg, may be given and then adjusted to maintain a leukocyte count of 3000 $\pm$ 500. If effective, such therapy is continued daily for 3 years.[10] The above course of treatment is modified with chlorambucil, 10 mg daily for 1 month orally, to be repeated every second month until the metastases are eliminated. Thereafter, courses are repeated every 2 or 3 months for 3 years.[10]

Embryonal Carcinoma, Teratocarcinoma and Choriocarcinoma

Single Drug Therapy (Mackenzie)[11]

Dactinomycin, 1.0 mg per day intravenously for 4 to 5 days, repeated monthly until 2 months after the cancer is completely gone. Additional courses are given every 2 months for three courses and then every 3 months for 2 years.

Double Drug Therapy (Golbey)[10]

Dactinomycin, 30 μg/kg per week intravenously, in one injection, and chlorambucil, 0.15 mg/kg per day orally, both drugs given until there is a fall in the leukocyte or platelet count (usually 4 to 8 weeks). Therapy is discontinued until the bone marrow recovers, and the course is then repeated for 3 years.

Triple Drug Therapy (Golbey)[10]

If there is no response to the combination of dactinomycin and chlorambucil, methotrexate, 2.5 to 5 mg per day orally, is added to the course of therapy. If methotrexate is contraindicated because of poor renal function, vincristine sulfate (Oncovin), 1 mg per week, is given intravenously.

Mithramycin

Kennedy[12] reported an 80 per cent response and a 25 per cent disease-free interval of 2 years after treating with mithramycin patients who had mixed testicular neoplasms. Mithramycin, 50 μg/kg per day, was given 3 times a week on alternate days. Hematologic, hepatic, and renal function was carefully monitored, and the course of therapy was continued until signs of toxicity developed (3 to 6 doses). Additional courses of therapy were given 2 to 4 weeks later. If no improvement was noted after two courses, the use of mithramycin was discontinued. If objective improvement occurred, a total of six courses, one month apart, was given. Alternate-day therapy caused less toxicity and yielded greater length of survival than that reported in an earlier series of patients given mithramycin daily. There were no deaths with alternate-day therapy (Tables 1 and 2).

Table 1.—*Comparison of the Results of Two Dose Schedules of Mithramycin in the Treatment of Advanced Testicular Neoplasms*[12]

	Daily	*Alternate Day*
Number of patients	21	23
Regression (%)	47	43
Duration of control (mean months)	6	16+
Survival (mean months)		
Responders	12.2	20+
Non-responders	4.3	5.7

Tables 1 and 2 from Kennedy, B. J.,[12] with permission.

TABLE 2.—*Comparison of the Incidence of Systemic Reactions with Two Dose Schedules of Mithramycin in the Treatment of Advanced Testicular Neoplasms*[12]

	Dose Schedule	
	*Daily** (%)	*Alternate-Day*† (%)
Anorexia	100	100
Vomiting	89	90
Fever	81	13
Irritability	29	34
Lethargy	47	26
Flushing	67	9
Facial swelling	33	4
Stomatitis	33	0
Epistaxis	59	0
Hemorrhage	43	0
Thrombocytopenia	52	4
Increased prothrombin time	72	17
Increased BUN	52	21
Increased LDH	100	100
Mortality	28.5	0

* Number of patients = 21.
† Number of patients = 23.

The data in these tables suggest that the renal, hepatic, and hematologic toxicity is great, and therefore a check of the platelet count, prothrombin time, lactate dehydrogenase (LDH) and blood urea nitrogen (BUN) before each subsequent dose of this drug is vital.

TUMORS ARISING FROM THE GENITOURINARY EPITHELIUM

Epithelial neoplasms of the renal pelvis, ureter, bladder and proximal urethra are derived from the same cell type (transitional or squamous), often are multicentric, and biologically behave similarly. In general, they are resistant to present-day chemotherapeutic agents.

Drugs that have been of some benefit in the treatment of bladder neoplasms are 5-fluorouracil, vinblastine, vincristine, cyclophosphamide, thio-TEPA, Streptonigrin, methotrexate, sarcolysin, Carzinophlin and mitomycin C. The most commonly used agent is 5-fluorouracil. Evaluation of the therapeutic effect of any drug is often difficult. In a recent double-blind study of patients with advanced bladder carcinoma, the group of patients treated with placebo responded better than a comparable group of patients treated with 5-fluorouracil.[13] Although systemic or perfusion chemotherapy has not been rewarding when used alone, some patients have responded to the combination of 5-fluorouracil and irradiation.[14,15]

Topical treatment of papillary lesions of the bladder that have not invaded beyond the subepithelium has resulted in complete destruction of the tumor in one-third of patients so treated, partial destruction in one third and no effect in one third.[16] The patient's fluid intake is restricted for 12 hours preceding the instillation. The treatment program consists of instilling into the bladder 60 mg of thio-TEPA in 60 ml of sterile water once a week for 4 weeks. The drug is retained in the bladder for 2 hours. Two weeks later, cystoscopy is performed, and the tumor effect evaluated. If the tumor has shrunk or if there is edema of the fronds, additional weekly courses are given for

2 to 4 weeks and any remaining tumor is fulgurated. Two to four more instillations are given after fulguration. Following this, instillations are continued monthly for a year. Prior to each instillation, the leukocyte count and the platelet count are determined to detect toxicity. Treatment is not given if the leukocyte count is less than 3,000 cu mm or the platelet count less than 50,000 cu mm.

Adenocarcinoma of the Kidney

It is difficult to evaluate the response of patients with metastases from adenocarcinoma of the kidney, since the course of the disease is exceedingly variable, the response to therapy may be delayed, and on rare occasions, spontaneous remissions have been observed.

Progestins

At the present, progestins are the preferred treatment for metastatic hypernephroma. Medroxyprogesterone acetate (Provera or Depo-Provera), 800 mg per week intramuscularly for 4 to 6 weeks, then 400 mg per week intramuscularly or 50 to 100 mg per day by mouth, or hydroxyprogesterone caproate, 50 mg by mouth twice a day, is given until objective regression or lack of tumor response is observed. Although subjective improvement may be noted earlier, it may take up to 13 months to detect objective signs.[17] Sixty-eight patients, reported in three separate series, treated with progestin or androgen, or both, showed an objective tumor response of 18 per cent.[17] If progestin therapy does not succeed, androgen therapy is tried.

Other chemotherapeutic agents have been used, but with only rarely favorable results (Tables 3 and 4). Corticosteroids have been effective in obtaining subjective improvement only.

Table 3.—*Summary of Chemotherapy of Metastatic Adenocarcinoma of the Kidney*[17]

Agents	*No. of Patients*	*Response* *Objective*	*Subjective*
Alkylating	19	1	1
Antimetabolite	19	–	2
Vinblastine	13	1	2
Dactinomycin	2	–	–
Corticosteroids	38	–	10
Progestins	16	2	–
Androgens	11	–	–

From Talley et al.,[17] with permission.

Table 4.—*Summary of Chemotherapy of Metastatic Adenocarcinoma of the Kidney*[18]

Agents	*No. of Patients*	*Objective Response*
Alkylating	79	7
Antimetabolite	83	11
Alkaloids	20	1
Antibiotics	46	4
Hormones	27	5
Miscellaneous	15	2

From Woodruff et al.,[18] with permission.

REFERENCES

1. Huggins, C.: Studies on prostatic cancer. *In* Immergut, M. A. (Ed.): Classical Articles in Urology. Springfield, Ill. Charles C Thomas, 1967, p. 232.
2. Nesbit, R. M. and Baum, W. C.: Endocrine control of prostatic carcinoma. J.A.M.A. 146:1317, 1950.
3. Fergusson, J. D.: Some aspects of the conservative management of prostate cancer. Proc. Roy. Soc. Med. 56:81, 1963.
4. Veterans Administration Cooperative Research Group: Carcinoma of the prostate: Treatment comparisons. J. Urol. 98:516, 1967.
5. Veterans Administration Cooperative Research Group: Estrogen treatment for cancer of the prostate: Early results with three doses of diethylstilbestrol and placebo. Cancer 26:257, 1970.
6. Scott, W. W. and Schirmer, H. K. A.: A new oral progestational steroid effective in treating prostatic cancer. Trans. Amer. Ass. Genitourin. Surg. 58:54, 1966.
7. Kaplan, E., Fels, I. G., Kotlowski, B. R., Greco, J. and Walsh, W. S.: Therapy of cancer of the prostate metastatic to the bone with ^{32}P-labeled condensed phosphate. J. Nucl. Med. 1:1, 1960.
8. Arduino, L.: Personal communication.
9. Prout, G. R. and Brewer, C. V. R.: Response of men with advanced prostatic carcinoma to exogenous administration of testosterone. Cancer 20:1871, 1967.
10. Golbey, R. B.: The place of chemotherapy in the treatment of testicular tumors. J.A.M.A. 213:101, 1970.
11. Mackenzie, A. R., Golbey, R. B. and Whitmore, W. F., Jr.: Exhibit, annual meeting of American Medical Association, 1967.
12. Kennedy, B. J.: Mithramycin therapy in advanced testicular neoplasms. Cancer 26:755, 1970.
13. Prout, G. R., Jr., Bross, I. D. J., Slack, N. H. and Ausman, R. K.: Carcinoma of the bladder: 5-fluorouracil and critical role of placebo. Cooperative Group Report I. Cancer 22:926, 1968.
14. Kaufmann, J. J., Langdon, E. A., Stein, J. J. and Burt, F. B.: Cancer of the bladder. Calif. Med. 101:334, 1964.
15. Woodruff, M. W., Murphy, W. T. and Hodson, J. M.: Further observations on the use of combination 5-fluorouracil and supervoltage irradiation therapy in the treatment of advanced carcinoma of the bladder. J. Urol. 90:747, 1963.
16. Veenema, R. J.: The role of thio-TEPA instillations in bladder cancer. J.A.M.A. 206:2725, 1968.
17. Talley, R. W., Moorhead, E. L., Tucker, W. G., San Diego, E. L. and Brennan, M. J.: Treatment of metastatic hypernephroma. J.A.M.A. 207:322, 1969.
18. Woodruff, M. W., Wagle, D., Gailani, S. D. and Jones, R., Jr.: The current status of chemotherapy for advanced renal carcinoma. J. Urol. 97:611, 1967.

Chemotherapy of Neoplasms of the Respiratory Tract

By Michael J. Mastrangelo, M.D.
and Arthur J. Weiss, M.D.

Cancer of the Head and Neck

NEOPLASMS OF THE HEAD AND NECK involve the skin, lip, buccal mucosa, gingivae, palate, floor of the mouth, tongue, tonsils, nasal cavity, nasopharynx, pharyngeal wall, larynx, paranasal sinuses, and thyroid and salivary glands. Most of these lesions are epidermoid in origin. The primary modalities of therapy are surgery and irradiation therapy. The response of head and neck neoplasms to chemotherapy is limited. Chemotherapy has, however, been used alone for palliative purposes and as an adjuvant to radiation or surgery or both.

The use of infusion chemotherapy alone or in combination with surgery and radiation therapy or both will be discussed by other authors in this volume. This discussion will be limited to the use of palliative systemic chemotherapy.

The available clinical data evaluating the efficacy of various chemotherapeutic agents in head and neck cancer are summarized in Table 1. The results of systemic chemotherapy are palliative but sometimes striking. Of the conventional drugs available, methotrexate is clearly the most effective, with an alkylating agent the drug of second choice. Dibromodulcitol also has produced some notable remissions. A new chemical agent, bleomycin,[14–16] has had extensive trial in Japan, and its efficacy in squamous cell carcinoma is promising. The data need further confirmation. This drug may cause serious side effects, primarily pulmonary fibrosis, and must be used only by those familiar with antineoplastic agents.

It must be emphasized that surgery or radiation therapy, or both, with or without infusion chemotherapy, are the therapeutic modalities of first choice. However, systemic chemotherapy can produce outstanding palliative results, though infrequently.

Cancer of the Lung

After several decades of intensive investigation, the control of bronchogenic carcinoma remains a frustrating problem. It was estimated that 57,000 men and 11,000 women would be discovered to have lung cancer during 1970.[17] About 50 per cent of these neoplasms will be inoperable at the time of diagnosis. Of those subjected to thoracotomy, only half will be actually resectable. The overall 5-year survival is about 5 per cent.[18]

The magnitude of the problem could perhaps be lessened by more effective prevention. Several extrinsic etiologic agents have been implicated in lung cancer, unlike most other human neoplasms.[19] Despite attempts to reduce exposure to these agents, the incidence of lung cancer in the male population has increased sharply in the last 20 years. The incidence of lung cancer in females is also rising sharply.[17] The value of chest X-ray surveys for early detection of lung cancer has proved to be slight. Mass roentgenographic surveys have been tried in the United States and Sweden, but the yield of curable cases is small.[20] The application of mass cytologic screening to

---

From the Division of Medical Oncology, Jefferson Medical College of Thomas Jefferson University, Philadelphia, Pennsylvania.

TABLE 1.—*Response of Head and Neck Tumors to Chemotherapy*

Drug	*Ref.*	*No. of Patients Type of Carcinoma*	*Response (No. of Patients)* Complete	Partial	No Change	*Symptomatic*	*No Response*
Dibromodulcitol	1	3 tonsil	2	1	—	—	0
		3 larynx	2	1	—	—	0
		1 pharynx	0	0	—	—	1
	2	3	0	0	—	1	2
Hydroxyurea	3	2 tongue	0	1	—	—	1
		1 larynx	0	0	—	—	1
	4	15	0	(40%)	—	(50%)	(50%)
Trimethylpurin-6-yl-ammonium chloride (NSC-51095)	5	1 larynx	0	0	—	—	1
6-Mercaptopurine	6	10	0	1	—	—	9
Hexamethylmelamine	7	36	0	3	16	—	17
Cyclophosphamide plus hexamethylmelamine	2	15	0	2	—	10	3
Methotrexate (oral)	8	8 squamous cell	1 (lip)	2 (floor of mouth, external auditory canal)	2 (soft palate, tongue)	—	3 (larynx, pharynx, alveolar ridge)
Methotrexate (intermittent, intravenous)	9	9 tongue	0	3	—	—	6
		3 larynx	0	3	—	—	0
		3 pharynx	0	1	—	—	2
Methotrexate (intravenous)	10	2 lip	0	2	—	2	—
		4 floor of mouth	0	1	—	2	—
		4 tongue	0	4	—	3	—
		1 soft palate	0	0	—	0	1
		2 tonsil	0	1	—	1	—
		2 antrum	0	0	—	0	2
		4 hypopharynx	0	3	—	2	—
		1 pyriform sinus	0	0	—	0	1
		13 larynx	0	9	—	8	—
		2 esophagus	0	0	—	1	—

Cyclophosphamide	11	9 larynx	0	3	—	—	6
		3 pyriform fossa	0	0	—	1	2
		1 postcricoid	0	1	—	—	0
		1 nasopharynx	0	1	—	—	0
		1 maxilla	0	1	—	—	0
		1 tongue	0	1	—	—	0
		1 tonsils	0	1	—	—	0
		3 pharynx	0	3	—	—	0
		1 melanoma	0	0	—	—	1
		1 middle ear	0	0	0	1 (?)	0
		5 glottis	0	0	0	0	5
Methotrexate and cyclophosphamide	12	5	0	1	0	—	4
Carbestrol	2	1	0	0	—	1	0
Porfiromycin	2	15	0	0	—	12	3
BCNU	2	11	1	1	—	7	2
Imidazole carboxamide	2	17	0	0	—	13	4
Methotrexate (amethopterin)	13						
(intravenous and oral)		10 tongue	0	6	—	—	4
		2 lip	0	1	—	—	1
		1 gingivae	0	0	—	—	1
		7 tonsils	0	2	—	—	5
		3 hypopharynx	0	2	—	—	1
		2 alveolar ridge	0	1	—	—	1
		1 antrum	0	1	—	—	0
		7 larynx	0	3	—	—	4
		3 oral cavity	0	1	—	—	2
		4 nasopharynx	0	1	—	—	3
		2 pyriform sinus	0	1	—	—	1
Bleomycin	14	10	0	2 (>50%) 3 (<50%)	—	—	5
	15	18	0	4	—	—	14
	16	32 maxilla	0	25	—	—	7
		1 nasal cavity	0	0	—	—	1
		22 oral cavity	0	17	—	—	5
		14 larynx	0	6	—	—	8
		2 pharynx	0	1	—	—	1

asymptomatic high-risk patients offers real promise for the detection of "truly early" lung cancer, but has not as yet achieved wide use.[21,22]

The therapeutic armamentarium to combat lung cancer consists of surgery, radiation therapy, and chemotherapy. Surgery remains the best therapy in operable cases, as it offers the greatest chance for cure. The best surgical results are achieved in the treatment of asymptomatic solitary pulmonary nodules. A series of 392 such patients was studied by the Veterans Administration and Armed Forces hospitals.[23] Of these 392 patients, 78.9 per cent had cancer confined to the lung and underwent so-called curative pulmonary resections. The 5-year survival rate was 38 per cent but only 19 per cent survived to the ninth year. Indeed, after as many as 10 apparently disease-free years, the risk of recurrence remains high. It is evident that relatively conservative surgical techniques are as effective as radical ones.[24] Little improvement can be expected in the survival rate in lung cancer as a result of improved surgical techniques, primarily because the main problem in lung cancer appears to be early dissemination of disease.[25]

Can lung cancer be cured by radiation alone? Hilton[26] treated 40 patients who appeared to be eligible for surgical resection with orthovoltage radiation therapy. He reported a 5-year survival rate of 22.5 per cent, with less than 5 per cent surviving 10 years. Since this is lower than the survival rate with surgery, surgery remains the treatment of choice in operable lung cancer. The early use of radiation as the only therapeutic modality in inoperable lung cancer has produced dismal results.[27–29] These poor results may have been related to the extent of disease. Wolf et al.[30] reported on 554 patients with localized (limited to a hemithorax) but clinically inoperable bronchogenic carcinoma who were randomly assigned to treatment with radiation or placebo. The median survival of patients given radiation therapy was 142 days as compared with 112 days for the placebo group. Thus, it would appear that for limited disease, radiation therapy offered a slight advantage over no therapy. The data are not as yet conclusive.

The routine use of preoperative radiation therapy as an adjuvant to the surgical treatment of bronchogenic carcinoma has been suggested in an attempt to improve the salvage rate from this disease. The Veterans Administration Surgical Adjuvant Cancer Chemotherapy Group[31] performed a prospective study of 311 patients, which failed to show any improvement in the salvage rate in the preoperative X-ray group over that obtained in the group treated by operation alone. In fact, a statistically significant adverse effect was recorded in the preoperative X-ray group in relation to operative morbidity and mortality. On the contrary, the role of radiation therapy in the treatment of superior vena caval obstruction, bronchial obstruction, hemoptysis, pathologic fractures, and pain secondary to neoplasia has been clearly established.[32,33]

With this background, it seems likely that any advance in the treatment of bronchogenic carcinoma must come from a systemic form of therapy. In 1948, Karnofsky et al.[34] reported their results on the use of nitrogen mustard (HN2; mechlorethamine) as palliative treatment of lung cancer. In 74 per cent of 35 patients, clinical improvement occurred as evidenced by alleviation of symptoms such as cough, dyspnea, hemoptysis, pain, weakness, and superior vena caval obstruction. In addition, regression of pulmonary metastatic nodules was noted. The improvement usually lasted from 2 weeks to 2 months, and further courses of HN2 were usually not as effective. This study prompted a host of subsequent studies with a variety of chemotherapeutic agents. In 1961, White[35] summarized the studies published to date and recorded over

TABLE 2.—*Proportion Surviving to Indicated Day*

Day	*Nitrogen mustard*	*Diethyl-stilbestrol*	*Inert compound*	*Testosterone propionate*	*Cortisone*	*Progesterone*
Point estimate						
30th	0.87	0.80	0.75	0.75	0.74	0.73
60th	0.75	0.58	0.62	0.62	0.46	0.51
90th	0.63	0.44	0.51	0.44	0.37	0.41
120th	0.51	0.33	0.46	0.37	0.26	0.33
150th	0.42	0.26	0.38	0.28	0.21	0.27
180th	0.39	0.25	0.30	0.22	0.18	0.23
90% Confidence interval estimate						
30th	0.78–0.93	0.72–0.87	0.66–0.82	0.66–0.82	0.65–0.82	0.64–0.81
60th	0.65–0.83	0.48–0.67	0.52–0.71	0.53–0.70	0.37–0.56	0.41–0.60
90th	0.53–0.73	0.35–0.54	0.42–0.61	0.36–0.53	0.28–0.47	0.32–0.51
120th	0.39–0.61	0.24–0.42	0.37–0.56	0.29–0.46	0.18–0.35	0.25–0.43
150th	0.32–0.52	0.19–0.36	0.29–0.48	0.20–0.36	0.14–0.30	0.19–0.36
180th	0.29–0.50	0.18–0.34	0.22–0.39	0.16–0.30	0.11–0.27	0.16–0.32

From Wolf et al.,[37] with permission.

100 with as many different agents or combinations of agents. Though the use of chemotherapy increased manyfold, the studies were, in general, poorly controlled.

The Veterans Administration Lung Cancer Study Group (VALCSG) began systematic attempts to evaluate the effects of chemotherapy on patients with inoperable bronchogenic carcinoma in 1958. Over 7,000 patients in 18 participating hospitals have been studied. Survival was used as an end point.[36] Because the disease occurs mostly in males, early trials of biologically active steroids versus HN2 and placebo were carried out. Wolf et al.[37] reported on 496 such patients randomly allocated to treatment for 3 months with HN2, diethylstilbestrol, testosterone, cortisone, progesterone and placebo (Table 2). Sixty-three per cent of the patients given HN2 were alive at the end of 90 days, as compared with 51 per cent of the patients receiving placebo and 37 per cent of the patients receiving cortisone. Mortality in the group treated with cortisone was highest during the second month of treatment. Table 3 shows that the median survival time for the control group was 93 days, as compared with 121 days for the group given HN2 and 56 days for the patients given cortisone. This was the first clear demonstration that HN2 favorably influenced survival in bronchogenic carcinoma.

TABLE 3.—*Median Survival Times and Estimated Mean Survival Times*

Therapy	*Survival* Median (days)	Estimated mean (days)
Nitrogen mustard	121	172
Diethylstilbestrol	75	138
Inert compound	93	138
Testosterone propionate	78	117
Cortisone	56	106
Progesterone	60	122

From Wolf et al.,[37] with permission.

TABLE 4.—*Percentage of Survival to Indicated Month*

	All Cases		*Squamous*		*Undifferentiated*		*Oat Cell*		*Adenocarcinoma*	
Month	*Inert compound*	*Cyclophos-phamide*	*Inert compound*	*Cyclophos-phamide*	*Inert compound*	*Cyclophos-phamide*	*Inert compound*	*Cyclophos-phamide*	*Inert compound*	*Cyclophos-phamide*
2	68	74	76	69	69	75	60	88	68	71
3	50	58	61	58	43	55	37	70	57	57
4	38	47	43	46	37	45	25	58	46	43
5	30	38	32	40	31	38	17	49	39	31
7	19	24	23	28	17	22	10	29	24	15
10	11	11	14	15	11	9	6	9	13	8
13	7	7	8	11	8	6	2	6	6	5
No. of patients treated	616	426	124	81	204	139	87	57	101	69

From Green et al.,[38] with permission.

Encouraged by the initial study with HN2, the VALCSG then conducted a randomized study to evaluate alkylating agents in bronchogenic carcinoma.[38] Nitrogen mustard, chlorambucil, oral cyclophosphamide, or intravenous cyclophosphamide was administered for 90 days. The patients were subdivided into limited (disease confined to a hemithorax) and extensive disease for further analysis, with survival being the end point. The median survival in days was 92 for the entire HN2 group, but only 76 for the placebo group. Analysis by extent of disease demonstrated that the increased survival was more prominent in the limited disease group. In addition in only squamous cell carcinoma did HN2 prolong life.

In patients with extensive disease treated with intravenous cyclophosphamide, the median survival time was 81 days versus 61 in the control group. Table 4 demonstrates that the improvement in survival rate was most marked in the oat cell category. Oral cyclophosphamide appeared to be ineffective in increasing survival time. The ease with which cyclophosphamide can be administered orally prompted a study in which a single intravenous course was followed by the oral preparation, but no improvement in survival time over placebo was noted. Though the oral preparation was given in total doses exceeding the amount given during a comparable period of intravenous administration, peak blood levels were undoubtedly higher via the intravenous route; this may account for the lack of effectiveness of the oral preparation.

After this study, the VALCSG studied the effects of 1,3-bis(2-chloroethyl)-1-nitrosourea (BCNU), imidazole carboxamide, methotrexate, streptonigrin and vinblastine.[36] The results with vinblastine and streptonigrin were believed to be inferior to those with placebo. The poor results with vinblastine were confirmed by Crosbie et al.[39] BCNU, imidazole carboxamide and methotrexate produced results comparable to those with placebo. Definitive evaluation will have to await more detailed reports.

The VALCSG also evaluated the efficacy of hydroxyurea (80 mg/kg every 3 days) in 170 patients with nonresectable bronchogenic carcinoma and found no difference in survival time between this group and a similar group of patients treated with cyclophosphamide (8 mg/kg per day intravenously for 5 days, repeated every 6 weeks).[40]

Considerable data are available concerning the effectiveness of chemotherapeutic agents in shrinking tumor masses. The objective measurement of pulmonary lesions is more difficult to evaluate than survival. In most studies, a greater than 50 per cent decrease (largest × the widest or perpendicular diameter) in mass size is used as the chief criterion for a favorable response. These data were recently reviewed in detail by Frost et al.[41] (Table 5).

HN2,[42-44] cyclophosphamide,[43,45] and methotrexate[46,47] are most effective, objective responses averaging around 30 per cent. Of the investigational drugs, BCNU[2,53] and dibromodulcitol[2] appeared to be the most effective. Procarbazine[48,56] and vincristine[49,57] were associated with objective regression in approximately 15 per cent of patients treated. Hexamethylmelamine, while not widely used, deserves further exploration. With a dosage of 12 mg/kg per day, a regression rate of 26 per cent was obtained; with dosage of 8 mg/kg per day, a 17 per cent remission rate was obtained. Also, it was noted that a high percentage of the patients treated did not progress during their treatment period.[50] Conversely, responses to methotrexate and procarbazine were usually short-lived. Hydroxyurea,[51,59,60] streptonigrin[61-63] and adriamycin[52,64] were only marginally effective. Tumor regression was short-lived, especially with hydroxyurea. This is interesting in light of the fact that this drug apparently is able to

TABLE 5.—*Objective Response of Measurable Lesions to Single Agents*

Treatment	*Patients entered*	*Percentage of patients responding*	*Patients responding**	*Reference*
Mechlorethamine	388	32	0–68†	42–44
Cyclophosphamide	340	28	10–52	43, 45
Methotrexate	127	24	5–32	46, 47
BCNU	38	16	11–30	53, 2
Dibromodulcitol	10	30	—	2
Procarbazine	103	20	10–50†	48, 56
Vincristine	29	17	12–50†	49, 57
Hexamethylmelamine	164	19	19–20	50, 58
Hydroxyurea	81	14	11–18	51, 59, 60
Streptonigrin	47	13	0–29	61–63
Adriamycin, daunorubicin	28	11	7–14	52, 64
Fluorouracil, FUDR	108	7	0–16	54, 65–67
Mercaptopurine	88	3	3–4	55, 68
Mitomycin C	49	8	—	69
Porfiromycin	26	7.5	—	2
Imidazole carboxamide	53	7.5	—	2
Placebo	35	6	—	70

* Range of response rates for the individual publications listed.
† Includes patients with high proportion of oat cell carcinomas.
Adapted from Frost et al.,[41] with permission.

prolong life. 5-Fluorouracil[54] and 6-mercaptopurine[55] were remarkably ineffective despite their wide acceptance for palliation of adenocarcinoma of the breast and bowel, and of leukemia, respectively. Mitomycin C,[69] porfiromycin,[2] and imidazole carboxamide[2] are only minimally effective.

An objective response rate of 6 per cent was found in a small series of patients with measurable disease treated with a placebo. These responses were short-lived.[70] Transiently static or slowly progressive disease in a small proportion of patients may occasionally contribute to benefits incorrectly ascribed to therapy.

Another use for chemotherapy is as an adjuvant to surgery. A cooperative study by 25 Veterans Administration hospitals evaluated a total of 1008 patients.[74] These patients were randomized into two groups. The treatment group received 6 mg/kg of cyclophosphamide administered into the pleural cavity at the close of the operation and the same dose intravenously on postoperative days 1, 2, 3, and 4. A second course was given in the fifth postoperative week consisting of 8 mg/kg intravenously for 5 days. A second group underwent the operative procedure but had no adjuvant chemotherapy. No significant increase in morbidity was noted that could be attributed to cyclophosphamide. However, of 414 patients who underwent apparently curative resections and who were randomized to receive cyclophosphamide, only 235 had the maximal protocol dosage. No increase in survival could be demonstrated in patients who had had either curative or palliative resections.

A current study is being undertaken using prolonged intermittent therapy.[72] Because no increase in survival could be demonstrated by the cyclophosphamide adjuvant study and because maximal chemotherapy could not be administered when started on the day of surgery, admission to the prolonged intermittent therapy protocol was more selective. An apparently curative resection was required. In addition, histologic examination of the specimen had to demonstrate one or more of the

TABLE 6.—*Response of Patients to Chemotherapy and/or Radiotherapy as Measured by Survival (Studies with Random Allocation of Patients)*

Treatment	*No. of Patients*	*Patient survival (months)* 50%	20%	*p*	*Ref.*
Radiation therapy	69	3.5	10.1		74
Radiation therapy and HN2	67	3.6	8.9	.05	
HN2 followed by radiation therapy	60	4.0	11.9		
Radiation therapy	115	4.5	13.3		73
Radiation therapy and 5-FU	113	4.4	10.5	.05	
Radiation therapy and dactinomycin	114	3.5	9.3		

Adapted from Frost et al.,[41] with permission.

following: (1) undifferentiated carcinoma, (2) blood vessel invasion, (3) lymphatic invasion, (4) involvement of visceral pleura, (5) positive lymph nodes, (6) tumor found in other tissues or organs removed, and (7) final pathologic classification: tumor extending beyond the lung. Thus, the study was limited to those patients with curative resection but a known high recurrence rate. Randomization was done on the fourteenth postoperative day to allow time for adequate histologic classification and to determine whether the patient was clinically able to undergo chemotherapy. The patients were randomized into one of three groups: control, no further antineoplastic therapy; or regimen A, cyclophosphamide intravenously, 8 mg per kilogram of body weight, for 5 consecutive days, to be repeated every 5 weeks for 18 months; or regimen B, the same dosage of cyclophosphamide alternated every 5 weeks with methotrexate given parenterally, 10 mg/day for 5 days, for a period of 18 months. Adequate numbers of patients have not yet been treated to provide statistically significant results.

Another use for chemotherapy is as an adjuvant to radiation therapy. The combination of radiation therapy with HN2, 5-fluorouracil and actinomycin showed no superiority over radiation therapy alone in random allocation studies performed by the Eastern Cooperative Oncology Group[73,74] (Table 6). The same conclusion was reached by others who compared radiation therapy alone with radiation therapy plus 5-fluorouracil,[75,76] cyclophosphamide[77] and HN2.[78]

Though the use of chemotherapy as an adjuvant to either radiation therapy or surgery would appear to be without merit at the present time, single-agent chemotherapy offers a definite though small improvement in survival. There is, however, reason for additional hope. Our experience with combination chemotherapy in leukemia and lymphomas and certain testicular tumors has stimulated the use of multiple-drug therapy in solid tumors.

The VALCSG[79] has compared the combination of cyclophosphamide, methotrexate and streptonigrin with cyclophosphamide alone. The patients on combination therapy received half the dose of each drug; a slight advantage with regard to the combination could be detected (Table 7). Mannes et al.[80] reported on the study of four regimens: (1) placebo; (2) cyclophosphamide alone; (3) cyclophosphamide, methotrexate (plus leucovorin) and vincristine; (4) cyclophosphamide, 5-fluorouracil, mitomycin C, procarbazine and vinblastine (Table 8). Alberto et al.[81] and Chanes and Bottomley[82] have reported a higher objective response rate for methotrexate-cyclophosphamide-procarbazine-vincristine and actinomycin-vincristine regimens; however, a critical evaluation of these results must await a more detailed publication.

TABLE 7.—*Percentage Alive on Indicated Day*

Day	*Placebo*	*Cytoxan = cyclophosphamide*	*Triple-drug therapy*
30	68.8	74.5	79.8
60	51.0	59.6	62.7
90	37.9	47.2	52.1
120	30.0	38.0	48.7

From Wolf,[79] with permission.

The VALCSG has begun a study to evaluate the effectiveness of three pairs of agents: (1) cyclophosphamide (not cell-cycle–sensitive) and methotrexate (cell-cycle–sensitive), (2) actinomycin D and vincristine, and (3) hydroxyurea and 1-(2-chloroethyl,3-cyclohexyl-1-nitrosourea) (CCNU) (CCNU crosses the blood-brain barrier). The initial results are encouraging.

One problem complicating bronchogenic carcinoma, malignant pleural effusions, occurs in about 50 per cent of patients. Although such effusions can on occasion be controlled by thoracentesis, generally more aggressive measures are required to control the distressing recurrence of fluid. The successful control of malignant pleural effusions can significantly increase the quality of life, but it rarely has any effect on the progress of the malignancy. As previously noted, in 1948 Karnofsky et al.[34] reported on the use of HN2 in the palliation of lung cancer. In this series, HN2 was administered intrapleurally to two patients, and in one the effusion did not recur. Since then intrapleural HN2 has been used extensively in the treatment of pleural effusions secondary to bronchogenic carcinoma[83] with a control rate of about 50 per cent. If there are no mitigating circumstances, a dose of 0.4 mg/kg is administered. Nitrogen mustard acts as both a sclerosing agent, producing an adhesive pleuritis, and a cytotoxic agent. By use of instillation, nausea, vomiting and leukopenia are diminished. Before instillation of the drug, most of the pleural fluid should be removed. The HN2 is given over a 5-minute period and the patient is then moved into various positions to disperse the drug. If control is not achieved and there are no persistent systemic toxic effects, the treatment can be repeated in 2 or 3 weeks.

Frequently the use of an antineoplastic agent is not advisable because of systemic toxicity. Quinacrine (Atabrine) can be used in these cases.[83,84] Quinacrine is cytotoxic to normal and neoplastic cells in tissue culture but this is not its mechanism of action in controlling malignant pleural effusions. The instillation of quinacrine into the pleural space produces a reactive adhesive pleuritis which is effective in obliterating the pleural cavity. The effectiveness of the drug is not related to the sensitivity of

TABLE 8.—*Response of Lung Cancer to Combination Chemotherapy*

Treatment	*No. of Patients*	*Median survival (months)*
Placebo	36	2.8
Cytoxan (cyclophosphamide)	36	5.1
Cytoxan and methotrexate with leucovorin and vincristine	47	7.5
Cytoxan and 5-fluorouracil and mitomycin C and procarbazine and vinblastine	78	6.5

the neoplasm, and a response rate of 75 per cent is anticipated. Quinacrine has the added advantage of producing no significant systemic effects which would interfere with concomitant chemotherapy. We favor removing as much pleural fluid as possible and instilling 200 to 400 mg of quinacrine. This dose is repeated daily or every other day for 3 to 5 doses until pleuritis is achieved. This is evidenced by pleuritic chest pain and fever, which may be as high as 103° F. During this interval, the formation of fluid may be accelerated and thoracentesis may be required. Quinacrine is a relatively safe drug but must be used with caution in patients with cerebral metastases, especially if cortisone is being administered concomitantly, for seizures have been reported when the drugs are used in combination. Dollinger et al.[84] treated 13 patients; in 9 (68 per cent) an objective response was noted. Only one had a recurrence of the effusion before death. Two patients were followed up, one 27 months without recurrence and the other 19½ months.

References

1. Sellei, C., Eckhardt, S., Horvath, I. P., Kralovanszky, J. and Institoris, L.: Clinical and pharmacologic experience with dibromodulcitol (NSC-104800), a new antitumor agent. Cancer Chemother. Rep. 53:377, 1969.
2. Sedransk, N.: Cumulative report of Phase I and Phase II studies conducted by the Central Oncology Group, National Cancer Institute, 1970.
3. Lerner, H. J., Beckloff, G. L. and Godwin, M. C.: Hydroxyurea (NSC-32065) intermittent therapy in malignant diseases. Cancer Chemother. Rep. 53:385, 1969.
4. Ariel, I. M.: Therapeutic effects of hydroxyurea. Cancer 25:705, 1970.
5. Phillips, R. W.: Further clinical studies of trimethylpurin-6-yl-ammonium chloride (NSC-51095) in malignant disease, with special emphasis on cancer of the urinary bladder. Cancer Chemother. Rep. 54:181, 1970.
6. Fink, D. J. and Foye, L. V.: 6-Mercaptopurine (NSC-755) given intermittently in high doses: Phase II study. Cancer Chemother. Rep. 54:31, 1970.
7. Wilson, W. L., Bisel, J. F., Cole, D., Rochlin, D., Ramirez, G. and Madden, R.: Prolonged low-dosage administration of hexamethylmelamine (NSC-13875). Cancer 25:568, 1970.
8. Huseby, R. A. and Downing, V.: The use of methotrexate orally in treatment of squamous cell carcinoma of the head and neck. Cancer Chemother. Rep. 16:511, 1962.
9. Papac, R., Levkowitz, E. and Bertino, J. R.: Methotrexate (NSC-740) in squamous cell carcinoma of the head and neck. II. Intermittent intravenous therapy. Cancer Chemother. Rep. 51:69, 1967.
10. Leone, L. A., Albala, M. M. and Rege, V. B.: Treatment of carcinoma of the head and neck with intravenous methotrexate. Cancer 21:828, 1968.
11. Harrison, D. F. N. and Tucker, W. N.: The role of chemotherapy in advanced cancer of the head and neck. Brit. J. Cancer 18:74, 1964.
12. Foley, J. F., Lemon, H. M. and Miller, D.: Low dosage methotrexate (NSC-740) and cyclophosphamide (NSC-26271) for solid tumors. Cancer Chemother. Rep. 54:41, 1970.
13. Papac, R. J., Jacobs, E. M., Foye, L. V. and Donohue, D. M.: Systemic therapy with amethopterin in squamous carcinoma of the head and neck. Cancer Chemother. Rep. 32:47, 1963.
14. Freireich, E. J. and Luce, J.: National Cancer Institute Special Meeting on Bleomycin, 1970, Appendix 6.
15. Krakoff, I. and Yagoda, A.: National Cancer Institute Special Meeting on Bleomycin, 1970, Appendix 7.
16. Rosenbaum, C. and Carter, S. K.: Clinical Brochure—Bleomycin (NSC-125066), National Cancer Institute, 1970, p. 24.
17. Silverberg, B. S. and Grant, R. N.: Cancer statistics. Cancer 20:10, 1970.
18. Roswit, B.: The outlook for the lung cancer patient. Hosp. Pract. 3:22, 1968.
19. Roe, F. J. C. and Walters, M. A.: Some unsolved problems in lung cancer etiology. Progr. Exp. Tumor Res. 6:126, 1965.
20. Boucot, K. R.: The value of chest x-ray surveys in the early detection of lung cancer. *In* Proc. 6th Nat. Cancer Cong. Philadelphia: J. B. Lippincott, 1970, pp. 813–819.
21. Davies, D. F.: A review of detection methods for the early diagnosis of lung cancer. J. Chronic Dis. 19:819, 1966.

22. Pearson, F. G., Thompson, D. W. and Delarue, N. C.: Experience with the cytologic detection, localization and treatment of radiologically undemonstrated bronchial carcinoma. J. Thorac. Cardiov. Surg. 54:371, 1967.
23. Steele, J. D. and Buell, P.: Survival in bronchogenic carcinomas resected as solitary pulmonary nodules,[20] pp. 835–839.
24. Boyd, D. P.: Is extended radical resection superior to lobectomy in treating resectable bronchial cancer? J.A.M.A. 195:1033, 1966.
25. Weiss, A. J.: Chemotherapy of lung cancer. *In* Brodsky, I. and Kahn, S. B. (Eds.): Cancer Chemotherapy. New York: Grune & Stratton, 1967.
26. Hilton, G.: British practice in radiotherapy. London: Butterworth and Co., 1955, p. 258.
27. The results of radium and X-ray therapy in malignant disease. Edinburgh: Livingstone, 1950, p. 52.
28. Dobbie, J. L.: The treatment of carcinoma of the lung. Brit. J. Radiol. 17:107, 1944.
29. Shorvon, L. M.: Carcinoma of the bronchus with especial reference to its treatment by radiotherapy. Brit. J. Radiol. 20:443, 1947.
30. Wolf, J., Patno, M. E., Roswit, B. and D'Esopo, N.: Controlled study of survival of patients with clinically inoperable lung cancer treated with radiation therapy. Amer. J. Med. 40:360, 1966.
31. Shields, T. W., Higgins, G. A., Lawton, R., Heilbrunn, A. and Keehan, R. S.: Preoperative x-ray therapy as an adjuvant in the treatment of bronchogenic carcinoma. J. Thorac. Cardiov. Surg. 59:49, 1970.
32. Rubin, P., Green, J., Holzwasser, G. and Gerle, R.: Superior vena caval syndrome. Radiology 81:388, 1963.
33. Poulter, C. A.: The place of radiation therapy in the management of lung cancer. *In* Cancer Management. Philadelphia: J. B. Lippincott, 1968, pp. 471–474.
34. Karnofsky, D. A., Abelmann, W. H., Craver, L. F. and Burchenal, J. H.: The use of nitrogen mustard in the palliative treatment of carcinoma: Cancer 1:634, 1948.
35. White, F. R.: The effects of drugs in human bronchogenic carcinoma. Cancer Chemother. Rep. 14:149, 1961.
36. Wolf, J.: Controlled trials in the treatment of carcinoma of the bronchus. In Tenth International Cancer Congress Abstracts. Houston, Tex.: Medical Arts Publishing Co., 1970, pp. 497–498.
37. Wolf, J., Spear, P., Yesner, R. and Patno, M. E.: Nitrogen mustard and the steroid hormones in the treatment of inoperable bronchogenic carcinoma. Amer. J. Med. 29:1003, 1960.
38. Green, R. A., Humphrey, E., Close, H. and Patno, M. E.: Alkylating agents in bronchogenic carcinoma. Amer. J. Med. 46:516, 1969.
39. Crosbie, W. A., Kamdar, H. H. and Belchen, J. R.: A controlled trial of vinblastine sulfate in the treatment of cancer of the lung. Brit. J. Dis. Chest 60:28, 1966.
40. Kaung, D. T., Sbar, S. and Patno, M. E.: Treatment of non-resectable cancer of the lung with hydroxyurea administered intermittently. Cancer Chemother. Rep. 55:87, 1971.
41. Frost, J. K., Feinstein, A. R., Higgins, G. A., Jr. and Selawry, O. S.: Lung cancer: Perspectives and prospects. Ann. Intern. Med. 73:1003, 1970.
42. Aronovitch, M., Meakins, J. F., Place, R., Kahana, L. M. and Groszman, M.: A controlled study with nitrogen mustard in inoperable bronchogenic carcinoma. Cancer 16:1072, 1963.
43. Barran, K. M., Helm, W. H. and King, D. A.: Bronchial carcinoma treated with nitrogen mustard and cyclophosphamide. Brit. Med. J. 2:685, 1965.
44. Levine, B. and Weisberger, A. A.: The response of various types of bronchogenic carcinoma to nitrogen mustard. Ann. Intern. Med. 42:1089, 1953.
45. Bergsagel, D. E., Robertson, G. L. and Hasselback, R.: Effect of cyclophosphamide on advanced lung cancer and the hematological toxicity of large, intermittent intravenous doses. Canad. Med. Ass. J. 98:532, 1968.
46. Andrews, M. C. and Wilson, W. L.: Phase II study of methotrexate in solid tumors. Cancer Chemother. Rep. 51:471, 1967.
47. Reed, L. J., Muggia, F. M., Klipstein, F. A. and Gellhorn, A.: Intermittent parenteral methotrexate therapy for carcinoma of the lung. Cancer Chemother. Rep. 51:475, 1967.
48. Samuels, M. L., Leary, W. V. and Howe, C. D.: Procarbazine in the treatment of advanced bronchogenic carcinoma of the lung. Cancer Chemother. Rep. 51:475, 1967.
49. Shaw, R. K. and Bruner, J. A.: Clinical evaluation of vincristine. Cancer Chemother. Rep. 42:45, 1964.
50. Wilson, W. L., Bisel, H. F., Cole, D., Rochlin, D., Ramirez, G. and Madden, R.:

Prolonged low dose administration of hexamethylmelamine. Cancer 25:568, 1970.
51. Slack, N. H. and Jones, R., Jr.: Single reversal trial of hydroxyurea in 91 patients with advanced cancer. Cancer Chemother. Rep. 54:53, 1970.
52. Kenis, Y. and Brule, G.: Preliminary clinical screening with daunorubicin. Europ. J. Cancer 6:155, 1970.
53. DeVita, V. T., Carbone, P. B., Owens, A. H., Jr., Gold, G. L., Krant, M. J. and Edmonson, J.: Clinical trials with 1,3-bis-(2-chloroethyl)-1-nitrosourea, NSC-409962. Cancer Res. 25:1876, 1965.
54. Weiss, A. J., Jackson, L. G. and Carabasi, R.: An evaluation of 5-fluorouracil in malignant disease. Ann. Intern. Med. 55:731, 1961.
55. Fink, D. and Foye, L. V., Jr.: 6-Mercaptopurine given intermittently in high doses. Cancer Chemother. Rep. 54:31, 1970.
56. Kenis, Y., DeSmedt, J. and Tagnon, H. J.: Action of natulan in 94 patients with solid tumors. Europ. J. Cancer 2:51, 1966.
57. Holland, J. F.: Data from the Eastern Oncology Group.[41]
58. De la Garcia, J. G., Carr, J. J. and Bisel, H. F.: Hexamethylmelamine in the treatment of primary cancer of the lung with metastasis. Cancer 22:571, 1968.
59. Bickers, J. N.: Phase II studies of hydroxyurea in adults: Carcinoma of the lung. Cancer Chemother. Rep. 40:45, 1964.
60. Bonadonna, G., Monfardini, S., Oldini, C. and DiPietro, S.: Clinical evaluation of hydroxyurea in advanced lung cancer. Tumori 53:331, 1967.
61. Humphrey, E. W. and Dietrich, F. S.: Clinical experience with the methyl ester of streptonigrin (NSC-45384): A pharmacologic study in six patients. Cancer Chemother. Rep. 33:21, 1963.
62. McCracken, S. and Aboody, A.: Continuous intravenous infusion of streptonigrin in patients with bronchogenic carcinoma. Cancer Chemother. Rep. 46:23, 1965.
63. Sullivan, R. D., Miller, E., Zurek, W. Z. and Rodriquez, F. R.: Clinical effects of prolonged intravenous infusion of streptonigrin in advanced cancer. Cancer Chemother. Rep. 33:27, 1963.
64. Bonadonna, G., DeLena, M. and Beritta, G.: Preliminary clinical screening with adriamycin in lung cancer. Europ. J. Cancer 7: 365, 1971.
65. Ansfield, F. and Curreri, A. R.: Further clinical studies with 5-fluorouracil. J. Nat. Cancer Inst. 22:497, 1959.
66. Moore, G. E., Bross, I. D. J., Ausman, R., Nadler, S., Jones, R., Jr., et al.: Effects of 5-fluorouracil in 389 patients with cancer. Cancer Chemother. Rep. 52:641, 1968.
67. Wilson, W. C., Bisel, H. F., Krementz, E. T., Lien, R. C. and Prohaska, J. V.: Further clinical evaluation of 2′-deoxy-5-fluorouridine. Cancer Chemother. Rep. 51:85, 1967.
68. Moore, G. E., Bross, I. D. J., Ausman, R., Nadler, S., Jones, R., Jr. et al.: Effects of 6-mercaptopurine in 290 patients with advanced cancer. Cancer Chemother. Rep. 52:655, 1968.
69. Whittington, R. M. and Close, H. R.: Clinical experience with mitomycin C. Cancer Chemother. Rep. 54:195, 1970.
70. Roswit, B., Patno, M. E., Rapp, R., Veinbergs, A., Feder, B., et al.: The survival of patients with inoperable lung cancer: A large-scale randomized study of radiation therapy versus placebo. Radiology 90:688, 1968.
71. Higgins, G. A., Humphrey, E. W., Hughes, F. A. and Keehn, R. J.: Cytoxan as an adjuvant to surgery for lung cancer. J. Surg. Oncol. 1:221, 1969.
72. Veterans Administration Surgical Adjuvant Cancer Chemotherapy Study Group protocol.
73. Hall, T. C., et al.: A clinical pharmacologic study of chemotherapy and x-ray therapy in lung cancer. Amer. J. Med. 43:186, 1967.
74. Krant, M. J., et al.: Comparative trial of chemotherapy and radiotherapy in patients with non-resectable cancer of the lung. Amer. J. Med. 35:363, 1963.
75. Carr, D. T., Childs, D. S. and Lee, R. E.: Radiotherapy plus 5-fluorouracil compared to radiotherapy alone for unresectable bronchogenic carcinoma. *In* Tenth International Cancer Congress Abstracts. Houston, Tex.: Medical Arts Publishing Co., 1970, pp. 512–513.
76. Von Essen, E. F., Fligerman, M. M. and Calabresi, P.: Radiation and 5-fluorouracil: A controlled clinical study. Radiology 81:1018, 1963.
77. Gollin, F. F., Ansfield, F. J. and Vermund, H.: Continual studies of combined chemotherapy and irradiation in inoperable bronchogenic carcinoma. Cancer Chemother. Rep. 51:189, 1967.
78. Levitt, S. H., Jones, T. K., Kilpatrick, S. J. and Bogardus, E. R.: Treatment of malignant superior vena caval obstruction. Cancer 24:442, 1969.
79. Wolf, J.: Report of a clinical trial of triple therapy in the treatment of inoperable

bronchogenic carcinoma. *In* Amer. Soc. Clin. Oncol. Abstracts, 1967.

80. Mannes, P., Derriks, R., Moens, R. and Heynen, E.: The polychemotherapy of inoperable bronchial cancer. *In* Tenth International Cancer Congress Abstracts. Houston, Tex.: Medical Arts Publishing Co., 1970, p. 450.
81. Alberto, P., Brunner, K., Martz, G. and Senn, H. J.: Treatment of bronchial cancer with simultaneous or sequential combination of methotrexate, cyclophosphamide, procarbazine and vincristine. *In* Tenth International Cancer Congress Abstracts. Houston, Tex.: Medical Arts Publishing Co., 1970, p. 469.
82. Chanes, R. E. and Bottomley, R. H.: A preliminary report on combined actinomycin D–vincristine in the treatment of human solid tumors. Proc. Amer. Ass. Cancer Res. 9:12, 1968.
83. Dollinger, M. R., Golbey, R. B. and Karnofsky, D. A.: Cancer Chemotherapy. Disease-A-Month, April, 1963, p. 72.
84. Dollinger, M. R., Krakoff, I. H. and Karnofsky, D. A.: Quinacrine (Atabrine) in the treatment of neoplastic effusions. Ann. Intern. Med. 66:249, 1967.

Soft-Tissue Sarcomas

By Bruce I. Shnider, M.D.

Tumors of the skin, ectodermal structures of the skin, and the lymph nodes develop from two primitive sources: the mesoderm and the neuro-ectodermal tissues of the peripheral nervous system. Out of the supportive and reticuloendothelial tissues arising from the mesenchyme develops a range of tumors known as soft-tissue sarcomas. The wide distribution of these tissues in the body makes it possible for such neoplasms to occur in almost any region of the body. Unfortunately, mesenchymal tumors do not always reproduce their prototype in a pure form, and as they become more undifferentiated, recognition and histologic identification become more difficult. The failure to properly classify the soft-tissue sarcomas, particularly the malignant ones, has led to a great deal of confusion concerning the distribution, frequency and responsiveness of these tumors to various forms of therapy. These mesenchymal neoplasms are among the least understood and most unsatisfactorily treated of the malignant tumors. Surgery, radiation therapy and chemotherapy are usually inadequately employed or resorted to too late to be effective.

In evaluating the chemotherapy of this group of malignancies, primary consideration will be given to the sarcomas listed in Table 1. Excluded from consideration are the sarcomas arising from bone, bone marrow and the nervous system, as well as those arising from the lymphoid or reticuloendothelial tissues of the lymph

Table 1.—*Soft-Tissue Sarcomas*

1. Fibrosarcoma
   (dermatofibrosarcoma protuberans)
2. Myxoma
3. Liposarcoma
4. Muscle tumors
   Leiomyosarcoma
   Rhabdomyosarcoma
5. Angiosarcomas
   Hemangioendothelioma
   Hemangiopericytoma
   Kaposi's
   Lymphangiosarcoma
6. Miscellaneous
   Synovial sarcoma
   Chondrosarcoma
   Malignant mesenchymoma
   Mesothelioma
   Undifferentiated
   Sarcoma botryoides
   Carcinosarcoma

From the Division of Medical Oncology, Department of Medicine, Georgetown University School of Medicine, Washington, D.C.

Supported in part by U.S. Public Health Service grants CA-08119 and CA-02824 from the National Cancer Institute, National Institutes of Health.

nodes or other body organs. As with other forms of cancer, soft-tissue sarcomas tend to metastasize at some time during their life cycle, characteristically through the blood stream to the lungs, liver or other viscera, and occasionally through the lymphatics to regional lymph nodes. In addition, they may infiltrate locally beyond the obvious zone of disease into surrounding organs. A knowledge of the route and metastatic potential of a particular sarcoma is essential to its proper therapeutic management.

Table 2 subclassifies these neoplasms into two groups: those with a high potential for malignancy which metastasize readily and those which are less malignant and are associated with infiltrative growth into surrounding tissues or, infrequently, metastases. In evaluating their responsiveness or lack of it, careful consideration must always be given to this potential for malignancy in determining the effectiveness of the treatment in producing regression of the tumor masses or in prolonging the survival of the patients undergoing treatment.

The best prospects of achieving a "cure" for a patient with a soft-tissue sarcoma lie in the hands of the therapist who makes the first attempt. This is usually the surgeon or, to a lesser degree, the radiation therapist. If the first attempt fails, the chances that subsequent attempts will succeed are markedly reduced. Usually, it is at this stage that chemotherapy is first considered. Regardless of which therapeutic modality is used first, no treatment should be undertaken without a biopsy, so that the physician can proceed armed with that knowledge. Without this information, treatment may not be radical enough initially or, at times, may be more drastic than is necessary. The curative approach to soft-tissue sarcomas requires that the treatment be aggressive, accurate and adequate. Accuracy in treatment depends upon a proper biopsy and its accurate pathologic interpretation, since the histologic characteristics may well influence the surgeon's decision as to the extent of the surgery. It may also indicate whether radiation therapy is the more appropriate primary treatment than surgery. Aggressive management depends upon the surgeon's knowledge and acceptance of the fact that soft-tissue sarcomas are potentially as malignant as any other variety of carcinoma.

Radiation therapy has a limited but important function in the management of these lesions. It is valuable as an adjunct to surgery in the radio-responsive neoplasms. On occasion, it may be used preoperatively to make a patient a more suitable candidate for surgery. At other times, it may be effective alone in the management of patients with localized angiosarcomas, liposarcomas and orbital rhabdomyosarcomas.

TABLE 2.—*Soft-Tissue Sarcomas*

Malignant (with high metastatic potential)
Undifferentiated fibrosarcoma and liposarcoma
Rhabdomyosarcoma
Malignant hemangioendothelioma and lymphangiosarcoma
Synovial sarcoma
Malignant mesenchymoma
Less Malignant (spread by infiltrative growth or, infrequently, metastasis)
Skin fibrosarcoma
Myxoma
Differentiated liposarcoma
Kaposi's sarcoma
Hemangiopericytoma (malignant)

Kaposi's sarcoma, malignant hemangiopericytomas and some of the differentiated myxoid liposarcomas or embryonal rhabdomyosarcomas are somewhat responsive to X-ray therapy. The other types of sarcomas generally require such large amounts of radiation that adjacent normal tissue may be compromised and systemic complications of therapy may develop. The effectiveness of radiation therapy can be enhanced by the cooperative planning of the surgeon, the pathologist and the chemotherapist for the over-all management of the patient and the sequential use of all therapeutic modalities.

The chemotherapeutic agents have become so widely used in the management of patients with disseminated malignancy that it is highly unlikely that any tumor has escaped a trial with some of the chemotherapeutic drugs. This applies as well for the soft-tissue sarcomas as interest in the use of chemotherapeutic agents as palliative therapy has increased. They have become especially useful when recurrence or metastasis follows surgery or radiotherapy or both. They are also of value when the tumor reaches such size or is so widely disseminated at the time of discovery that the more common conventional methods of treatment cannot be utilized. Despite this wide use, the proper assessment of the value of chemotherapeutic agents in the therapy of these tumors has been difficult, because most of the available data consists of reports based upon the treatment of single cases or extremely small series of cases.

Despite this growing interest and the large number of drugs that have been tried therapeutically after primary surgery or radiation therapy, or both, sarcomas of the soft tissues tend to be highly malignant and to offer a discouraging therapeutic and prognostic outlook. The overall 5-year survival has been reported by James[1] as 39.4 per cent in over 1,200 cases of soft-tissue sarcoma evaluated. Table 3 lists the reported 5-year survival figures for some of the soft-tissue sarcomas and demonstrates the wide variation in survival depending upon the malignancy potential and metastatic pattern of the neoplasm.

Over 40 different chemotherapeutic drugs have been used in the treatment of various soft-tissue sarcomas, either as single agents or in combination. Table 4 lists the general classes of drugs and the two-, three- or four-drug combinations used in clinical trials. Few of these drugs have been given to sufficient numbers of patients, so that therapeutic activity cannot be satisfactorily evaluated. Nonetheless, a knowledge of the drugs given and the types of responses seen may be valuable to the physician responsible for the management of the patient even though the numbers of cases treated with any single agent or combination of agents may not be statistically significant.

An increasing number of trials have been made with alkylating agents such as

TABLE 3.—*Five-Year Survival with Soft-Tissue Sarcomas*[1]

Type	%
Rhabdomyosarcoma	20.8–35
Liposarcoma	25–40
Synovial sarcomas	27.5–37
Fibrosarcoma	48
(desmoid variety)	95
Dermatofibrosarcoma	88–96
Neurofibrosarcoma	35.7
Leiomyosarcoma	39.6
Kaposi's sarcoma	45.9

TABLE 4.—*Types of Chemotherapeutic Agents Previously Used in Treating Soft-Tissue Sarcomas*

Single drug therapy	*Combination therapy*
Alkylating agents	Cyclophosphamide and prednisone
Cyclophosphamide	Actinomycin D and nitrogen mustard
Chlorambucil	Actinomycin D and vincristine
(1,3,bis(β-chloroethyl)-1-nitrosourea	Thio-TEPA and testosterone
Dihydroxybusulfan	Triaziquone and nitrogen mustard
Mechlorethamine	Vincristine and cyclophosphamide
Melphalan	
Meturedepa	5-Fluorouracil, cyclophosphamide and thio-TEPA
Thio-TEPA	
Procarbazine	Cyclophosphamide, actinomycin D and vincristine
Triaziquone	
Cariolisine	Cyclophosphamide, thio-TEPA and melphalan
1-Acetyl-2-picolinohydrazine	
Antimetabolites	Mitomycin C, melphalan and vincristine
Fluorodeoxyuridine	
Fluorouracil	Methotrexate, cyclophosphamide, vincristine and 5-fluorouracil
Methotrexate	
6-Mercaptopurine	5-Fluorouracil, vinblastine, hydroxyurea and triethylenemelamine
Cytosine arabinoside	
6-Azauridine	Actinomycin D, 5-fluorouracil, thio-TEPA, X-ray
Plant alkaloids	
Vinblastine	Mitomycin C, cyclophosphamide, thio-TEPA and chromomycin
Vincristine	
Vinglycinate sulfate	Mitomycin C, 5-fluorouracil, thio-TEPA, fluoxymesterone
Antibiotics	
Mithramycin	
Mitomycin C	
Daunomycin	
Azotomycin	
Actinomycin D	
Bleomycin	

cyclophosphamide, chlorambucil, phenylalanine, mustard, meturedepa, triaziquone (Trenimon), and cariolisine. From these trials, some relative therapeutic order of activity can be determined. In 1967, Haddy et al.[2] gave cyclophosphamide, 30 mg per kilogram of body weight, intravenously in divided doses at 8-hour intervals to 13 patients with rhabdomyosarcoma. They noted a "good response" of 50 per cent or better regression in tumor size in 6 of the 13 patients, and a "partial response" of 25 to 50 per cent tumor regression in 4 patients. Samuels and Howe,[3] evaluating the response to cyclophosphamide in Ewing's sarcoma, noted a complete regression of tumor in 2 of 11 patients, and a partial regression in 5 of 11 patients given oral and parenteral drug. Cittadini,[4] Mannheimer,[5] and Sutow,[6] testing the effect of cyclophosphamide in a composite group of 45 patients with undifferentiated soft-tissue sarcoma, noted over 50 per cent regression in 13 patients and a 25 to 50 per cent regression in 9 additional patients. The dosage varied from an initial 1 gram of drug intravenously, followed by oral maintenance of 100–200 mg per day, to 30 mg/kg per week for a total of 4 weeks by either the intravenous or oral route.

Moore et al.,[7] reporting for the Eastern Clinical Drug Evaluation Program, found that chlorambucil, 0.2 mg/kg per day for 42 days, produced only one complete objective response and partial objective responses in 6 of 28 patients with connective-tissue sarcoma treated in the protocol study. In Kaposi's sarcoma, Kyalwazi[8,9] noted 52 per cent complete regression and 43 per cent partial regression in a group of 21 patients treated with triaziquone, 550 μg twice a week. In these patients, complete disappearance of nodules and edema, and return of skin texture to normal were noted in the patients who had complete regressions, whereas in the patients with partial regression, the nodules partially or completely disappeared but the edema persisted. Triaziquone was not effective in the treatment of florid Kaposi's sarcoma. The Eastern Clinical Drug Evaluation Program[10] gave meturedepa to 13 patients with soft-tissue sarcoma, and noted a partial objective response in only one of 13 patients. Romieu[11] reported an increase in survival time in 3 patients with fibrosarcoma, 1 patient with myxosarcoma and 1 patient with rhabdomyosarcoma treated with cariolisine of a group of 8 patients with soft-tissue sarcomas. The drug, 15–50 mg, was administered by intra-arterial perfusion. In all patients reported, disease was confined to the upper or lower extremities.

In the group of chemotherapeutic antibiotics, actinomycin D has been the one most widely used in soft-tissue sarcomas. Daunomycin, mithramycin and mitomycin C have also been tried, but to a lesser degree. Sagerman et al.,[12] Burrington,[13] Edland,[14] and James et al.[15] found a response rate of approximately 50 per cent in the rhabdomyosarcomas treated with actinomycin D. Rhabdomyosarcomas of the orbit had a slightly higher response rate. The dosage most widely used was 0.5 mg per day for 5 to 12 days. Malkasian[16] and Cupps et al.[17] found actinomycin D fairly effective in the management of leiomyosarcoma, fibrosarcoma, liposarcoma and undifferentiated sarcomas, and reported a high response rate for these tumors, with remissions lasting from 3 to 10 months. Kyalwazi[8,9] found a better than 50 per cent response rate in Kaposi's sarcoma of the florid variety in patients receiving actinomycin D. Carter[18] and Moore et al.,[19] reporting on the effectiveness of mitomycin C in the management of rhabdomyosarcoma and undifferentiated sarcoma, found response rates of 4 of 11 patients and 2 of 32 patients, respectively. Tan,[20] utilizing daunomycin in the treatment of patients with rhabdomyosarcoma, reported objective responses in 8 of 20 patients and 3 of 5 patients with undifferentiated sarcoma. Only 1 of 3 patients with fibrosarcoma receiving mithramycin had a 50 per cent or better response after 8 days of treatment.[21] Hreshchyshyn[22] noted a response in 7 of 20 patients with uterine sarcoma who received actinomycin D in the usual standard dosage of 75 γ/kg over a 5-day period, with courses being repeated once every 3 to 4 weeks.

Vincristine is the only member of the plant alkaloid group of chemotherapeutic agents to undergo any extensive trial in the soft-tissue sarcomas. Sutow et al.[23] and Selawry et al.[24] reported 13 complete responses and 5 partial responses in a group of 32 patients with rhabdomyosarcoma who were treated with vincristine. The dosage varied from 0.02 mg/kg for 5 days, then 0.05 mg weekly in Sutow's series to 0.8 to 2.5 γ/M^2 in Selawry's series. Among the angiosarcomas, 3 of 5 patients treated responded in the series reported by Urbach and Feinerman,[25] Sutow et al.,[23] and Burgoon and Soderberg.[26] Two of 7 patients with Ewing's sarcoma showed a partial response[23,24] and 11 of 37 patients with undifferentiated sarcoma were said to show good partial response after being treated with vincristine. No responses were noted in liposarcomas, and only an occasional response was seen in the leiomyosarcomas.

The only active antimetabolites are methotrexate and fluorouracil. Van Dyk et al.[27] and Malkasian et al.[16] reported a 70 per cent response rate among leiomyosarcoma patients treated with 5-fluorouracil, but a much lower response rate in the undifferentiated sarcomas treated with fluorodeoxyuridine. Sullivan et al.[28] reported 5 of 16 undifferentiated sarcomas responding to the oral and parenteral administration of methotrexate. Andrews and Wilson[29] and Wiltshaw[30] noted a much lower response rate in the undifferentiated sarcomas that they treated with methotrexate. The leiomyosarcomas and fibrosarcomas were much more responsive, with 4 of 11 patients responding in the former category and 5 of 8 in the latter category. Papac[31] and Talley et al.,[32] using cytosine arabinoside in a variety of dose schedules, reported partial responses in 2 of 12 soft-tissue sarcomas treated with this agent. No responses in the soft-tissue sarcomas have been seen with the purine antagonists or with a variety of pyrimidine antagonists other than fluorouracil.[33]

Because of the unresponsiveness to single agents, many combinations of chemotherapeutic drugs have undergone clinical evaluation for the therapy of soft-tissue sarcomas. Among the most effective have been combinations of actinomycin D or an alkylating agent with a variety of less active compounds. Lawton et al.,[34] using 5-fluorouracil, methotrexate, vinblastine and hydroxyurea (Hydrea) reported a mean survival time of 16 months for 7 of 9 undifferentiated sarcomas responding to this combination. Malkasian et al.[16] reported a response rate of over 50 per cent in 7 of 13 leiomyosarcomas treated with actinomycin D, 5-fluorouracil, thio-TEPA and cyclophosphamide. Nelson[35] and Goodwin et al.[36] reported 11 of 24 rhabdomyosarcomas responding to a combination of actinomycin D and mechlorethamine. The mean survival for this group was 3.2 years. In the combined series of Grosfeld et al.,[37] James et al.,[15] and Hayes et al.,[38] 73 patients with rhabdomyosarcoma were given actinomycin D and vincristine. A regression in tumor masses of 50 per cent or better was noted in 20 patients. When cyclophosphamide was added to this combination, Pratt[39] was able to achieve a response rate of approximately 80 per cent in patients with widely disseminated rhabdomyosarcoma. Their survival time varied from 4.5 to 18 months. Malkasian et al.,[16] using three alkylating agents, cyclophosphamide, thio-TEPA and L-sarcolysine (melphalan), reported 7 of 7 leiomyosarcomas responding objectively. For Kaposi's sarcoma, Kyalwazi[8,9] combined intra-arterial mechlorethamine with oral triaziquone to produce a 100 per cent response rate. One of the highest rates of response to combination chemotherapy has been reported by Knock et al.[33] With administration of oxophenarsine, heparin, malonate and fluoride, they reported 14 objective responses in a group of 17 undifferentiated sarcomas. When 5-fluorouracil, cyclophosphamide and hydroxyurea were added, there were 24 objective responses in another group of 28 similar tumors.

In all the series reported the responses have, in general, been no longer than 12 months in duration, and retreatment with the same therapy or new forms of therapy has not been effective. Another problem in assessing the value of combination therapy has been the great variety of definitions of response and the variable criteria for determining the effectiveness of the chemotherapeutic drugs being tested.

Tables 5 through 8 tabulate the soft-tissue sarcomas and the drugs reported to be most effective as palliative forms of therapy. The dosages listed are those most frequently employed in producing the response rates listed in these tables. In general, the responses seen tended to be transient, without significant changes in survival times. In some instances, chemotherapy was given in conjunction with or after radiation therapy; in other instances, the chemotherapeutic agent was administered prior to surgery or X-ray therapy. As will be noted from these tabulations, the soft-tissue

TABLE 5.—*Chemotherapeutic Drugs Currently Most Effective in Soft-Tissue Sarcomas*

Tumor	*Drug(s)*	*Dosage*	*Response*	*Comments (Ref.)*
Fibrosarcoma	Methotrexate	2.5–10 mg/day divided doses for 2–15 days OR 0.2 mg/kg IV days 1 and 4; then 0.1 mg/kg every other day for 4 doses; repeat every 42 days	5/7	Response transient. No change in survival.[29,30]
	Actinomycin D	15 γ/kg daily IV for 5 days; repeat in 21–28 days; or 0.5 mg daily for 5–12 days	2/7	Therapy usually given after X-ray therapy.[16,17]
Myxosarcoma	Actinomycin D	0.25–0.5 mg/day IV } for 5 days	3/7	Response of short duration. Moderate toxicity.[16]
	5-FU	15 mg/kg/day IV } for 5 days		
	Sarcolysin (melphalan)	8 mg/day IV } for 5 days		
	Cytoxan	400 mg IV once		
Liposarcoma	Actinomycin D	5.1 γ/kg/day for 12 days	2/5	Response of short duration (3–4 mos.).[17]

TABLE 6.—*Chemotherapeutic Drugs Currently Most Effective in Soft-Tissue Sarcomas of Muscle Origin*

Tumor	*Drug(s)*	*Dosage*	*Response*	*Comments (Ref.)*
Leiomyosarcoma	Methotrexate	0.2–0.4 mg/kg IV 2 times a week	4/11	Remissions 2 months or more.[29,30]
	Actinomycin D	0.5 mg IV daily for 5–12 days	12/27	Remissions temporary. Usually followed by X-ray therapy.[22,14]
	Vincristine (VCR)	1.4 mg/m²/week; dose was reduced when toxicity developed	2/2	Neurotoxicity frequent side effect. Transient response.[24,40]
	Cyclophosphamide Sarcolysin (melphalan) Thio-TEPA	35–50 mg a day for 4 doses 8 mg/day until toxicity 45 mg/wk IV	7/9	Exact criteria for response not clear.[16]
	Actinomycin D 5-FU Thio-TEPA Cyclophosphamide	0.25–0.5 mg IV a day } for 5 days 15 mg/kg/day IV } for 5 days 45 mg IV } for 5 days 400 mg IV	7/13	Cyclic therapy every month. Response criteria not clear.[16]
Rhabdomyosarcoma	Actinomycin D	15 γ/kg/day IV for 5 days; or 1.5–3.0 mg/m² in 4 divided doses over 8–14 days	23/24	2 or more courses before responses are evident.[17,37,38,12,41]
	Cyclophosphamide	30 mg/kg p.o. or IV in 3 divided doses at 8 hr. intervals for 1 day	10/25	Duration 8–36 weeks.[2]
	Vincristine	1.5 mg/m²/wk IV; or 0.8–2.5 γ/m² IV daily	17/21	Duration 1–28 months.[24]
	Mitomycin C	250 γ/kg/day for 5–10 days	5/12	Duration 3 months.[18,19]
	Daunomycin	1 mg/kg/day IV for 6–8 days	5/10	Over 50% regression. Duration not given.[20]
	Actinomycin D and Mechlorethamine	15 γ/kg/day IV for 5 days 30 mg single intra-arterial dose	10/24	Mean survival 3 years, 2.5 months.[35,39]
	Actinomycin D and Vincristine	15 γ/kg IV for 5 days with 2 week drug-free interval; then VCR 0.05 mg/kg weekly for 6 weeks; repeat cycle	12/14	Repeat courses required to obtain maximum remission.[37,38]
	Actinomycin D, Oral methotrexate and Cyclophosphamide	15 γ/kg/day IV for 5 days 1.25 mg q.i.d. 6 to 10 days Intra-arterial infusion	5/9	Lesions of orbit; 5 patients alive and well.[12,39]

TABLE 7.—*Chemotherapeutic Drugs Currently Most Effective in Soft-Tissue Angiosarcomas*

Tumor	*Drug(s)*	*Dosage*	*Response*	*Comments (Ref.)*
Hemangiosarcoma	Vincristine	2 mg IV twice weekly; or 1.5 mg/m^2 every other week	3/7	Neurologic side effects common. Short-lived remissions.[26,25]
	Vincristine and Cyclophosphamide	1.5 mg/m^2 every 2 weeks; 300 mg/m^2 given on alternate weeks	1/2	10 months free of disease.[25]
Kaposi's	Triaziquone (Trenimon)	0.2 mg IV every 2 days to total of 2.6 mg; or 550 μg p.o. twice weekly	12/21—complete remission 9/21—partial remission	Complete regression of nodules and edema. Partial—nodules regress, but edema persists.[8,9]
	Actinomycin D	500 μg/day for 5 days	13/24—complete remission 5/24—partial remission	Complete regression of nodules and edema. Partial—nodules regress, but edema persists.[8,9]
	Sarcolysin (melphalan)	30–50 mg/week IV	3/7	Subjective remission only.[42]
Lymphangiosarcoma	Cyclophosphamide	200 mg p.o./day until toxicity	1/4	Complete response for 6 months.[43]
	Thio-TEPA	30–60 mg/week IP or IV depending on status of disease	1/4	Good regression for up to 2 years.[43]

TABLE 8.—*Chemotherapeutic Drugs Currently Most Effective in Miscellaneous Soft-Tissue Sarcomas*

Tumor	*Drug(s)*	*Dosage*	*Response*	*Comments (Ref.)*
Connective tissue	Chlorambucil	0.2 mg/kg/day for 42 days	7/28	One complete and 6 partial responses of 2-3 months' duration.[7]
Synovial	Cyclophosphamide	300 mg days 1 and 5	Regression in 1 patient for 27 months	Repeat courses every week. Patient received 30 courses of drug.[44]
	Vincristine	0.025 mg/kg days 2 and 5		
	Methotrexate	0.5 mg/kg days 1 and 5		
	5-Fluorouracil	10 mg/kg days 1 and 5		
Mesenchymoma	Methotrexate	0.2 mg/kg IV for 4 days. 0.1 mg/kg IV on day 6 for 4 doses; repeat on day 42	1/2	50% decrease in pulmonary lesions.[29]
Undifferentiated	Methotrexate	0.2 mg/kg IV days 1 and 4, then 0.1 mg every other day for 4 doses; repeat on day 42 or 5 mg/24 hrs by continuous infusion	11/42	Duration 40–260 days.[28,30]
	Vincristine	0.02 to 0.05 mg/kg/wk; or 0.05 to 0.075 mg/kg/wk	6/20	Neurotoxicity. Duration not given,[16,23,24]
	Cyclophosphamide	15–30 mg/kg IV in 1–3 injections; or 400 mg/day for 10 days at 4–6 week intervals; or 30 mg/kg/wk until relapse	14/44	Duration 2–8 months.[12]
	Actinomycin D	5 γ/kg/day for 12 days	5/12	Duration 3–4 months.[17]
	Combination therapy	Using above drugs plus prednisone	2/14	High toxicity. Palliation, with little objective regression.[44,15]

sarcomas are relatively resistant to chemotherapy. The exceptions appear to be Kaposi's sarcoma, embryonal rhabdomyosarcoma, and selected undifferentiated sarcomas. These are generally responsive to single agents given sequentially or combinations of chemotherapeutic drugs.

For the present, the most effective drugs available to the physician for general therapy are actinomycin D, vincristine, cyclophosphamide and triaziquone. Next in order of effectiveness are methotrexate, mitomycin C and daunomycin. Combinations of these same drugs also appear to merit consideration.

In general, however, the results of chemotherapy of these tumors are disappointing and discouraging at present. The search for new and more effective single agents or combinations continues. A number of Phase I and II studies[45-47] are in progress. Whether these studies will be more rewarding in developing new drugs for the treatment of these sarcomas remains to be determined. Possibly, at a similar symposium in the near future, the prospects for patients with these neoplasms will be brighter and our chemotherapeutic arsenal will consist of more effective weapons than are available today.

Acknowledgment

The author wishes to acknowledge with thanks the valuable assistance of Barry D. Herman, Terrence J. Lee, Richard A. Walsh and Joseph E. Cronkey, and Mrs. Lois Rosenberger in the preparation of this chapter.

References

1. James, A. G.: Cancer Prognosis Manual, 2d ed. American Cancer Society, 1966.
2. Haddy, T. B., Nora, A. H., and Sutow, W. W.: Cyclophosphamide treatment for metastatic soft tissue sarcoma. Amer. J. Dis. Child. 114:301, 1967.
3. Samuels, M. L. and Howe, C. D.: Cyclophosphamide in the management of Ewing's sarcoma. Cancer 20:961, 1967.
4. Cittadini, G.: Problemi di cancerologia Clinica: Lo shock citostatico con ciclofosfamide. Minerva Med. 57:1715, 1966.
5. Mannheimer, E., Karrer, K., Boeckl, O. and Priesching, A.: Hochdosierte zytostatische Therapie und autologe Knochenmarks re-infusion bei malignen tumoren. Munchen. Med. Wschr. 109:1808, 1967.
6. Sutow, W. W.: Cyclophosphamide in Wilms' tumor and rhabdomyosarcoma. Cancer Chemother. Rep. 51:407, 1967.
7. Moore, G. E., Bross, I. D. J., Ausman, R., Nadler, S., Jones, R., Jr., et al.: Effects of chlorambucil (NSC-3088) in 374 patients with advanced cancer. Eastern Clinical Drug Evaluation Program. Cancer Chemother. Rep. 52:661, 1968.
8. Kyalwazi, S. K.: Kaposi's sarcoma. E. Afr. Med. J. 46:459, 1969.
9. Kyalwazi, S. K.: Chemotherapy of Kaposi's sarcoma: Experience with Trenimon. E. Afr. Med. J. 45:17, 1968.
10. Moore, G. E., Bross, I. D. J., Ausman, R., Nadler, S., Jones, R., Jr. et al.: Effects of meturedepa (NSC–51325) in 233 patients with advanced cancer. Eastern Clinical Drug Evaluation Program. Cancer Chemother. Rep. 52:667, 1968.
11. Romieu, C. and Pujol, H.: La chemioterapia regionale con circolazione extracorporea. Minerva Med. 56:1993, 1965.
12. Sagerman, R. H., Cassady, J. R. and Tretter, P.: Radiation therapy for rhabdomyosarcoma of the orbit. Trans. Amer. Acad. Ophthal. Otolaryng. 72:849, 1968.
13. Burrington, J. D.: Rhabdomyosarcoma of the paratesticular tissues in children. J. Pediat. Surg. 4:503, 1969.
14. Edland, R. W.: Embryonal rhabdomyosarcoma. Amer. J. Roentgen. 93:671, 1965.
15. James, D. H., Jr., Hustu, O. and Wrenn, E. L., Jr.: Childhood malignant tumors: Concurrent chemotherapy with dactinomycin and vincristine sulfate. J.A.M.A. 197:1043, 1966.
16. Malkasian, G. D., Jr., Mussey, E., Decker, D. G. and Johnson, C. E.: Chemotherapy of gynecologic sarcomas. Cancer Chemother. Rep. 51:507, 1967.

17. Cupps, R. E., Ahmann, D. L. and Soule, E. H.: Treatment of pulmonary metastatic disease with radiation therapy and adjuvant actinomycin D. Cancer 24:719, 1969.
18. Carter, S.: Mitomycin C. Cancer Chemother. Rep. 53:99, 1968.
19. Moore, G. E., Bross, I. D. J., Ausman, R., Nadler, S., Jones, R., Jr., et al.: Effects of mitomycin C (NSC-26980) in 346 patients with advanced cancer. Eastern Clinical Drug Evaluation Program. Cancer Chemother. Rep. 52:675, 1968.
20. Tan, C., Tasaka, H. and Yu, K. P.: Daunomycin, an antitumor antibiotic, in the treatment of neoplastic disease. Cancer 20:333, 1967.
21. Baum, M.: A clinical trial of mithramycin in the treatment of advanced malignant disease. Brit. J. Cancer 22:176, 1968.
22. Hreshchyshyn, M. M.: Experiences with chemotherapy in gynecologic cancer. N.Y. J. Med. 64:2431, 1964.
23. Sutow, W. W., Berry, D. H. and Haddy, T. B.: Vincristine sulfate therapy in children with metastatic soft tissue sarcoma. Pediatrics 38:465, 1966.
24. Selawry, O., Holland, J. F. and Wolman, I. J.: Effect of vincristine on malignant tumors in children. Cancer Chemother. Rep. 52:497, 1968.
25. Urbach, F. and Feinerman, L.: Angiosarcoma. Arch. Derm. 99:774, 1969.
26. Burgoon, C. F., Jr. and Soderberg, M.: Angiosarcoma. Arch. Derm. 99:773, 1969.
27. Van Dyk, J. J., Clarkson, B. D., Duschinsky, R., Keller, O., La Sala, E. and Krakoff, I. H.: Clinical evaluation of 5-bromo-5-fluoro-6-methoxy-dihydro-2′-deoxyuridine. Cancer Res. 27:2129, 1967.
28. Sullivan, R. D., Miller, E. and Zurek, W. Z.: Re-evaluation of methotrexate as an anticancer drug. Surg. Gynec. Obstet. 125: 819, 1967.
29. Andrews, N. C. and Wilson, W. T.: Phase II study of methotrexate (NSC-740) in solid tumors. Cancer Chemother. Rep. 51:471, 1967.
30. Wiltshaw, E.: Methotrexate in treatment of sarcomata. Brit. Med. J. 2:142, 1967.
31. Papac, R. J.: Clinical and hematologic studies with 1-β-D-arabinosylcytosine. J. Nat. Cancer Inst. 40:997, 1968.
32. Talley, R. W., O'Bryan, R. M., Tucker, W. G. and Loo, R. U.: Clinical pharmacology and human antitumor activity of cytosine arabinoside. Cancer 20:809, 1967.
33. Knock, F. E., Galt, R. M. and Renaud, O. V.: Clinical cancer chemotherapy aimed at potential cell regulators. Arch. Surg. 100:167, 1970.
34. Lawton, R. L., Latourette, H. B. and Collier, R. G.: Simultaneous high-energy irradiation and chemotherapy. Arch. Surg. 91: 155, 1965.
35. Nelson, A. J., III: Embryonal rhabdomyosarcoma: Report of twenty-four cases and study of the effectiveness of radiation therapy upon the primary tumor. Cancer 22:64, 1968.
36. Goodwin, W. E., Mims, M. M. and Young, H. H., II: Rhabdomyosarcoma of the prostate. J. Urol. 99:651, 1968.
37. Grosfeld, J. L., Clatworthy, H. W., Jr. and Newton, W. A., Jr.: Combined therapy in childhood rhabdomyosarcoma. J. Pediat. Surg. 4:637, 1969.
38. Hayes, D. M., Mirabal, V. Q. and Patel, H. R.: Rhabdomyosarcoma of the spermatic cord. Surgery 65:845, 1969.
39. Pratt, C. B.: Response of childhood rhabdomyosarcoma to combination chemotherapy. J. Pediat. 74:791, 1969.
40. Smart, R., Ottoman, E., Rochlin, B., Hornes, J., Silva, A. R. and Goepfert, H.: Clinical experience with vincristine (NSC-67574) in tumors of the CNS and other malignant diseases. Cancer Chemother. Rep. 52:733, 1968.
41. Soule, E. H., Geitz, M. and Henderson, E. D.: Embryonal rhabdomyosarcoma of the limbs and limb-girdles. Cancer 23: 1336, 1969.
42. Falkson, G. and Falkson, H. C.: A clinical trial with sarcolysin. S. Afr. Med. J. 41:224, 1967.
43. Tragus, E. T., and Wagner, D. E.: Current therapy for postmastectomy lymphangiosarcoma. Arch. Surg. 97:839, 1968.
44. Constanzi, J. J. and Coltman, C. A., Jr.: Combination chemotherapy using cyclophosphamide, vincristine, methotrexate and 5-fluorouracil in solid tumors. Cancer 23:589, 1969.
45. Carter, S.: Azotomycin. Cancer Chemother. Rep. 52:207, 1968.
46. Lessner, H. E.: BCNU (1,3,bis(β-chloroethyl)-1-nitrosourea): Effects on advanced Hodgkin's disease and other neoplasia. Cancer 22:451, 1968.
47. Armstrong, J. G., Dyke, R. W., Fouts, P. J., Hawthorne, J. J., Jansen, C. J., Jr., and Peabody, A. M.: Initial clinical experience with vinglycinate sulfate, a molecular modification of vinblastine. Cancer Res. 27:221, 1967.

Chemotherapy of Brain Tumors

By B. J. KENNEDY, M.D.

THE MANAGEMENT OF PATIENTS with primary brain tumors has been altered dramatically during the past 10 years. Although the prognosis is still grim, the earlier recognition of brain tumors, more accurate diagnostic procedures, and new treatments are factors that are improving the outlook for these patients.

The impact of primary brain tumors on the number of deaths in the United States is seen by the 1970 estimates of tumors of the central nervous system: 12,000 new patients and 7,900 anticipated deaths. These represent 3 per cent of the annual number of deaths from cancer in the United States.

With respect to age, the significance of these tumors is even more dramatic. Among tumors causing death in children in both sexes under 15 years, central nervous system (CNS) tumors rank second; from ages 15 to 34 years they rank third in males and fifth in females; and from ages 34 to 54 CNS tumors rank fourth in males.

Within the medical profession there prevails a general attitude of discouragement, especially in regard to glioma tumors. Not infrequently, after the initial diagnosis and therapy, the patients are placed in nursing homes for terminal care. Recent advances in the treatment of glioblastoma multiforme have prompted new looks at the total management of brain tumors in general.

INCIDENCE OF INTRACRANIAL TUMORS

The reporting of incidence of intracranial tumors varies widely because of differences in surgical practices with the increasing removal of metastatic lesions by some surgeons, in diagnostic techniques, in morphologic interpretation, in genetic factors, and in the attraction of specialty clinics or consulting physicians for certain types of neoplasms. Thus, any given series is an unreliable indicator of tumor incidence in the general population.

In a review of over 15,000 intracranial tumors culled from several reports, the range of incidence can be noted (Table 1).[1,2] The gliomas are numerically the most import-

TABLE 1.—*Incidence of 10 Most Common Intracranial Tumors*[1,2]

Tumor	*Ranges* (%)
Gliomas	31–49
Meningiomas	9–18
Pituitary adenomas	3–18
Sarcomas	1–6
Arteriovenous malformations	2–4
Hemangioblastomas	1–2
Craniopharyngiomas	1–4
Neurinomas	1–9
Granulomas, etc.	1–7
Metastatic tumors	3–25

From the Section of Oncology, Department of Medicine, University of Minnesota School of Medicine, Minneapolis, Minnesota.

Supported in part by grants CA-08101, CA-05158, and CA-08832 from the National Cancer Institute, National Institutes of Health.

TABLE 2.—*Incidence of Intracranial Gliomas*[1-5]

Tumor	*Frequence* (%)
Glioblastoma multiforme	51.3
Astrocytoma	24.5
Ependymoma	6.4
Oligodendroglioma	5.5
Spongioblastoma unipolare	3.4
Mixed gliomas	3.4
Astroblastoma	2.1
Medullo-epithelioma	1.1
Unclassified	1.8

Zimmerman series, 1,633 patients.[1]

ant of the primary brain neoplasms in man, with reported ranges between 31 and 49 per cent. All are malignant because they are invasive, but the degree of malignancy varies widely. Seldom do they metastasize extracranially spontaneously. The astrocytoma and glioblastoma multiforme tumors represent 72 to 89 per cent of the glioma tumors and thus constitute the most common type of brain tumor (Table 2).[1-5] The glioblastoma multiforme tumors represent the astrocytoma grade III or IV used in some series. This is based on the concept that this tumor is of astrocytic origin and represents the more malignant form of the tumor classified as grade I or II. More recently the number of glioblastoma multiforme tumors reported has increased because of the better recognition of glioblastoma and because a second biopsy of a previous diagnosed astrocytoma often reveals criteria for the diagnosis of glioblastoma.

DIAGNOSIS

An earlier diagnosis of glioblastoma multiforme should result in greater therapeutic accomplishments. Adults suffering from their first convulsion or epileptiform episode, adults under 50 who have had a "stroke" or have undergone a change in personality, or who have previously unnoticed neurologic symptoms indicative of cerebral involvement must alert the physician to the possibility of a brain tumor. The sequence in an untreated, rapidly growing brain tumor is frequently focal symptoms, followed by symptoms of increased intracranial pressure such as headache, vomiting, and blurred vision, later stupor or coma, and finally death.

EVALUATION OF TUMORS OF THE CENTRAL NERVOUS SYSTEM (CNS)

The evaluation of the site and size of a brain tumor is important in the initial diagnosis as well as assessment of alterations in the size of the lesion as induced by radiation therapy or chemotherapy. No specific test has proved totally effective; hence, several approaches are necessary in the description of a lesion.

The history and recording of changes in symptoms provide a significant clue to the presence of a cerebral lesion and the measurement of subjective improvement often denoting real objective improvement.

The neurologic examination supplies one of the most significant methods for evaluating the brain tumor. A comprehensive examination by the same examiner repeated at regular intervals provides data that can be interpreted with great accuracy. Furthermore, it takes into consideration the damage to normal brain tissue when the tumor has been removed or destroyed. The neurologic examination includes a thorough ophthalmoscopic evaluation. The assessment of intracranial pressure constitutes a measurement of the course of the tumor as well as the presence and degree of cerebral edema. The extent of papilledema, bulging of the craniotomy site, elevation of bone flaps, and the clinical course are utilized as aids in measurement. Psychometric tests provide a recorded measurement of personality trends. Demonstration of the localization or size of a lesion is aided by skull roentgenograms, electroencephalograms, brain scans, angiograms and pneumoencephalograms. Although skull roentgenograms and EEG's reflect the presence of abnormalities and localization, they are of little value in the assessment of the course of a tumor. Pneumoencephalograms in some instances may demonstrate a lesion, but repeated examination is a more formidable task. In many cases the test is contraindicated. Angiography has improved the demonstration of abnormal anatomy and physiology by selective catheterization techniques. Although successful in localizing tumors in 76 per cent of cases, repeated angiograms for evaluation of the course of a tumor are difficult.

The brain scan has provided localization data for brain tumors and an objective means of estimating tumor volume. Advances in localization of brain lesions have been due to improvements in instrumentation and new radiopharmaceutical agents. The localization of brain tumors depends upon a significant count-rate differential between the uptake of isotope-labeled protein by tumor and edematous brain and the uptake by the surrounding normal brain. Although effective in demonstrating localization of tumors 80 per cent of the time,[6] the brain scan for evaluation of the course of a tumor has been ineffective. A comparison of subtle changes is difficult, if not impossible. In no case has improvement in the brain scan been noted without clinical improvement. The interpretation of the brain scan becomes less meaningful once a craniotomy has been performed, with surgical resection of tumor. The minuscule changes in recurrent tumor growth become almost impossible to describe. Perhaps improvements in technique will make possible better assessment of tumor size.

The techniques for following the course of brain tumors are especially important in the new chemotherapeutic treatments. No single method permits adequate assessment of the effects of therapy upon a brain tumor. Consequently, the best approach is the judicious opinion of a good clinician interpreting the clinical course, physical examination, and several diagnostic procedures.[7]

The introduction of therapy has two major effects on the patients: (1) a temporary improvement of the patient's condition regardless of the effect on survival; because of subjective or measurable improvement the patient's period of survival is made more useful; and (2) alteration of expected survival because of the favorable effect on the tumor by therapy. The date of diagnosis is used to compute survival time. In malignant gliomas survival data have been surprisingly uniform. Therefore, in a large group of patients, a significant change in survival data will be detected early. Such data provide an effective means for evaluating the normal course of a glioblastoma multiforme and the alterations induced by therapy.

Brain Tumor Therapy

The natural history of glioblastoma multiforme of the brain indicates that the duration of the disease is 7 to 14 months from the first symptom until death.[8] In the past, the outlook for glioblastomas has been so poor that most neurologists and many neurosurgeons advocated that no effort be made to remove them. If these tumors were not removed, or were inadequately removed, no patients improved. The advent of new therapies, however, demonstrates that patients can improve and some live longer. Surgery, radiation therapy, chemotherapy, or combinations of these are all playing roles in changing therapeutic concepts in brain neoplasms.

Surgery

Today, a surgical procedure is necessary for the final accurate premortem diagnosis of glioblastoma multiforme and may be helpful in the treatment of many. A biopsy through a small craniotomy may prove to be all that can be justified. Usually, however, an attempt at major surgical extirpation is preferred. The surgical mortality associated with glioblastoma multiforme in the decade 1944 to 1954 was almost 50 per cent; at present it is less than 3 per cent.[5]

It has been amply shown that the length of effective survival of patients with glioblastoma multiforme has been substantially increased when it is possible to carry out major surgical removal of the neoplasm, especially as a precursor to other forms of treatment.

Surgical procedures are extremely valuable to relieve increased intracranial pressure. When the brain tumor cannot be removed totally, extirpation of the tumor bulk is desirable. With the exception of deep midline tumors, glioblastomas should be approached with the knowledge that the most radical surgical procedure consistent with maintaining neurologic function will be attended by a low operative mortality and will result in improved survival. Only about one-third of glioblastomas are located so that they can be surgically removed by radical operation.

Radiation Therapy

The length of survival and quality of recovery of patients who have undergone radiation therapy for glioblastomas are better than was formerly expected. Patients whose tumors cannot be extirpated completely should have radiation therapy as well as those whose tumors cannot be removed at all. When radiation is used postoperatively, it is difficult to relate the effects of treatment to one or the other; hence, survival data are important. Traveras[8] reported that 89 patients who had a single biopsy and no radiation therapy died sooner than those receiving only radiation therapy. Most of the patients were dead three months after simple biopsy. All were dead in 18 months. Patients having a partial resection plus radiation therapy had a better survival curve (43 per cent lived 9 months) than those who had a biopsy followed by radiation therapy (29 per cent lived 9 months). In addition, partial removal of tumor provided decompression, with a rapid improvement in the neurologic status. It was emphasized that a patient must live 30 days if the course of radiation therapy is to be considered completed.

Bouchard[9] recently reported on 176 patients with glioblastoma treated mainly with surgery and radiation therapy. Of these, 77 (44 per cent) survived more than 1 year, 33 (19 per cent) more than 2 years, 23 (13 per cent) more than 3 years, and 13 (7.4 per cent) more than 5 years. He concluded that radiation therapy used postoperatively produced better results. These values were not far different from those of Jelsma and Buey,[5] who reported that 13 per cent of the patients treated by radical resection and radiation therapy were alive 2 years after operation.

The efficacy of radiation therapy is limited by the damaging consequences of radiation to the normal brain. When doses of 6,000 to 9,000 r are delivered to the brain, severe damage appears at 8 to 26 months.

The interpretation of various reports is confused by the mixture of types of brain neoplasms in data results and the various stages of the disease compared at the time of treatment. It is apparent that more carefully randomized studies are necessary. However, it seems that radiation therapy increases survival of patients with glioblastomas, but offers no hope of cure. Even when radiation therapy is combined with radical surgical resection, survival beyond two years is uncommon.

Chemotherapy

Remarkable advances have been made in the field of cancer chemotherapy. The peculiarities of the central nervous system require certain modifications of the chemotherapeutic principles applied to other tumor systems. During the past 20 years sporadic reports of the efficacy of chemotherapeutic agents in the treatment of glioblastoma multiforme have sparked an interest in the potentialities of this treatment modality.

In a review of the literature of 145 patients with glioblastoma multiforme treated by chemotherapy, it was concluded that the survival figures with chemotherapy were not significantly better than those with surgery or radiotherapy or both.[10] However, the comparison in this manner is truly invalid, since the case materials were neither homogeneous nor randomized.

It is apparent from the review that chemotherapy of glioblastoma multiforme had a favorable effect on the disease. Symptomatic relief occurred with reduction in severity of headaches, improved level of consciousness, decrease in paresis or dysphasia, improved motion, and improved ability to care for oneself. Objective improvement was noted with disappearance of tumor masses or of papilledema, and resolution of neurologic abnormalities.

In a comprehensive review of the chemotherapy of brain tumors, Shapiro and Ausman[11] emphasized that the prognosis for the patient with malignant tumor has not improved even with the introduction of neurosurgical techniques and radiation therapy. Furthermore, they contended that there is little possibility of improving the surgical or radiation therapies of malignant brain tumors. They emphasized that although attempts to prolong survival of such patients by chemotherapy have had little success to date, with new knowledge of the biology of tumor cells, the reaction of the host, and the pharmacology of chemotherapeutic agents, chemotherapy offers an encouraging approach to the control of brain cancer and prolongation of survival.[11]

The selection of chemotherapeutic agents for brain tumors is influenced by the nature of the blood supply to the brain and by the fact that the central nervous system is protected by the mysterious blood-brain barrier. A drug should have certain characteristics to be considered for brain tumor therapy. The drug preferably should be able to pass the blood-brain barrier and enter the tumor in sufficient concentration to be effective.[12] To penetrate normal brain tissue, a drug should be lipid-soluble and of small molecular size. Yet we know little of the requirement for a drug to enter the growing tumor within the brain in which the surrounding blood-brain barrier may be modified.

The conduct of early clinical evaluation of drugs in brain tumors points up the need for more effective methods of study, including the development of experimental model systems. Some have been reported.[13–16] Kennedy et al.,[16] working with mithramycin, pointed out that current animal tumor systems for detecting the antitumor effectiveness of that agent would fail to show its antitumor activity.[16] This should be a cause for concern on the part of investigators interested in animal screening studies, and is a further possibility in the study of animal model systems in primary brain tumors. Mouse gliomas that have been introduced for study are more nearly like a metastatic than a primary tumor. Hence, the approach to the effective use of chemotherapeutic agents in the treatment of glioblastoma multiforme should involve multiple factors in the investigation, not dependence on any one system.

One recognizes the handicaps in developing chemotherapy of brain tumors. The lack of a suitable animal model and of meaningful drug selection for specific tumors are problems comparable to those in other solid tumor systems. The greatest obstacle to successful brain tumor chemotherapy is our inability to measure tumor mass and, therefore, response or lack of response to therapy. The clinician's judgment of the response is only a crude estimate of the tumor's behavior, and length of survival is no guide to the response of an individual patient. Nevertheless, attempts are under way to combat these problems and meet the requirements for chemotherapy of primary brain tumors.

Current Chemotherapeutic Agents

Techniques of Drug Administration

Multiple methods for administering chemotherapeutic agents are available in the treatment of primary brain tumors. The oral, parenteral, and intravenous methods are comparable to other forms of chemotherapy. Unique to the brain tumors are the introduction of agents into a brain tumor cyst, intrathecal administration, and intravascular drug administration by regional perfusion or intra-arterial therapy. The technique of administration may be single repeated injections, constant drip infusion, or perfusion of the ventricular system. The different techniques result from the different rationale as to the mode of access of the drug to the CNS tumor. Whether the blood-brain barrier is a factor is not clear. Hence, each drug used requires testing to determine whether it enters the tumor.

Mithramycin

Mithramycin (Mithracin) was introduced for the treatment of cerebral neoplasms because of the CNS agitation noted during its administration to patients with disseminated embryonal cell carcinoma of the testis and because of the apparent delayed uptake of tritiated mithramycin by brain tissue. This suggested that mithramycin crosses the blood-brain barrier. The first clinical study of its effectiveness, reported by our laboratory, detailed a dramatic response of one patient with glioblastoma and neurologic improvement in others.[17] Mithramycin was shown to inhibit the synthesis of ribonucleic acid (RNA).[15,16] In tissue culture it is an effective compound against certain human glioblastomas.[7,18] In a glioma tumor in C57 black mice, mithramycin significantly inhibited the growth of the tumor.[16] In contrast, mithramycin would not be detected as an antitumor agent in the current system for screening agents for antitumor activity.

Our initial clinical report was followed by further confirmation of the clinical effectiveness of mithramycin.[19,20] These observations created a new interest in the chemotherapy of glioblastoma multiforme.

In January 1967, the Brain Tumor Chemotherapy Study Group was established under the auspices of the chemotherapy program of the National Cancer Institute. Mithramycin was selected for randomized study.[21] Both treatment and control groups received optimal conventional therapy including surgery and radiation therapy. Mithramycin, 25 μg/kg, was infused intravenously over a 6-hour period for 21 days or until toxicity intervened. Two further courses of chemotherapy lasting 12 days were undertaken at 6-week intervals if the patient's tolerance of toxicity permitted. Of 96 patients, the treated patients had a median survival of 103 days and the untreated controls 117 days. It was concluded that the toxicity of this agent outweighed its potential benefits.

Unfortunately, this study used what is now regarded as a toxic dose of mithramycin. In view of the newer methods of administration of mithramycin in alternate-day dosages, further exploration of this agent is warranted.[22]

The dangers of discarding effective antineoplastic agents because of their toxicity is demonstrated by another study in which mithramycin was administered by continuous carotid artery infusion.[18] Although antitumor activity was noted, it was concluded that the overall morbidity controverted the significance of the isolated favorable responses.

Study of a glioma tumor in mice suggested that there was an additive effect when mithramycin and radiation therapy were administered concomitantly.[15] Clinical studies under way may not confirm this concept. However, the clinical problems encountered in the assessment of therapeutic results in this group of patients emphasize the need for careful randomization and matching of clinical materials before making sweeping condemnations of any chemotherapeutic regimen.

Although mithramycin does have antitumor activity in glioblastoma multiforme, the clinical results with its use alone are not encouraging for practical therapy. Further study of the methods of administration and combination with radiation therapy is warranted.

Vincristine Sulfate

Vincristine sulfate (Oncovin) has been studied in the therapy of primary brain tumors because of its affinity for nervous tissue demonstrated by side effects of palsies, paresthesias, ophthalmoplegia, and paraplegia.

Vincristine sulfate was administered intra-arterially in a small group of patients immediately after surgical decompression.[23,24] The results have not been striking.

BCNU

1,3-Bis(2-chloroethyl)-1-nitrosourea (BCNU), being highly soluble in lipids, is able to ford the blood-brain barrier and gain access to the cerebral spinal fluid and bloodstream simultaneously. BCNU inhibits ribonucleic acid and DNA, and produces greater inhibition of nucleic acid than of protein synthesis. It functions as an alkylating agent. In an experimental animal system, BCNU significantly prolonged the life span of mice bearing intracerebral tumors from 10 to 137 per cent.[14] In this same system, cyclophosphamide less consistently increased survival, and mithramycin and methotrexate not at all.

In clinical trials BCNU has been shown to be effective against brain tumors.[25] Objective improvements occurred in 7 of 18 patients with glioblastoma and 4 of 6 with astrocytoma.

Partial responses were reported in 10 of 16 patients with gliomas.[12] Three dose schedules were employed: 50 to 60 mg/m^2 intravenously once weekly, 20 to 30 mg/m^2 thrice weekly, and 80 mg/m^2 for 3 days. The total dose per patient ranged from 300 to 975 mg/m^2. Myelosuppressive toxicity was encountered at a high rate. Because of thrombocytopenia, a great number of patients needed platelet transfusions.

Miscellaneous Agents

A variety of other agents have been employed in the management of gliomas. Methotrexate,[26] nitrogen mustard,[27] bromouridine and 8-azaguanine[11] are among those of interest. None seem to warrant a high recommendation for practical clinical therapy.

Corticosteroids

Cerebral edema is a major problem with brain tumors. This appears to be related to hemorrhage, necrosis, and compression of surrounding blood vessels and brain tissue. The edema is predominantly intracellular.

The administration of massive doses of corticosteroids will produce rapid reduction of signs and symptoms of increased intracranial pressure. Maximal improvement occurs in a few days. The attainment and maintenance of clinical improvement are dose-dependent. Dexamethasone, 10 mg intravenously, followed by 4 mg every 6 hours, is an effective dose. Equivalent doses of other corticosteroids are also beneficial.

The results of corticosteroid therapy are correlated directly with the reduction of cerebral edema.

References

1. Zimmerman, H. M.: Brain tumors: Their incidence and classification in man and their experimental production. Ann. N.Y. Acad. Sci. 159:337–359, 1969.
2. Conrad, F. G., Myers, P. and Buckley, R.: Glioblastoma multiforme. Minn. Med. 52:491–497, 1969.
3. Cushing, H.: Intracranial tumors. Springfield, Ill.: Charles C Thomas Co., 1932.
4. Courville, C. B.: Intracranial tumors: Notes upon a series of 300 verified cases with some current observations pertaining to their mortality. Bull. Los Angeles Neur. Soc. Suppl. 2, July, 1927.
5. Jelsma, R. and Buey, P. C.: Treatment of glioblastoma multiforme of the brain. J. Neurosurg. 27:400, 1967.
6. Tator, C. H., Morley, T. P. and Paul, W.: The pursuit of selectivity and refinement in the radioisotopic diagnosis of intracranial tumors. Ann. N.Y. Acad. Sci. 159:533–551, 1969.
7. Bering, E. A., Jr., Wilson, C. B. and Norrell, H. A., Jr.: The Kentucky conference on brain tumor chemotherapy. J. Neurosurg. 27:1–10, 1967.
8. Taveras, J. M., Thompson, H. G. Jr., and Pool, J. S.: Should we treat glioblastoma multiforme? Amer. J. Roentgenol. 87: 473–479, 1962.
9. Bouchard, J.: Radiation therapy in the management of primary brain tumors. Ann. N.Y. Acad. Sci. 159:563–570, 1969.
10. Batzdorf, U.: Chemotherapy of glioblastoma multiforme: An appraisal. Bull. Los Angeles Neur. Soc. 31:164–176, 1966.
11. Shapiro, W. R. and Ausman, J. I.: The chemotherapy of brain tumors: A clinical and experimental review. *In* Plum, I. F. (Ed.): Recent Advances in Neurology. Philadelphia: F. A. Davis Company, 1969, pp. 149–235.
12. Walker, M. D. and Hurwitz, B. S.: BCNU (1,3-Bis(2-chloroethyl)-1-nitrosourea) (NSC-409962) in the treatment of malignant brain tumor—A preliminary report. Cancer Chemother. Rep. 54:263–272, 1970.
13. Ausman, J. I., Shapiro, W. R. and Rall, D.: Studies on the chemotherapy of experimental brain tumors: Development of an experimental model. Cancer Res. 30:2394–2400, 1970.

14. Shapiro, W. R., Ausman, J. I. and Rall, D. P.: Studies on the chemotherapy of experimental brain tumors: Evaluation of 1,3-bis (2-chloroethyl)-1-nitrosourea, cyclophosphamide, mithramycin, and methotrexate. Cancer Res. 30:2401–2413, 1970.
15. McNulty, T. B., Dirks, V. A., Yarbro, J. W. and Kennedy, B. J.: Combination chemotherapy with radiation and mithramycin or actinomycin D in a transplanted mouse glioma. Cancer 23:1273–1279, 1969.
16. Kennedy, B. J., Yarbro, J. W., Kickertz, V. and Sandberg-Wollheim, M.: Effect of mithramycin on a mouse glioma. Cancer Res. 28:91–97, 1968.
17. Kennedy, B. J., Brown, J. H. and Yarbro, J. W.: Mithramycin (NSC-24559) therapy for primary glioblastomas. Cancer Chemother. Rep. 48:59–63, 1965.
18. Mealey, J., Jr., Chen, T. T. and Pedlow, E.: Brain tumor chemotherapy with mithramycin and vincristine. Cancer 26:360–367, 1970.
19. Ranshoff, J., Martin, B., Medrek, T. J., Harris, M. N., Golomb, F. M. and Wright, J. C.: Preliminary clinical study of mithramycin (NSC-24550) in primary tumors of the central nervous system. Cancer Chemother. Rep. 49:51–56, 1965.
20. Ranshoff, J., Hochwald, G. and Martin, B. F.: Chemotherapy of primary malignant central nervous system tumors. Ann. N.Y. Acad. Sci. 159:591–598, 1969.
21. Medical News: Neurosurgeons collaborate in study of brain. J.A.M.A. 210:240–241, 1969.
22. Kennedy, B. J.: Mithramycin therapy in advanced testicular neoplasms. Cancer 26:755–766, 1970.
23. Owens, G., Javid, R., Belmusto, L., Bender, M. and Blau, M.: Intra-arterial vincristine therapy of primary gliomas. Cancer 18: 756–760, 1965.
24. Owens, G.: Chemotherapy of brain tumors. Progr. Neurol. Surg. 1:190–201, 1966.
25. Wilson, C. B., Boldrey, E. B., and Enot, K. J.: 1,3-Bis (2-chloroethyl)-1-nitrosourea (NSC-409962) in the treatment of brain tumors. Cancer Chemother. Rep. 54:273–281, 1970.
26. Norrell, H. and Wilson, C.: Brain tumor chemotherapy with methotrexate given intrathecally. J.A.M.A. 201:15–17, 1967.
27. Owens, G.: Intra-arterial chemotherapy of primary brain tumors. Ann. N.Y. Acad. Sci. 159:603–607, 1969.

Toxic Effects of Cancer Chemotherapy Agents on the Nervous System

By A. Charles Winkelman, M.D. and
Elliott L. Mancall, M.D.

DERANGEMENTS OF NEURAL FUNCTION attending the use of chemotherapeutic agents in the treatment of systemic malignancy are not unanticipated in view of the remarkable sensitivity of both the central and the peripheral nervous system to the action of a wide variety of noxious agents. The paucity of reports of neurologic disease occurring in such circumstances is therefore curious. The explanation of this discrepancy is not immediately apparent, but a number of contributory factors may be suggested. Most cytotoxic agents cross the blood-brain barrier poorly, if at all; thus, the nervous system, or at least its central component, may be shielded from the direct toxic effects of these drugs. Further, the patient may be too ill as a result of the basic disease process and its immediate complications to permit detailed neurologic evaluation, particularly if the neurologic manifestations are relatively minor. Finally, the patient may die before neurologic complications of therapy might appear, or the therapy itself may exert such systemic toxicity that extended use may prove impossible. If the validity of all such factors is presumed, it is nonetheless likely that the sparsity of pertinent case records reflects, to a greater or lesser degree, a lack of awareness of the features of the many neurologic disorders which appear in this patient population; a review of data currently available in this regard therefore seems appropriate.

So that disorders of this type may be viewed in proper perspective, attention must first be drawn to those neurologic problems which may develop in the patient with malignant disease entirely unrelated to the use of chemotherapeutic agents per se. It is clear that the accurate formulation of neurologic disease in any such patient depends upon the appropriate consideration and logical exclusion of these various conditions, which may be briefly summarized as follows:

1. *Metastatic Disease.* The occurrence of solitary or multiple nodular metastases as expanding mass lesions in the meninges or within the nervous parenchyma itself is so well known as to require little or no additional comment. The great rarity of intramedullary lesions within the spinal cord and brain stem is particularly noteworthy. Less widely appreciated is diffuse invasion of the leptomeninges by neoplastic cells, in so-called carcinomatosis or lymphomatosis of the meninges. This presents most commonly as a subacute or chronic meningitis, with signs of meningeal irritation, involvement of cranial nerves, and signs of increased intracranial pressure; lymphocytic pleocytosis in the spinal fluid and hypoglycorrachia are characteristically encountered. Isolated infiltration of peripheral or cranial nerves or of spinal roots by neoplastic cells may also appear, although rarely, and poses at times a major diagnostic problem.

From the Division of Neurology, Department of Medicine, Hahnemann Medical College and Hospital, Philadelphia, Pennsylvania.

Supported in part by Developmental Training Grant No. 1 T08 NB10056 from the National Institute of Neurological Diseases and Stroke, National Institutes of Health.

2. *Remote Effects of Visceral Malignancy.* A number of neurologic diseases have been defined as reflections of tumor growth elsewhere in the body whose occurrence bears no discernible relation to metastatic deposits as such. Carcinoma of the lung, breast, and ovary are most frequently implicated in a causal sense. The pathogenesis of these disorders is not known; some as yet undefined defect in neural metabolism induced or conditioned by the associated malignancy is often postulated as an underlying cause. Improvement in the neurologic abnormalities may be noted after removal of the primary tumor. The not uncommon appearance of these entities before the underlying malignant disease itself has become manifest merits particular attention. Included in this group are the following:

a. *Carcinomatous Myopathy*[1,2] This presents with muscle weakness and wasting often associated with pain and tenderness. The pelvic and shoulder girdles and the proximal muscles of the extremities are involved characteristically in a symmetrical fashion; bulbar muscles may also be affected. The tendon reflexes may be lost early or late in the course; sensation is ordinarily preserved. In rapidly evolving cases, myoglobinuria may appear. Both the clinical and pathologic features are identical with those of polymyositis;[3] it is probably best to look upon this myopathy as a particular form of polymyositis indistinguishable from that disorder as recognized in other contexts.

b. *Lambert-Eaton Syndrome.*[4] This is a syndrome of muscle weakness and fatigability associated with extreme hypersensitivity to curare. Often likened to myasthenia gravis, it occurs most commonly with carcinoma of the lung. It differs from true myasthenia by virtue of sparing of the bulbar and ocular muscles, which are commonly involved in myasthenia; absence of consistent response to anticholinesterase agents, as is characteristic of myasthenia; and improvement in muscle strength and activity with repetitive stimulation, the reverse of what obtains in the myasthenic. Guanidine is said to be useful therapeutically.

c. *Carcinomatous Neuropathy.*[5,6] Ordinarily appearing as a distal and symmetrical polyneuropathy, this generally involves the lower extremities earlier and more severely than the upper. It may be purely motor, purely sensory, or mixed, and often is associated with myopathic features, the combination being referred to as *carcinomatous neuromyopathy.* The peripheral nerves may also be the site of frank hemorrhage, either within the sheath or in the substance of the nerves or spinal roots themselves, as found in patients with leukemia and others with overt bleeding tendencies. Allusion has already been made to the occurrence of neoplastic infiltrates in the nerves as well.

d. *Carcinomatous Myelopathy.*[7] This is a very rare, intensely necrotizing process involving the spinal cord. It presents clinically as an acutely evolving flaccid areflexic paraplegia associated with a symmetrical and ascending segmental sensory loss and sphincter paralysis. The disease predominates in the thoracic cord; when the cervical enlargement is involved, the arms may be affected. Death ensues within a matter of days or weeks. The absence of spontaneous pain and of vertebral tenderness and the characteristically ascending clinical course assist in distinguishing this entity from the much more common epidural metastatic deposits. Clinical and pathologic features of amyotrophic lateral sclerosis have also been described in patients harboring malignancy;[8,9] the concurrence of the two disorders here is probably coincidental and without meaningful causal relation.

e. *Carcinomatous Cerebellar (Spinocerebellar) Degeneration.*[10] Characterized pathologically by degeneration of the cerebellar cortex, and, on occasion, of other parts of the neuraxis as well, this is evidenced clinically by a subacutely evolving syndrome of ataxia involving the trunk and the limbs in a fairly symmetrical fashion. Tremors, dysarthria, and various abnormalities of ocular motility including nystagmus, oscillopsia, and skew deviation are common. Pyramidal tract signs and sensory abnormalities may appear, and dementia is frequent. The slowly evolving course and the absence of headache, papilledema, or other signs of increased intracranial pressure serve to set this apart clinically from metastatic disease of the posterior fossa. *Dementia* may also develop as an isolated neurologic abnormality in the patient with cancer; its pathologic substrate cannot ordinarily be defined, but in a few patients changes of so-called *limbic encephalitis* have been described.

3. *Radiation Myelopathy*.[11,12] This is sometimes found in the patient with malignant disease, almost always after radiation therapy when the lower cervical or upper thoracic spine or both have been included in the treated zones. Signs of involvement of these portions of the cord are recognized clinically, the manifestations generally developing subacutely and in an asymmetrical fashion; at times a typical Brown–Séquard syndrome is observed. There is usually a delay of some months after the course of radiation therapy before the neurologic signs appear. The disorder is self-limited, and clinical recovery is not rare. It is probably due to vascular occlusion as a result of radiation damage to the meningeal vessels; multiple infarcts may be evident within the cord substance.

4. *Infection*. The occurrence of sepsis, often involving unusual organisms, is commonplace in the debilitated patient, and meningitis is not uncommon; the development of *Torula* meningitis is particularly well known in this connection. In recent years yet another disorder of presumed infectious origin has been recognized, particularly in patients suffering from chronic lymphatic leukemia and Hodgkin's disease, viz., *progressive multifocal leukoencephalopathy*,[13,14] a disease of white matter generally looked upon as a slow virus infection of the nervous system with a virus of the papova group.[15,16] Although it is not ordinarily pathogenetic, at least as regards the central nervous system, the responsible viral agent apparently becomes capable of producing recognizable disease in patients whose immunologic capability is diminished. The disorder is characterized clinically by the development of dementia, pyramidal tract signs, and visual abnormalities, particularly homonymous hemianopsia. Additional neurologic signs appear as the disease progresses, since virtually all parts of the neuraxis may be involved. Once established, the disease proceeds inexorably, death ensuing within weeks or months. Pathologically, one observes scattered throughout the white matter demyelinating lesions which tend to enlarge and coalesce to form extensive zones of loss of myelin. Axons are relatively well preserved. Bizarre changes in astrocytes and inclusion material within enlarged oligodendrocytes are characteristically seen on histologic examination. The presumption of viral etiology is based upon electron microscopic observations of particulate aggregates which appear identical to those of the papova-polyoma type of viruses.

Specific Toxicity of Individual Chemotherapeutic Agents

Vinca Alkaloids

Vincristine (Oncovin) and vinblastine (Velban) adversely affect both the hematopoietic and the nervous system, though not equally so. The side effects of vinblastine involve primarily the bone marrow; in contrast, the therapeutic use of vincristine is limited by its prominent neurotoxic effects, and this agent is thus of greater neurologic significance.[17] The toxic manifestations of vincristine, particularly as regards the peripheral nervous system, are clearly a dose-related phenomenon.[17,18] Many individuals exhibit no symptoms with a dosage of 2 mg per square meter given once weekly, although at this level the deep tendon reflexes may be observed to be absent. At somewhat higher doses, many, if not most, patients experience mild paresthesias. In the case of cranial nerve palsies, on the other hand, a much wider range of drug (from 2.6 mg to 136 mg) may be administered before symptoms appear.[19] In patients with hepatic insufficiency, the neurologic complications, in particular the peripheral neuropathies, tend to be more severe, even with small doses.

Vincristine exerts its neurotoxic effects principally upon the peripheral nervous system[20] and, to a lesser degree, the autonomic nervous system; the central nervous system enjoys relative immunity. In the peripheral neuropathy which appears, the legs tend to be affected earlier and more severely than the arms. Depression or loss of the deep tendon reflexes is observed initially; paresthesias in the extremities are noted very early, in some cases on the first day of treatment. Pain, sensory loss, weakness, and atrophy then appear. A disturbance of ambulation, characterized by such terms as "broad-based" and "steppage," is often noted, and undoubtedly is a consequence of the weakness and sensory loss; it is sometimes interpreted as a sign of cerebellar dysfunction, but with little justification. The electrophysiologic observation of normal conduction velocities and sparing of the H reflex, noted in some patients, would suggest localization of the disease process to the muscle spindle.[18]

Alterations of cranial nerve function are also encountered in patients receiving vincristine, although less often than is polyneuropathy. Cranial nerve palsies generally develop somewhat later than the peripheral neuropathy; although signs of ocular motor paresis have been noted as early as two weeks after institution of therapy in a few cases, the onset of such palsies is often delayed until 10 weeks or longer.[19] The most common cranial nerve deficits are ocular, and are characterized by ptosis, paresis of upward gaze, and varying combinations and degrees of ophthalmoplegia. The pupil is always spared. Other cranial nerves involved include the trigeminal, as manifested by absent corneal reflexes or paroxysmal pain in the jaw, or both, and the facial, with unilateral or bilateral impairment. The signs of cranial nerve dysfunction in most instances disappear following reduction or discontinuance of vincristine. The time required for recovery is variable, ranging from as early as 2 weeks to as long as 4 to 5 months; in contrast, symptoms of vincristine-induced peripheral neuropathy diminish much more rapidly, often within 1 week after cessation of therapy. It should be pointed out that ocular abnormalities similar to those described here may be found in patients with leukemia who have not received vincristine[19]; however, the temporal relationship of these changes to the initiation of therapy, the regression of the symptoms following reduction or discontinuance of the drug, and the presence of other signs of vincristine toxicity such as alopecia, peripheral neuropathy, constipation, nausea and vomiting, support the concept that the cranial nerve palsies are in fact vincristine-induced in most cases. Unfortunately no pathologic studies are available to assist in identifying the precise anatomic substrate of these symptoms.

The autonomic nervous system is also generally involved. Constipation is the most common symptom, occurring in most if not all patients. Incontinence, bladder atony, difficulty in beginning micturition, and hypotension are additional signs of autonomic dysfunction found in some individuals.

Depression,[21] insomnia,[22] agitation, psychotic states, hallucinations and convulsions[23] have been described in patients treated with vincristine, particularly those receiving protracted therapy, and presumably represent central neurotoxic responses. Nausea and vomiting commonly associated with the use of this drug have been considered by some to be an additional manifestation of central toxicity, presumably reflecting direct action on the emetic mechanisms in the medulla.

Antimetabolites

Methotrexate (aminopterin), a folic acid antagonist, produces mental depression, peripheral neuropathy and bladder dysfunction. Somnolence and confusion occur in 10 to 15 per cent of patients receiving the drug; in such patients bilateral slowing is noted in the electroencephalogram.[24] Seizures have also been described. Systemic toxic reactions have been reduced by the concurrent use of folinic acid. Curiously, the intrathecal use of methotrexate appears to produce less toxic side effects than its systemic use.[25]

The antipyrimidine *5-fluorouracil* produces on occasion an acute cerebellar syndrome,[26,27] the development of which appears dose-related. Clinical abnormalities become evident within 2 to 20 weeks after institution of therapy; dysarthria, head nodding, ataxia of trunk and limbs, and dysmetria are noted. Seizures and optic neuritis have also been described.[28] Disappearance of signs follows within one to two days after therapy is stopped. Pathologic studies in man have demonstrated chromatolysis of neurons in the olivary and dentate nuclei and reduction in number of the cerebellar granule cells. The intravenous administration of 5-fluorouracil and the cisternal injection of the pyrimidine antagonist fluorotic acid have both been followed by similar cerebellar difficulties in the experimental animal.

Alkylating Agents

When utilized systemically, this group of drugs seems to have only minimal adverse effect in the nervous system. On the other hand, *nitrogen mustard* is highly toxic when administered via the carotid artery for direct perfusion therapy of brain tumors.[29] Immediately or soon after the perfusion, convulsions and cerebral edema appear; long-term therapy is associated with deafness, ophthalmoplegia and depression, features which evolve in a progressive fashion and which are usually irreversible.

Sarcolysin, when administered intra-arterially, has been noted to induce peripheral neuropathy, in one reported series appearing one to two months after therapy was completed.[30]

Cyclophosphamide (Cytoxan) appears to have little potential for inducing neurologic disease as such, but ataxia has been reported in a few instances.[31]

Busulfan (Myleran), a nonmustard alkylating agent, has been implicated in the production of agitation, irritability and convulsions when given in high doses.[29] A disturbance in neuromuscular transmission has recently been recorded.[32]

Antineoplastic Antibiotics

Actinomycin D has few, if any, consistent neurotoxic effects. Mental depression has, however, been noted at times.

Miscellaneous Agents

Methylhydrazine (procarbazine) is a monoamine oxidase inhibitor whose use has been associated with adverse effects on the central and the peripheral nervous systems.

Psychological disturbances such as depression, somnolence, restlessness and even psychosis may occur, and ophthalmoplegia with pupillary sparing has been noted. Postural hypotension and polyneuropathy have been described, the latter occurring in as high as 20 per cent of patients so treated.[33]

Dimethylacetamide, a drug with antitumor activity but no longer in clinical use, merits brief comment in this context. Patients receiving doses of this agent in excess of 300 mg/kg were noted to become lethargic, depressed and confused on the second and third day of treatment.[34] By the fourth and fifth day, the patients developed vivid visual hallucinations and, to a lesser degree, auditory hallucinations. Electroencephalographic changes were associated with the psychic disturbance, serial studies indicating generalized slowing which was maximal when the hallucinations were most marked. The symptoms subsided upon withdrawal of the drug, the electroencephalogram also reverting to normal.

Steroids, when used over prolonged periods of time, may produce myopathy characterized by symmetrical weakness and at times atrophy, without pain or sensory disturbance, and involving primarily the girdle and proximal limb musculature. The weakness usually improves as steroids are reduced. On occasion, polyneuropathy has also been ascribed to the use of catabolic steroids.

References

1. Brain, W. R. and Henson, R. A.: Neurological syndromes associated with carcinoma: The carcinomatous neuromyopathies. Lancet 2: 972, 1958.
2. Henson, R. A., Russell, D. S. and Wilkinson, M.: Carcinomatous neuropathy and myopathy: A clinical and pathological study. Brain 77:82, 1954.
3. Walton, J. N. and Adams, R. D.: Polymyositis. Baltimore: Williams and Wilkins, 1958.
4. Lambert, E. H., Rooke, E. D., Eaton, L. M. and Hodgson, C. H.: Myasthenic syndrome associated with bronchial neoplasm: Neurophysiology studies. *In* Viets, H. R. (Ed.): Myasthenia Gravis. Springfield, Ill.: Charles C Thomas, 1961.
5. Denny-Brown, D.: Primary sensory neuropathy with muscular changes associated with carcinoma. J. Neurol. Neurosurg. Psychiat. 11:73, 1948.
6. Croft, P. B. and Wilkinson, M.: The incidence of carcinomatous neuromyopathy, with special reference to carcinoma of the lung and breast. *In* Brain, L. and Norris, F. (Eds.): The Remote Effects of Cancer on the Nervous System. New York: Grune & Stratton, 1965, p. 44.
7. Mancall, E. L. and Rosales, R. K.: Necrotizing myelopathy associated with visceral carcinoma. Brain 87:639, 1964.
8. Rowland, L. P. and Schneck, S. A.: Neuromuscular disorders associated with malignant neoplastic disease. J. Chronic Dis. 16:777, 1963.
9. Norris, F. H., Jr. and Engel, W. K.: Carcinomatous amyotrophic lateral sclerosis. *In* Brain, L. and Norris, F. (Eds.): The Remote Effects of Cancer on the Nervous System. New York: Grune & Stratton, 1965, p. 24.
10. Brain, W. R., Daniel, P. M. and Greenfield, J. G.: Subacute cortical cerebellar degeneration and its relation to carcinoma. J. Neurol. Neurosurg. Psychiat. 14:59, 1951.
11. Stevenson, L. D. and Eckhardt, R. E.: Myelomalacia of the cranial portion of the spinal cord, probably the result of roentgen therapy. Arch. Path. 39:109, 1945.
12. Alajouanine, T., Lhermitte, F., Cambier, J. and Gautier, J. C.: Memoires originaux: les lésions post-radiothérapiques tardives du système nerveux central (à propos d'une observation anatomo-clinique de myelopathie cervicale). Revue Neurol. 1:105, 1961.
13. Åström, K. E., Mancall, E. L. and Richardson, E. P., Jr.: Progressive multifocal leukoencephalopathy: A hitherto unrecognized complication of chronic lymphatic leukaemia and Hodgkin's disease. Brain 81:93, 1958.
14. Richardson, E. P., Jr.: Progressive multifocal leukoencephalopathy. *In* Brain, L. and Norris, F. (Eds.): The Remote Effects of Cancer on the Nervous System. New York: Grune & Stratton, 1965, p. 6.

15. ZuRhein, G. M.: Polyoma-like virions in a human demyelinating disease. Acta Neuropathol. 8:57, 1967.
16. Dayan, A. D.: Progressive multifocal leukoencephalopathy. *In* Whitty, C. W. M., Hughes, J. T. and MacCallum, F. O. (Eds.): Virus Diseases and the Nervous System. Oxford: Blackwell Scientific Publications, 1969, p. 199.
17. Carbone, P. P., Bono, V., Frei, E., III and Brindley, C. O.: Clinical studies with vincristine. Blood 21:640, 1963.
18. Sandler, S. G., Tobin, W. and Henderson, E. S.: Vincristine induced neuropathy. Neurology 19:367, 1969.
19. Albert, D. M., Wong, V. G. and Henderson, E. S.: Ocular complications of vincristine therapy. Arch. Ophthal. 78:709, 1967.
20. Moress, G. R., D'Agostino, A. N. and Jarcho, L. W.: Neuropathy in lymphoplastic leukemia treated with vincristine. Arch. Neurol. 16:377, 1967.
21. Karon, M. R., Freireich, E. J. and Frei, E., III: A preliminary report in vincristine sulfate: A new active agent for the treatment of acute leukemia. Pediatrics 30:791, 1962.
22. Council on Drugs: Antineoplastic agents: Vincristine sulfate (Oncovin). J.A.M.A. 191:751, 1965.
23. Lassman, L. P., Pearce, G. W. and Gang, T.: Sensitivity of intracranial gliomas to vincristine sulfate. Lancet 1:296, 1965.
24. Brewer, J. I., Gerbie, A. B., Dulkant, R. E., Nagle, R. G. and Torok, E. E.: Chemotherapy in trophoblastic disease. Amer. J. Obstet. Gynec. 90:566, 1964.
25. Lampkin, B. C., Higgins, G. R. and Hammond, D.: Absence of neurotoxicity following massive intrathecal administration of methotrexate. Cancer 20:1780, 1967.
26. Weiss, A. J., Jackson, L. G. and Carabasi, R.: An evaluation of 5-fluorouracil in malignant disease. Ann. Intern. Med. 55: 731, 1961.
27. Moertel, C. G., Reitmeir, R. J., Balton, C. F. and Phorten, R. G.: Cerebellar ataxia associated with fluorinated pyrimidine therapy. Cancer Chemother. Rep. 41:15, 1964.
28. Riehl, J. L. and Brown, W. J.: Acute cerebellar syndrome secondary to 5-fluorouracil therapy. Neurology 14:961, 1964.
29. Boesen, E. and Davis, W.: Cytotoxic Drugs in the Treatment of Cancer. London: Arnold, 1969.
30. Rochlin, D. B. and Smart, C. R.: Isolation perfusion: Evaluation of 249 cases. Surgery 56:834, 1964.
31. Haddy, T. B., Nora, A. H., Sutow, W. W. and Vietti, T. J.: Cyclophosphamide treatment for metastatic soft tissue sarcoma. Amer. J. Dis. Child. 114:301, 1967.
32. Djaldetti, M., Pinkhas, J., DeVries, A., Kott, E., Joshua, H. and Dollberg, L.: Myasthenia gravis in a patient with chronic myeloid leukemia treated by busulfan. Blood 32:336, 1968.
33. Samuels, M. L., Leary, W. V., Alexandrian, R., Howe, C. D. and Frei, E., III: Clinical trials with procarbazine in malignant lymphoma and other disseminated neoplasia. Cancer 20: 1187, 1967.
34. Weiss, A. J., Mancall, E. L., Koltes, J. A., White, J. C. and Jackson, L. G.: Dimethylacetamide: A hitherto unrecognized hallucinogenic agent. Science 136:151, 1962.

III. BONE MARROW PHYSIOLOGY AND PROTECTION

Chemotherapy and Erythropoiesis

By ALLAN J. ERSLEV, M.D.

THE RATE OF RED CELL PRODUCTION is exceedingly sensitive to changes in the metabolic environment of the bone marrow. This is most easily observed in patients with chronic hemolytic anemia in whom changes in red cell production almost immediately are translated into changes in red cell count or red cell mass. In these patients, brief infections or minor surgery may cause a profound anemia due to temporary cessation of red cell production.[1] In patients with normal red cell life span such erythropoietic changes undoubtedly occur in response to changes in the "milieu interior," but are much more difficult to recognize. Ferrokinetic studies such as serum or red cell iron turnover are of some help, but of more importance clinically are measures which can be followed serially. The best of these are the reticulocyte count and the serum iron concentration. Unfortunately, these tests have still not received their deserved recognition as routine checks on the rate of red cell production, and we still rely primarily on the insensitive but automated red cell count, hematocrit and hemoglobin concentration.

In patients receiving chemotherapy, it is of special importance to monitor the rate of red cell production accurately. It will not only provide clues as to the development of complications such as infections, tissue injury or hemorrhages, but it will also indicate the overall cellular response to the chemotherapeutic agents. The erythron from the nebulous stem cells to the highly differentiated erythrocytes is a circumscribed, self-perpetuating biologic unit, and it serves admirably as a model for the effect of chemotherapeutic agents on other less accessible cellular systems.

NORMAL ERYTHROPOIESIS

Nucleated red cells are characterized both morphologically and biochemically by their synthesis of hemoglobin (Fig. 1). Because of the progressive accumulation of hemoglobin molecules, they are not capable of cellular renewal but depend on a continuous influx of cells from an earlier compartment, the so-called stem cell pool. The morphologic identity of cells in this pool has not been firmly established but it has been suggested that they resemble mature lymphocytes.[2] The differentiation to recognizable nucleated red cells could occur via a "blast transformation" akin to the transformation of lymphocytes to immunologically committed cells. The differentiation of erythroid stem cells is believed to be triggered by the renal hormone erythropoietin,[3] which is released in response to tissue hypoxia; its effect on stem cell adjusts the functional activities of the erythron to the need for oxygen in the tissues.

It has been proposed that erythropoietin acts on stem cells during their G_1 phase and causes a derepression of that gene sequence which is responsible for the formation

From the Cardeza Foundation, Department of Internal Medicine, Jefferson Medical College of the Thomas Jefferson University, Philadelphia, Pennsylvania.

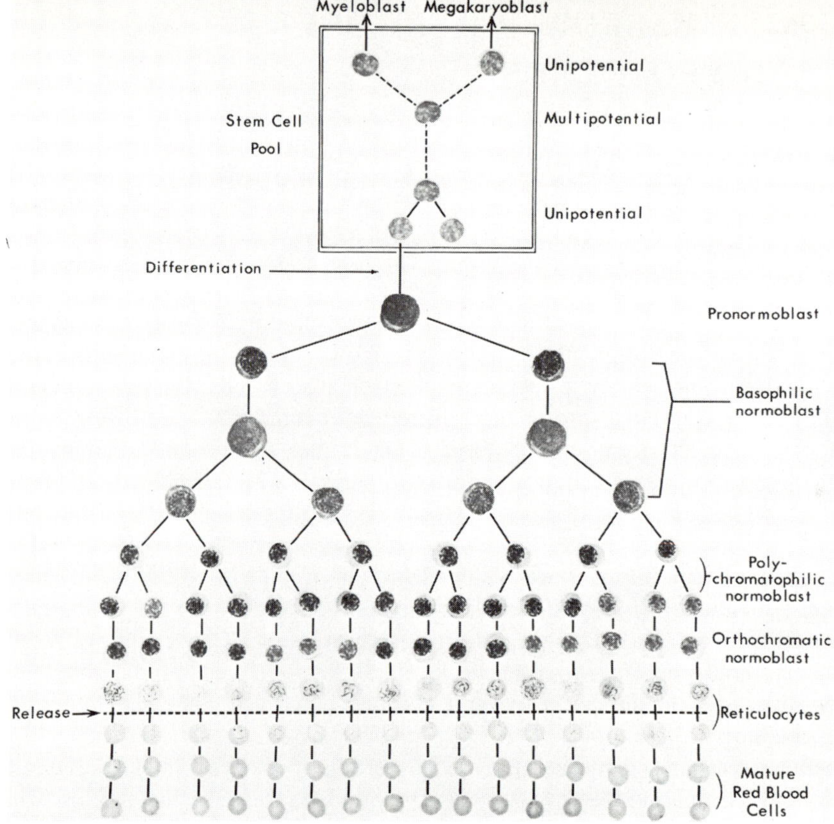

FIG. 1.—Schematic outline of the stem cell pool and the nucleated red cell compartment.

of "erythroid" messenger RNA. This hypothesis has been supported by in vitro studies which have shown an increase in the synthesis of RNA 15 minutes after the addition of erythropoietin.[4] Actinomycin D, a known inhibitor of DNA synthesis, prevented this effect.

The stem cells responsive to erythropoietin appear to move continuously through a regenerative cycle. The length of the G_1 phase depends on the total mass of stem cells providing autoregulation of the pool size.[5] Although this pool has many functional feedback links with other stem cell pools, it is believed that distinct pools exist for stem cells committed to erythroid cells, myeloid cells and megakaryocytes. These pools can adjust their functional capacity, but if they are injured by radiation or chemotherapeutic drugs, they apparently are being replenished from an earlier multipotential stem cell compartment.[6] The existence of such stem cells has been postulated by clinicians for years to explain the pancytosis of polycythemia vera or the pancytopenia of aplastic anemia. Definite demonstration of their existence was provided by the spleen colonization technique of Siminovitch et al.[7] The so-called colony-forming unit probably represents a multipotential stem cell triggered to intense proliferation by being transplanted into a host depleted of bone marrow. Under normal conditions, these cells must exist in a resting G_0 phase since large amounts of tritiated thymidine or hydroxyurea (suicide technique) fail to diminish the number of colony-forming units while they almost eliminate the erythropoietin-sensitive stem cells.[8]

The earliest recognizable erythroid cell is a pronormoblast. It is a large cell programmed to synthesize hemoglobin and divide three to four times during a period of 4 to 5 days. Although division entails DNA synthesis, there is a stepwise reduction in nuclear volume. This nuclear condensation finally results in a compact, inactive pycnotic nucleus which is extruded. Concomitantly and independently of the mitotic divisions, the nucleated red cells incorporate iron, synthesize protoporphyrin and globin and assemble the characteristic hemoglobin molecules. These activities continue for several days after the inactivation and extrusion of the nucleus indicating the presence of long-lived messenger RNA. The cells are released from the bone marrow; a few days later ribosomes and mitochondrias disappear and the cells transform into mature circulating erythrocytes.

The Effect of Chemotherapeutic Agents on Erythropoiesis

In a number of important reviews, Karnofsky and coworkers[9,10] have attempted to categorize chemotherapeutic agents according to their action on proliferating cells. Most of the known actions have been established by in vitro studies of cell cultures and of cell free systems. In vitro studies of nucleated red cells and reticulocytes have been particularly rewarding and provided much information about the pharmacology of chemotherapeutic agents. In vivo studies of erythropoiesis have also been of great importance since the effect of various metabolites and antimetabolites often is clearly reflected by changes in the morphology of the nucleated red cells and in the number of reticulocytes. However, it is important to remember that the erythron has only a limited number of functional and morphologic options. If sensitive to a chemotherapeutic agent, it can either respond by a production of defective "megaloblastoid" cells or by a reduction in the number of cells produced. It frequently does both, and it seems likely that the difference between these responses merely is quantitative, with early or mild nuclear injury causing the formation of megaloblasts and later or more severe injury causing bone marrow suppression.

Megaloblastosis

All drugs that are cancer chemotherapeutic have either a direct or indirect injurious effect on the synthesis and metabolism of DNA. Even the drugs with a primary action on RNA or protein metabolism (actinomycin D, L-asparaginase, puromycin) will have secondary actions on DNA, actions which probably are more important therapeutically and certainly more visible morphologically. The common feature of all these drugs is that they will cause megaloblastic transformation of the erythroid population. Studies on B_{12} and folic acid metabolism indicate that such a transformation is caused by an "unbalanced growth," impairment of DNA synthesis without or with less impairment of RNA and protein synthesis.[11] Since the megaloblast in the deficiency anemias resembles those in the marrows of patients treated with chemotherapeutic drugs, it is assumed that the mechanism is the same and that the common fundamental defect lies in the replication of DNA.

Functionally, the megaloblastic marrows behave the same regardless of etiology, and one observes the characteristic ineffective erythropoiesis with low reticulocyte counts and low iron utilization despite erythroid hyperplasia. In the drug-induced cases, the serum levels of folic acid and B_{12} are normal or even increased, and there is no hematologic response to treatment with these vitamins. Eventually the bone marrow becomes hypoplastic, with a reduced number of erythroid cells and a low serum iron turnover.

Bone Marrow Hypoplasia

It has been estimated that about 50 per cent of hypoplastic or aplastic anemias are drug induced or drug related. This statistic, however, does not include patients in whom hypoplastic anemia is found as an expected side effect of the use of cancer chemotherapeutic agents. If such cases were included, hypoplastic anemia would probably be one of the most important iatrogenic diseases. Hypoplastic anemia is characterized by general bone marrow suppression, but occasionally bone marrow aspiration discloses intense erythroid hyperplasia. Since low reticulocyte counts, increased transfusion requirements, prolonged half-life of ^{59}Fe and decreased iron utilization indicate generalized suppression, such bone marrow samples probably represent remnants of active marrow, so-called "hot pockets." Occasionally, these "hot pockets" herald bone marrow regeneration, but more often they are the last vestiges of active red marrow.

The underlying defect of bone marrow suppression is believed to reside in the stem cells. Every agent capable of interfering with DNA metabolism may cause damage to the proliferating capacity of the stem cell pool. It has been proposed that the sequence of events involves initial mitotic suppression of the erythropoietin sensitive stem cells which normally are in slow but steady generative cycle. This presumably calls forth a compensatory response by the dormant multipotential stem cells; they go into cycle and are promptly suppressed by the toxic agent. The result is an initial erythroid hypoplasia (usually associated with megaloblastoid transformation) and subsequently general bone marrow hypoplasia and pancytopenia.

The severity of stem cell suppression is usually dependent on the dosage and length of exposure. The drugs commonly used for cancer chemotherapy will all cause such suppression despite different modes of action on nucleic acid metabolism. Some drugs are reputed to have more bone marrow toxicity than others, but these differences are not clear-cut and may be more related to individual responsiveness than to specific pharmacologic action.

Although the anemia and pancytopenia caused by bone marrow suppression usually are reversible, it is not certain that this normalization reflects complete anatomic restoration of the suppressed and injured stem cell pool. It is possible that a reduced number of stem cells can maintain a normal cell count in the circulating blood merely by shortening their regenerative cycle. This would obviously mean that such bone marrow has less reserve to withstand subsequent injury and is more vulnerable to the development of a self-sustaining and irreversible aplastic anemia. On the other hand, it has been suggested that this dreaded complication is unrelated to amount or length of drug exposure, but is caused by a constitutional hypersensitivity to the drug or to a chance injury of a vital chromosomal segment in stem cells.

The pathogenesis of chloramphenicol-induced aplastic anemia can be used as a model. Chloramphenicol causes a reversible suppression of the erythron, presumably because of injury to the mitochondrias.[12] However, in a few cases, chloramphenicol causes an irreversible bone marrow aplasia. This latter complication is apparently not related to the amount of drug ingested and is probably not a dose-related toxicity reaction.[13] A more likely explanation is that the development of aplastic anemia demands a constitutional metabolic abnormality rendering the stem cells excessively sensitive to the action of chloramphenicol. However, it is also possible that the vacuolization which regularly occurs in bone marrow cells of patients treated with chloramphenicol may delete chromosomal segments involved in cellular renewal.[14] This kind of injury would make aplastic anemia a disease of bad luck and would also suggest that prolonged and intensive therapy may increase the odds that nuclear damage will involve vital areas in the cellular genome. A similar explanation has been proposed for patients in whom the exposure to bone marrow toxic agents has led to the development of leukemia. In such cases the chromosomal injury presumably does not sterilize the stem cell but rather liberates it from the proliferative constraint of physiologic control mechanisms. Recently it has been suggested that irreversible damage to "vascular stem cells" may be responsible for the development of sustained aplastic anemia.[15] Such damage may lead to changes in the "vascular microenvironment" and interfere with bone marrow regeneration.

These considerations and speculations have to be kept in mind when the potential dangers of bone marrow suppression are assessed after administration of cancer chemotherapeutic agents. Does it merely indicate a reversible and intended suppression of the proliferative capacity of cells or is it a preamble to the development of an irreversible bone marrow aplasia? No final answer can be given, but it behooves the physician to remember that prolonged therapy is probably more apt to cause irreversible aplasia than is brief exposure to drugs and that careful monitoring of the bone marrow activity is advisable to keep the inherent risks within reasonable limits.

Steroid hormones, particularly androgens and cortisones, are used widely in the chemotherapy of cancer and have been shown to have powerful effects on erythropoiesis. Although androgens were known to be mildly erythropoietic, Kennedy was the first to show that clinically significant erythrocytosis may occur in women treated with testosterone for breast cancer.[16] Since then numerous studies have established androgens as both erythro- and myelo-stimulating agents.[17] The effect on red cell production is presumed to be mediated by the release of endogenous erythropoietin. However, erythropoietin titers in many responsive patients are high even before treatment, and it has been suggested that direct stimulation of the erythroid cells must occur in order to explain the erythropoietic response. Certainly, the associated general myelostimulating effect so frequently observed must be caused by a mechanism unrelated to erythropoietin. Adrenal steroids can also cause stimulation of the bone marrow, and high leukocyte and platelet counts are not uncommon in patients treated with such compounds.

Conclusions

The erythropoietic tissue responds to cancer chemotherapeutic agents by a megaloblastic transformation of normoblasts and by a reversible suppression of the proliferative capacity of erythropoietin sensitive stem cells. If treatment is sustained, the stem cell injury becomes irreversible leading to bone marrow hypoplasia, anemia and eventually a life-threatening pancytopenia. Since the object of cancer chemotherapy is to eradicate certain proliferating cellular clones, some suppression of the erythron in treated patients is almost inevitable. Consequently, if carefully monitored, this bone marrow response may be a valuable guide in the use of cancer chemotherapeutic drugs and may not necessarily be an unwanted or dangerous complication.

References

1. Erslev, A. J. and McKenna, P. J.: Effect of splenectomy on red cell production. Ann. Intern. Med. 67:990, 1967.
2. Cladkowicz, G., Bennett, M. and Shearer, G. M.: Pluripotent stem cell function of the mouse marrow "lymphocyte". Science 144:866, 1964.
3. Erslev, A. J.: The role of erythropoietin in the control of red cell production. Medicine 43:661, 1964.
4. Krantz, S. B. and Goldwasser, E.: On the mechanism of erythropoietin induced differentiation. II. The effect on RNA synthesis. Acta Biochim. Biophys. 103:325, 1965.
5. Kretchmar, A. L.: Erythropoietin: Hypothesis of action tested by analog computer. Science 152:367, 1966.
6. Stohlman, F., Jr.: Regulation of red cell production. *In* Greenwalt, T. J. and Jamieson, G. A. (Eds.): Formation and Destruction of Blood Cells. Philadelphia: J. B. Lippincott, 1970.
7. Siminovitch, L., McCulloch, E. A. and Till, J. E.: The distribution of colony-forming cells among spleen colonies. J. Cell. Comp. Physiol. 62:327, 1963.
8. Becker, A. J., McCulloch, E. A., Siminovitch, L. and Till, J. E.: The effect of differing demands for blood cell production on DNA synthesis by hematopoietic colony-forming cells of mice. Blood 26:296, 1965.
9. Karnofsky, D. A. and Clarkson, B. D.: Celullar effects of anti-cancer drugs. Ann. Rev. Pharmacol. 3:357, 1963.
10. Dowling, M. D., Krakoff, J. H. and Karnofsky, D. A.: Mechanism of action of anticancer drugs. *In* Cole, W. H. (Ed.): Chemotherapy of Cancer. Philadelphia: Lea and Febiger, 1970.
11. Beck, W. S., Hook, S. and Barnett, B. H.: The metabolic functions of vitamin B_{12}. I. Distinctive modes of unbalanced growth behavior in *Lactobacillus leishmanii.* Biochem. Biophys. Acta 55:455, 1962.
12. Martels, O. J., Manijan, D. R., Smith, V. S. and Yunis, A. A.: Chloramphenicol and bone marrow mitochondria. J. Lab. Clin. Med. 12:927, 1969.
13. Yunis, A. A. and Bloomberg, G. R. Chloramphenicol toxicity: Clinical features and pathogenesis. Progr. Haematol. 4:138, 1968.
14. Castaldi, G. and Mitus, W. J.: Chromosome vacuolization and breakage. Arch. Intern. Med. 121:177, 1968.
15. Knospe, W. H., Blom, J. and Crosby, W. H.: Regeneration of locally irradiated bone marrow. II. Induction of regeneration in permanently aplastic medullary cavities. Blood 31:400, 1968.
16. Kennedy, B. J. and Gilbertson, A. S.: Increased erythropoiesis induced by androgenic-hormone therapy. New Eng. J. Med. 256:719, 1953.
17. Sanchez-Medal, L., Gomez-Leal, A., Duarte, L. and Rico, M. G.: Anabolic androgenic steroids in the treatment of acquired aplastic anemia. Blood 34:283, 1969.

Chemotherapy and Leukokinetics

By DANE R. BOGGS, M.D. AND PAUL A. CHERVENICK, M.D.

MOST CHEMOTHERAPEUTIC AGENTS used in the treatment of malignant neoplastic diseases are also fairly nonspecific cell poisons. Most particularly, they are damaging to the cellular compartments which are active in production of new cells such as the lining cells of the gut and the cells of the hematopoietic system. Therefore, all such chemotherapeutic agents have a predictable dose related hematopoietic toxicity. In other chapters in this volume, the effects of chemotherapeutic agents on platelets and their precursors and upon red cells and their precursors are considered. In this chapter we shall consider the effect of chemotherapy upon blood neutrophils and the stem cells for the hematopoietic system and give brief consideration to its effect upon other leukocytes.

Some understanding of normal cell kinetic patterns is essential for the intelligent use of chemotherapy. The pattern of proliferation, the time required for cell production, cell distribution and life span of hematopoietic cells are germane to the design of chemotherapy trials. With an understanding of the physiology of these cellular systems, the seemingly mysterious "delayed" toxicity of some drugs begins to make sense. For instance, after a single dose of a cell-poisoning drug, neutropenia should not develop for a week or more if the marrow is normal. The duration of the neutropenia will be dependent upon whether the agent is cycle active or non-cycle active in nature. This discussion is designed to provide the reason for this type of statement and is divided into the following parts:

Normal stem cell kinetics; normal neutrophil kinetics; the effects of chemotherapeutic agents upon these classes of cells; methods of predicting the degree of normal cell toxicity induced by chemotherapeutic agents; and the chemotherapeutic effects on other leukocyte systems.

NORMAL STEM CELL KINETICS

Since the hematopoietic cells of the blood are constantly being lost and must be replaced, the replacement system (stem cell system) for normal hematopoietic tissue must have two distinguishing characteristics: (1) a stem cell must be capable of self replication, and (2) it must also be capable of differentiation into more mature cells. In a stem cell compartment of stable size, for each cell which differentiates, another stem cell must be produced by self replication in order to maintain compartment size.[1]

Pluripotential Stem Cells

There is now excellent evidence that in man and in the mouse there is a single cellular compartment capable of giving rise to megakaryocytes, red cell precursors, neutrophil precursors and eosinophil precursors. Evidence for this cell in man comes

---

From the Department of Medicine, University of Pittsburgh School of Medicine, Pittsburgh, Pennsylvania.

Supported in part by research grant No. AM14352-02 from the National Institute of Arthritis and Metabolic Diseases and by research grant No. T479A from the American Cancer Society.

primarily from chromosome studies in patients with chronic myelocytic leukemia, since the typical form of this disease in most patients is manifested by a defect in chromosome 21.[2] Whang and coworkers[3] found this chromosomal defect not only in neutrophil precursors but also in erythrocytic precursors and probably in megakaryocytes. The absence of this defect in other cells such as lymphocytes clearly indicates that it is not an inherited chromosomal defect. Furthermore, the presence of this defect in these three cell lines of bone marrow origin suggests that the defect arises in a cell which is a common stem cell for these three precursors. In addition, there is ancillary evidence suggesting a clonal evolution of chronic myelocytic leukemia.[4] In paroxysmal nocturnal hemoglobinuria there is also evidence for a common defect in neutrophils, platelets and erythrocytes.[5] Thus, in these diseases, it seems reasonable to suggest that the difficulty began in a single stem cell, that this stem cell was pluripotential for neutrophils, erythrocytes and megakaryocytes, and that this single abnormal cell successfully competed with normal hematopoietic stem cells, thus repopulating the bone marrow.

Similarly, if the mouse's hematopoietic system is severely damaged by irradiation, regeneration of the system is primarily from a pluripotential hematopoietic stem cell. Till and McCulloch[6] demonstrated that if mice were lethally irradiated and injected with syngeneic bone marrow, macroscopic nodules were present on the spleen some ten days later. Examination of these nodules revealed them to be composed of erythrocytic, neutrophilic or megakaryocytic tissue, or all three. Later studies from their laboratory clearly demonstrated that these began from a single cell and that these colonies were indeed clones.[7] Thus, in the mouse a method is available to study this pluripotential hematopoietic stem cell known as the colony-forming unit cell (CFU cell).

There are two general methods by which spleen colonies may be studied in the mouse. The first is the above mentioned transplantation method, in which tissue from spleen, bone marrow, washings from the peritoneal cavity, buffy coat cells from the blood, or fetal liver are transplanted into a lethally irradiated recipient.[8] The recipient spleen forms colonies from the transplanted material. In the second or endogenous spleen colony method, the mouse is sublethally irradiated so that his colony forming cell compartment is severely reduced, but not eliminated, and the hematopoietic system is regenerated from these surviving cells. In this circumstance colonies are also visible on the spleen some ten days after irradiation and the number of colonies is inversely proportional to the dosage of whole-body irradiation delivered to the animal.

The CFU cell system is probably at rest in the ordinary steady state. For instance, Becker and coworkers[9] exposed cells to "suicidal" doses of tritiated thymidine prior to cell transplant and produced little, if any, decrease in the number of colony-forming cells noted in the recipient. This would suggest that this cell is either in a state of G_0 generative cycle or else is in an exceedingly long generative cycle equivalent to G_0 state. If extremely severe damage (700 R or more of whole-body irradiation) is induced in the stem cell compartment of the mouse there is evidence that regeneration may be from a stem cell more primitive than the CFU cell. In this circumstance cytogenic evidence suggests that lymphocytes are also derived from such a stem cell.[10] Thus, we have evidence that there are concatenated stem cell systems of increasing maturity. It is apparent that since severe damage to this system is required before the stem cell also pluripotential for lymphocytes comes into play, this cell, like the CFU cell, must be in G_0 state or in an exceptionally long generative cycle.

Pattern of Regeneration of Depleted Stem Cell Compartments in the Mouse

We have studied the rate of regeneration of colony forming unit cells after this compartment is damaged by irradiation.[8,11,12] Because of a variety of difficulties attending the transplant system,[8] we have chosen to restrict our studies to regeneration of endogenous colonies. Mice were given a single dose of whole-body irradiation to reduce the stem cell compartment. At intervals of one, two, three, four or more days thereafter, a second dose of whole-body irradiation was given and the number of spleen colonies ten days after the second irradiation was measured. In this system, spacing the second irradiation at increasing intervals would have no influence upon the number of colonies until regrowth of the colony-forming system occurred. That is, if there is no regrowth for the first three days, animals given an initial 350 R followed by 350 R on days 1, 2 or 3, should all have the same number of colonies ten days later. Conversely, if the colony-forming compartment was growing during the interval between the first and second exposures to irradiation, the number of colonies present would increase as the irradiation was spaced further apart. Irradiation kills cells in an exponential fashion, so that the compartment is reduced by a fixed percentage rather than by an absolute number of cells.[13] The summation of a number of such studies is illustrated in Figure 1. In 11 experiments in which the initial irradiation was 300 R or more, there was a rapid increase in colonies, indicating that regrowth began almost immediately after reduction of the compartment. The mean colony-doubling time in these experiments was 16 hours. However, when the initial irradiation dose was 200 R or less, a much slower doubling time was observed.

These studies suggested that the severely reduced compartments (300 or more R) regrew at a faster rate than the less severely damaged compartments (200 R or less).

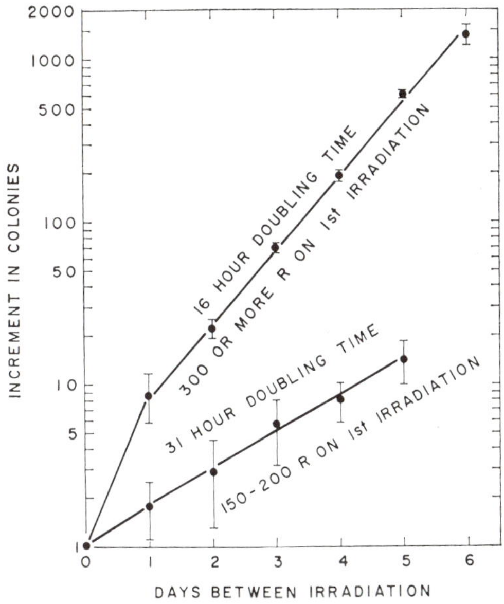

FIG. 1.—Recovery of the pluripotential hematopoietic stem cell compartment following whole-body irradiation. Mice were given two irradiation exposures at varying intervals. The number of colonies present on the spleen was measured 10 days after the second irradiation.

One explanation for such a difference was to suggest that differentiation was still occurring from the compartment which was not too severely damaged, whereas, with greater damage, compartment regrowth had to precede the onset of differentiation.

To further investigate this hypothesis, studies of the time of onset of differentiation following whole-body irradiation in relation to dose of irradiation were carried out by exposing groups of mice to various levels of whole-body irradiation. Each day thereafter a subgroup was injected with radioactive iron and killed to determine when an increased rate of uptake of radioactive iron into marrow, spleen and red blood cells occurred. Results of one such experiment are shown in Figure 2. As shown in this figure, the group given 200 R had an increasing iron uptake as soon as the value could be measured, suggesting that erythropoiesis was never completely interrupted. With 400 R there was a period during which no increase was observed, followed by a rapidly increasing iron uptake, and after 600 R an even longer period of basal iron uptake was observed. In all such experiments, as the dose of irradiation was increased, there was a longer period during which iron uptake remained at a baseline level before it suddenly increased.

A summation of all such experiments suggested that erythropoiesis is interrupted at approximately 200 R and that for each further increase of 100 R of whole-body irradiation, there is a lag of approximately 1.6 days before erythropoiesis begins. These data tend to support the previous suggestion that in a severely damaged system,

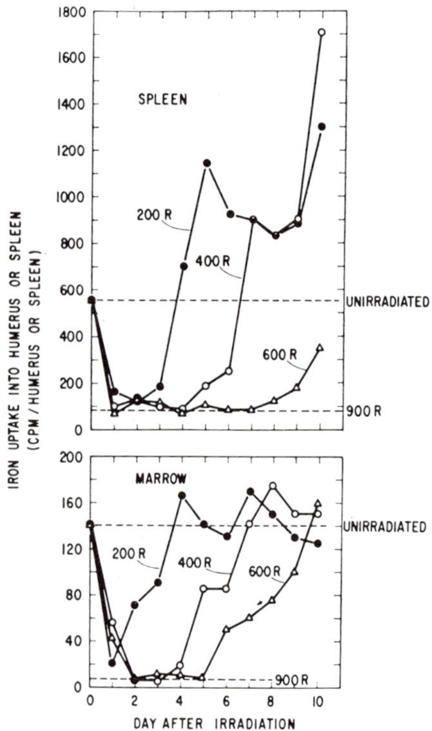

FIG. 2.—The relation between the dose of whole-body irradiation and the time of resumption of erythropoiesis. Mice were exposed to varying levels of irradiation, and at daily intervals thereafter groups were injected with radioactive iron and then killed; iron uptake into the spleen (upper figure) and the marrow (lower figure) was determined.

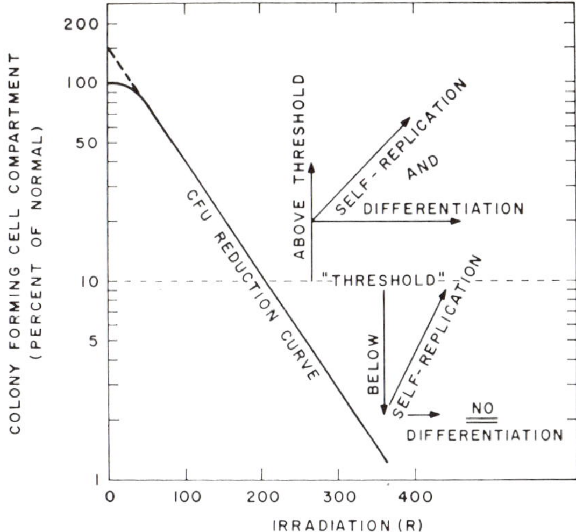

FIG. 3.—A suggested model for hematopoietic recovery following irradiation. A "threshold" is suggested, below which stem cell replication without differentiation is also occurring, so that the doubling time for self-replicating stem cells slows. The threshold is placed at 10 per cent of normal, since that is the approximate reduction obtained by 200 R.

repopulation of the stem cell compartment must precede significant differentiation. This model for recovery of a damaged stem cell compartment is illustrated in Figure 3.

Radiation survival is primarily dependent upon regeneration of neutrophils and megakaryocytes, since the usual cause of hematopoietic postirradiation death is infection due to neutropenia or bleeding due to thrombocytopenia. We carried out further experiments to determine whether cells differentiated into these three compartments at a fixed rate or whether the compartment was subject to competing stimuli. In these experiments the rate of erythropoietic demand was changed by inducing polycythemia either by hypertransfusion or in posthypoxic mice; or by accelerating the demand for erythropoiesis by bleeding mice or injecting erythropoietin.[14] In such animals the total number of neutrophils and neutrophil precursors in the humerus was measured at 7 and 10 days following irradiation (Table 1).

In the animals in which demands for erythropoiesis were virtually absent because of plethora, a larger than normal number of neutrophils and neutrophil precursors was

TABLE 1.—*Effect of Altered Rates of Erythropoiesis on Marrow Granulocytes after* 400 *R Whole-Body Irradiation*

Procedure	*Absolute number of granulocytes per humerus** (*% of control*)
Increased erythropoiesis	
Bleeding + 400 R	52
Erythropoietin + 400 R	80
Decreased erythropoiesis	
Hypertransfusion + 400 R	170
Hypoxia + 400 R	235

* The absolute number of granulocytes was determined 10 days after irradiation; control animals had an average of 3×10^6 cells per humerus.

present. Conversely, when an unusual demand for erythropoiesis was superimposed, as represented by the bled or erythropoietin treated mice, a reduced number of neutrophils and neutrophil precursors was observed. These results are compatible with the hypothesis that output from the stem cell compartment is subject to competing demands and that there is a possibility of experimental manipulation of the output of the various differentiated compartments.

Mature Stem Cells

If we are to assume that the CFU cell in the normal state is in a virtual state of G_0, then some other source for the constant replacement of blood cells must be found. There are studies to suggest that this source is stem cells which are more mature and more differentiated than the CFU cell and perhaps unipotential for a single cell line. Such cells are the (still partially hypothetical) erythropoietin-sensitive cell, for which there is significant but indirect evidence separating this cell system from the CFU system.[15,16] Perhaps more definitive evidence is found for the separation of a cell which can give rise to granulocytes from the CFU cell. If mouse bone marrow[17] or, for that matter, human bone marrow[18] or human peripheral blood[19] is cultured in a semisolid medium with a proper feeder layer or conditioned media, colonies of granulocytic and mononuclear cells arise from marrow or peripheral blood. When marrow from the WWv mouse with a known severe defect in the CFU cell compartment is used for transplantation experiments, no macroscopic colonies are observed and only very tiny microscopic colonies can be seen. However, when its marrow is placed in a soft gel medium in vitro, a normal concentration of colonies of normal size is observed.[20] This strongly suggests that in this animal the more mature stem cell which gives rise to granulocytes is intact, while the CFU cell compartment is faulty, thus providing direct evidence for two distinct compartments.

Stem Cell Model

Figure 4 depicts a proposed model for the stem cell system.[1] In normal circumstances red cells, platelets and neutrophils are maintained in balance by mature, perhaps unipotential stem compartments. If these compartments are damaged or if there is an unusual demand for cells, these more mature compartments are replenished by the multipotent CFU cell compartment, which is ordinarily at rest. When both of these

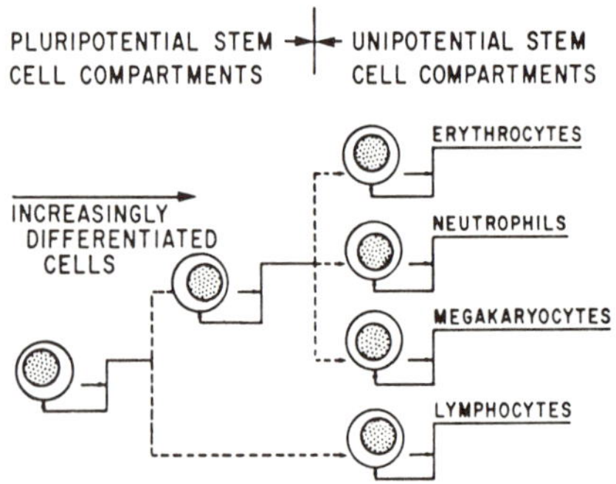

FIG. 4.—A suggested model for the hematopoietic stem cell compartments. The dashed lines indicate pathways which operate only when compartments are stressed. From Winkelstein and Boggs,[1] with permission.

compartments are severely damaged or under conditions of extreme stress, a still more primitive compartment is brought into play, which is also capable of feeding the lymphocyte compartment. In normal steady-state conditions the lymphocyte constitutes its own stem cell compartment, since these cells are capable of division giving rise to more lymphocytes. It is apparent that the exact structure of the stem cell compartments is not presently known, but from the information available we can make certain generalizations which may be of some use in designing chemotherapeutic experiments, as will be discussed later.

Normal Neutrophil Kinetics

Blood Neutrophil Compartment[21,22]

In a normal steady state, the blood neutrophil compartment is maintained by the inflow from the bone marrow balancing the outflow to tissues and body cavities (Fig. 5). The average neutrophil spends only ten hours in the blood, and loss from the blood is a random function. That is, the neutrophil which has just entered the blood from the marrow is as likely to leave on its first circulatory circuit as is one which has been around for many hours. This rapid rate of turnover indicates that on the average, the mass of blood neutrophils is replaced two and a half times each day. The determination of the concentration of neutrophils in venous blood samples can be somewhat misleading since in normal circumstances, approximately one-half of blood neutrophils are marginated on the walls of capillary or postcapillary venules. Thus, one underestimates the number of neutrophils in the blood by such a determination of concentration.

Neutropenia can be brought about by one of three mechanisms or combinations of these mechanisms: (1) decreased production, with reduced outflow from the bone marrow; (2) increased destruction of neutrophils so that marrow production is overwhelmed; or (3) an increase in the proportion of marginated neutrophils. Since increased margination does not require any change in inflow from the bone marrow, the number of immature neutrophils in the blood does not change. One of the most

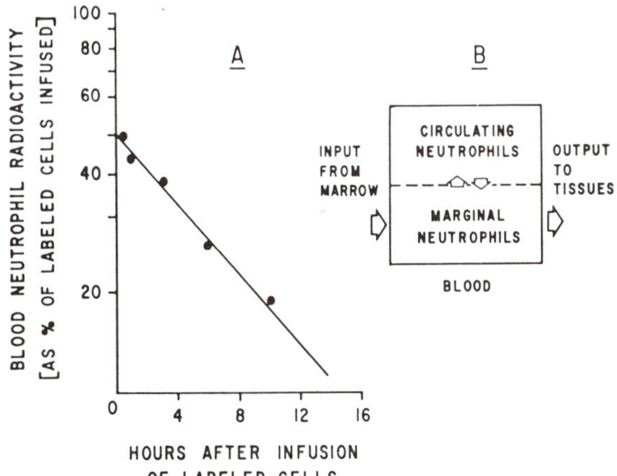

Fig. 5.—Blood neutrophil kinetics. The curve of radioactivity (5A) is that obtained after infusion of autologous neutrophils labeled with radioactive diisopropylfluorophosphate. From Winkelstein and Boggs,[1] with permission.

useful determinations in explaining the change in neutrophil concentration of the blood is a ratio of band to segmented neutrophils. If there is a sudden inflow from the bone marrow, the band:segmented ratio will increase. Thus, if neutropenia is accompanied by a very few bands, it is not considered as functionally severe as neutropenia in which almost all neutrophils of the blood are bands.

Marrow Neutrophil Compartment

Morphologic examination of the bone marrow reveals a continuum of neutrophil maturation in which, for functional descriptive purposes, three subcompartments may be distinguished (Fig. 6). The production pool consists of those cells capable of undergoing mitosis, myeloblasts, promyelocytes and myelocytes. The postmitotic maturation pool consists of metamyelocytes, bands and segmented neutrophils. A further subdivision of the maturation pool separates the effective storage pool (marrow granulocyte reserve of Craddock[23]) of band and segmented neutrophils from the metamyelocytes which are not readily released to the blood. In the average normal subject there are at least 15 times as many band and segmented neutrophils in the bone marrow as there are in the blood. This reserve can be released to the blood upon demand, and such demand is probably controlled by a circulating humoral releasing factor.[24] Therefore, this storage pool constitutes an effective means of rapidly delivering a large number of neutrophils to a site of infection and can supply the blood with extra cells until production has time to catch up to increasing demands. With a normal marrow structure, and even with extreme neutropenia, it is unusual for cells less mature than a band to be released to the blood. Thus, with neutropenia due to increased peripheral cell loss, we see a preserved production pool as well as metamyelocytes, but very few bands and segmented neutrophils are seen in the marrow. This is the circumstance often termed "maturation arrest," a misnomer, in our opinion. An explanation for this morphologic picture which seems more reasonable than "arrest" is that with the increased demands for cells in the blood, as is assumed to occur with most instances of neutropenia, as soon as a neutrophil matures to the band stage it is released to the blood and the storage pool is completely exhausted.

In the average normal subject, a period of approximately 11 days is required for a myelocyte to divide, mature into a segmented neutrophil, enter and then leave the blood. However, it must be realized that much of this time is spent within the storage pool. If there is an increased demand for cells or if the storage pool is attenuated, then the time required for a myelocyte to mature and enter the blood can be markedly reduced.

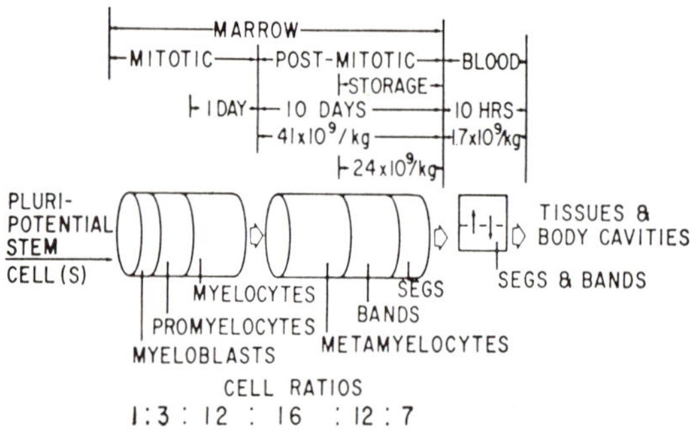

FIG. 6.—A model of the total neutrophil system. From Boggs,[22] with permission.

The exact structure of the production compartment is as yet undetermined. For instance, it is not known if the myeloblast or, for that matter, the promyelocyte or myelocyte, is capable of acting as a stem cell. Conversely, it is possible that the stem cell is as yet unidentified and that all of these compartments are merely doubling compartments. The generation time for the normal myelocyte is probably of the order of 24 hours. Whether increased production is accomplished by decreasing generation time, increasing feed-in from the stem cell compartment or combinations of these events is unknown.

The normal site of production for neutrophils is the production pool of the bone marrow (see Fig. 6). After the last mitosis at the myelocyte state, a further period of maturation occurs. Normally the mature cells spend a significant length of time in a storage pool of the bone marrow. From this they are released to the blood for but a brief transit and then migrate out of the blood vessels into tissues and body cavities. There, they presumably provide a cleansing function by phagocytic activities as well as being immediately available for migration from the blood into beginning inflammatory exudates. The "functional home" of the neutrophil is clearly beyond the blood in tissues, body cavities, and beginning exudates. In the absence of a normal number of neutrophils available for migration into such sites, infections are more frequent and are abnormally severe, since they cannot be contained and localized by the rapid entrance of neutrophils into exudates.

EFFECTS OF CHEMOTHERAPEUTIC AGENTS ON STEM CELLS AND NEUTROPHILS

The ideal cancer chemotherapy agent would be one which did not affect normal cells, but would either kill neoplastic cells or lead to a decrease in their production. Although a few agents, such as certain hormones, vincristine and asparaginase, have minimal effect upon normal hematopoietic cells, most chemotherapeutic agents have straight dose-related hematopoietic toxicity. Certain patients are sensitive to even the agents enumerated above. For instance, we have observed a few patients whose normal bone marrow cells were eradicated by a single dose of asparaginase; other investigators have made similar observations.[25]

To understand the effects of chemotherapeutic agents upon hematopoietic cells, it is important to know whether they are cycle-active or noncycle-active. A cycle-active drug affects only cells which are in an active generative cycle. Most of these act as inhibitors of DNA synthesis, such as hydroxyurea, or as mitotic inhibitors, such as vinblastine. Noncycle-active agents, such as x-irradiation and various alkylating agents, will damage cells in an active mitotic cycle but will also have severe effects upon potentially dividing cells. Still other agents, such as 6-mercaptopurine and cyclophosphamide, have effects which are intermediate between the two, but are probably more active upon cells which are in a generative cycle.[26]

This distinction between cycle-active and noncycle-active becomes most important when it is remembered that the normal pluripotential stem cell compartment is not in a generative cycle. Thus, in the purest type of system which one can devise, namely, a single dose of a cycle- or noncycle-active agent, quite different effects upon normal cell level are observed. The neutrophil concentration after administration of a single dose of vinblastine sulfate (cycle-active) or a single dose of nitrogen mustard (noncycle-active) to normal dogs is shown in Figure 7. Both these agents led to comparable degrees of neutropenia; however, the neutropenia due to nitrogen mustard was of

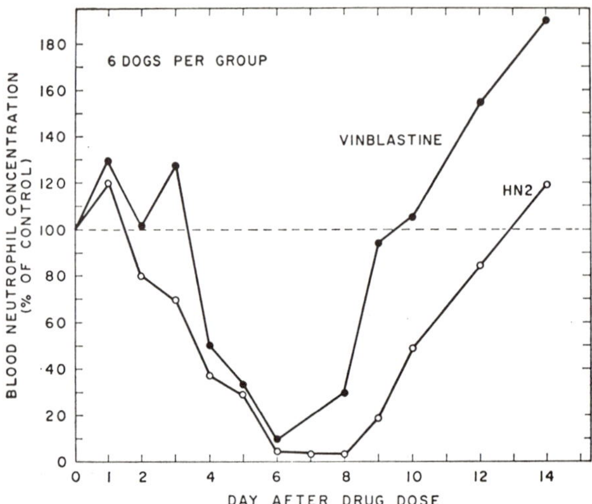

FIG. 7.—The differing effects of a single dose of vinblastine or nitrogen mustard upon blood neutrophil concentration.[27]

longer duration, and recovery was significantly slower than in the neutropenia due to vinblastine. Vinblastine, a cycle-active agent, would not be expected to significantly damage the pluripotential stem cell compartment when given in a single dose. Therefore, regeneration of identifiable compartments could be accomplished very rapidly from this intact back-up system. This was evidenced by study of the bone marrow of such dogs, in which a return of myeloblasts, promyelocytes and myelocytes occurred quickly and the neutropenia was brief.[27] Conversely, nitrogen mustard would damage the pluripotential stem cell compartment. Therefore, before the mature compartment could fully recover, a certain amount of self-replication would be demanded in the stem cell compartment and, thus, a slower recovery would be expected.

The above difference in drug effect on neutrophil kinetics is not limited completely to effects on the proliferating compartments.[27] Note the difference in pattern of onset of neutropenia between these two drugs (see Fig. 7); with vinblastine sulfate, neutrophil levels were maintained for 3 days, but more gradually developing neutropenia occurred with nitrogen mustard. Kinetic study of these two situations indicated that after vinblastine sulfate the storage pool of the marrow was able to feed into the blood at a regular rate until it was exhausted, whereas feed-in from the storage pool was gradually reduced by nitrogen mustard. A possible explanation for these two differences is that nitrogen mustard also damages the structural characteristics of the marrow as well as the proliferation compartments, leading to a damaged output from the storage pool system.

The difference in activity of these two drugs in single doses in dogs is also supported by human chemotherapeutic studies. Vinblastine can be given every 7 to 10 days without producing progressive toxicity in most patients, suggesting that the damage can be repaired in man within this time. This is reasonable considering the time parameters of the marrow neutrophil system. Conversely, a much longer period (some weeks) is required between doses of nitrogen mustard if repair of the system is to occur. If nitrogen mustard is given at 7- to 10-day intervals, at a dose which will induce a degree of neutropenia comparable to that after vinblastine, the neutrophil system may become exhausted. This presumably reflects repetitive damage to the pluripotential stem cell pool.

We do not ordinarily administer chemotherapeutic drugs in single doses. The effect on neutrophils and stem cells of regularly repeated dosages is much more complex. We have attempted to illustrate this in a theoretical situation in Figure 8, which shows the effect of a repeated single dose of a DNA-inhibiting cycle-active agent upon the stem cell system, the marrow mitotic pool, the marrow storage pool and the blood neutrophil compartment. This theoretic dose of drug is sufficient to destroy any cells which are in an active generative cycle. It is assumed that DNA synthesis accounts for one-half of the cycle.

With the first dose, the stem cell compartment is only very slightly reduced, since only a small proportion is in DNA synthesis. The marrow mitotic pool is reduced by half, since half of it is in DNA synthesis. Neither the marrow storage pool nor the blood is immediately affected. By the time the second dose is administered, the stem cell pool has hypertrophied slightly in response to the damage in the more mature compartments; half of it is now in DNA synthesis, and with the second dose half of it is destroyed. Again the marrow mitotic pool is reduced by half, and since it had not fully regenerated, it is smaller than after the first dose. The marrow storage pool again is not affected by the second dose, but is smaller than normal because of reduced feed-in from the marrow mitotic pool and continued output to the blood. Since significant storage remains, the blood has not been affected. By the time of the third dose, some regeneration has occurred in the stem compartment, but it is not back to normal and half is still in DNA synthesis. Therefore, it is again reduced by half and the same is true for the marrow mitotic pool. Again because of continued normal feed-in to the blood and subnormal feed-in from the marrow mitotic pool, the marrow storage pool is now rather small. However, it is still maintaining the blood at a near-normal size. By the time the next dose is due, disaster has struck. There is severe neutropenia because the storage pool has become completely exhausted and feed-in into the blood has been markedly reduced.

If we are correct in our hypothesis that a severely reduced stem cell pool will not differentiate until it is reconstituted to a certain size, it is possible that feed-in from that pool to the marrow mitotic pool would cease at some point in Figure 8 and a still longer delay would be required before recovery of blood cells occurred.

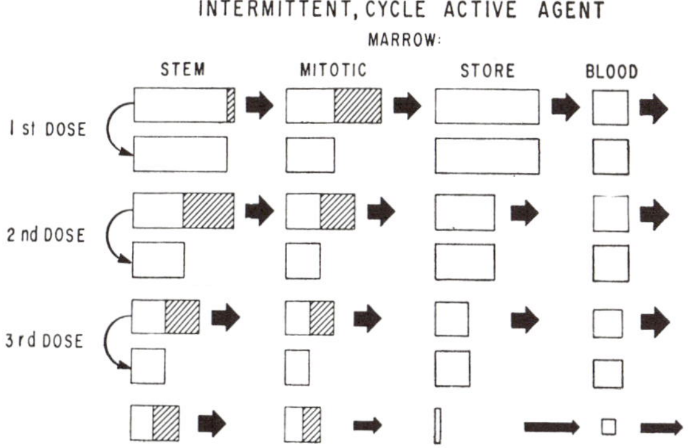

FIG. 8.—The effect of repeated doses of a cycle-active agent on the neutrophil system. The drug is assumed to act only on cells in DNA synthesis (shaded area of compartments).

The main practical point to be considered from this type of kinetic diagram is the insensitivity of blood neutrophil level to the degree of damage occurring in the system. It cannot be emphasized too strongly that the last compartment in which damage appears is the blood compartment. Thus, by the time neutropenia appears, there has already been severe damage to the entire system.

If the time between doses of the drug shown in Figure 8 were to be lengthened until complete repair and even over-shoot in the stem cell and marrow mitotic compartment had occurred between doses, neutropenia would not develop or would at most be transient. The storage pool serves as an effective buffer between the production compartment and the blood. The question which remains is whether a spaced dose of chemotherapeutic agents can be found which will obviate serious long-term damage to the neutrophil system, but will still have effective antitumor activity. As previously noted, the ideal chemotherapeutic agent would be one which affected tumor cells but not normal cells. Lacking such agents, we can exploit studies of differences in generative times of tumor cell populations and normal cell populations.

Various studies suggest that many tumor cell populations in man have a slower generative cycle than do normal hematopoietic cells.[28] In this case these differences can be exploited, even though slight, by properly timed doses of cell-killing chemotherapeutic agents. A theoretic graph of the effect of such timing is illustrated in Figure 9.

In Figure 9, we have assumed that we are dealing with a normal hematopoietic cell population with a generation time (doubling time) of 24 hours. Generation and doubling times are the same, assuming there is no cell loss in the compartment and all cells are in cycle. In this system the tumor which we are attacking has a longer generation and doubling time (36 hours) than the normal cell compartment (24 hours). We

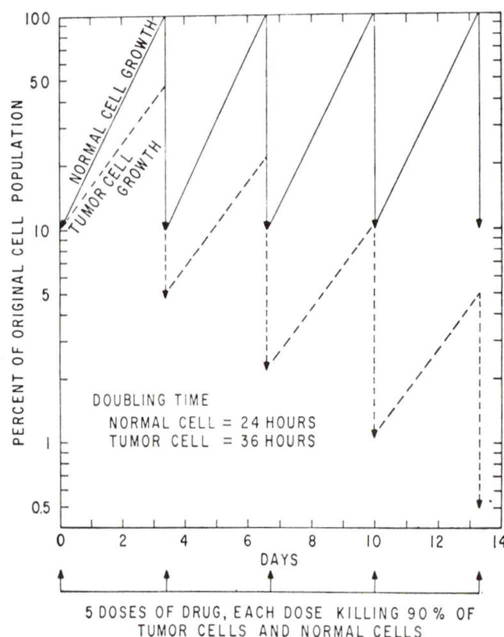

FIG. 9.—Differential effect of an antitumor agent given in repeated doses on normal cells and tumor cells.

are administering a noncycle-active drug which will reduce both the normal cell population and the tumor cell population to 10 per cent of its original value with each dose. By timing the dosage to approximately three and a half days, the normal cell population returns to baseline levels between doses, whereas the tumor cell population with its slower growth rate does not attain these levels. Yet the proportional reduction with each dose leads to a progressive decrease in total tumor cell population. By these means the normal cell population is never reduced to more than 10 per cent of its starting value, whereas, following the fifth dose, the tumor cell population is reduced to less than 1 per cent of its original value. This type of therapy has been effective in murine leukemia[29] and may form the basis for the effectiveness of certain intermittent therapeutic regimens in man. However, it must be remembered that a number of assumptions, all of which are unproved, are built into this type of theoretic design:

1. The normal hematopoietic system can repair itself from chemotherapeutic damage with equal facility following an infinite number of doses. Studies attempting to exhaust the recovery potential of the murine hematopoietic system are equivocal in their results,[30] but most investigators have the clinical impression that in man the more exposure to chemotherapeutic agents the patient has, the less capable is his bone marrow of recovering.
2. The rate of tumor-cell growth remains constant for tumor-cell populations of various sizes. There is evidence in certain murine tumors that the rate of growth decreases as the size of the tumor increases.[29] Thus, it is possible that as the tumor is reduced in size, its rate of regrowth may accelerate and equal or exceed that of normal tissue. Similarly, in man, there is evidence that many leukemic cells are not growing.[28]
3. The overall assumption that a tumor can be destroyed simply by killing the cells of which it is composed.

However, this type of consideration gives strong emphasis to efforts designed to measure not only normal cell generation and doubling times but tumor cell generation and doubling times in man.

Methods of Predicting Degree of Hematopoietic Toxicity

Normal stem cell assays in man are still in their infancy and at the present time are limited to determining what is probably a stem cell for granulocytic and monocytic tissue in human marrow and blood.[19] However, as more thorough and sophisticated assays for this class of cell become available, it may become the most important means of determining how susceptible a patient is to the hematologic ravages of chemotherapy.

At present there are methods available for determining the relative size of the neutrophil system at the beginning of chemotherapy or during courses of chemotherapy. As should be evident from the preceding discussion of normal neutrophil kinetics and of the effect of chemotherapy on neutrophils, merely measuring the concentration of neutrophils in venous blood samples is entirely unsatisfactory as a means of assessing the size of the neutrophil system. If a careful look at a blood smear is coupled with blood neutrophil concentration measurements, a bit more information can be obtained. If the predominant cell on blood smears is a band rather than a segmented neutrophil, then in all probability the marrow storage pool is markedly reduced in size and the patient is likely to develop severe neutropenia even at chemotherapeutic doses calculated to be benign.

Perhaps the most widely used method of assessing the size of the marrow neutrophil storage pool is measuring the blood neutrophil response after the injection of endotoxin or etiocholanolone.[31,32] If there is an existing storage pool which is functionally normal, there will be an increase in concentration of blood neutrophils after injection of either drug. However, the primary disadvantage of these techniques, as we see them, is that they do not give a measure of the size of the storage pool. If there is no response, one can be relatively certain that the store is functionally absent. However, there is no guaranty that a store significantly reduced in size would not feed out enough neutrophils to provide a normal blood neutrophil rise in response to endotoxin or etiocholanolone. Thus, these crude tests can determine whether or not there is a storage pool, but give a little assessment of its size.

Careful examination of a marrow aspirate probably gives as much information as the above tests, if not more, and is probably less traumatic to the patient than the repeated venipunctures required for the above tests. If the store is absent, it is visually absent, that is, the marrow has very few bands and segmented neutrophils. If the patient is not anemic, the myeloid:erythroid ratio gives further semiquantitative information. If band and segmented neutrophils constitute at least 30 per cent of total neutrophils (and neutrophil precursors) in the marrow and if the myeloid:erythroid ratio is more than 2 to 1 in a nonanemic patient, then in all probability a normal-size marrow store is present. However, in the usual patient given chemotherapy, anemia is generally present, and with anemia the myeloid:erythroid ratio cannot be expected to give quantitative data. In this circumstance, an independent means of measuring marrow size is desired. The most simple and probably most reliable test of marrow mass is a plasma iron turnover which can be related to total erythroid cell production in the marrow. Finch and coworkers[33] have demonstrated that in the absence of marked iron overload and with the exception of the patient who is producing few or no red cells, there is a fairly good correlation between plasma iron turnover and number of nucleated red cell precursors in the bone marrow. If an estimate of total nucleated red cell precursors is obtained from the relatively simple measure of plasma iron turnover, then the myeloid:erythroid ratio of a marrow aspirate can be placed in more meaningful perspective and a rough quantitation of total marrow neutrophil mass can be computed from the M:E ratio.

The coupling of a needle biopsy of the marrow with examination of a smear from a marrow aspirate gives additional information. In a good biopsy specimen, if the cellular portion of the marrow exceeds the fat spaces, or if it is equal to the fat spaces, then one can be reasonably sure that a normal marrow mass is present. However, the main problem in interpreting marrow biopsies is whether this small sample is representative of the entire marrow. There is reasonably good evidence that cell ratios are constant from one portion of the active marrow to another in man, with the exception of diseases such as multiple myeloma. However, there are no studies which assure us that the overall cellularity of the marrow as measured by biopsy is similar from one site to another.

Chemotherapeutic Effects on Other Leukocytic Systems

The effects of chemotherapeutic agents upon lymphocytes and monocytes, and perhaps upon eosinophils and basophils, are unquestionably of significant consequence to the patient. However, we have not considered these cells in detail for two reasons: (1) The kinetics of these cell types in man is as yet only partially understood, and (2) there are no reliable means of measuring the effects of chemotherapy upon these cellular systems. However, some brief consideration concerning the lymphocytic and monocytic systems is certainly justified.

Monocytes are excellent phagocytes moving into the tissues from blood and there becoming macrophages. Monocytes arise from the bone marrow from as yet unidentified precursors[34] and probably have a common origin with the neutrophil.[21] In addition to killing offending organisms, they play a role in the development of the immune response. Antigen is processed by macrophages, and a product of this processing, whether antigen or a related product, stimulates antibody formation by the lymphocytic system.[1] Most chemotherapeutic agents, if delivered in sufficient dosage, reduce the number of monocytes, but the clinical consequences of this effect have not been clearly delineated.

In an oversimplified view,[1] the function of the lymphocyte is to form antibodies, humoral antibodies as represented by circulating immunoglobulins, and cell-bound antibodies such as those involved in skin hypersensitivity reactions and in tissue transplantation rejection. Generalizing from studies in animals, one can state that the lymphocytes which are produced in the bone marrow migrate through the thymus, where they are acted upon either by thymic lymphocytes or by thymic factors. These modified immunocytes thereafter move into peripheral lymphocytic tissues, where they form the functioning immunocyte system.

Most small lymphocytes of the blood are cells with an exceedingly long life span.[35] Actually, "life span" is a misnomer since the lymphocyte is capable of being its own stem cell and producing two identical progenitors by cell division. However, as judged by chromosomal studies in patients subjected to irradiation, the average intermitotic interval for the small blood lymphocyte is probably two years or more.[35] Blood lymphocytes constantly recirculate, leaving the blood through specialized postcapillary endothelial networks in lymph nodes where they make up the cuff of small lymphocytes surrounding the germinal follicles of the node. Leaving the nodes, they are picked up by lymphatics and reenter the blood through the thoracic duct.

The recirculation of lymphocytes can be modified by a variety of means. A decrease in the concentration of blood lymphocytes accompanies almost any stress phenomenon and follows almost all varieties of chemotherapy as an acute response. There is little or no evidence to suggest that this transient type of lymphopenia represents either a decrease in lymphocyte production or an increase in lymphocyte destruction. It may represent simply a redistribution of lymphocytes. Any factor which induces a change in the recirculatory pattern of this cell will produce a profound effect upon blood lymphocyte concentration, since the overwhelming majority of small lymphocytes are not in the blood but are on the recirculatory phase in the tissues. For this reason, interpretation of lymphopenia per se is exceedingly difficult.

Many chemotherapeutic agents lead to reduced antibody formation, and indeed this characteristic has been utilized in employing these agents for immune suppression in nonmalignant diseases. Antibody production by lymphocytes, whether of the cell bound or humoral variety, probably depends on some variation of the following: Antigen with or without modification by macrophages stimulates the small lymphocyte to proliferate into a blast-like stage. The cell divides and produces progeny capable of producing antibody to the offending antigen. If of a cell-bound nature, the cell remains a lymphocyte in morphologic appearance and carries the antibody. If of a humoral nature, the cell converts to a plasma cell which produces and releases immunoglobulins. If this is a new antigen in the experience of the host, this new information is coded into a previously uncommitted immunologically competent small lymphocyte. If the host has prior experience with the antigen, a small lymphocyte carrying the memory for antibody production to that antigen is stimulated. The first, or primary, response is more delayed than the secondary antibody response. In either event, cell proliferation is probably required, and all chemotherapeutic agents which reduce capacity for cell proliferation in all probability have some influence upon the potential immune response. Quantitation of this effect in man lags behind our understanding of the effects of chemotherapy upon the neutrophil system. This lag in understanding does not necessarily imply a difference in the importance of the two mechanisms.

It may prove that chemotherapeutic damage to the immune system is of greater long range importance than damage to the neutrophil system. As a theoretical example, let us consider the possibility that the normal immune system is in the process of trying to contain and banish the offending tumor which has invaded its province. By administering overly vigorous chemotherapy we may not only reduce the size of existing tumor tissue, but also reduce the ability of the immune system to cope with tumor tissue. Perhaps the occasional apparent cures resulting from chemotherapy[36] represent reduction of tumor size to a level where the host can control it rather than killing all cells by chemotherapy per se.

Chemotherapy is a two-edged sword with respect to treatment of cancer. If it is ever to be considered curative, it must reduce the tumor cell population either to zero or to a degree where the host is able to manage the cancer with its own defense system. If reduction of the tumor cell population to zero is the aim, then enough normal cells must be preserved to allow the host to survive, and of course, the inciting factor leading to the original malignant proliferation must have disappeared for the cancer to be cured. Alternatively, if one assumes that at least certain patients have developed some degree of resistance to their own tumor, and that they can be helped by reducing the tumor population to the point that they can handle it themselves, then severe damage to the immune system must be avoided.

References

1. Winkelstein, A. and Boggs, D. R.: White Cell Manual. Seattle: University of Washington Press, 1970.
2. Sandberg, A. A. and Hossfeld, D. K.: Chromosomal abnormalities in human neoplasia. Ann. Rev. Med. 21:379, 1970.
3. Whang, J., Frei, E., III, Tjio, J. H., Carbone, P. P. and Brecker, G.: The distribution of the Philadelphia chromosome in patients with chronic myelogenous leukemia. Blood 22:664, 1963.
4. Fialkow, P. J., Lisker, R., Detter, J., Giblett, E. R. and Zavala, C.: 6-Phosphogluconate dehydrogenase: Hemizygous manifestation in a patient with leukemia. Science 163:194, 1969.
5. Aster, R. H. and Enright, S. E.: A platelet and granulocyte membrane defect in paroxysmal nocturnal hemoglobinuria: Usefulness for the detection of platelet antibodies. J. Clin. Invest. 48:1199, 1969.
6. Till, J. E. and McCulloch, E. A.: A direct measurement of the radiation sensitivity of normal mouse bone marrow cells. Radiat. Res. 14:213, 1961.
7. Becker, A. J., McCulloch, E. A. and Till, J. E.: Cytological demonstration of the clonal nature of spleen colonies derived from transplanted mouse marrow cells. Nature 197:452, 1963.
8. Boggs, D. R. and Chervenick, P. A.: Hematopoietic stem cells. *In* Greenwalt, T. J. and Jamieson, G. A. (Eds.): Formation and Destruction of Blood Cells. Philadelphia: J. B. Lippincott, 1970, pp. 240–255.
9. Becker, A. J., McCulloch, E. A., Siminovitch, L. and Till, J. E.: The effect of differing demands for blood cell production on DNA synthesis by hematopoietic colony-forming cells of mice. Blood 26:296, 1965.

10. Wu, A. M., Till, J. E., Siminovitch, L. and McCulloch, E. A.: Cytological evidence for a relationship between normal hematopoietic colony-forming cells and cells of the lymphoid system. J. Exp. Med. 127:455, 1968.
11. Chervenick, P. A. and Boggs, D. R.: Pattern of hematopoietic stem cells repopulation. Clin. Res. 17:114, 1969.
12. Chervenick, P. A. and Boggs, D. R.: A kinetic model of hematopoietic stem cell repopulation and differentiation. J. Clin. Invest. 48:47A, 1969.
13. Marsh, J. C., Boggs, D. R., Bishop, C. R., Chervenick, P. A., Cartwright, G. E. and Wintrobe, M. M.: Factors influencing hematopoietic spleen colony formation in irradiated mice. I. The normal pattern of endogenous colony formation. J. Exp. Med. 126:835, 1967.
14. Chervenick, P. A. and Boggs, D. R.: The effect of altered rates of erythropoiesis upon granulocytopoiesis. J. Clin. Invest. 47:19A, 1968.
15. Kubanek, B., Ferrari, L., Tyler, W. S., Howard, D., Jay, S. and Stohlman, F.: Regulation of erythropoiesis. XXIII. Dissociation between stem cells and erythroid response to hypoxia. Blood 32:586, 1968.
16. Porteous, D. D. and Lajtha, L. G.: On stem-cell recovery after irradiation. Brit. J. Haemat. 12:177, 1966.
17. Bradley, T. R. and Metcalf, D.: The growth of mouse bone marrow cells *in vitro*. Aust. J. Exp. Biol. Med. Sci. 44:287, 1966.
18. Pike, B. L. and Robinson, W. A.: Human bone marrow colony growth in agargel. J. Cell. Physiol. 76:77, 1970.
19. Chervenick, P. A. and Boggs, D. R.: *In vitro* growth of granulocytic and mononuclear colonies from blood of normal individuals. Blood 37:131, 1971.
20. Bennett, M., Cudkowicz, G., Foster, R. S., Jr. and Metcalf, D.: Hemopoietic progenitor cells of W anemic mice studied in vivo and in vitro. J. Cell. Physiol. 71:211, 1968.
21. Athens, J. W.: Blood: Leukocytes. Ann. Rev. Physiol. 25:195, 1963.
22. Boggs, D. R.: The kinetics of neutrophilic leukocytes in health and in disease. Seminars Hemat. 4:359, 1967.
23. Craddock, C. G., Perry, S. and Lawrence, J. S.: The dynamics of leukopenia and leukocytosis. Ann. Intern. Med. 52:281, 1960.
24. Boggs, D. R., Chervenick, P. A., Marsh, J. C., Cartwright, G. E. and Wintrobe, M. M.: Neutrophil releasing activity in the plasma of dogs injected with endotoxin. J. Lab. Clin. Med. 72:177, 1968.
25. Ho, D. H., Whitecar, J. P., Luce, J. K. and Frei, E.: L-Asparagine requirement and the effect of L-asparaginase on the normal and leukemic human bone marrow. Cancer Res. 30:466, 1970.
26. Bruce, W. R., Meeker, B. E. and Valeriote, F. A.: Comparison of the sensitivity of normal hematopoietic and transplanted lymphoma colony-forming cells to chemotherapeutic agents administered in vivo. J. Nat. Cancer Inst. 37:233, 1966.
27. Boggs, D. R., Athens, J. W., Cartwright, G. E. and Wintrobe, M. M.: The different effects of vinblastine sulfate and nitrogen mustard upon neutrophil kinetics in the dog. Proc. Soc. Exp. Biol. Med. 121:1085, 1966.
28. Mauer, A. M. and Fisher, V.: Characteristics of cell proliferation in four patients with untreated acute leukemia. Blood 28: 428, 1966.
29. Simpson-Herren, L. and Harris, L. H.: Kinetic parameters and growth curves for experimental tumor systems. Cancer Chemother. Rep. 52:143, 1970.
30. Boggs, D. R., Marsh, J. C., Chervenick, P. A., Cartwright, G. E. and Wintrobe, M. M.: Factors influencing hematopoietic spleen colony formation in irradiated mice. III. The effect of repetitive irradiation upon proliferative ability of colony-forming cells. J. Exp. Med. 126:871, 1967.
31. Wolfe, S. M., Rubenstein, M., Mulholland, J. H. and Alling, D. W.: Comparison of hematologic and febrile response to endotoxin in man. Blood 26:190, 1965.
32. Kimball, H. R., Vogel, J. M., Perry, S. and Wolff, S. M.: Quantitative aspects of pyrogenic and hematologic responses to etiocholanolone in man. J. Lab. Clin. Med 69:415, 1967.
33. Finch, C. A., Deubelbeiss, K., Cook, J. D., Eschbach, J. W., Harker, L. A., et al.: Ferrokinetics in man. I, II, III. Medicine 49:17, 1970.
34. Volman, A. and Gowans, J. L.: The origin of macrophages from bone marrow in the rat. Brit. J. Exp. Path. 46:62, 1965.
35. Ford, W. L. and Gowans, J. L.: The traffic of lymphocytes. Seminars Hemat. 6:67, 1969.
36. Burchenal, J. H. and Murphy, M. L.: Long-term survivors in acute leukemia. Cancer Res. 25:1491, 1965.

Chemotherapy and Thrombopoiesis

By Jack Levin, M.D.

MEGAKARYOCYTES HAVE BEEN RECOGNIZED as the source of circulating platelets since the beginning of the twentieth century.[1] However, intensive study of megakaryocytopoiesis and platelet production did not begin until the 1960s. It is now recognized that platelets are non-nucleated but are structured pieces of megakaryocytes that enter the circulation after megakaryocytes mature and demarcation of the cytoplasm into platelets has occurred. Studies of the kinetics of platelet production indicate that the cells recognized as megakaryocytes do not replicate and that maintenance of the megakaryocyte pool is dependent upon entry into this pool of new cells from a yet unidentified population of precursor cells.[2,3] However, DNA synthesis occurs in immature megakaryocytes (endoreduplication) resulting in polyploid cells.[4-6] These cells usually, but not always, contain a multilobed (or segmented) nucleus.[3-5,7] Recognizable megakaryocytes usually have ploidy levels of 8N, 16N, or 32N (diploid cells are 2N), based on measurements of DNA content.[2,4-6] Megakaryocytes at any level of polyploidy are capable of undergoing cytoplasmic maturation with subsequent production of platelets.[2,3,5,6] The nonreplicating but polyploid nature of megakaryocytes makes them unique among the elements of the bone marrow.

Many experimental studies in rodents and dogs have demonstrated that production of platelets by megakaryocytes normally reflects the level of circulating platelets. Thrombocytopenia produced either by exchange transfusion or administration of platelet antiserum is followed by increased production of platelets, and subsequently platelet levels rise to greater than normal ("rebound thrombocytosis").[8-11] Increased platelet production is associated with an increase in the number and size of megakaryocytes,[7,11-13] their rate of maturation,[10,12,14,15] and the influx of precursor cells into the pool of identifiable megakaryocytes.[10,12-14] Conversely, thrombocytosis produced by hypertransfusion of platelets is followed by rebound thrombocytopenia, which has been interpreted as secondary to suppression of platelet production.[16-19] Reduction of the number of megakaryocytes 3 to 4 days after induction of thrombocytosis,[17] and a decrease in megakaryocyte number and size after 4 to 10 days of thrombocytosis[7] also suggest decreased thrombopoiesis. Furthermore, suppression of platelet production in these circumstances has been suggested by decreases in the rate of appearance of radioactively labeled platelets in the circulation after the administration of $Na_2{}^{35}SO_4$ or selenomethionine-^{75}Se (^{75}SeM), isotopes that are incorporated into megakaryocyte cytoplasm.[20] It appears that thrombopoiesis is not totally suppressed by sustained thrombocytosis, just as erythropoiesis is not uniformly suppressed by polycythemia.[21,22]

Both stimulation and suppression of thrombopoiesis in rats, after production of thrombocytopenia or thrombocytosis, respectively, are detectable only after a delay of approximately 24 hours.[11,13,15,17] Adjustment in the rate of thrombopoiesis

---

From the Department of Medicine, The Johns Hopkins University School of Medicine and Hospital, Baltimore, Maryland.

Carried out under Contract NYO-1208-109 between the United States Atomic Energy Commission and The Johns Hopkins University, and supported in part by Graduate Training Grant No. TI-AM-5260 from the National Institute of Arthritis and Metabolic Diseases, U.S. Public Health Service.

apparently occurs at the level of megakaryocytic precursors or Stage I megakaryocytes,[7,11,13] and subsequently a population of megakaryocytes that has been altered in number, ploidy, size, and rate of maturation can be identified in the bone marrow. Maximal rebound thrombocytosis or rebound thrombocytopenia, after induction of thrombocytopenia or thrombocytosis, occurs approximately 6 days after alteration of the platelet levels of rabbits and rats.[11,17,19] This period of time is that required for two consecutive populations (cohorts) of megakaryocytes to enter the marrow pool, mature, and release platelets.[23,24]

Limited but similar data have been obtained in humans. The administration of ^{3}HTdr to one patient resulted in a gradual increase of the fraction of labeled megakaryocytes in the marrow, with the maximal labeled fraction (50 per cent) occurring at 6 days.[16] The administration of $Na_2{}^{35}SO_4$ or ^{75}SeM to humans resulted in the gradual appearance of labeled platelets in the circulation, with maximal levels reached approximately 6 to 9 days after administration of the isotope.[25-27] This is compatible with initial incorporation of $Na_2{}^{35}SO_4$ or ^{75}SeM into the cytoplasm of megakaryocytes, maturation of these cells, and then release of the labeled platelets into the circulation. Harker has demonstrated alterations in megakaryocyte number and size in abnormal hematologic states characterized by thrombocytopenia or thrombocytosis, and has shown a correlation between megakaryocyte mass and platelet turnover,[28,29] except in states of ineffective thrombopoiesis. The average megakaryocyte volume in patients with idiopathic thrombocytopenic purpura was increased, and the magnitude of change was inversely related to the platelet count.[29] In contrast, patients with reactive thrombocytosis had megakaryocytes that were smaller in volume than normal cells.[28]

These observations suggest that there is an effective feedback mechanism by which the rate of thrombopoiesis is affected by the level of the circulating platelet mass. Odell et al.[13] and Ebbe et al.[15,30] have suggested that the time lag between alteration of platelet levels and detection of altered megakaryocytopoiesis reflects either mechanisms effective at the level of precursor cells, or a delay in the production of a humoral substance (thrombopoietin) which is responsible for altered thrombopoiesis, or both. Recent studies in animals and humans have provided evidence for the existence of such humoral regulators of platelet production.[19,31-34]

Agents Which Affect Thrombopoiesis

There are many mechanisms by which therapeutic agents cause thrombocytopenia. The varied group of substances that are utilized as antitumor drugs usually do so by direct depression of bone marrow function, in particular, of thrombopoiesis. This is presumably the result of depression, not only of cells identifiable as megakaryocytes, but also of megakaryocytic precursors. These toxic effects often provide opportunities to confirm data obtained from experimental studies of platelet production, or to learn new facts about thrombopoiesis in man.

Antitumor Agents

Acute thrombocytopenia, produced by antitumor agents, often is followed by rebound thrombocytosis, with platelet levels occasionally exceeding 1,000,000/mm^3.[35] The administration of cytosine arabinoside by acute intravenous injection is followed by maximal thrombocytopenia 12 days later, and by maximal rebound thrombocytosis at 22 days.[36] Folic acid antagonists produce maximal thrombocytopenia

9 to 15 days after administration, with a subsequent rebound thrombocytosis.[37,38] Rebound thrombocytosis, after therapy with amethopterin was started, reached a maximum at about 18 to 22 days, or 7 to 10 days after thrombocytopenia.[38] In contrast, a large dose of mechlorethamine (nitrogen mustard), a noncycle-active agent, although producing maximal thrombocytopenia at 10 to 15 days, was not associated with rebound thrombocytosis.[39] Noncycle-active agents injure cells regardless of their stage in the mitotic cycle (including resting phase, or nonproliferating cells). Cycle-active (or cycle-dependent) drugs are antimetabolic agents that exert their primary effects on cells in a specific stage of thc generation cycle.

These data strongly suggest that these agents damage megakaryocytic precursors and megakaryoblasts, thus decreasing the input of new platelets into the circulation. Maximal depression of platelet levels, 10 to 15 days after administration of drug, is compatible with estimations of the life span of human platelets.[40,41] The occurrence of rebound thrombocytosis approximately 10 days after thrombocytopenia supports the concept of a feedback mechanism in humans, and possibly represents the response to thrombocytopenia of a cohort of megakaryocytes that have been synchronized, as suggested by Lampkin et al.[42]

Some drugs apparently suppress myelopoiesis and thrombopoiesis equally, but this is not always the case. Large doses of mechlorethamine have produced similar degrees of depression of these hematopoietic elements,[39] as has total-body irradiation.[43] However, the administration of small doses of mechlorethamine on alternate days produced thrombocytopenia in only 20 per cent of cases, whereas anemia and leukopenia occurred in 58 to 87 per cent of the patients studied.[44] Cyclophosphamide, another noncycle-active agent, produces relatively less thrombocytopenia than leukopenia, but, paradoxically, does produce rebound thrombocytosis.[45]

In general, cycle-active agents seem to depress both erythroid and myeloid elements to a significantly greater degree than they do platelet precursors. A striking example of the disparity of the effects of cytosine arabinoside on white blood cells and platelets has been reported by Burke et al.,[36] who observed maximal platelet depression at the same time relative leukocytosis occurred, followed by rebound thrombocytosis concomitant with maximal leukopenia. Frei et al.[35] reported greater depression of white blood cells than platelets in 88 cases given cytosine arabinoside in 1-, 2-, or 4-day infusions (Table 1). Single doses of cytosine arabinoside caused slight leukopenia without thrombocytopenia, whereas the same total amount administered in divided daily doses produced greater thrombocytopenia with little additional leukopenia (Table 2).[46] Vincristine, administered intravenously once weekly, produced leukopenia in 25 per cent of the cases, but no instances of thrombocytopenia attributable to the drug were recorded.[47]

TABLE 1.—*Effect of Cytosine Arabinoside upon White Blood Cells and Platelets* (222 *Trials*)

Incidence of depression			
White blood cells/mm³		*Platelets/mm³*	
3,000–5,000	< 3,000	50,000–200,000	< 50,000
35	31	26	13

Cytosine arabinoside was administered by a single rapid intravenous injection or in a continuous infusion lasting 24, 48, or 96 hours. Hematopoietic suppression increased as the duration of administration was lengthened, and marked leukopenia was more common than thrombocytopenia. Modified from Frei et al.[35]

TABLE 2.—*Effect of Cytosine Arabinoside upon White Blood Cells and Platelets* (8 *Trials*)

	Maximal depression	
	Daily	*Single dose*
WBC/mm³	3,850	4,790
Platelets/mm³	72,300	237,200

Cytosine arabinoside (maximal total dose 50 mg/kg) was administered either daily for 4 to 10 days, or in a single dose. Repeated daily doses produced significant thrombocytopenia. Modified from Talley and Vaitkevicius.[46]

Experimental studies by Morse and Stohlman[48] demonstrated that doses of vincristine that severely depress erythropoietic activity cause little change in the rate of thrombopoiesis. These studies showed no significant changes in the differential counts or morphology of megakaryocytes in rats given vincristine, despite concomitant depopulation of marrow erythroid elements. The continued differentiation of precursor cells into the megakaryocytic pool indicated that vincristine did not halt differentiation of "committed" stem cells into megakaryoctyic precursors. The authors therefore concluded that there were different immediate precursor cells for these cell lines. This is supported by observations that erythropoietin does not produce thrombocytosis.[12,18]

Studies in animals have provided additional understanding of mechanisms by which antitumor agents suppress thrombopoiesis. Incorporation of selenomethionine-^{75}Se (^{75}SeM) into platelets was decreased in rabbits that received mechlorethamine one, two, or four days before the administration of ^{75}SeM (Fig. 1).[19] A brief peak of radioactivity in the circulating platelets was observed during a period of

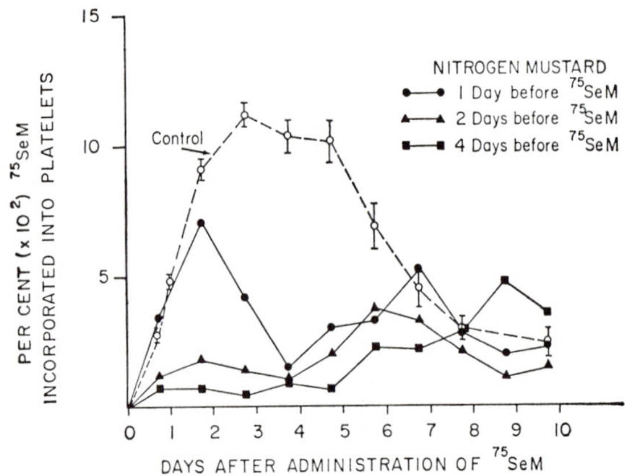

FIG. 1.—Effect of nitrogen mustard upon incorporation of ^{75}SeM into platelets. Two rabbits received a single dose of nitrogen mustard one day before ^{75}SeM (●). Initial dose of nitrogen mustard was given 2 days before ^{75}SeM to 2 animals (▲), and 4 days before ^{75}SeM to 3 animals (■). The mean is shown. The experimental groups significantly differed from normal animals until day 7. Appearance of ^{75}SeM in platelets of normal animals is shown by open circles and hatched line. In each group, administration of nitrogen mustard in a dose sufficient to cause thrombocytopenia (see Fig. 2) resulted in a decrease of incorporation of ^{75}SeM into platelets. ^{75}SeM subsequently reappeared in circulating platelets when marrow function was reestablished. A short period of thrombocytosis which occurred 24 to 48 hours after administration of nitrogen mustard was reflected, in one group (●), by a brief peak of appearance of ^{75}SeM in circulating platelets. From Evatt and Levin,[19] with permission of The Rockefeller University Press.

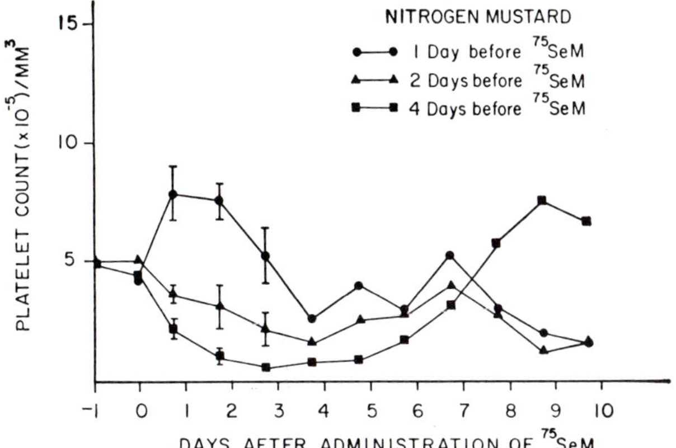

FIG. 2.—Effect of nitrogen mustard upon peripheral platelet counts. The mean ±1 SE is shown for each of the 3 groups of animals, where significant differences existed. Thrombocytopenia occurred with each dosage schedule, and there was good correlation between alteration in peripheral platelet counts and appearance of ^{75}SeM in circulating platelets.

relative thrombocytosis which occurred 24 to 48 hours after the administration of mechlorethamine in one group of animals (Fig. 2). In the other two groups of animals, significant levels of the isotope did not appear in the circulating platelets for 5 to 6 days (see Fig. 1). In each experimental group, there was a delayed or secondary increase in the level of ^{75}SeM in platelets, 6 to 10 days after administration of the isotope, which correlated with the platelet counts (Figs. 1, 2, and 3). The increase in percentage of ^{75}SeM associated with platelets, as the platelet count was rising, indicated entry into the circulation of a heavily tagged population of new platelets. Presumably ^{75}SeM, which did not appear in circulating platelets at the usual times (i.e., 2 to 4 days), remained available in the marrow within megakaryocytes or their precursors that were not productive, and subsequently appeared in the circulating platelets when megakaryocyte function was reestablished.

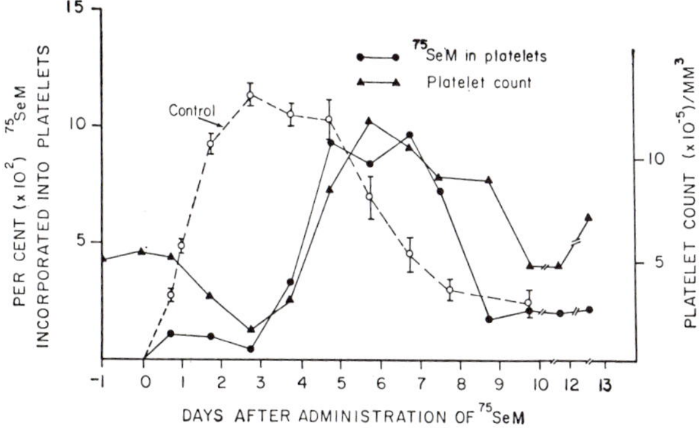

FIG. 3.—Effect of nitrogen mustard upon incorporation of ^{75}SeM into platelets and peripheral platelet counts. One animal that had received nitrogen mustard 2 days before ^{75}SeM manifested an unusual rebound phenomenon, with a period of marked thrombocytosis after thrombocytopenia. Delayed appearance of ^{75}SeM, after the dose of nitrogen mustard, was seen during this recovery period. Appearance of ^{75}SeM in platelets of normal animals is shown by open circles and hatched line. From Evatt and Levin,[19] with permission of The Rockefeller University Press.

Lindell and Zajicek[49] demonstrated that maximal reduction in the number of megakaryocytes in the femurs of rats that had received total body irradiation did not occur until 5 to 7 days following irradiation, which suggested that the damage had occurred to megakaryocyte precursors, and not primarily to cells that already were in the pool of recognizable megakaryocytes. Furthermore, the irradiation of one femur produced the same changes in that area as when the animals had received total-body irradiation, indicating that during the period of observation, the irradiated marrow had not been recolonized by stem cells from the nonirradiated areas of the body.[49]

Ebbe and Stohlman[30] have demonstrated that the induction of acute thrombocytopenia either immediately before or after exposure to irradiation partially protects mice against the thrombocytopenic effects of 200 to 400 R of total-body irradiation. Elson reported that production of thrombocytopenia with a rapidly acting nitrogen mustard partially protects animals against the thrombocytopenic effects of subsequently administered busulfan.[43] Both groups[30,43] concluded that bone marrow stimulation, before the maximal depressive action of busulfan or irradiation, had been protective.

Other antitumor agents (e.g. vincristine and vinblastine) may produce thrombocytosis *without* prior thrombocytopenia. This was observed in 13 of 40 cases after weekly intravenous injections of vincristine,[47] and also has been reported by Hwang et al.[50] and Robertson and McCarthy.[51] There did not appear to be a significant interval of time between initiation of drug therapy and development of thrombocytosis, and cessation of drug seemed to be associated with an immediate drop in the platelet count to pretreatment levels. Thrombocytosis also has been observed in rats after administration of vincristine.[51,52] The mechanisms which account for these changes are unclear, but it has been suggested that certain dose levels may stimulate thrombopoiesis.[52]

Another agent has been shown to result in cyclical changes in the levels of some circulating blood cells. Kennedy[53] has reported that patients treated with hydroxyurea may show oscillatory changes in the levels of circulating white blood cells and platelets. No changes were observed either in reticulocyte counts or hemoglobin levels. These observations support the suggestion of Morley et al.[54,55] that the kinetics of normal marrow function may be cyclical, and provide additional evidence that the committed stem cells of the three hematopoietic cell lines differ significantly from each other.

Other Agents

There are other mechanisms by which drugs or other agents produce thrombocytopenia without suppression of platelet production by megakaryocytes (Table 3). Many drugs, including quinidine, novobiocin, digitoxin, stibophen, and apronalide (Sedormid), have been shown to produce thrombocytopenia secondary to an antigen-antibody reaction.[56–59] The prerequisite components for this phenomenon include the drug, a plasma protein with which the drug binds, antibody to the drug-protein complex, and platelets. Platelets are involved only secondarily, by providing a surface upon which the antigen-antibody complex can adhere.[58] Rechallenge of sensitive individuals with the offending drugs results in recurrent thrombocytopenia.[58–61] Agglutination and lysis of platelets from the patient or normal donors, inhibition of clot retraction, and complement fixation often can be demonstrated in vitro, in the presence of the drug and serum of an affected person that contains the antibody.[58–66]

The nature of the antibody appears to be the main factor in determining whether thrombocytopenia, leukopenia or hemolytic anemia is produced in the susceptible patient.[58] The antibody shows a striking specificity for the drug against which it is active, since quinine cannot be substituted for quinidine[63] nor digitoxigenin or digoxin for digitoxin.[59] In rare instances, the production of antibodies against *donor* platelets can result in the occurrence of delayed thrombocytopenia (post-transfusion purpura), which takes place when antigen-antibody complexes, containing donor platelets, or fragments thereof, adhere to the platelets of the recipient.[58]

Infection (usually with gram-negative organisms),[67,68] malignancy,[69,70] and hemolytic reactions to blood transfusion[71,72] can result in intravascular coagulation that produces both thrombocytopenia and hypofibrinogenemia. Endotoxin or red cell stroma may be the precipitating triggers of the first and last examples,[68,71,72] but the mechanism by which some tumors produce intravascular coagulation remains unclear. The production of a thromboplastic substance by tumor cells has been suggested as a possible cause.[68] In other instances, turbulent blood flow in vascular tumors is believed to result in sequestration and destruction of platelets sufficient to produce systemic thrombocytopenia.[73,74] The rapid transfusion of large volumes of blood that does not contain viable platelets can produce thrombocytopenia by dilution of circulating platelets.[75] Ristocetin, an antibiotic, produces thrombocytopenia in man and rabbits as a result of a direct, dose related effect on circulating platelets.[76] Lysis of platelets can be demonstrated in vitro, by addition of the drug to saline suspensions of platelets.[76] It also has been suggested that mithramycin (NSC-24559) causes qualitative changes in circulating platelets (and damages the terminal vascular bed) in addition to production of thrombocytopenia secondary to hematopoietic depression.[77,78]

The different mechanisms by which thrombocytopenia can be produced without depression of thrombopoiesis should be considered in the evaluation of any patient receiving antitumor agents. Thrombocytosis can be present in patients with malignant disease before therapy.[79,80] The mechanism of thrombocytosis in malignant disease is not understood, and it is not known whether such patients are more resistant to the production of thrombocytopenia by antitumor agents. Harker and Finch[28] have demonstrated overproduction of platelets in patients with thrombocytosis associated with myeloproliferative disorders, suggesting a defective feedback mechanism.

TABLE 3.—*Production of Acute Thrombocytopenia without Suppression of Thrombopoiesis*

Agent	*Mechanism*	*Reference*
Quinidine*	Immunologic	62, 63
Blood transfusion	Immunologic (post-transfusion purpura)	58
Blood transfusion	Intravascular coagulation (hemolytic transfusion reaction)	71, 72
Infection	Intravascular coagulation (? endotoxin)	67, 68
Malignancy	Intravascular coagulation	68
Blood transfusion	Dilution of circulating platelets	75
Ristocetin	Direct toxic effect on circulating platelets	76

* Many other drugs produce thrombocytopenia by this mechanism. (See text.)

Discussion

The effects of antitumor agents upon thrombopoiesis in man and animals strongly support the concept of a feedback mechanism that is responsive to levels of circulating platelets. Rebound thrombocytosis may be due in part to synchronization of megakaryocytes that are stimulated by the state of thrombocytopenia during the stages of DNA synthesis. Megakaryocytes that mature during a period of thrombocytopenia have increased ploidy and cytoplasmic mass, and probably produce more platelets per megakaryocyte.[4,7,11,28,29] The time required for the development of thrombocytopenia and rebound thrombocytosis following administration of antitumor agents provides additional evidence that platelet life span in man is approximately 10 days. A similar, or perhaps shorter, period is required for the maturation of megakaryoblasts into platelet producing, mature megakaryocytes.

The dissociation between the production of reticulocytopenia, of leukopenia, and of thrombocytopenia by antitumor agents[35,47,53,78,81,82] is most compatible with the existence of biologically different, committed precursors for these three hematopoietic cell lines, with resultant variations in sensitivity to antitumor agents. Such observations also indicate that an important effect of therapeutic doses of most marrow-suppressive drugs is upon committed stem cells, rather than affecting the uncommitted or pluripotential stem cells. The administration of ^{75}SeM to rabbits when megakaryocyte function had been severely depressed has provided evidence that megakaryoblasts or their precursors were capable of incorporating and storing this amino acid until function was recovered.[19]

In some studies single infusions of cytosine arabinoside, a cycle-active drug which blocks DNA synthesis, produced relatively little thrombocytopenia.[35,46] Only megakaryocytic precursors and immature megakaryocytes appear to engage in DNA synthesis[3,6]; thus, most of the megakaryocyte population escaped damage, because the duration of drug effect was not sufficient to significantly alter input of new cells into the megakaryocyte compartment. However, when the duration of treatment was extended, significant thrombocytopenia occurred.[46]

Another partial explanation for the relative resistance of megakaryocytes to many antitumor drugs is that the thrombopoietin sensitive cell may be in a resting (or nonsynthetic) state, and therefore is not susceptible to the action of ionizing radiation or drugs that cause similar damage.[30] Observations that support this concept are the effects on thrombopoiesis of single doses of irradiation or noncycle-active drugs that affect both proliferating and nonproliferating cells; and the increased sensitivity of mice to irradiation after induction of chronic thrombocytopenia, which presumably increases megakaryocyte flux.[30]

Megakaryocytes are unique in that they are polyploid, and do not undergo cellular division. This complex state of high ploidy, in addition to an unknown microenvironment, may account for some of the differences observed. Increased ploidy perhaps alters drug uptake. The large amount of DNA present in megakaryocytes may provide these cells with a reserve capability permitting partial loss of DNA or synthetic ability, while retaining the potential to produce some platelets.

References

1. Robb-Smith, A. H. T.: Why the platelets were discovered. Brit. J. Haemat. 13:618, 1967.
2. Odell, T. T., Jr., and Jackson, C. W.: Megakaryocytopoiesis. *In* Stohlman, F., Jr. (Ed.): Hemopoietic Cellular Proliferation. New York: Grune & Stratton, 1970, pp. 278–284.

3. Ebbe, S.: Megakaryocytopoiesis. *In* Gordon, A. S. (Ed.): Regulation of Hematopoiesis. Vol. II. New York: Appleton-Century-Crofts, 1970, pp. 1587–1610.
4. Odell, T. T., Jr. and Jackson, C. W.: Polyploidy and maturation of rat megakaryocytes. Blood 32:102, 1968.
5. Paulus, J-M.: DNA metabolism and development of organelles in guinea-pig megakaryocytes: A combined ultrastructural, autoradiographic and cytophotometric study. Blood 35:298, 1970.
6. Odell, T. T., Jr., Jackson, C. W. and Friday, T. J.: Megakaryocytopoiesis in rats with special reference to polyploidy. Blood 35:775, 1970.
7. Harker, L. A.: Kinetics of thrombopoiesis. J. Clin. Invest. 47:458, 1968.
8. Craddock, C. G., Adams, W. S., Perry, S., and Lawrence, J. S.: The dynamics of platelet production as studied by a depletion technique in normal and irradiated dogs. J. Lab. Clin. Med. 45:906, 1955.
9. Matter, M., Hartmann, J. R., Kautz, J., DeMarsh, Q. B. and Finch, C. A.: A study of thrombopoiesis in induced acute thrombocytopenia. Blood 15:174, 1960.
10. Odell, T. T., Jr., McDonald, T. P. and Asano, M.: Response of rat megakaryocytes and platelets to bleeding. Acta Haemat. 27:171, 1962.
11. Ebbe, S., Stohlman, F., Jr., Overcash, J., Donovan, J. and Howard, D.: Megakaryocyte size in thrombocytopenic and normal rats. Blood 32:383, 1968.
12. Ebbe, S.: Megakaryocytopoiesis and platelet turnover. Series Haemat. 1:65, 1968.
13. Odell, T. T., Jr., Jackson, C. W., Friday, T. J. and Charsha, D. E.: Effects of thrombocytopenia on megakaryocytopoiesis. Brit. J. Haemat. 17:91, 1969.
14. Odell, T. T., Jr. and Kniseley, R. M.: The origin, life span, regulation and fate of blood platelets. *In* Tocantins, L. M. (Ed.): Progress in Hematology. Vol. III. New York: Grune & Stratton, 1962, pp. 203–217.
15. Ebbe, S., Stohlman, F., Jr., Donovan, J. and Overcash, J.: Megakaryocyte maturation rate in thrombocytopenic rats. Blood 32:787, 1968.
16. Cronkite, E. P., Bond, V. P., Fliedner, T. M., Paglia, D. A. and Adamik, E. R.: Studies on the origin, production and destruction of platelets. *In* Johnson, S. A., Monto, R. W., Rebuck, J. W., and Horn, R. C., Jr. (Eds.): Blood Platelets. Boston: Little, Brown, 1961, pp. 595–609.
17. Odell, T. T., Jr., Jackson, C. W. and Reiter, R. S.: Depression of the megakaryocyte-platelet system in rats by transfusion of platelets. Acta Haemat. 38:34, 1967.
18. de Gabriele, G., and Penington, D. G.: Physiology of the regulation of platelet production. Brit. J. Haemat. 13:202, 1967.
19. Evatt, B. L. and Levin, J.: Measurement of thrombopoiesis in rabbits using ^{75}selenomethionine. J. Clin. Invest. 48:1615, 1969.
20. Levin, J.: Humoral control of thrombopoiesis. *In* Greenwalt, T. J. and Jamieson, G. A. (Eds.): Formation and Destruction of Blood Cells. Philadelphia: J. B. Lippincott, 1970, pp. 143–150.
21. Stohlman, F., Jr.: Some aspects of erythrokinetics. Seminars Hemat. 4:304, 1967.
22. Schooley, J. C. and Garcia, J. F.: Suppression of erythropoiesis in the plethoric rat by antierythropoietin. Proc. Soc. Exp. Biol. Med. 133:953, 1970.
23. Ebbe, S. and Stohlman, F., Jr.: Megakaryocytopoiesis in the rat. Blood 26:20, 1965.
24. Cooney, D. P. and Smith, B. A.: Maturation time of rabbit megakaryocytes. Brit. J. Haemat. 11:484, 1965.
25. Vodopick, H. A. and Kniseley, R. M.: Sulfur-35 studies in man: Platelet survival and plasma and urinary radioactivity assayed by beta liquid scintillation spectrometry. J. Lab. Clin. Med. 62:109, 1963.
26. Najean, Y. and Ardaillou, N.: The use of ^{75}Se-methionin for the in vivo study of platelet kinetics. Scand. J. Haemat. 6:395, 1969.
27. McIntyre, P. A., Evatt, B. L., Hodkinson, B. A. and Scheffel, U.: Selenium-75 selenomethionine as a label for erythrocytes, leukocytes, and platelets in man. J. Lab. Clin. Med. 75:472, 1970.
28. Harker, L. A. and Finch, C. A.: Thrombokinetics in man. J. Clin. Invest. 48:963, 1969.
29. Harker, L. A.: Thrombokinetics in idiopathic thrombocytopenic purpura. Brit. J. Haemat. 19:95, 1970.
30. Ebbe, S. and Stohlman, F., Jr.: Stimulation of thrombocytopoiesis in irradiated mice. Blood 35:783, 1970.
31. Penington, D. G.: Isotope bioassay for "Thrombopoietin." Brit. Med. J. 1:606, 1970.
32. Harker, L. A.: Regulation of thrombopoiesis. Amer. J. Physiol. 218:1376, 1970.
33. Shreiner, D. P. and Levin, J.: Detection of thrombopoietic activity in plasma by stimulation of suppressed thrombopoiesis. J. Clin. Invest. 49:1709, 1970.

34. Cooper, G. W., Cooper, B. and Chung, C-Y.: Demonstration of a circulating factor regulating blood platelet production using ^{35}S-sulfate in rats and mice. Proc. Soc. Exp. Biol. Med. 134:1123, 1970.
35. Frei, E., III, Bickers, J. N., Hewlett, J. S., Lane, M., Leary, W. V. and Talley, R. W.: Dose schedule and antitumor studies of arabinosyl cytosine (NSC-63878). Cancer Res. 29:1325, 1969.
36. Burke, P. J., Serpick, A. A., Carbone, P. P. and Tarr, N.: A clinical evaluation of dose and schedule of administration of cytosine arabinoside (NSC 63878). Cancer Res. 28: 274, 1968.
37. Holland, J. F.: Symposium on the experimental pharmacology and clinical use of antimetabolites. VIII. Folic acid antagonists. Clin. Pharmacol. Ther. 2:374, 1961.
38. Ogston, D., Dawson, A. A. and Philip, J. F.: Methotrexate and the platelet count. Brit. J. Cancer 22:244, 1968.
39. Sensenbrenner, L. L. and Owens, A. H., Jr.: The effects of mechlorethamine on bone marrow function and iron metabolism in man. Johns Hopkins Med. J. 121:162, 1967.
40. Aster, R. H. and Jandl, J. H.: Platelet sequestration in man. I. Methods. J. Clin. Invest. 43:843, 1964.
41. Shulman, N. R., Marder, V. J. and Weinrach, R. S.: Similarities between known antiplatelet antibodies and the factor responsible for thrombocytopenia in idiopathic purpura. Physiologic, serologic and isotopic studies. Ann. N. Y. Acad. Sci. 124:499, 1965.
42. Lampkin, B. C., Nagao, T., and Mauer, A. M.: Drug effect in acute leukemia. J. Clin. Invest. 48:1124, 1969.
43. Elson, L. A.: Comparison of the physiological response to radiation and radiomimetic chemicals. Pattern of blood response. *In* de Hevesy, G. C., Forssberg, A. G. and Abbatt, J. D. (Eds.): Advances in Radiobiology. Springfield, Ill.: Charles C Thomas, 1957, pp. 372–375.
44. Dameshek, W., Weisfuse, L. and Stein, T.: Nitrogen mustard therapy in Hodgkin's disease. Blood 4:338, 1949.
45. Colvin, O. M.: Unpublished observations.
46. Talley, R. W. and Vaitkevicius, V. K.: Megaloblastosis produced by a cytosine antagonist 1-β-D-arabinofuranosylcytosine. Blood 21:352, 1963.
47. Carbone, P. P., Bono, V., Frei, E., III and Brindley, C. O.: Clinical studies with vincristine. Blood 21:640, 1963.
48. Morse, B. S. and Stohlman, F., Jr.: Regulation of erythropoiesis. XVIII. The effect of vincristine and erythropoietin on bone marrow. J. Clin. Invest. 45:1241, 1966.
49. Lindell, B., and Zajicek, J.: The effect of whole-body X-irradiation on the megakaryocytic system in rat femur. *In* de Hevesy, G. C., Forssberg, A. G. and Abbatt, J. D. (Eds.): Advances in Radiobiology. Springfield, Ill., Charles C Thomas, 1957, pp. 376–381.
50. Hwang, Y. F., Hamilton, H. E., and Sheets, R. F.: Vinblastine-induced thrombocytosis (Letter to the editor). Lancet 2:1075, 1969.
51. Robertson, J. H. and McCarthy, G. M.: Periwinkle alkaloids and the platelet-count. Lancet 2:353, 1969.
52. Robertson, J. H., Crozier, E. H. and Woodend, B. E.: The effect of vincristine on the platelet count in rats. Brit. J. Haemat. 10:331, 1970.
53. Kennedy, B. J.: Cyclic leukocyte oscillations in chronic myelogenous leukemia during hydroxyurea therapy. Blood 35:751, 1970.
54. Morley, A.: A platelet cycle in normal individuals. Australasian Ann. Med. 18: 127, 1969.
55. Morley, A., King-Smith, E. A. and Stohlman, F., Jr.: The oscillatory nature of hemopoiesis. *In* Stohlman, F., Jr. (Ed.): Hemopoietic Cellular Proliferation. New York: Grune & Stratton, 1970, pp. 3–14.
56. Harrington, W. J.: The purpuras. Disease-A-Month, July 1957.
57. Crosby, W. H. and Kaufman, R. M.: Drug-induced blood dyscrasias. IV. Thrombocytopenia. J.A.M.A. 189:417, 1964.
58. Shulman, N. R.: A mechanism of cell destruction in individuals sensitized to foreign antigens and its implications in autoimmunity. Ann. Intern. Med. 60:506, 1964.
59. Young, R. C., Nachman, R. L., and Horowitz, H. I.: Thrombocytopenia due to digitoxin. Amer. J. Med. 41:605, 1966.
60. Day, H. J., Conrad, F. G. and Moore, J. E.: Immunothrombocytopenia induced by novobiocin. Amer. J. Med. Sci. 236:475, 1958.
61. Kahn, H. R. and Brod, R. C.: Thrombocytopenia due to stibophen. Arch. Intern. Med. 108:496, 1961.
62. Larson, R. K.: The mechanism of quinidine purpura. Blood 8:16, 1953.
63. Shulman, N. R.: Immunoreactions involving platelets IV. Studies on the pathogenesis of thrombocytopenia in drug purpura using

test doses of quinidine in sensitized individuals; their implications in idiopathic thrombocytopenic purpura. J. Exp. Med. 107:711, 1958.
64. Ackroyd, J. F.: The pathogenesis of thrombocytopenic purpura due to hypersensitivity to Sedormid (allyl-isopropyl-acetyl-carbamide). Clin. Sci. 7:249, 1949.
65. Ackroyd, J. F.: The role of complement in Sedormid purpura. Clin. Sci. 10:185, 1951.
66. Bigelow, F. S. and Desforges, J. F.: Platelet agglutination by an abnormal plasma factor in thrombocytopenic purpura associated with quinidine ingestion. Amer. J. Med. Sci. 224:274, 1952.
67. Rosner, F. and Ritz, N. D.: The defibrination syndrome. Arch. Intern. Med. 117:17, 1966.
68. Deykin, D.: The clinical challenge of disseminated intravascular coagulation. New Eng. J. Med. 283:636, 1970.
69. Pittman, G. R., Senhauser, D. A. and Lowney, J. F.: Acute promyelocytic leukemia. Amer. J. Clin. Path. 46:214, 1966.
70. Merskey, C., Johnson, A. J., Kleiner, G. J. and Wohl, H.: The defibrination syndrome: Clinical features and laboratory diagnosis. Brit. J. Haemat. 13:528, 1967.
71. Krevans, J. R., Jackson, D. P., Conley, C. L. and Hartmann, R. C.: The nature of the hemorrhagic disorder accompanying hemolytic transfusion reactions in man. Blood 12:834, 1957.
72. Rock, R. C., Bove, J. R. and Nemerson, Y.: Heparin treatment of intravascular coagulation accompanying hemolytic transfusion reactions. Transfusion 9:57, 1969.
73. Sutherland, D. A. and Clark, H.: Hemangioma associated with thrombocytopenia. Amer. J. Med. 33:150, 1962.
74. Thatcher, L. G., Clatanoff, D. V. and Stiehm, E. R.: Splenic hemangioma with thrombocytopenia and afibrinogenemia. J. Pediat. 73:345, 1968.
75. Jackson, D. P., Krevans, J. R. and Conley, C. L.: Mechanism of the thrombocytopenia that follows multiple whole blood transfusions. Trans. Ass. Amer. Physicians 69:155, 1956.
76. Gangarosa, E. J., Johnson, T. R. and Ramos, H. S.: Ristocetin-induced thrombocytopenia: Site and mechanism of action. Arch. Intern. Med. 105:107, 1960.
77. Monto, R. W., Talley, R. W., Caldwell, M. J., Levin, W. C. and Guest, M. M.: Observations on the mechanism of hemorrhagic toxicity in mithramycin (NSC-24559) therapy. Cancer Res. 29:697, 1969.
78. Kennedy, B. J.: Metabolic and toxic effects of mithramycin during tumor therapy. Amer. J. Med. 49:494, 1970.
79. Marchasin, S., Wallerstein, R. O. and Aggeler, P. M.: Variations of the platelet count in disease. Calif. Med. 101:95, 1964.
80. Levin, J. and Conley, C. L.: Thrombocytosis associated with malignant disease. Arch. Intern. Med. 144:497, 1964.
81. Levin, J. and Cluff, L. E.: Endotoxemia and adrenal hemorrhage. J. Exp. Med. 121:247, 1965.
82. Burke, P. J., Owens, A. H., Jr., Colsky, J., Shnider, B. I., Edmonson, J. H., et al.: A clinical evaluation of a prolonged schedule of cytosine arabinoside (NSC-63878). Cancer Res. 30:1512, 1970.

Bone Marrow Transplantation: Immunologic Considerations and Current Status

By J. WAYNE STREILEIN, M.D.

INTEREST IN HUMAN BONE MARROW TRANSPLANTATION as a clinically useful procedure has grown tremendously over the past several years, and many of the patients who have received these transplants have suffered from hematologic or other forms of malignant disease. Although the role of bone marrow transplantation as a therapeutic maneuver in clinical medicine is unclear at this point in time, the potentialities such therapy offers are enormous. It is appropriate, therefore, that this topic should be included in a volume devoted to cancer chemotherapy.

Radiation sickness, an often fatal disorder that can be induced in men and animals by exposure to high doses of x-irradiation, became the object of intense experimental effort after World War II. On the basis of studies carried out in experimental animals, it was found that animals receiving lethal whole-body x-irradiation within a broad dose range (300 to 1000 rads) died primarily from the effects of bone marrow failure induced by the x-rays. Moreover, it was shown that for this dose range, a fatal outcome for exposed animals could be circumvented by the provision of hematopoietic stem cells in suspensions of bone marrow cells from another animal of the same species. It was clear from these data that cells within a bone marrow suspension, when injected intravenously, are capable of seeking out and ultimately repopulating an x-ray–suppressed marrow cavity.

In light of this experimental work, intensive efforts were made in the late 1950s and early 1960s to bring this new information to bear on appropriate problems in clinical medicine. Investigators such as Mathé[1] and Thomas[2] conducted these clinical experiments; the uniformly disappointing nature of their results dampened enthusiasm for bone marrow transplantation at these and other centers during the middle 1960s. However, within the past three years increasing numbers of bone marrow transplants have again been performed, and it is appropriate to identify the reasons for this renewed clinical interest.

First, during this period significant improvements have been made in the general area of tissue typing. In addition, increased experience with older forms of immunosuppression, as well as the advent of new and different types of immunosuppressive therapy, has held hope for improved results. Last, our understanding of the pathogenesis of graft-versus-host disease is undergoing a revolution which is providing a new horizon of therapeutic possibilities for control.

IMMUNOLOGIC CONSIDERATIONS IN BONE MARROW TRANSPLANTATION

To understand the problems associated with bone marrow transplantation, it is essential that the basic principles of transplantation immunology be kept firmly in mind. It is now well established that grafts of tissues and cells between individuals of

---

From the Department of Medical Genetics, University of Pennsylvania School of Medicine, Philadelphia, Pennsylvania.

Supported in part by grant No. AI 01700 from the U.S. Public Health Service and by the Markle Foundation.

an outbred population of the same species are regularly and completely rejected. The only exception to this rule occurs when the donor and the recipient of the tissue in question are identical twins.

The rejection process is initiated when the recipient, or, in reality, his immunologically competent lymphocytes, recognizes certain antigenic determinants on the homografted tissue as foreign. These so-called transplantation antigens incite within the host a specific immune response which is manifest in the production of specifically sensitized lymphoid cells and specific isoantibody. By one or another means, these products of the immune response are able to bring about the rejection of the homograft.

Since homografts from most somatic tissues are rejected in homologous hosts, it is generally believed that transplantation antigens are expressed on most cells, including those of the bone marrow and lymphatic tissues. As in cross-matching for the transfusion of whole blood, it is reasonable to expect that if the transplantation antigens of donor and recipient of a potential bone marrow transplant could be matched, rejection of the graft might be prevented, or at least considerably delayed.

Histocompatibility Testing in Man

Man is probably like the mouse and other mammalian species studied to date in that a large number of genetic loci seem to be responsible for the expression of a variety of transplantation antigens on cellular surfaces. However, not all transplantation antigens are of equal potency; some are obviously stronger than others. In man, two genetic loci are of crucial importance to the survival of a tissue homograft. The isohemagglutinin locus which determines the ABO blood group antigens is one locus,[3] and serologic typing for these antigenic specificities is a routine clinical laboratory procedure. The other main histocompatibility locus, the HL-A, whose definition has been accomplished only within the past 6 years,[4] is exceedingly complex and rivals the H-2 locus of the mouse in this regard. In 1954, Dausset et al. described an anti-leukocyte antibody in the serum of a multiply-transfused patient.[5] Since that time, an ever-increasing number of antigenic specificities have been described on peripheral blood leukocytes and many of these leukocytic antigens appear to be governed by alleles at the HL-A locus. To date, 13 specificities have been widely recognized by serologic methods in different laboratories throughout the world and have been given numerical designation by the World Health Organization.[6] As seen in Table 1, the HL-A locus appears to be made up of two subloci,[7] the LA series, at which specificities 1, 2, 3, 9, 10 and 11 are found; and the Four series, at which specificities 5, 7, 8, 12, and 13 are recognized. In addition, there are at least 14 other specificities regularly identified in various laboratories, and doubtless these will shortly achieve WHO designation as bona fide specificities. Moreover, evidence exists that suggests that a third sublocus may be associated with HL-A.[8] Although at present it is not possible to identify all of the specificities at this locus, it is clear that most specificities,

Table 1.—*Major Locus for Human Histocompatibility*

HL-A Specificities determined serologically at	
Sublocus LA	Sublocus Four
1–2–3–9–10–11	5–7–8–12–13
40–59–63–66	50–51–52–53–54–55–57–58–60

TABLE 2.—*Haplotype Analysis*

Results of Serotyping		*Chromosomal Assignment*
		A 1,8
Mother	1,2,8	B 2
		C 3,7
Father	1,3,5,7	D 1,5
Children	1,3,7,8	AC
	1,5,8	AD
	2,3,7	BC
	1,2,5	BD

especially those reflecting high gene frequencies in the population, are already detectable.

Despite an incomplete knowledge of all specificities at the HL-A locus, workable means have been sought to determine HL-A identity for donor-recipient pairs with the limited sera now available. One method which is called "haplotyping" is illustrated in Table 2. Every person has one pair of autosomal chromosomes bearing alleles at the HL-A locus. It has been reasoned from empiric data that the HL-A region on each of these chromosomes will determine one specificity from the LA series and one from the Four series, such that the maximal number of specificities any individual could express on his somatic cells would be two specificities from each sublocus. Since our ability to detect all specificities is at present incomplete, there may be empty spaces in certain individuals indicating either homozygosity at one sublocus or the presence of an unknown, as yet undetectable, specificity. To accomplish haplotyping, i.e. match patients for the antigens determined by this region, parents and children within a family are serotyped for their individual HL-A specificities.

Obviously, reasonably large families are essential for this type of analysis. On the basis of the segregation of individual specificities among the offspring, it is usually possible to identify each parental chromosome by recognizing that certain HL-A specificities segregate together. Having determined the HL-A specificities carried on each of the four parental chromosomes, it is then possible to determine the HL-A locus bearing chromosomal origins of each offspring. Two siblings who are thus demonstrated to have received identical chromosomes from each parent are then said to be haplotype-identical. In this case, even if all the specificities at the HL-A locus cannot be tested for, since these siblings have each received pairs of identical chromosomes, their HL-A genotype must also be identical. Obviously, no parent-child combination could result in haplotype identity, nor can a similar analysis be carried out on unrelated individuals. On theoretical grounds, 25 per cent of siblings should be haplotype identical.

Another empiric check on HL-A identity of potential donor and recipient is the mixed leukocyte culture test, recently developed.[9] In this procedure, peripheral blood leukocytes from donor and recipient are mixed and placed in tissue culture. Bach[10] has shown that if donor and recipient possess different alleles at the HL-A locus, their respective lymphocytes will be mutually stimulated to undergo mitosis (as measured by their incorporation of tritiated thymidine). The lymphocytes from HL-A identical pairs are mutually nonstimulatory in mixed leukocyte culture, irrespective of whether these individuals may be disparate at several non-HL-A histocompatibility loci.

Since so much effort is being expended in order to establish HL-A identity for donor and recipient of bone marrow transplant, it is reasonable at this point to discuss why it is desirable to obtain this degree of tissue matching.

Graft-versus-Host Disease in Man

A bone marrow graft differs from heart and kidney grafts not only by virtue of its being a cellular suspension rather than a solid tissue graft. In addition to the progenitors of red cells, granulocytes, and platelets, an aspirate of bone marrow contains immunologically competent lymphoid cells as well as their progenitors. Experimentally, when immunologically competent cells are inoculated into homologous hosts whose own immune response has been blunted (e.g. with x-ray), they may recognize the alien transplantation antigens on the tissues of the host, and, reacting immunologically against them, set up a graft-versus-host (GvH) reaction which is often lethal for the host.[11]

From work with inbred rodent strains, it appears that when donor and host in such a situation differ at the major histocompatibility loci for that species (such as the HL-A locus in man), severe lethal graft-versus-host disease can be expected. On the contrary, when donor and host differ at only minor histocompatibility loci, much less severe GvH disease develops. Extrapolating from mouse to man, it would be expected that if donor and recipient of a bone marrow transplant were identical at the HL-A locus, tolerable or at least controllable GvH disease might be achieved.

Before leaving these considerations of graft-versus-host disease, there is one other matter of significance to discuss—a matter that has particular relevance to the question of bone marrow transplantation in patients with hematologic malignancies. There is a growing body of experimental evidence that casts doubt on the traditional views of the pathogenesis of this disease. Since transplantation antigens are present on most tissues of the body, it was originally assumed that attacking donor lymphoid cells could strike their targets at random, and that all tissues were at equal risk of this destructive immunologic process. However, experience with GvH disease in man and other mammals over the past 15 years has indicated that this is not the case.

As can be seen in Table 3, only lympho-hematopoietic tissues are regularly and uniformly involved in the GvH process. This realization, along with related information, has led to the generation of an altered hypothesis regarding the pathogenesis of GvH disease: The primary and perhaps the only specific targets of the immunologic attack in GvH disease are host lymphoid cells. The extent to which destruction is brought to nonlymphoid tissues—such as skin, gut, liver, and perhaps even erythro-

Table 3.—*Graft-versus-Host Disease: Resume of Tissues Affected and Their Relative Incidences*

Always	*Often*	*Rarely*
Lymphatic:	Skin and mucous membranes	Muscle
Nodes	Gastrointestinal tract-lining epithelium	Bone
Spleen	Liver	Endocrine glands
Thymus		Nervous system
Hematopoietic		
Reticuloendothelial system		

cytic and granulocytic precursors—is a reflection of "innocent bystander" killing, a nonspecific sequela to the primary immune event, the interaction of donor and host lymphoid cells.[12] Whether of local or systemic type, the GvH reaction in many ways mimics the mixed leukocyte interactions that occur in vitro.[13] The implications of this hypothesis for the rationale of employing bone marrow transplantation in hematologic malignancies will now be explored.

Potential Roles for Bone Marrow Transplantation in the Therapy of Hematologic Malignancies

There is the old, rather naive notion that the way to treat leukemia is to eradicate from the patient, by means of x-ray or chemotherapy, or both, all leukemic cells. Since such therapy might be expected to destroy utterly the patient's hematopoietic capacity as well, provision of homologous bone marrow aspirate would reconstitute the patient, thus effecting a cure.

It would be impertinent to point out that there is no therapeutic regimen yet devised that is capable of eradicating all malignant cells without simultaneously eradicating the patient as well. Consequently, if bone marrow transplantation has any potential usefulness, it must be sought under some other theoretical guise.

Bone marrow transplantation, as it is currently employed, is a significant and aggressive clinical maneuver. Without speculating on any mysterious mechanisms, a nonspecific remission might be expected on occasion in leukemic patients undergoing this procedure in somewhat the same manner in which vigorous shaking of an errant alarm clock may sometimes set it to ticking again.

More importantly, the GvH process may prove useful in controlling the leukemic process per se. This idea was originally advanced by Mathé,[14] and with the newer ideas on the pathogenesis of GvH disease as a background, two mechanisms which might be efficacious in GvH disease suggest themselves:

1. If the specific targets of the immunologic attack in GvH disease are lymphoid cells, it would be reasonable to expect that leukemic lymphoid cells might share with normal lymphocytes the role of target for the attacking donor cells by virtue of the transplantation antigens expressed on their surfaces. Experimental evidence in support of this idea has been reported recently from Owens' laboratory in Baltimore[15] and by Glasspiegel and his colleagues in Milwaukee.[16] In the hands of both groups of investigators, mouse lymphoid leukemic cells were completely destroyed by GvH reactions which, although of significant intensity, failed to kill the murine hosts.

2. Even if the only targets of the immunologic attack in GvH disease are lymphoid cells, this interaction of donor and host lymphoid cells which has been shown to be capable of destroying indifferent epidermal cells could be imagined to result in the nonspecific destruction of other "innocent bystander" cells, in this case leukemic cells. Although no direct evidence is at hand with regard to the eradication of myeloid leukemia in experimental animals with GvH disease, our work[17] and that of Sensenbrenner and Santos[18] indicates that hematopoietic stem cells for erythrocytes, granulocytes and platelets may indeed be destroyed nonspecifically by a contiguous GvH process.

Implicit in both of these suggestions is the assumption that in bone marrow transplantation at the clinical level, a *mild* GvH reaction can be obtained, i.e. one sufficiently strong to destroy leukemic cells preferentially, yet sufficiently mild so as to be tolerable to the patient. Whether this hoped-for state can be achieved is a prime question being asked by clinical investigators now embarking on programs of human bone marrow transplantation.

Current Status of Human Bone Marrow Transplantation

From the viewpoint of genetics, two kinds of marrow transplants are possible in man: isogeneic grafts, which are carried out between identical twins, and allogeneic grafts, which are conducted between any two members of the human population who are not identical twins. Immunologically, these two types of transplants differ markedly in their expectations for success and so it is logical to consider them separately.

Thomas and his colleagues compiled the world experience with isogeneic bone marrow transplants in man and presented this material at a recent meeting of the Experimental Hematology Society.[19] To date, 13 such transplants have been performed on two types of patients: patients with idiopathic, drug-induced or x-ray–induced bone marrow failure; and patients with end-stage hematologic malignancy, usually leukemia. Irrespective of the reason for transplantation, a successful engraftment of identical twin bone marrow was obtained in every case. In those patients suffering from bone marrow failure alone, the transplant was life saving, and records of follow-up periods ranging from 3 to 10 years with continued good health of the recipients attest to the efficacy of this form of treatment. Patients with leukemia fared less well with bone marrow grafts, and though there was no graft-versus-host disease with which to contend, each patient either succumbed to the original leukemia process with little evidence of remission, or died of intercurrent infection which could be attributed directly to prior intensive chemotherapy for their disease. Thus the conclusions from this series are clear: For patients with bone marrow failure unassociated with malignant disease who have identical twins, bone marrow transplantation is likely to be curative. Alternatively, patients who have leukemia fare little better whether or not they are subjected to bone marrow transplantation from healthy identical twins.

With regard to allogeneic bone marrow transplants, Bortin[20] has recently compiled a collection of all such transplants performed in the world and recorded during the period 1958 to 1968. In this diverse series, patients with a variety of malignant and nonmalignant disease were used as recipients. During this interval, methods of immunosuppression and of chemotherapy for malignancy had undergone a revolution. Consequently, it is more difficult to discern a pattern in this compilation than in the isogeneic series. Nonetheless, what does emerge is interesting and informative: (1) In patients with aplastic anemia for whatever reason or with nonhematologic malignancies, very few marrow transplants appeared to "take," that is, only 15 of 104 patients exhibited evidence of engraftment. Naturally, very little therapeutic advantage could possibly have accrued to these patients from the procedure. (2) In patients with leukemia or with disorders of immunologic deficiency, the incidence of marrow graft "takes" was much higher (51 of 84 in the former, 12 of 15 in the latter). It is suspected that the higher incidence of engraftment among leukemic patients as opposed to patients with aplastic anemia or nonhematologic malignancies reflects the often demonstrated immunologic deficiency which these patients exhibit, whether from chemotherapy or from the disease process itself. (3) Among patients obtaining a viable graft, graft-versus-host disease regularly developed, and was usually lethal in leukemic patients. There is a suggestion in the data that less severe GvH disease occurred in patients who had had grafts for disorders of immunologic deficiency.

Clearly, procedural difficulties had to be solved before the basic question regarding the usefulness of allogeneic bone marrow transplantation for hematologic malignancies could be answered. Improved means of preparing the recipient for the allograft were essential. Better tissue typing and donor-recipient matching seemed essential. Some means had to be sought to control the unruly graft-versus-host disease which was generally destroying the patient before any beneficial effects of the transplant could occur. About four years ago a Cooperative Group in Bone Marrow Transplantation was formed from various centers around the world, and an attempt was made to develop reasonably standard protocol so that results could be compared among centers throughout the world. As means of tissue typing rapidly gained sophistication, it was decided that wherever possible only HL-A identical, haplotype-identical, mixed leukocyte culture negative sibling pairs would be engrafted. Santos[21] developed a method of recipient preparation based on his and other experimental work in rodents in which the recipient received one unit of whole donor blood intravenously five days before grafting, followed by large doses of cyclophosphamide. The rationale for this procedure was to stimulate recipient immune competent cells to donor antigens and then destroy these cells with cytotoxic drugs during their most vulnerable period, 24 to 48 hours after antigen exposure. Variations on immunosuppression at this point included large doses of methotrexate or whole-body x-irradiation, and even antilymphocyte globulin. In addition, beginning two days after the grafting procedure, the recipient was placed on low maintenance doses of cyclophosphamide or methotrexate in an effort to ward off GvH disease.

It is still probably too early to tell how these changes in procedure have affected clinical results. For what it is worth, 11 grafts were performed during 1969 that approximated this type of protocol.[21] All were haplotype-identical sibling pairs. They included a preponderance of patients with acute leukemia, but a few patients with disorders of immunologic deficiency were also studied. Engraftment was obtained in 7 of these cases; severe, lethal GvH disease occurred in 4. More recently, workers at the National Cancer Institute have reported on 9 HL-A matched sibling pairs in whom leukemia was the underlying disorder; 7 obtained viable grafts, but only 5 developed significant GvH disease.[22] For the optimist, a trend is indeed visible in these early findings. The likelihood of obtaining a successful engraftment is very high now, and there seems to be less significant graft-versus-host disease. It is still much too early to make any useful statements about the usefulness of the procedure as a therapeutic maneuver for human leukemia.

Discussion

Clinical bone marrow transplantation as it is currently practiced is neither "fish nor fowl" as a therapeutic procedure. It is carried out by an enthusiastic cadre of clinical investigators who are riding the crest of an optimistic wave borne by only suggestive preliminary data. Consequently, a prediction of its ultimate place in clinical therapy would be imprudent and very likely incorrect. Clearly, bone marrow transplantation offers some hope as a potentially important tool in the therapeutic armamentarium of the physician caring for patients with hematologic malignancies. However, its ultimate role will depend upon further advances and refining of contemporary tissue typing, improvement in immunosuppression regimens, and gathering sophistication in the clinical care of these desperately ill patients by judicious use of reverse isolation rooms, leukocyte transfusions, and antibiotics. Most importantly, its ultimate utility will depend upon an expanded understanding of the graft-versus-host process, especially with regard to our ability to control it, and to direct its destructive potential preferentially toward the leukemic disease.

References

1. Mathé, G., Bernard, J., Schwarzenberg, L., Larrieu, M. J., Lalanne, C. M., et al.: Treatment of leukemic subjects in remission by total-body irradiation followed by homologous bone marrow transfusion. Rev. Franc. Etud. Clin. Biol. 4:675, 1959.
2. Thomas, E. D., Lochte, H. L. and Ferrebee, J. W.: Irradiation of the entire body and marrow transplantation: Some observations and comments. Blood 14:1, 1959.
3. Rapaport, F. T., Dausset, J., Barge, A. and Hors, H.: ABO erythrocyte antigens in transplantation: Sensitization to skin allografts with soluble A substance. *In* Proceedings of First International Congress of the Transplantation Society. Copenhagen: Munksgaard, 1967, p. 311.
4. Dausset, J., Ivanyi, P. and Ivanyi, D.: Tissue alloantigens in the human: Identification of a complex system (Hu-1). *In* Histocompatibility Testing. Copenhagen: Munksgaard, 1967, p. 51.
5. Dausset, J. and Nenna, A.: Presence d'une leucoagglutine dans le serum d'un cas d'agranulocytose chronique. C. R. Soc. Biol. 146:1539, 1952.
6. W.H.O. Terminology Report. *In* Histocompatibility Testing. Baltimore: Williams and Wilkins, 1970, p. 4.
7. Kissmeyer-Nielsen, F., Svejgaard, A. and Hauge, M.: Genetics of the human HL-A transplantation system. Nature 219:1116, 1968.
8. Sandberg, L., Thorsby, E., Kissmeyer-Nielsen, F. and Lindholm, A.: Evidence of a third sublocus within the HL-A chromosomal region. *In* Histocompatibility Testing. Baltimore: Williams and Wilkins, 1970, p. 165.
9. Bach, F. and Hirschorn, K.: Lymphocyte interaction: A potential histocompatibility test in vitro. Science 143:813, 1964.
10. Bach, F.: Transplantation: Pairing of donor and recipient. Science 168:1170, 1970.
11. Billingham, R. E.: The biology of graft-versus-host reactions. Harvey Lect. 62:21, 1968.
12. Streilein, J. W. and Billingham, R. E.: An analysis of graft-versus-host disease in Syrian hamsters. I. The epidermolytic syndrome: Description and studies on its procurement. J. Exp. Med. 132:163, 1970.
13. Wilson, D. B. and Elkins, W. L.: Proliferative interaction of lymphocytes in vitro and in vivo: Manifestations of immunologic competence. *In* Proceedings of Third Leukocyte Culture Conference. New York: Appleton-Century-Crofts, 1969, p. 391.
14. Mathé, G. and Amiel, J. L.: Immunotherapy, new method of treatment of leukaemias. Nouv. Rev. Franc. Hemat. 4:211, 1964.
15. Owens, A. H.: Effect of graft-versus-host disease on the course of L1210 leukemia. Exp. Hemat. 20:43, 1970.
16. Glasspiegel, J. S., Saltzstein, E. C., Rimm, A. S., Giller, R. H. and Bortin, M. M.: Graft versus leukemia: Adoptive immunotherapy for the eradication of murine leukemia (in press.)
17. Streilein, J. W.: Common pathogenesis for the lesions of GvH disease. Transplant. Proc. 3:418, 1971.
18. Sensenbrenner, L. L. and Santos, G. W.: Effect of syngeneic and allogeneic lymph node cells on spleen colony-forming units. Fed. Proc. 29:785, 1970.
19. Thomas, E. D., Rudolph, R. H., Fefer, A., Storb, R., Buckner, C. D. and Neiman, P. E.: Isogeneic marrow grafting in man (in press).
20. Bortin, M. M.: A compendium of reported human bone marrow transplants. Transplantation 9:571, 1970.
21. Congdon, C. C.: Cooperative group on bone marrow transplantation in man. Exp. Hemat. 20:97, 1970.
22. Graw, R. G., Yankee, R. A., Leventhal, B. G., Rogentine, G. N., Herzig, G. P., et al.: Graft-versus-host disease complicating HL-A matched bone marrow transplantation (in press).

Hypersplenism and Chemotherapy

By Leif G. Suhrland, M.D.

THE SPLEEN AND ITS STRUCTURE, function and circulation have been the subjects of considerable controversy for many years. Some of the disagreement has arisen because the human spleen has no exact counterpart in other animals. There is enough species variation, both structurally and functionally, to make direct transfer of information from animals to humans inapplicable. In addition, the study of splenic function is complicated by the fact that this organ shares many cellular components with other organs and tissues. However, during the last decade, through the careful work of Weiss, Jandl, Aster, Weed, Bowdler, Murphy and many others, much of the mystique has been replaced by scientific observations, and a clarification of the role of the spleen in health and disease has resulted.

Since the purpose of this volume is to expand our basic knowledge of malignant neoplastic disease, it seems particularly relevant to increase our understanding of an organ that frequently becomes involved, directly or indirectly, in the cancer process. The association of the spleen with alterations in cellular elements of peripheral blood has been known for more than a half century. Yet we have only recently cast aside some misconceptions surrounding this organ by elucidating its normal and abnormal functions. The title of this chapter suggests that we may be dealing with an exaggeration of processes that occur naturally within the spleen. Therefore, a brief review of current knowledge concerning the structure and function of the spleen may help us to understand conditions of hematologic and immunologic importance.

The spleen is essentially a vascular organ composed of three main components: vascular channels, lymphatic tissue, and phagocytic cells.

Other components such as autonomic nerve supply, connective tissue framework and lymphatic drainage channels, are important structurally, but less so functionally in man. Since it is within this vascular structure that both cellular as well as non-cellular elements of the blood are modified, the pathways that these elements traverse will be described.

Blood enters the splenic artery from the celiac axis at a flow rate normally about 150 ml/min (Fig. 1). From the splenic arteries, blood courses through trabecular arteries and enters the white pulp as central arteries. Here, arterioles are given off, to terminate in the white pulp, where is is thought that some plasma skimming occurs, concentrating red cells in the central artery. This artery, as it penetrates the red pulp, becomes the artery of the pulp, branching into many smaller arterioles. The blood is then finally collected in the splenic sinuses of the red pulp. Some uncertainty still exists regarding these latter connections. Between the splenic sinuses are the so-called splenic cords of Billroth, a reticular meshwork of the pulp which may provide a principal route of flow. At any rate, blood is finally collected in the pulp vein and thence to the splenic vein outside the organ to the portal circulation. During this transit period, which may range from 20 seconds to 2 minutes in the normal spleen, red cells are subjected to a variety of stresses, both metabolic and physical. It is also during this

---

From the Department of Medicine, College of Human Medicine, Michigan State University, East Lansing, Michigan.

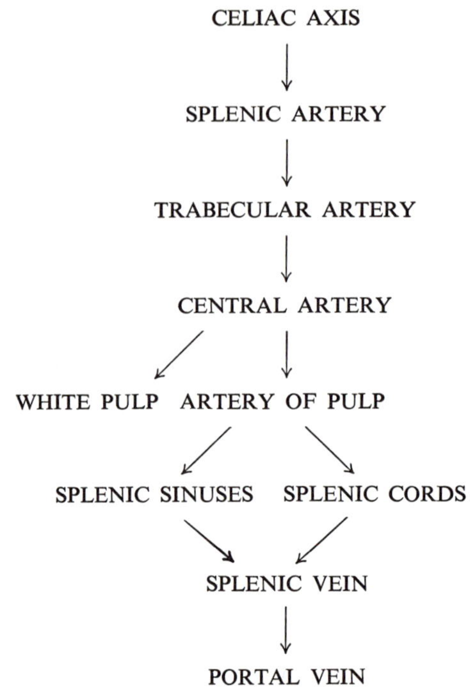

FIG. 1.—Diagrammatic representation of splenic circulation.

period that blood cells are exposed to numerous different types of phagocytic cells lining the sinuses, where fragmentation and destruction may occur.

This concept of the splenic circulation, although incomplete and perhaps oversimplified, may provide a background for a brief review of splenic functions in man. In general, it is possible to classify these into three main categories: production, destruction, and storage or pooling.

PRODUCTION

Normally, after the newborn period, the spleen is not a site of extramedullary hematopoiesis. Lymphopoiesis, however, does occur but only on a limited scale, and contributes very little to the total lymphocyte economy except through recirculation of these cells. On the other hand, the spleen is intimately involved in antibody formation, but even here its role is dependent upon the type and route of entry of antigenic material. Blood-borne particulate antigens are more likely to be trapped and to produce a specific antibody response. Still a mystery is how the message of this antigenic material is transferred from the phagocytes to immunocompetent cells.

DESTRUCTION

A major function of the spleen is removing particulate material from the blood. This capability is enhanced by the unique circulatory system found within the spleen, as previously described. Thus red cells, leukocytes and platelets when altered even to mild degrees may be readily removed from the circulation. Bacteria and other particulate material likewise may be phagocytized in the spleen. Metastatic carcinoma to the spleen is not common, although microscopic foci of tumor cells frequently are found. This suggests that the spleen normally provides an adequate filtering system, but a hostile environment inhibits further proliferation.

As the spleen enlarges, normal phagocytic function may become more pronounced and frequently involves only the red cells. Sequestration and destruction of leukocytes may occur, but is less readily demonstrable.

Storage or Pooling

Man, unlike some animals, has little capacity to store red cells in the spleen. Normally, the red cell content in the spleen is only 20 to 40 ml. However, in pathologic states with splenomegaly, the capacity to pool red cells may be increased to approximately 20 per cent of the total circulating red cell mass. Transit time may be considerably prolonged, thus effectively removing this red cell mass from the peripheral circulation.

Pooling of platelets in the normal spleen, on the other hand, may account for up to one-third of the total platelet mass. In splenic enlargement this pool size may be markedly increased up to 90 per cent of the platelet mass and may occur with only minimal enlargement of the spleen.

Although the spleen may be considered a major source for the recirculation of lymphocytes, a leukocyte pool probably is small, if one exists at all. In addition, under pathologic states with splenomegaly, the presence of such a pool of leukocytes has not been demonstrated in the human spleen. However, it is quite likely that a splenic pooling of cells may be an important mechanism in the development of peripheral cytopenias associated with splenomegaly.

The term *hypersplenism* has been popularized by Dameshek and Doan and encompasses a variety of unrelated disorders with certain findings in common. The characteristic findings for this condition are (1) an enlarged spleen, (2) a reduction in one or more cellular elements of the blood, and (3) normal or hyperplastic bone marrow.

Splenectomy in this disorder tends to correct the blood cytopendia. Although the mechanisms causing the reduction in peripheral blood counts are not completely understood, an exaggeration of the normal functions of the spleen appears to be the most likely explanation. These are destruction and pooling, or a combination of the two functions. Another mechanism has been proposed by some workers in which the spleen elaborates a humoral substance that inhibits the release of cells from the bone marrow. Isolation and characterization of this substance have not been reported, and consequently this remains in the hypothetical stage.

It is obvious that when hypersplenism intervenes in the course of a malignant neoplastic disease, the resulting cytopenia influences subsequent therapy, whether radiation or chemotherapy. Therefore, consideration will be given to four general areas: prevention, early recognition, treatment, and the influence of treatment on subsequent chemotherapy.

The development of hypersplenism in the lymphomas and leukemias is difficult to predict but occurs with such frequency that consideration might be given to a prophylactic splenectomy. This, of course, is being done in various centers in this country in the treatment of Hodgkin's disease as an adjunct to clinical staging. Results of these studies must await an adequate trial with proper controls.

Early recognition of splenomegaly is now possible through the development of new techniques in radiography and nuclear medicine, adding another dimension to physical diagnosis. In addition to the early detection of splenic enlargement, differentiation must be made between the effects of treatment and hypersplenism. An adequate bone marrow examination is essential.

When diagnostic criteria for hypersplenism have been satisfied, choices for subsequent treatment are limited. Radiation therapy to the spleen has not been very effective, and chemotherapy is usually restricted by the cytopenia. Splenectomy is the recommended procedure provided the patient can withstand major surgery. In addition, blood component products should be readily available with adequate facilities and personnel for handling postoperative complications. Hemorrhage and infection are the most common causes of postoperative mortality. After a successful splenectomy, with the return of peripheral blood counts toward normal, further treatment of the underlying disease with chemotherapy may be possible. Reports from this country and Europe suggest that patients with lymphosarcoma or chronic lymphatic leukemia with hypersplenism are more likely to benefit from splenectomy than are patients with the other lymphomas and leukemias. However, the groups are too small and varied to draw any firm conclusions. Furthermore, lack of proper controls should add caution to the final interpretation of these studies.

BIBLIOGRAPHY*

1. Aster, R. H.: Pooling of platelets in the spleen: Role in the pathogenesis of "hypersplenic" thrombocytopenia. J. Clin. Invest. 45:645, 1966.
2. Blaustein, A.: The Spleen. New York: McGraw-Hill, 1963.
3. Bowdler, A. S.: The spleen: Structure and function. Brit. J. Hosp. Med. 1:8, 1970.
4. Comas, F. V., Andrews, G. A. and Nelson, B.: Spleen irradiation in secondary hypersplenism. Amer. J. Roentgen. 104:668, 1968.
5. Crosby, W. H., Whelan, T. J. and Heaton, L. D.: Splenectomy in the elderly. Med. Clin. N. Amer. 50:1533, 1966.
6. Dameshek, W. and Gunz, F.: Leukemia. New York: Grune & Stratton, 1964.
7. Doan, C. A.: The spleen: Its structure and function. Postgrad. Med. 43:126, 1968.
8. Gomer, M. M. R., Silverstein, M. N. and ReMine, W. H.: Indication for splenectomy in hematologic diseases. Surg. Gynec. Obstet. 129:129, 1969.
9. Holt, J. M. and Witts, L. J.: Splenectomy in leukemia and reticulosis. Quart. J. Med. 35:369, 1954.
10. Jandl, J. H.: The spleen and reticuloendothelial system. *In* Sodeman, W. A. and Sodeman, W. A., Jr. (Eds.): Pathologic Physiology. Philadelphia: W. B. Saunders, 1967.
11. Jandl, J. H. and Aster, R. H.: Increased splenic pooling and pathogenesis of hypersplenism. Amer. J. Med. Sci. 253:383, 1967.
12. Meeker, W. R., DePerio, R., Grace, J. T. and Stutzman, L.: The role of splenectomy in malignant lymphoma and leukemia. Surg. Clin. N. Amer. 47:1163, 1967.
13. Mittelman, A., Stutzman, L. and Grace, J. T.: Splenectomy in malignant lymphoma and leukemia. Geriatrics 23:142, 1968.
14. Murphy, J. R.: Erythrocyte metabolism. J. Lab. Clin. Med. 60:86, 1962.
15. Norday, A. and Neset, G.: Splenectomy in hematologic diseases. Acta Med. Scand. 183:117, 1968.
16. Rubenstroth-Bauer, G.: The role of humoral splenic factors in the formation and release of blood cells. Seminars Hemat. 2:229, 1965.
17. Strumia, M. D., Strumia, P. V. and Bassert, D.: Splenectomy in leukemia: Hematologic and clinical effects on 34 patients and review of 299 published cases. Cancer Res. 26:519, 1966.
18. Weed, R. and Weiss, L.: The relationship of red cell fragmentation occurring within the spleen to cell destruction. Trans. Ass. Amer. Physicians 79:426, 1966.
19. Weiss, L.: The spleen. Seminars Hemat. 2:205, 1965.
20. Wenneberg, E. and Weiss, L.: The structure of the spleen and hemolysis. Ann. Rev. Med. 20:29, 1969.

*Specific references have been omitted, since the text alludes to general publications from many of the authors listed.

Replacement of Platelets and Granulocytes in Patients with Myelosuppression

By John P. Whitecar, Jr., M.D., David S. deJongh, M.D., and Emil J Freireich, M.D.

MYELOSUPPRESSION is a commonly encountered complication of the modern treatment of patients with cancer, resulting from the malignant cells that crowd out the normal hematopoietic organ or the specific agents used in treating the disease.

Because of the rapid development of specific agents and improved techniques, effective therapy is now available for many tumors. This has led to the prolongation of useful life for the patient. Therefore, regardless of the cause, aggressive and effective supportive measures must be utilized to assist the patient through periods of myelosuppression. Successful control and eradication of the underlying neoplastic disease frequently depend on the ability of the patient to survive the period of myelosuppression.

Acute leukemia is a model of all diseases with myelosuppression, whether due to bone marrow infiltration with malignant cells or to therapeutic manipulation. Patients with acute leukemia die almost exclusively as a result of bone marrow failure associated with the disease, resulting in either hemorrhage or infection.

Indications for Replacement Therapy

The deficiency of any substance is an indication for its replacement. However, when the deficiency may be transient in nature or there is a measurable risk related to its replacement, replacement is indicated only when the deficiency reaches the level at which there is a high probability of serious consequences. A quantitative relation exists between the level of the circulating platelet and granulocyte counts and the risk of hemorrhage and infection, respectively. Ideally, both of these formed elements should be administered to maintain the circulating concentration of both cell types above the level known to cause potentially serious consequences.

In the case of platelets, such capability now exists and, in fact, is routinely utilized. In one study, when the platelet count was less than 1,000/cu mm, hemorrhage was observed on 92 per cent of the days; on 30 per cent of the days gross hemorrhage occurred (Table 1).[1] In contrast, when the platelet count was greater than 100,000/cu mm, hemorrhage was present on less than 1 per cent of the days, and gross hemorrhage occurred on only 0.07 per cent of the days. Since gross bleeding includes the life-threatening forms of hemorrhagic complication, maintenance of a platelet count greater than 20,000/cu mm is usually associated with the elimination of a major threat to life. Therefore, in patients without apparent hemorrhage, maintenance of a platelet count above 20,000/cu mm by replacement therapy will be associated with a minimum frequency of severe hemorrhage. Hemorrhage does occur, however, in patients with platelet counts greater than 20,000 and in those instances transfusion would also be indicated. If hemorrhage occurs in patients with

---

From the Departments of Developmental Therapeutics and Clinical Pathology, The University of Texas M. D. Anderson Hospital and Tumor Institute at Houston, Houston, Texas.

TABLE 1.—*Relation Between Platelet Count and Hemorrhage in Patients with Acute Leukemia*[1]

Platelet count (× 10^3 *per cu mm*)	*Days with any hemorrhage* (%)	*Days with gross hemorrhage* (%)
<1	92	30
1–3	79	11
3–5	66	7
5–10	54	4
10–20	38	2
20–50	16	0.8
50–100	8	0.3
>100	<1	0.07

From Gaydos, Freireich and Mantel,[1] with permission.

platelet counts greater than 100,000 whose platelets are otherwise normal, most likely there is another cause for the hemorrhage.

A similar quantitative relation exists between the frequency and severity of infection and the level of circulating granulocytes (Table 2).[2] When the absolute granulocyte count was less than 100/cu mm, more than 50 per cent of the days were associated with identified infection and 15 per cent of the days were accompanied by disseminated severe infection. When the circulating granulocyte count is greater than 1,000/cu mm, however, the number of days associated with identified infection was reduced to 9 per cent, and only 1 per cent of the days were associated with disseminated infection. Obviously, the goal should be to maintain the circulating granulocyte concentration in excess of 1,000/cu mm throughout the patient's course of therapy. Unfortunately, at the present time such resources are not available, and granulocyte transfusions, for the most part, are restricted to patients with identified infection.

TABLE 2.—*Relation Between Granulocyte Level and Infection*[2]

Granulocyte count per cu mm	*Fever without proved infection**	*Identified infection**	*Disseminated infection**
<100	9	53	15
100–500	8	36	6
500–1000	8	20	2
1000–1500	7	9	1
>1500	4	10	1

* Percentage of days spent at each granulocyte level.
From Bodey et al.,[2] with permission.

CRITERIA FOR EFFECTIVE TRANSFUSION

When erythrocytes are transfused, a simple measurement of the post-transfusion hemoglobin concentration or hematocrit reveals the effectiveness of the transfusion in replacing the deficient formed elements. However, the platelet and the granulocyte are unique and differ from the erythrocyte in two important ways: the volumes of distribution are markedly different,[3] and normal granulocyte and platelet function require that they be destroyed while carrying out their physiologic roles. Three methods are available to evaluate the effectiveness of transfusion of platelets and granulocytes. In patients who are bleeding or who have infections, cessation of hemorrhage and lysis of fever with clearing of infection are indisputable evidence of the effectiveness of the transfused elements. For research purposes, labeling of the cells with ^{51}Cr or $DF^{32}P$ will permit measurement of the number of transfused cells present in the circulation of the recipient at any time after transfusion. This technique will distinguish between the transfused cells and the endogenous cells of the recipient. However, for clinical purposes, in the absence of hemorrhage and infection, a platelet count and granulocyte count increment is ordinarily measured 1 hour after and 20 hours after a transfusion. Although this will not identify the exact survival time of the transfused cells, it will measure the duration of protection against hemorrhage or infection and therefore indicate the requirements in terms of dose and frequency of replacement.

Survival of Transfused Cells

The half-life of platelets and granulocytes in normal subjects is 4 to 8 days[4] and 4 to 8 hours,[5] respectively. In severely thrombocytopenic patients, however, the half-life of circulating platelets is only 1 to 2 days. The survival of granulocytes from patients with chronic myelocytic leukemia (CML) appears to be longer than those from normal donors and may be related to the transfusion of immature granulocytes which mature in the recipient.[6] The half-life of transfused granulocytes (CML) is less than 10 hours.

Survival data indicate that transfusion of platelets is required every 2 or 3 days and granulocytes daily to maintain effective circulating levels.

Collection of Cells for Transfusion

Platelets may be harvested from any unit of fresh whole blood. However, plasmapheresis is a more satisfactory technique because at least two units may be collected from a donor at a single session and the erythrocytes may be returned to the donor, making it possible for him to donate as frequently as twice a week. To date the only known limitation on platelet donation is the loss of protein associated with the plasmapheresis, and this may be obviated by returning the plasma to the donor.[7] Tissue typing of both the donor and the recipient has been useful in donors refractory to random platelet transfusion. The post-transfusion increment and the survival of transfused platelets were greater in cases where the donor-recipient pairs were "histocompatible."[8] However, there is no evidence at present of a similar advantage in unrelated "histocompatible" donor pairs. Since most adult patients require at least a 4-unit transfusion of platelets, the recent development of the 4-unit plasmapheresis technique[9] will permit a single donor-recipient pairing, thereby effecting optimal control of the transfusion variables. A unit of platelets is defined as the platelets obtained from 1 unit of whole blood, whether the platelets are transfused as a unit of fresh whole blood, platelet-rich plasma or platelet concentrates.

In the past, platelet transfusion practice was limited by the need to utilize only fresh preparations, preferably within 6 hours of collection. Since the demonstration that platelets should be processed and stored at room temperature for maximal preservation, stored platelets are now used routinely in many centers. Platelets may be stored for 24 to 48 hours and still be reasonably effective in patients with severe thrombopenia.[10] This storage should be carried out at 22° C. Storage temperatures higher or lower than 22° C result in shorter platelet survival time.[11]

Granulocytes may be prepared from whole-blood collections, but the buffy coats of 30 to 50 units are required to achieve an adequate dose of granulocytes for a granulocytopenic child.[6] Granulocytes may also be collected by a routine plasmapheresis technique similar to that used for platelet collection. However, this technique is useful only when the donor has an exceedingly high circulating granulocyte count, as is seen in patients with chronic myelogenous leukemia. In order to collect granulocytes more effectively from either CML or normal donors, the IBM Blood Cell Separator has been utilized by continuous flow separation of the major blood components, with selection of the component desired and the return of the remainder to the donor.[12] The cell separator is even more efficient at collecting chronic myelogenous leukemia granulocytes. When CML granulocytes from closely matched donors by histocompatibility testing are used, the post-transfusion increment is higher.[13] However, techniques for utilizing granulocytes from normal people are rapidly being developed and may soon become established.

Results of Therapy

Since the introduction of platelet transfusion for patients with thrombopenia secondary to acute leukemia, the incidence of deaths associated with hemorrhage was decreased from 85 per cent to 30 per cent.[14] Although all hemorrhage has been reduced, the reduction in severe hemorrhage has been most marked. The transfusion of both fresh and stored platelets has resulted in the rapid cessation of hemorrhage in those patients in whom thrombopenia was responsible.[15] However, 30 per cent of the deaths of patients with acute leukemia are accompanied by major hemorrhage, and many of these patients have evidence of disseminated intravascular coagulation (DIC). DIC activates the fibrinolytic system, resulting in the presence of degradation products of fibrinogen with anticoagulant activity. In these patients heparinization is required as well as replacement of platelets.

Granulocyte transfusions from donors with chronic myelogenous leukemia are clearly effective in reducing fever in as many as 50 per cent of the recipients. These granulocytes have been demonstrated in the bone marrow of patients with marrow hypoplasia, in sites of inflammation,[16] and have been identified engulfing bacteria at the site of infection.[17] The ability of transfusion to achieve this result is dependent on the dose of granulocytes.

The ideal therapy would be the establishment of a temporary myeloid homograft to assist the patient during the period of myelosuppression. Such myeloid homografts have occurred in patients receiving chronic myeloid leukemia granulocytes in the past.[16] The recent demonstration of the ability to harvest cells from the peripheral blood of normal donors which have the capability of forming myeloid colonies in vitro indicates that such a therapeutic triumph may be at hand.[18]

References

1. Gaydos, L. A., Freireich, E. J, and Mantel, N.: The quantitative relationship between platelet count and hemorrhage in patients with acute leukemia. New Eng. J. Med. 266:905, 1962.
2. Bodey, G. P., Buckley, M., Sathe, Y. S. and Freireich, E. J: Quantitative relationships between circulating leukocytes and infection in patients with acute leukemia. Ann. Intern. Med. 64:328, 1966.

3. Freireich, E. J: Replacement of platelets and granulocytes by transfusion. *In* Brodsky, I. and Kahn, S. B. (Eds.): Cancer Chemotherapy. New York: Grune & Stratton, 1967, p. 288.
4. Gardner, F. H. and Cohen, P.: Platelet life span. Transfusion 6:23, 1966.
5. Athens, J. W., Haab, O. P., Raab, S. O., Mauer, A. M., Ashenbrucker, H., et al.: Leukokinetic studies. IV. The total blood circulating and marginal pools and the granulocyte turnover rate in normal subjects. J. Clin. Invest. 40:989, 1961.
6. Yankee, R. A., Freireich, E. J, Carbone, P. P. and Frei, E., III: Replacement therapy using normal and chronic myelogenous leukemia leukocytes. Blood 24:844, 1964.
7. Kliman, A., Carbone, P. P., Gaydos, L. A. and Freireich, E. J: Effects of intensive plasmapheresis on normal blood donors. Blood 23:647, 1964.
8. Yankee, R. A., Grumet, F. C. and Rogentine, G. N.: Platelet transfusion therapy: Selection of donors by lymphocyte HLA typing. New Eng. J. Med. 281:1208, 1969.
9. Yankee, R. A.: Personal communication.
10. Murphy, S., Sayar, S. N. and Gardner, F. H.: Storage of platelet concentrates at 22°C. Blood 35:549, 1970.
11. Murphy, S. and Gardner, F. H.: Platelet preservation. Effect of storage temperature on maintenance of platelet viability: Deleterious effect of refrigerated storage. New Eng. J. Med. 280:1094, 1969.
12. Freireich, E. J, Judson, G. and Levin, R. H.: Separation and collection of leukocytes. Cancer Res. 25:1516, 1965.
13. Graw, R. G., Jr., Eyre, H. J., Goldstein, I. M. and Terasaki, P. I.: Histocompatibility testing for leukocyte transfusion. Lancet 2:77, 1970.
14. Hersh, E. M., Bodey, G. P., Nies, B. A. and Freireich, E. J: Causes of death in acute leukemia. J.A.M.A. 193:105, 1965.
15. Whitecar, J. P., Jr. and Freireich, E. J: Unpublished observations.
16. Freireich, E. J, Levin, R. H., Whang, J., Carbone, P. P., Bronson, W. and Morse, E. E.: The function and fate of transfused leukocytes from donors with chronic myelocytic leukemia in leukopenic recipients. Ann. N.Y. Acad. Sci. 113:1081, 1964.
17. Eyre, H. J., Goldstein, I. M., Perry, S. and Graw, R. G., Jr.: WBC transfusions: Function of transfused granulocytes from donors with chronic myelocytic leukemia (CML). Proc. Amer. Ass. Cancer Res. 11:24, 1970.
18. McCredie, K. B., Hersh, E. M. and Freireich, E. J: Cells capable of colony formation in the peripheral blood of man. Science 171:293, 1971.

Management of Infectious Complications During Cancer Chemotherapy

By Gerald P. Bodey, M.D.

The survival of many patients with malignant diseases has been prolonged by the use of chemotherapeutic agents. However, many of these agents cause substantial toxicity, including myelosuppression, immunosuppression and gastrointestinal ulceration. Maximal antitumor activity is seldom achieved without at least moderate toxicity. Hence, many cancer patients are predisposed to infection because of their disease or its therapy. Now that effective therapy is available for some tumors, the successful management of infectious complications has become increasingly important.

Most infections occurring in cancer patients are caused by gram-negative bacilli.[1] *Escherichia coli*, *Klebsiella* sp. and *Pseudomonas* sp. are responsible for most episodes of septicemia at our institution. During the 3-year period ending in 1969, 85 per cent of the 493 episodes of septicemia were caused by gram-negative bacilli. The incidence of septicemia in patients with metastatic carcinoma was 2.4 per 100 hospital admissions (Table 1), which is six times higher than the incidence in a general hospital.[2] The highest incidence was in patients with leukemia, 45 episodes per 100 admissions. *E. coli* was responsible for the largest proportion of episodes of septicemia in patients with lymphoma, multiple myeloma and metastatic carcinoma, whereas *Pseudomonas* sp. septicemia was most common in leukemic patients.

Cancer patients with impaired host defense mechanisms are susceptible to a wide variety of infectious diseases that are encountered infrequently in most other patients. Serious *Salmonella* infections, clostridial septicemia and listeriosis are a few of the unusual bacteria infections seen in these patients. Disseminated cytomegalovirus

Table 1.—*Incidence of Septicemia in Cancer Patients at University of Texas M. D. Anderson Hospital*

Organism	*Incidence per 100 admissions in patients with* Solid tumors	*Lymphoma and myeloma*	*Leukemia*
Gram-positive cocci	0.3	1.1	5.7
Gram-negative bacilli	1.9	6.9	36.4
E. coli	0.6	3.4	10.0
Pseudomonas	0.4	1.1	10.7
Klebsiella	0.4	0.8	7.1
All septicemia	2.4	8.4	45.0
Average Yearly Admissions	3320	262	140

From Bodey,[1] with permission of Year Book Medical Publishers.

From the Department of Developmental Therapeutics, The University of Texas M. D. Anderson Hospital and Tumor Institute at Houston, Houston, Texas. Dr. Bodey is a Scholar of The Leukemia Society of America, Inc.

Supported in part by USPHS grants CA 10042-05 and CA 05831 from the National Cancer Institute.

and herpes infections, toxoplasmosis and *Pneumocystis carinii* pneumonia occasionally occur in cancer patients and present difficult diagnostic and therapeutic problems.[3–5] The rate of systemic fungal infections has increased during the last decade in association with the use of more effective antitumor and antibacterial therapy.[6,7] Although most of these infections are caused by *Candida* spp., aspergillosis, nocardiosis and cryptococcosis are not uncommon. The diagnosis of these infections is difficult because the organisms seldom can be cultured from sites of infection ante mortem. *Candida* spp. is cultured from the blood of less than 30 per cent of patients with disseminated candidiasis. Pulmonary infiltrates are seen on chest roentgenograms of only 50 per cent of patients with pulmonary fungal disease. It is becoming increasingly apparent that until better diagnostic procedures become available, a therapeutic trial with an antifungal agent such as amphotericin B is necessary for patients in whom the diagnosis of fungal infection is suspected but cannot be proved.

Fever in most cancer patients indicates infection. Patients with lymphoma are the main exception, since nearly 50 per cent of febrile episodes are due to their malignant disease.[8] In patients with acute leukemia, who frequently have granulocytopenia, over 70 per cent of febrile episodes are due to documented infection. These patients are unable to produce an adequate inflammatory response, and may have urinary tract infection without pyuria, meningitis without cerebrospinal fluid pleocytosis, and pneumonia without physical signs or pulmonary infiltrates on chest X-ray films.

Infection is likely to disseminate widely and rapidly in patients with granulocytopenia. Septicemia occurred in 35 per cent of 40 pediatric patients with pneumonia (Table 2) and was confirmed by autopsy examination.[9] None of the patients with granulocyte counts greater than 1000/cu mm had septicemia, as compared with 64 per cent of the patients with granulocyte counts less than 1000/cu mm. Eight of the 10 patients with granulocyte counts less than 100/cu mm had septicemia in association with their pneumonia.

The rapid spread of infection in granulocytopenic patients is illustrated by the clinical course of a 46-year-old woman with acute myelogenous leukemia whose temperature reached 102°F after a platelet transfusion (Fig. 1). Antibiotic therapy was not instituted because she had no other signs or symptoms of infection. Eight hours later she became hypotensive and coarse rales were heard in both lungs. She died 6 hours later despite the rapid intravenous injection of 3 gm of cephalothin and 5 gm of carbenicillin. Autopsy examination revealed extensive pneumonia of the middle lobe of the right lung and foci of gram-positive cocci in the kidneys, ovaries and adrenals. *Staphylococcus aureus* was cultured from two blood specimens obtained shortly before death.

Since infections may cause rapid death in cancer patients, antibiotics must be administered promptly at the onset of fever, before the infecting organism is identified.

TABLE 2.—*Role of Granulocytopenia in Pneumonia and Septicemia*

Granulocyte count/cu mm	*Percentage of patients with* Pneumonia	Pneumonia and Septicemia	*Total*
>1000	100	0	18
<1000	36	64	22
< 100	20	80	10

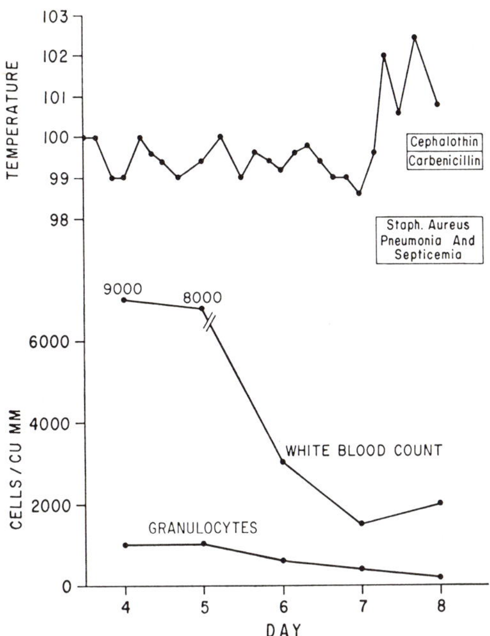

FIG. 1.—Clinical course of a 46-year-old woman with acute myelogenous leukemia who died very rapidly after the onset of *Staphylococcus aureus* septicemia.

Antibiotics must be selected that provide broad-spectrum activity against gram-positive cocci and gram-negative bacilli, including *Pseudomonas* sp. Some antibiotics which are very active against organisms in vitro, are only minimally effective against infections in granulocytopenic patients. For example, the polymyxins are very active against *Pseudomonas* sp. in vitro, but seldom are effective in the treatment of infections occurring in granulocytopenic patients. During the 3-year period ending June 1968, 67 cancer patients at our institution had *Pseudomonas* septicemia.[10] Only 24 per cent of the 46 patients who received a polymyxin antibiotic responded to this therapy. The response rate for patients receiving no antipseudomonal antibiotic was 14 per cent. Twenty-two of the 46 patients already were receiving a polymyxin antibiotic when *Pseudomonas* sp. was cultured from their blood. The response to the polymyxins was related to the patients' ability to produce granulocytes in response to their infection. Of the patients whose granulocyte count increased during the week after onset of septicemia, 58 per cent survived. Of those patients whose granulocyte count either decreased or remained unchanged, only 8 per cent survived.

A major advance in the treatment of *Pseudomonas* infections was the introduction of carbenicillin, a new semisynthetic penicillin.[11] Although the in vitro activity of this drug is only marginal against *Pseudomonas* sp., it has minimal toxicity and can be administered in very high doses. We administered carbenicillin to 39 patients during 43 episodes of *Pseudomonas* infections (Table 3). The response rate was 88 per cent, although 21 per cent of the patients either relapsed when therapy was discontinued or died of other causes before their infection was completely eradicated. Carbenicillin was effective regardless of the site of infection, the status of the patients' host defenses or granulocyte reserves. The poor results obtained by some investigators with this antibiotic are due to the administration of inadequate doses or failure to initiate

TABLE 3.—*Effect of Carbenicillin Against* Pseudomonas *sp. Infections*

Type of infection	*Episodes*	*Response* Complete	*Partial*	*Relapse*	*Failure*
Pneumonia	11	7	0	2	2
Cellulitis	7	4	1	1	1
Septicemia alone*	18	13	2	2	1
Miscellaneous	7	5	1	0	1
All septicemia	31	20	4	4	3
Total	43	29	4	5	5

* Includes 7 patients with ecthyma gangrenosum but negative blood cultures.

antibiotic therapy promptly at the onset of infection.[12] Carbenicillin is also effective against most *Proteus* spp. infections and some *E. coli* infections. It is ineffective against *Klebsiella* sp. and nonpigmented *Serratia* sp., and superinfections caused by these organisms occur in about 15 per cent of granulocytopenic patients receiving carbenicillin.[13]

The effectiveness of carbenicillin is illustrated by the clinical course of a 62-year-old man who underwent treatment for acute myelogenous leukemia (Fig. 2). He became febrile while receiving cloxacillin for a *Staphylococcus aureus* skin abscess. Physical examination was unremarkable, but *Pseudomonas* sp. was cultured from his blood. He was treated with carbenicillin, his fever promptly subsided and the infection was eradicated, despite the fact that his granulocyte count never exceeded 1000/cu mm.

Gentamicin sulfate is being used widely at present because of its broad-spectrum activity. The drug is very effective in the therapy of most gram-negative bacilli infections.[14] Infections caused by nonpigmented *Serratia* sp. have become a serious problem at our institution, and gentamicin is the only antibiotic that is active against this organism. This drug has two important advantages over other aminoglycoside antibiotics. Cross-resistance between gentamicin and other aminoglycosides is only unilateral, that is, organisms which become resistant to gentamicin also become resistant to the other aminoglycosides, but the converse is not true. Second, transfer

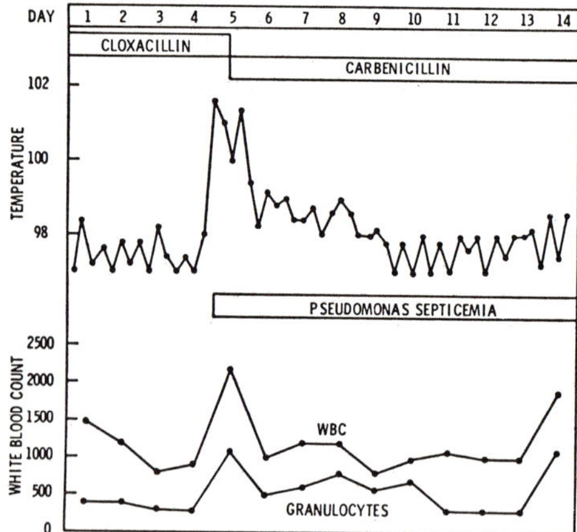

FIG. 2.—Clinical course of a 62-year-old man with acute myelogenous leukemia in whom *Pseudomonas* septicemia developed; the infection responded to carbenicillin therapy.

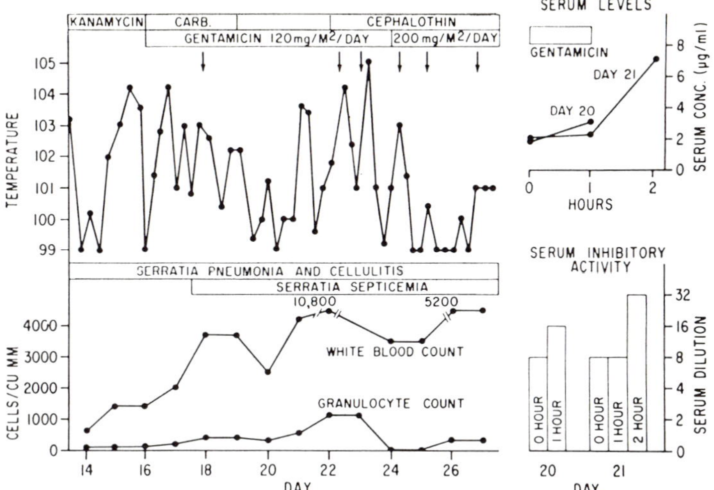

FIG. 3.—Clinical course of a 37-year-old woman with acute myelogenous leukemia in whom *Serratia* infection developed; the infection failed to respond to gentamicin even though the organism remained sensitive in vitro.

of resistance from one organism to another has not been observed for gentamicin.

Although gentamicin is a notable addition to our antibiotic armamentarium, it is only minimally effective in the treatment of infections occurring in patients with granulocytopenia. We have used gentamicin in the treatment of 27 cancer patients with infections caused by the *Klebsiella-Enterobacter-Serratia* group.[15,16] The response rate was 64 per cent for the patients with granulocyte counts greater than 500/cu mm, but only 31 per cent for the patients with granulocyte counts less than 500/cu mm.

Figure 3 illustrates the clinical course of a 37-year-old woman with acute leukemia who failed to respond to gentamicin therapy. Cellulitis in extensive areas, and myositis of the face, neck, arms and thigh developed; cephalothin, kanamycin and carbenicillin were administered. The lesions progressed and pneumonia developed. After multiple culture attempts, *Serratia* sp. resistant to all antibiotics except gentamicin was cultured from an area of cellulitis. Therapy was initiated with 120 mg/m^2/day gentamicin intravenously, and her cellulitis improved. However, *Serratia* sp. was cultured repeatedly from blood specimens and her pneumonia progressed. The dose of gentamicin was increased to 200 mg/m^2/day, but she died of her infection. Her granulocyte count remained under 500/cu mm except after transfusions of white blood cells. All the isolates of *Serratia* sp. cultured from this patient were sensitive in vitro to 0.39 μg/ml gentamicin. On two occasions, her serum inhibited the organism in vitro at a dilution of 1:8 just before she received a dose of gentamicin, and at a dilution of 1:32 when serum concentration reached its peak.

PREVENTION OF INFECTION

Since there is a high incidence of infection in patients undergoing cancer chemotherapy, and the fatality rate from these infections is substantial, methods for preventing infection are being investigated. Prophylactic measures must be directed against both the organisms in the hospital environment and the organisms comprising the patient's endogenous flora. During the past 5 years we have been investi-

TABLE 4.—*Antibiotic Regimens*

Oral regimens Antibiotics	Dosage	*Topical regimens* Antibiotic	Concentration in Aerosol (cc)	Concentration in Ointment (gm)
Antibacterial Agents		Neomycin sulfate	100 mg	50 mg
Regimen A		Nystatin	—	25,000 units
Paromomycin sulfate	500 mg	Vancomycin hydrochloride	10 mg	5 mg
Polymyxin B sulfate	70 mg	Polymyxin B sulfate	5 mg	2.5 mg
Vancomycin hydrochloride	250 mg			
or Regimen B				
Gentamicin sulfate*	200 mg			
Vancomycin hydrochloride	250 mg			
Antifungal Agents				
Amphotericin B†	500 mg			
or Nystatin	3.6 million units			

All antibiotics except nystatin were given in flavored solution every 4 hours. Nystatin was given as 6 tablets and 6 cc suspension every 4 hours.
* Supplied by Schering Corp. as Garamycin syrup.
† Supplied by E. R. Squibb and Sons as Preparation AJS.

gating a prophylactic program which includes the use of isolation units, to protect against nosocomial contamination, and antibiotic regimens to eliminate the endogenous microbial flora.

Two types of patient isolators are being utilized. One unit, the Life Island, is a bed enclosed in a plastic tent (Fig. 4).[17] The other unit is a laminar air flow room (Fig. 5).[18] Both units provide filtered air from which 99.99 per cent of viable particles are removed. In the Life Island, there are 13 air exchanges per hour and air flow is turbu-

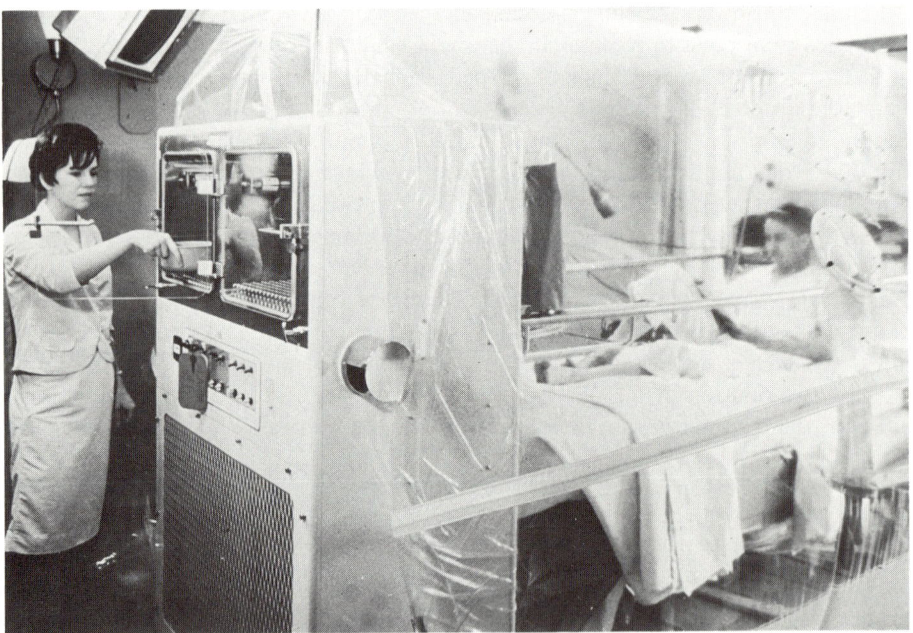

FIG. 4.—Life Island unit.

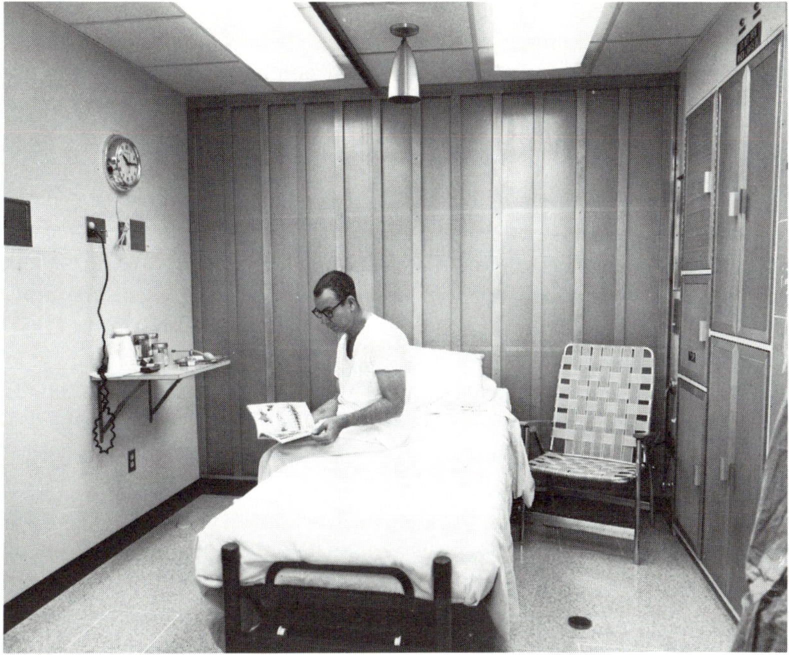

FIG. 5.—Laminar air flow room.

lent. In the laminar air flow room, there are 386 air exchanges per hour and air flow is unidirectional. Procedures can be performed on patients in the Life Island through plastic sleeves on the side of the canopy. Personnel entering the laminar air flow rooms must wear sterile apparel. Both types of units are cleaned and fogged with germicidal agents prior to the patients' occupancy. Patients admitted to both types of isolation units are put on prophylactic oral and topical antibiotic regimens (Table 4) and are given germicidal soap baths. The two oral antibacterial antibiotic regimens are similar in activity and patient tolerance. All items entering the units, including the patients' food, are presterilized by steam or gas autoclaving.

The units are monitored for microbial contamination during the patients' occupancy. In contrast with regular hospital rooms, both types of units substantially reduce the microbial population of the patients' environment, as measured by air and surface sampling (Table 5). Air contamination is 60-fold less in the Life Island

TABLE 5.—*Environmental Cultures of Protected Environment Units*

	LAF rooms*	*Life Islands*	*Hospital rooms*
Air samples			
Number of samples	417	225	26
Organisms/1000 cu ft of air	6	60	3518
Surface samples			
Number of samples	480	1096	—
% sterile samples	91	70	—
Floor samples			
Number of samples	570	—	48
Median organisms/sq ft	50	—	6000

* Laminar air flow.
From Bodey, G. P. and Rodriguez, V.,[19] with permission of Year Book Medical Publishers.

units and 600-fold less in the laminar air flow rooms than in regular hospital rooms. Over 90 per cent of surface samples from the laminar air flow rooms and 70 per cent from the Life Island units are sterile. Microbial contamination of the floors of the laminar air flow rooms and regular hospital rooms is quantitated by swabbing one-foot squares before daily cleansing procedures. Microbial contamination of floor samples in the laminar air flow rooms is 100-fold less than in regular hospital rooms. Only 2 per cent of environmental cultures obtained from laminar air flow rooms and 20 per cent from Life Island units contain organisms that are highly pathogenic, such as *E. coli*, *Pseudomonas* sp., and *Candida* spp. These organisms, introduced into the room by the patients, are eventually eliminated by the cleansing procedures. Nearly 50 per cent of cultures obtained from regular hospital rooms contain highly pathogenic organisms.

Thirty-eight studies have been conducted on 34 patients who remained in the units for a median of 56 days (range 7 to 216 days). Their ages ranged from 13 to 68 years. Eighty-one per cent of the patients tolerated the confinement without difficulty. Six patients who occupied Life Island units manifested psychologic problems which necessitated their removal from the units. All of these patients were seriously ill with complications such as azotemia and infection. Their psychologic problems improved only when these underlying physical disorders were corrected.

Antibiotic regimens were initiated for 35 of the 38 patients. The regimens had to be changed in only three patients, who experienced severe abdominal pain or persistent vomiting. Culture specimens from the patients' ears, nose, throat, skin, urine and stool were obtained before entry into the units and at least weekly thereafter. The types of organisms which persisted despite the antibiotic regimens are shown in Table 6. Fungi or highly pathogenic bacteria were consistently present in the nose and ears of less than 35 per cent of the patients. Fungi were consistently cultured from the stools of 46 per cent of the patients and highly pathogenic bacteria from the stools of 20 per cent of the patients. Fungi persisted in the throats of 51 per cent of the patients and highly pathogenic bacteria in 31 per cent.

Twenty-eight patients with acute leukemia received conventional chemotherapeutic agents, including combinations of vincristine, prednisone, 6-mercaptopurine, methotrexate, arabinosyl cytosine and cyclophosphamide. A group of control patients was selected for comparison who had undergone the same chemotherapeutic regimens and who were similar with respect to age, morphologic diagnosis, prior therapy, and extent of disease. The median survival time from the onset of therapy was 33 weeks for patients in the protected environments compared with 24 weeks for the control group. Fifteen of the 28 protected environment patients and 16 of the 28 control patients had complete remission. However, the duration of remission was

TABLE 6.—*Effect of Antibiotic Regimens on Patients' Microbial Flora*

	Percentage of patients having				
Site	*No organisms*	*No pathogens*	*Fungi*	*No bacterial pathogens*	*Total no. of patients*
Nose	34	66	6	72	35
Ears	30	80	13	93	30
Throat	0	20	49	69	35
Stool	29	34	46	80	35

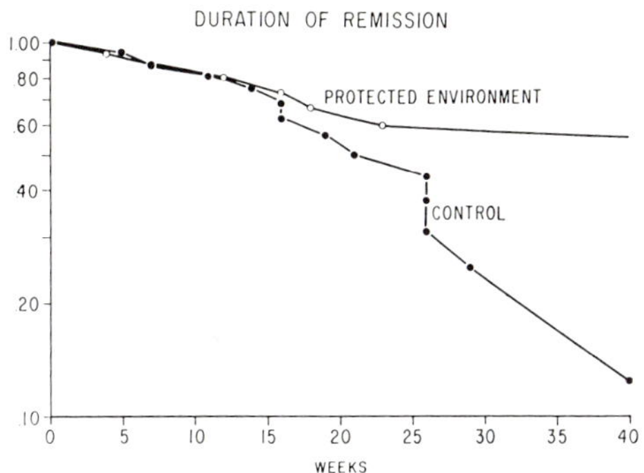

FIG. 6.—Comparison of duration of remission of patients with acute leukemia who received chemotherapy in protected environment units with duration of remission of a corresponding control group.

significantly longer for patients in the protected environment (Fig. 6). The median duration of remission was 40 weeks for the protected environment group compared with 21 weeks for the control group. Many former patients are still in remission. The superior results in the protected environment group are due, at least in part, to the fact that these patients received more intensive chemotherapy. The average maximal dose administered was 50 per cent higher for the patients in the protected environment units.

Since the patients in the protected environment units received more intensive chemotherapy, they spent a greater proportion of their remission induction period with severe granulocytopenia. These patients had granulocyte counts of less than 500/cu mm 54 per cent of their time in comparison with 37 per cent of the control group. The incidence of infections was determined relative to the duration of time spent at various levels of circulating granulocytes, and expressed as number of episodes per 1,000 days (Table 7). The incidence of both local and severe infection was lower in the protected environment group than in the control group. This was true even at normal granulocyte levels.

These studies indicate that patients undergoing cancer chemotherapy are able to tolerate antibiotic prophylaxis and confinement in protected environment units. The program results in a substantial reduction in the patients' microbial burden. Intensive chemotherapy can be administered and results in longer remissions. Although the incidence of infection has been reduced, new antibiotic regimens must be developed if the risk of infection is to be completely eliminated.

TABLE 7.—*Incidence* of Infection Related to Level of Circulating Leukocytes*

Granulocyte Level	*Local infection*		*Severe infection*	
	P.E.†	*C.*†	*P.E.*	*C.*
< 500	12	12	7	17
500–1500	9	15	4	3
> 1500	10	14	0	24

* Expressed as number of episodes per 1,000 days spent at granulocyte level.
† P.E. = protected environment; C. = control.

References

1. Bodey, G. P.: Infections and cancer: Natural history, diagnosis and treatment. *In* Clark, R. L. et al. (Eds.): Oncology, 1970. Vol. 3, Diagnosis and Management of Cancer: General Considerations. Chicago: Year Book Medical Publishers (in press).
2. McCabe, W. R. and Jackson, G. G.: Gram negative bacteremia. Arch. Intern. Med. 110:847, 1962.
3. Bodey, G. P., Wertlake, P. T., Douglas, G. and Levin, R. H.: Cytomegalic inclusion disease in patients with acute leukemia. Ann. Intern. Med. 62:899, 1965.
4. Vietzke, W. M., Gelderman, A. H., Grimley, P. M. and Valsamis, M. P.: Toxoplasmosis complicating malignancy: Experience at the National Cancer Institute. Cancer 21:816, 1968.
5. Esterly, J. A. and Warner, N. E.: *Pneumocystis carinii* pneumonia. Arch. Path. 80:433, 1965.
6. Bodey, G. P.: Fungal infections complicating acute leukemia. J. Chron. Dis. 19:667, 1966.
7. Casazza, A. R., Duvall, C. P. and Carbone, P. P.: Infection in lymphoma: Histology, treatment and duration in relation to incidence and survival. J.A.M.A. 197:710, 1966.
8. Boggs, D. R. and Frei, E., III: Clinical studies of fever and infection in cancer. Cancer 13:1240, 1960.
9. Bodey, G. P. and Hersh, E. M.: The problem of infection in children with malignant disease. *In* Neoplasia in Childhood (Proceedings of the 12th Annual Clinical Conference at The University of Texas M. D. Anderson Hospital and Tumor Institute at Houston, Houston, Texas). Chicago: Year Book Medical Publishers, 1969, pp. 135–154.
10. Whitecar, J. P., Jr., Bodey, G. P. and Luna, M.: *Pseudomonas* septicemia in patients with malignant diseases. Amer. J. Med. Sci. 260: 216, 1970.
11. Acred, P., Brown, D. M., Knudsen, E. T., Rolinson, G. N. and Sutherland, R.: New semi-synthetic penicillin active against *Pseudomonas pyocyanea*. Nature 215:25, 1967.
12. Hoffman, T. A. and Bullock, W. E.: Carbenicillin therapy of *Pseudomonas* and other gram-negative bacillary infections. Ann. Intern. Med. 73:165, 1970.
13. Bodey, G. P., Rodriguez, V. and Luce, J. K.: Carbenicillin therapy of gram-negative bacilli infections. Amer. J. Med. Sci. 257:408, 1969.
14. Martin, C. M., Cuomo, A. J., Geraghty, M. J., Zager, J. R. and Mandes, T. C.: Gram-negative rod bacteremia. J. Infect. Dis. 119:506, 1969.
15. Bodey, G. P., Rodriguez, V. and Smith, J. P.: *Serratia* species infections in cancer patients. Cancer 25:199, 1970.
16. Rodriguez, V., Whitecar, J. P., Jr., and Bodey, G. P.: Therapy of infections with the combination of carbenicillin and genta. micin. Antimicrob. Agents Chemother- 9:386, 1969.
17. Bodey, G. P., Hart, J., Freireich, E. J, and Frei, E., III: Studies of a patient isolator unit and prophylactic antibiotics in cancer chemotherapy. Cancer 22:1018, 1968.
18. Bodey, G. P., Freireich, E. J, and Frei, E., III: Studies of patients in a laminar air flow unit. Cancer 24:972, 1969.
19. Bodey, G. P. and Rodriguez, V.: Prevention and treatment of infections in cancer patients. *In* Oncology, 1970. Vol. 3, Diagnosis and Management of Cancer: General Considerations. Chicago: Year Book Medical Publishers (in press).

The Effects of Androgens on Cancer Chemotherapy

By ISADORE BRODSKY, M.D., S. BENHAM KAHN, M.D.
AND JAMES F. CONROY, D.O.

TO EFFECTIVELY TREAT SOLID TUMORS and hematologic malignancies, dosages of chemotherapeutic drugs producing marrow suppression frequently are required. The dose-response relation for both alkylating agents and antimetabolites is steep.[1]

In a group of patients with lymphoma, a two-fold increase in the dose of folic acid antagonists or an alkylating agent caused a two and one-half to five-fold difference in the proportion of patients evidencing objective responses. However, with the increase in dosage there was also a rise in the proportion of patients manifesting toxicity.[2,3] This problem has become particularly acute with the advent of high-dose, large-field and experimental "prophylactic" radiation therapy for Stage III Hodgkin's disease. Such extensive radiation therapy seriously limits the subsequent use of chemotherapy because of suppression of the bone marrow reserve.[4,5] We agree with Lacher[5] that the whole question of initial aggressive radiation therapy for the treatment of Stage III Hodgkin's disease must be carefully reevaluated.

The development of drugs with a better therapeutic index is essential. However, for the present, methods capable of controlling the toxic effects of chemotherapeutic agents would also permit the administration of larger doses, which would presumably lead to a higher proportion of objective responses. The chief toxic effect that limits further administration of chemotherapeutic drugs is bone marrow suppression. Suppression of erythrocyte activity can be easily managed, at least initially, with blood transfusions, but suppression of marrow granulopoiesis and of thrombopoiesis presents more difficult problems. Leukopenia (WBC < 3000/cu mm) frequently is associated with infection and thrombocytopenia with bleeding. Leukopenia is the most frequently encountered toxic effect of chemotherapeutic drugs. The most important techniques being used to control the side effects of marrow suppression by chemotherapeutic drugs and radiation therapy are: (1) Platelet transfusions to control thrombocytopenia.[6] (2) Transfusions of leukocytes to control drug-induced leukopenia.[7] (3) Prophylactic antibiotics; reverse isolation and Life Islands.[8] (4) Marrow stimulation with androgens.[9,10] (5) Bone marrow transplantation.[11] (6) Extracorporeal irradiation of the blood.[12]

At Hahnemann Medical College, for the past 9 years, we have studied the effects of androgen therapy on the marrow suppressive effects of chemotherapy and radiation therapy. The androgen used most often in our studies has been testosterone enanthate (Delatestryl).[9,10,13]

Balance studies indicate that the primary metabolic effect of testosterone is the induction of an anabolic state, as indicated by retention of nitrogen, phosphorus, potassium, and sulfur in proportions that exist in the protoplasm.[14] The hormone

---

From the Department of Medicine, Division of Hematology and Medical Oncology, Hahnemann Medical College and Hospital, Philadelphia, Pennsylvania.

Supported in part by Clinical Cancer Training Grant CA08024 from the National Cancer Institute, National Institutes of Health.

is metabolized and excreted as urinary 17-ketosteroid compounds.[14,15] Metabolic balance studies have demonstrated variations in anabolic effects between short-acting and long-acting testosterone esters.[15,16] A short-acting steroid ester, testosterone propionate, after a single injection of 600 mg, caused nitrogen retention of 1.02 gm per day, with a total duration of anabolic effect of only 12 days.[16] In contrast, the long-acting steroid ester testosterone enanthate, after a single injection of 700 mg, caused nitrogen retention of 1.76 gm per day.[16] The anabolic activity persisted for 33 days, as compared with 12 days for testosterone propionate. This dose of testosterone enanthate also induced a significant retention of calcium and phosphorus, whereas a similar dose of testosterone propionate did not.[16] Reifenstein and Howard[16] indicated that the anabolic effect of a single injection of testosterone enanthate approached that achieved by the daily administration of such short-acting steroid compounds as methyltestosterone and testosterone propionate. It is conceivable that larger doses of testosterone enanthate will cause even greater metabolic effects. Because of its greater anabolic activity per milligram steroid compound, testosterone enanthate has been used in our studies in preference to the short-acting esters.

It is well documented that testosterone administration stimulates erythropoiesis in man,[9,10,17,18] but the mechanism of action by which this stimulation occurs is still unknown. Present experimental evidence indicates that testosterone causes a rise in the erythrocyte mass by direct stimulation of marrow erythropoiesis in a manner analogous to, but not entirely similar to, erythropoietin. Nathan and Gardner[19] have shown that it is unlikely that the effect of testosterone on erythrocyte production is merely a consequence of a generalized anabolism with a secondary enhancement of erythrocyte cell production. They demonstrated that in the female rat the erythropoietic response to androgen was independent of the effects of the hormone on body composition.[19] Pharmacologic doses of testosterone can also stimulate granulopoiesis and thrombopoiesis.[9,13,20,21] Donati and Gallagher[22] demonstrated that testosterone enanthate stimulated erythropoiesis, granulopoiesis and thrombopoiesis in the rat and had a protective effect on the hematologic suppression that occurred after the administration of 10, 25, 100 or 250 μc of ^{32}P. At higher doses of radioactivity, this particular effect was lost.

In our studies the chief emphasis was placed on the possibility that testosterone, by effecting granulopoiesis, would permit the administration of larger doses of cancer chemotherapeutic agents in patients with solid tumors and hematologic malignancies. The effect of androgen on erythropoiesis was also evaluated.

To evaluate the effect of androgens on the duration and total dosage of chemotherapy, a randomized group of patients should be obtained and carefully matched as to age, sex, type, and extent of tumor. One group would then receive chemotherapy and the other group would receive chemotherapy plus testosterone. The data could then be evaluated for statistical significance. In such an experiment the most difficult problem would be the selection of patients exactly comparable in the clinical severity of the disease. For example, inoperable carcinoma of the stomach with metastasis to the lungs might tolerate more chemotherapy than an inoperable carcinoma with metastasis to the liver. To date such a study has not been performed in patients. The time certainly appears ripe to launch a large scale cooperative venture to evaluate the possible benefits of testosterone and other anabolic steroids as adjuncts to chemotherapy and radiation therapy. Recently Lahiri et al.[23] found that testosterone enanthate was a useful adjunct to chemotherapy in the treatment of 118 patients with advanced cancer. However, there was no control group receiving chemotherapy alone.

In our studies at Hahnemann, because of the small number of suitable patients and the difficulty in obtaining two cases of carcinoma simultaneously with the same extent of disease, each subject was used as his or her own control. In addition, because of the nature of marrow involvement in each group, the data on patients with solid tumors and hematologic malignancies are presented separately.

Ten patients with solid tumors—5 adenocarcinomas of the large bowel, 3 adenocarcinomas of the breast, 1 squamous cell carcinoma of the cervix, and 1 liposarcoma—received first a course of chemotherapy, followed by 6 to 8 weeks of testosterone enanthate in a dose of 600 mg intramuscularly weekly. The drugs used were either 5-fluorouracil (5-FU) or cyclophosphamide (Cytoxan). Subsequently, the same course of chemotherapy was repeated exactly. Marrow function was evaluated by means of serial leukocyte counts, ferrokinetics, bone marrow aspiration, and pyrogen tests immediately after the first course of chemotherapy, and the second course of chemotherapy after administration of testosterone enanthate.[9] The pyrogen stimulation test is used to evaluate the marrow granulocyte reserve.[23] In this test Piromen—a *Pseudomonas* lipopolysaccharide endotoxin, 25 μg—is injected intravenously. Normal subjects challenged by endotoxin characteristically show a fall in the leukocyte count at 1 to 1.5 hours. Then, within 3 to 5 hours, there is a rise of 2500/cu mm or more in the absolute granulocyte count, as compared with the control level before injection. A depressed response indicates a decrease in the marrow granulocytic reserve.[24] This is usually associated with increased sensitivity to chemotherapeutic drugs from the standpoint of the early development of severe leukopenia.

Table 1 shows the results of therapy in ten patients with solid tumors. The data represent the ratios of the average initial white blood cell count (WBC_i) and the

TABLE 1.—*Results in Treating Solid Tumors with Chemotherapy Before and After Administration of Testosterone*

Case no.	*Type of carcinoma*	*Before testosterone* WBC_f/WBC_i*	*After testosterone* WBC_f/WBC_i*	*Chemotherapy*† *(gm)*	*Agent*
1.	Colon	0.18	0.36	3	5-FU
2.	Colon	0.13	0.20	7	5-FU
3.	Colon	0.20	0.65	3.5	5-FU
4.	Colon	0.22	0.53	4.5	5-FU
				3.2	Cyclophos.
5.	Colon‡	0.08	0.10	4	5-FU
6.	Breast	0.29	0.56	4.5	5-FU
7.	Breast	0.19	0.63	5	5-FU
8.	Breast‡	0.16	0.25	4.5	5-FU
9.	Liposarcoma	0.13	0.42	3.2	Cyclophos.
10.	Cervix‡	0.03	0.12	2.5	Cyclophos.
		Median 0.17	Median 0.39		
		Mean 0.16	Mean 0.38		

* WBC_f = lowest white blood cell count after completion of course of chemotherapy.
WBC_i = average white blood cell count before start of chemotherapy.
Fall in white blood cell count expressed as fraction of initial white blood cell count after identical courses of cancer chemotherapy before and after testosterone (WBC_f/WBC_i).
† Identical course (daily dose × time) given before and after testosterone; 5-FU = 5-fluorouracil; Cyclophos. = cyclophosphamide.
‡ Previous pelvic irradiation of 3,000 rads or more.

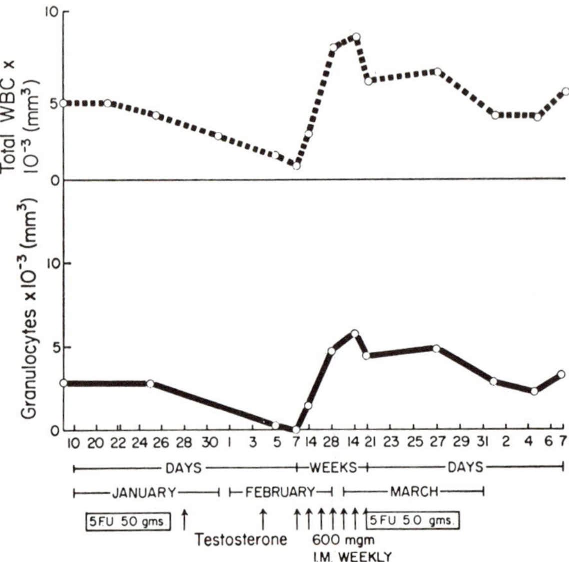

FIG. 1.—Course of a patient with adenocarcinoma of the breast treated with 5-fluorouracil (5-FU) and testosterone.

lowest WBC count obtained (WBC_f) after identical courses of chemotherapy before and after treatment with testosterone. The ratio is WBC_f/WBC_i. The pretestosterone ratio was less than 0.25, with the exception of one case. After treatment with testosterone and an identical course of cancer chemotherapy, 6 of 10 patients had ratios in excess of 0.25. The pretreatment mean was 0.16, with a median of 0.17. After administration of testosterone and an identical course of chemotherapy, the mean was 0.38, with a median of 0.39. A typical case treated in this manner is presented in Figure 1.

In Table 2 are presented seven cases of either multiple myeloma or lymphosarcoma

TABLE 2.—*Results of Chemotherapy in Treating Patients with Lymphoma or Multiple Myeloma Before and After Administration of Testosterone*

Case no.	*Diagnosis*	*Before testosterone* WBC_f/WBC_i*	*After testosterone* WBC_f/WBC_i*	*Chemotherapy*†	
1.	Multiple myeloma	0.17	1.70	28 mg	U.M.
2.	Multiple myeloma	0.22	0.97	76 mg	L-PAM
3.	Multiple myeloma	0.10	0.74	218 mg	L-PAM
4.	Multiple myeloma	0.17	0.75	36 mg	L-PAM
5.	Multiple myeloma	0.39	0.73	120 mg	L-PAM
6.	Lymphosarcoma	0.14	0.67	2.5 gm	Cyclophos.
7.	Lymphosarcoma	0.50	0.50	3.7 gm	Cyclophos.
		Median 0.17	Median 0.74		
		Mean 0.24	Mean 0.87		

* WBC_f = lowest white blood cell count after completion of course of chemotherapy.
WBC_i = average white blood cell count before start of chemotherapy.
Fall in white blood cell count expressed as fraction of initial white blood cell count after identical courses of chemotherapy before and after testosterone (WBC_f/WBC_i).
† Identical course (daily dose × time) given before and after testosterone; U.M. = Uracil mustard; L-PAM = L-phenylalanine mustard; Cyclophos. = cyclophosphamide.

treated in a manner identical to that in the solid tumor cases. The chemotherapeutic drugs used for the patients with myeloma were either uracil mustard (1 case) or melphalan (4 cases). The two patients with lymphosarcoma were treated with cyclophosphamide. Before administration of testosterone enanthate and after the first course of chemotherapy, the mean WBC_f/WBC_i ratio was 0.24, with a median of 0.17. After treatment with testosterone enanthate and an identical course of chemotherapy, the median WBC_f/WBC_i ratio was 0.74, with a mean of 0.87. A typical case treated in this manner is presented in Figure 2.

An analysis of the data for both the solid tumors and the multiple myeloma-lymphosarcoma group indicates that administration of testosterone enanthate decreases the leukocyte cytotoxic effects of the chemotherapeutic agents. The data are presented graphically in Figure 3. The degree of protection is greater in the hematologic malignancies than in the solid tumors. It is recognized that this represents a small series, but the trend has been consistent. It is possible that in the cases of multiple myeloma and lymphosarcoma the first course of chemotherapy produced an objective remission with a decrease in marrow infiltration of either plasma cells or abnormal lymphocytes. Therefore, it is possible that the second course of chemotherapy was better tolerated because of improved marrow function. However, several

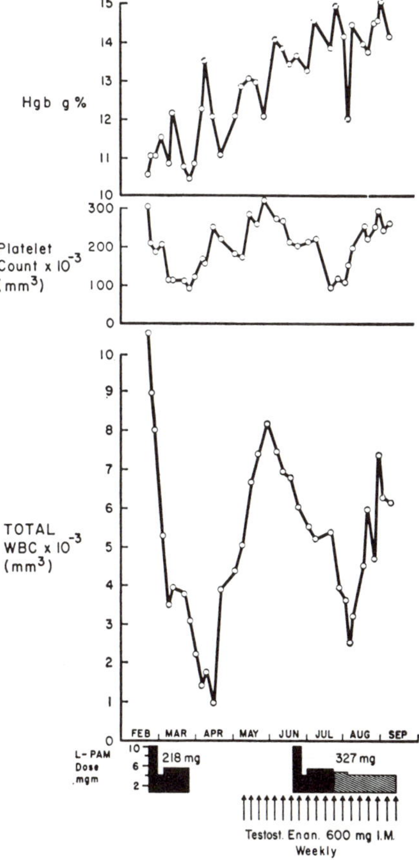

FIG. 2.—Course of a patient with multiple myeloma treated with melphalan (L-PAM) and testosterone.

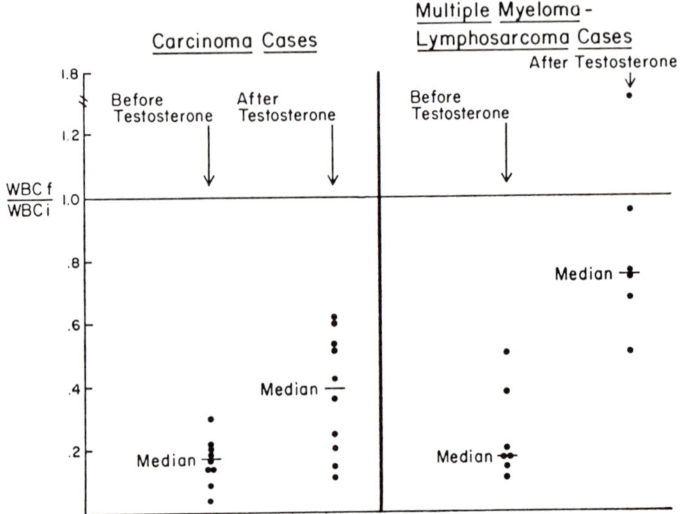

FIG. 3.—Records of a decrease in the leukocyte count of patients with solid tumors or multiple myeloma or lymphosarcoma after identical courses of chemotherapy expressed as fraction of initial leukocyte count before and after testosterone.

patients did not show an objective response to the first course of chemotherapy and yet showed improvement from the standpoint of a decrease in the leukocyte count after the second course of chemotherapy. We initially treated one patient with multiple myeloma to toxic levels (leukocyte count <3000 and platelet count <112,000) with a combination of melphalan (6 mg per day) and testosterone enanthate (600 mg weekly). This therapeutic regimen produced a 30 per cent decrease in the abnormal myeloma protein. The objective response was associated with clinical improvement, as manifested by a cessation of bone pain. Following marrow recovery, melphalan in the same dose (6 mg) was administered without testosterone until the white blood cell count was <3000/cu mm. During the first course of chemotherapy with testosterone, 222 mg (3.7 mg/kg) of melphalan was administered. During the second course without testosterone 206 mg (3.4 mg/kg) of melphalan was given before leukopenia developed. Without testosterone during the second course of chemotherapy a smaller total dose of melphalan was given, even though there had been significant improvement in marrow function after the first course of chemotherapy with testosterone.

The results indicate that the combined use of testosterone and chemotherapy may be most successful in cases of multiple myeloma and the lymphoproliferative disorders. During treatment of multiple myeloma with melphalan, serious hematologic toxicity frequently is encountered.[10] Melphalan in a daily dose of 0.2 mg/kg caused leukopenia in 50 per cent of patients with multiple myeloma who received a total dose of 1.8 to 9.4 mg/kg (median 3.0 mg/kg). Hematologic toxicity resulting in leukopenia, thrombocytopenia, and a fall in hemoglobin concentration greater than 2.0 gm/100 cc was observed in 22 of 34 patients given courses of melphalan; its administration was continued until the WBC fell below 3000/cu mm.[10] Osserman and Takatsuki[25] reported that suppression of leukopoiesis appeared to be an unavoidable counterpart of the tumor-suppressive action of melphalan. The leukocyte count was considered the best index of adequate dosage.[25] In our series the median total toxic dose with melphalan and testosterone was 6.1 mg/kg,[10] compared with

TABLE 3.—*Chemotherapy in Multiple Myeloma*

Patient no.	*Without testosterone enanthate 1st course chemotherapy** *mg*	*mg/kg*	*With testosterone enanthate 2nd course chemotherapy* *mg*	*mg/kg*	*Total dose of testosterone enanthate* *gm*
1.	28	0.36	147	1.9	10.8
2.	76	1.5	235	4.7	11.4
3.	216	4.4	372	7.5	11.4
4.	38	0.65	118	2.2	10.0
5.	120	2.5	242	5.0	14.0
Mean	96	1.9	223	4.3	

* Patient 1 was treated with uracil mustard and patients 2 to 5 were treated with melphalan. Chemotherapy was continued until WBC was 3,000/cu mm.

3.0 and 3.3 mg/kg reported by Bergsagel et al.[26] and Brook et al.[27] In our group of 5 cases, a second course of chemotherapy given with testosterone permitted a higher total dose of either uracil mustard or melphalan to be given before significant leukopenia developed. The data are presented in Table 3.

Another consideration in the use of combination chemotherapy and testosterone is that once marrow suppression has occurred, recovery will be quicker in patients receiving testosterone than in patients not treated with testosterone. Bergsagel et al. indicated that doses of melphalan causing moderate leukopenia resulted in marrow suppression for 6 to 10 weeks.[26] Our results are similar.[10] However, in 10 treatment courses with a combination of melphalan and testosterone enanthate, recovery from leukopenia varied between 1 and 4 weeks, with a median recovery time of 3 weeks.

The cancer patients did not have marrow involvement with tumor cells, but three patients had had previous X-ray therapy. In these cases where exposures were more than 3000 rads to the pelvic area, pyrogen stimulation tests indicated depression in marrow granulocytic reserve. The use of testosterone did not lessen the leukocyte cytotoxic effects of the second course of chemotherapy (Table 1, cases 5, 8, 10).

The effect of testosterone enanthate (600 mg per week for 6 weeks) on the hemoglobin concentration, packed cell volume, and red blood cell mass is presented in Table 4. The red blood cell mass was calculated from chromium (^{51}Cr) tagging red

TABLE 4.—*Effect of Testosterone Enanthate (T.E.) on Erythropoiesis*

Diagnosis	*Hb gm %* *Pre-T.E.*	*Post-T.E.*	*PCV %* *Pre-T.E.*	*Post-T.E.*	*RBC mass (ml)* *Pre-T.E.*	*Post-T.E.*	*Increase in RBC mass (%)*
1. Multiple myeloma	10.1	14.2	33	44	1370	2123	55
2. Multiple myeloma	13.1	17.6	43	53	2858	4485	57
3. Multiple myeloma	12.8	13.4	39	44	1206	1944	61
4. Lymphoma	6.6	11.5	22	38	1248	1813	45
5. Lymphoma	10.6	11.3	35	40	1080	1664	54
6. Lymphoma	10.6	13.2	33	40	1869	2266	21
7. Liposarcoma	10.5	10.5	35	35	1478	1452	−2
8. Ca colon	10.5	9.0	36	32	1302	1165	−10
9. Ca colon	13.6	12.8	43	41	2631	3879	47
10. Ca cervix	9.4	12.2	29	38	1297	1697	31
11. Acute leukemia	9.8	5.3	30	17	805	911	2

Abbreviations: Hb = hemoglobin; PCV = packed cell volume; RBC = red blood cell; Ca = carcinoma.

cells or extrapolation of the radioactive iron (^{59}Fe) clearance curve back to zero time.[28] In 8 of 11 cases there was a significant rise in the RBC mass after administration of testosterone enanthate.

In addition to their possible role in bone marrow stimulation and protection, androgens can directly influence the course of certain solid tumors and hematologic malignancies. Objective remissions are produced by androgens in approximately 21 per cent of postmenopausal women with carcinoma of the breast.[29] Bloom[30] reported favorable results in patients with metastatic adenocarcinoma of the kidney treated with androgens. Gardner and Pringle[31] reported clinical improvement in four out of eight patients with multiple myeloma treated with testosterone enanthate alone, but the only evidence for an objective response was a rise in the hemoglobin concentration.

Our results in the treatment of multiple myeloma also indicate that testosterone singly can cause subjective improvement with a rise in the RBC mass. Testosterone, through its anabolic and marrow stimulating effects, probably acts synergistically with such effective alkylating agents as melphalan in the treatment of multiple myeloma. It is too early to speculate on a possible prolongation in life expectancy with combined testosterone and melphalan therapy. Anemia is frequently a major complication in cases of lymphoma and chronic lymphatic leukemia. Etiologic factors include bone marrow suppression secondary to lymphocytic infiltration, bleeding, hypersplenism, and hemolysis. In some cases the anemia responds dramatically to androgen therapy (Table 4, cases 4–6). Kennedy[32] reported a similar effect of androgens in the treatment of lymphosarcoma and chronic lymphatic leukemia. It has been our impression that testosterone administration in some cases of lymphosarcoma was associated with a decrease in lymphadenopathy and splenomegaly suggesting lympholysis. West[33] reported favorable results with massive androgen therapy in 11 of 20 patients with chronic lymphatic leukemia. Stimulation of erythropoiesis was predominant, but in some cases stimulation of granulopoiesis and thrombopoiesis was also noted. In other cases androgen therapy induced lympholysis.[33]

The mechanism by which androgens in pharmacologic doses can directly influence the course of leukemia, lymphoma, multiple myeloma and, in our experience, also Hodgkin's disease, is poorly understood. A direct effect on lymphocyte metabolism has already been suggested. This hypothesis is supported by work in experimental animals. Wettstein-Frey and Craddock[34] demonstrated that administration of testosterone to normal female rats caused increased erythropoiesis and granulocytosis associated with decrease in total nucleated cells in the bone marrow because of a sharp drop in marrow lymphocytes. A similar type of reciprocal reduction in marrow lymphoid cells and increase in hematocrit was noted by Yoffey[35] after hypoxic stimulation of erythropoiesis. Such experiments support the concept that a small lymphocytic type cell might function as the pluripotential hematopoietic stem cell. The thymus is also depleted of lymphocytes following androgen administration.

However, androgens, in contradistinction to the adrenal corticosteroids, do not have a lympholytic effect in that the volume of peripheral lymphatic tissue is maintained.[34–36] We agree with Wettstein-Frey and Craddock that the main effect of androgens is accelerated differentiation of marrow lymphoid cells into erythroid and granulocyte cell lines and thymus lymphoid cells into immunologically active cells in the periphery. Therefore, in the lymphomas, multiple myeloma, and Hodgkin's disease, androgens may have a direct effect on the neoplastic lymphocyte per se. Since lymphocyte metabolism among the different lymphoproliferative disorders is extremely variable, the effects of androgen therapy may also show great variation.[37]

The androgens may be effective in a nonspecific manner by increasing the immune response of the host to the neoplasm. This is an important consideration in view of the great stress now being placed on host factors and immunotherapy in the pathogenesis and treatment of neoplasia.

A final example of the effectiveness of androgens in the treatment of hematologic disorders is a rare case of cyclic neutropenia.[21] This condition is characterized by episodes of neutropenia or agranulocytosis, monocytosis, mucosal ulcers, malaise and fever, recurring approximately every 21 days and lasting 4 to 7 days. Between cycles the patient is in excellent health. The causes of this condition are unknown. Morley and Stohlman[38] have suggested that the basic cause of cyclic neutropenia is bone marrow suppression leading to the more obvious identification of a double feedback mechanism that controls granulopoiesis. One loop alters proliferation of stem cells, whereas the second affects maturation and release of cells into the blood stream.

Approximately 42 cases of cyclic neutropenia have been observed. Thus far only splenectomy and the administration of adrenal steroids have at times lessened the severity of the symptoms, but no therapy has influenced the periodic neutropenia. We reported a case in which androgen therapy (testosterone enanthate) caused subjective and objective improvement by significantly decreasing the severity of the periodic neutropenia.[21] The results of therapy are shown in Figure 4. During the control period from November 1962 to mid-February 1963, agranulocytosis occurred at 3-week intervals. Testosterone enanthate, 600 mg per week, was started in March 1963, and after 6 to 8 weeks of treatment a definite change in the pattern of the illness occurred; the granulocyte count was always above 500/cu mm. During this period the patient was asymptomatic. Splenectomy was performed in August 1963 and testosterone was stopped. A relapse immediately ensued. Testosterone was restarted in January 1964,

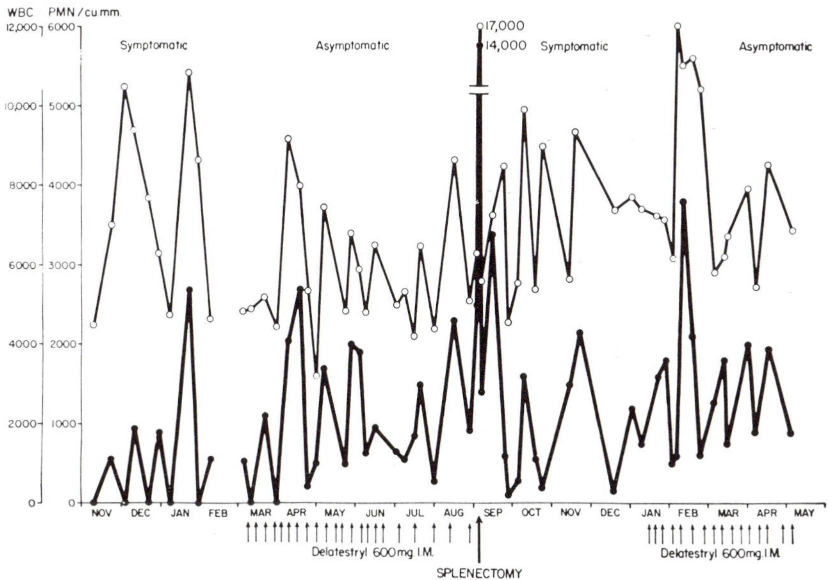

FIG. 4.—Course of a patient treated for cyclic neutropenia with testosterone.

with resultant clinical and hematologic improvement. The effect of testosterone on the marrow granulocytic reserve was documented by pyrogen stimulation tests.

An interesting aspect of this study was the effect of androgens on marrow lymphocytes and peripheral blood lymphocytes and monocytes. The increase in marrow granulocyte reserve was associated with a sharp decrease in marrow lymphocytes. On the basis of present knowledge, one might conclude that lymphocytes in bone marrow were being converted to erythroid and, in particular, myeloid precursors. This would in part overcome the marrow suppression and ameliorate the severity of the cyclic neutropenia.

The important side effects associated with administration of testosterone have been (1) local pain at the site of injection, 10 per cent of cases; (2) acneform eruptions; (3) increased libido in males and females; (4) masculinization in females, associated with hirsutism and deepening of the voice; (5) fluid retention; (6) prostatic hypertrophy; (7) increased sensitivity to heat; and (8) hyperuricemia.[39] The chief point of concern is the masculinization of female patients. In one case deepening of the voice was irreversible. On several occasions we have been forced to discontinue the hormone because of excessive and intolerable increase in the libido in a female. Fluid retention is easily controlled with diuretics; this is a greater problem in females than in males. Nathan and Gardner[19] noted more fluid retention in female rats than in male rats treated with androgens. The case of cyclic neutropenia developed 2+ prostatic hypertrophy, but there were no symptoms of urinary obstruction. The development of marked hyperuricemia occasionally has been reported in patients with myelofibrosis treated with androgens.[39] This complication was not noted in our series. In general, massive parenteral androgen therapy is better tolerated, with less dangerous side effects, than high doses of adrenal corticosteroids.

Obviously, many questions remain to be answered, such as the dosage of androgens; evaluation of other anabolic androgens, such as nandrolone phenpropionate (Durabolin), combination chemotherapy, androgen therapy, and immunotherapy; and the effects of combined adrenal corticosteroid treatment and androgen therapy on the course of certain lymphoproliferative disorders. The antitumor efficacy of nandrolone phenpropionate was equal to or greater than testosterone propionate in advanced breast cancer.[40] Nandrolone phenpropionate also had a protective effect on the bone marrow when administered concomitantly with chlorambucil.[41] At Hahnemann we

TABLE 5.—*Effect of Nandrolone Phenpropionate (N.P.—Durabolin) on Erythropoiesis*

Diagnosis	*Hb gm %* Pre-N.P.	*Hb gm %* Post-N.P.	*PCV %* Pre-N.P.	*PCV %* Post-N.P.	*RBC mass (cc)* Pre-N.P.	*RBC mass (cc)* Post-N.P.	*Increase in RBC mass (%)*
1. Multiple myeloma	8.2	11.2	32	35	1134	1312	16
2. Lymphoma	8.6	8.2	28	28	814	1337	64
3. Lymphoma	10.2	10.3	33	34	736	1389	89
4. Lymphoma	13.6	14.0	40	42	1040	1365	31
5. Mesenchymal sarcoma	13.2	13.2	40	39	2808	1958	−30
6. Breast Ca	13.8	14.1	40	45	1293	1979	53
7. Breast Ca	14.2	11.8	40	36	1248	1355	9
8. Myelofibrosis	10.6	13.4	34	40	2048	2921	43
9. P.N.H.	8.2	11.2	32	35	1134	1312	16

Abbreviations: Hb = hemoglobin; PCV = packed cell volume; RBC = red blood cell; Ca = carcinoma; P.N.H. = paroxysmal nocturnal hemoglobinuria.

have recently evaluated the effect of nandrolone phenpropionate on erythropoiesis. The hormone was administered in a dose of 100 mg intramuscularly weekly for 6 weeks (total dose 600 mg) (Table 5). The percentage increase in red cell mass was similar to that obtained with testosterone enanthate in a dose of 600 mg intramuscularly weekly (see Table 4). The masculinizing side effect in this small series was substantially less than that observed with testosterone enanthate. These results are encouraging, and indicate that it may be possible to develop an anabolic agent unassociated with masculinizing side effects on the one hand and bone marrow stimulation and lymphocyte mobilization on the other.

References

1. Frei, E., III: Breast cancer. Ann. Intern. Med. 63:334, 1965.
2. Brindley, C. O., Salvin, L. G., Potee, K. G., Lipowska, B., Shnider, B. I., et al.: Further comparative trial of triethylene thiophosphoramide and mechlorethamine in patients with melanoma and Hodgkin's disease. J. Chron. Dis. 17:19, 1964.
3. Frei, E., III, et al.: Clinical studies of dichloromethotrexate (NSC 29630). Clin. Pharmacol. Ther. 6:160, 1965.
4. Curran, R. E. and Johnson, R.: Tolerance to chemotherapy after prior irradiation for Hodgkin's disease. Ann. Intern. Med. 72:505, 1970.
5. Lacher, M. J.: Chemotherapy of Hodgkin's disease. (This volume.)
6. Freireich, E. J, Kliman, A., Gaydos, L. A., Mantel, N., and Frei, E., III: Response to repeated platelet transfusion from the same donor. Ann. Intern. Med. 59:277, 1963.
7. Freireich, E. J, Levin, R. H., Whang, J., Carbone, P. P., Bronson, W. and Morse, E. E.: The function and fate of transfused leukocytes from donors with chronic myelocytic leukemia in leukopenic recipients. Ann. N.Y. Acad. Sci. 113:1081, 1964.
8. Schwarz, S., Colvin, M., Himmelsbach, C. K., and Frei, E., III: The effect of bacterial suppression and reverse isolation on intensive cancer chemotherapy. Clin. Res. 13:48, 1965.
9. Brodsky, I., Dennis, L. H. and Kahn, S. B.: Testosterone enanthate (NSC-17591) as a bone marrow stimulant during cancer chemotherapy: Preliminary report. Cancer Chemother. Rep. 34:59, 1964.
10. Brodsky, I., Dennis, L. H., DeCastro, N. A., Brady, L. and Kahn, S. B.: Effect of testosterone enanthate and alkylating agents on multiple myeloma. J.A.M.A. 193:874, 1965.
11. Streilein, J. W.: Bone marrow transplantation. (This volume.)
12. Cronkite, E. P., Jansen, C. R., Ma ther G. C., Nielsen, L., Usenik, E. A., et al.: Studies on lymphocytes. I. Lymphopenia produced by prolonged extracorporeal irradiation of the circulation of the blood. Blood 20:203, 1062.
13. Brodsky, I. and Kahn, S. B.: The effect of androgens on cancer chemotherapy. *In* Brodsky, I. and Kahn, S. B. (Eds.): Cancer Chemotherapy. New York: Grune & Stratton, 1967, pp. 275–287.
14. Reifenstein, E. C., Jr., Albright, F. and Wells, S. L.: The accumulation, interpretation, and presentation of data pertaining to metabolic balances, notably those of calcium, phosphorus, and nitrogen. J. Clin. Endocr. 5:367, 1945.
15. Reifenstein, E. C., Jr., Howard, R. P., Turner, H. H. and Lowrinmore, B. S.: Studies comparing the effects of certain testosterone esters in man. J. Amer. Geriat. Soc. 2:293, 1954.
16. Reifenstein, E. C., Jr. and Howard, R. P.: Protein-anabolic effectiveness in postmenopausal and senile osteoporosis of a single injection of the long-acting steroid ester, testosterone enanthate. Metabolism 7: 364, 1958.
17. Gardner, F. H. and Pringle, J. C., Jr.: Androgens and erythropoiesis. II. Treatment and myeloid metaplasia. New Eng. J. Med. 264:103, 1961.
18. Kennedy, B. J.: Stimulation of erythropoiesis by androgenic hormones. Ann. Intern. Med. 57:917, 1962.
19. Nathan, D. G. and Gardner, F. H.: Effects of large doses of androgen on rodent erythropoiesis and body composition. Blood 26:411, 1965.
20. Shahidi, N. T. and Diamond, L. K.: Testosterone induced remission in aplastic anemia of both acquired and congenital types. New Eng. J. Med. 264:953, 1961.

21. Brodsky, I., Reimann, H. and Dennis, L. H.: Treatment of cyclic neutropenia with testosterone. Amer. J. Med. 38:802, 1965.
22. Donati, R. M. and Gallagher, N. I.: Reversion by testosterone (NSC-9700) of radiation induced hematologic depression in rats. Cancer Chemother. Rep. 50:649, 1966.
23. Lahiri, S., Piro, S., Nevinny, H., Biano, G., and Hall, T.: Testosterone enanthate (TE) in the supportive care of the cancer patient. Proc. Amer. Ass. Cancer Res. 11:46, 1970.
24. Fink, M. E. and Calabresi, P.: The granulocyte response to an endotoxin (Pyrexal) as a measure of functional marrow reserve in cancer chemotherapy. Ann. Intern. Med. 57:732, 1962.
25. Osserman, E. F. and Takatsuki, K.: Plasma cell myeloma: gammaglobulin synthesis and structure. Medicine 42:357, 1963.
26. Bergsagel, D. E., Sprague, C. C. and Ross, S. W.: Evaluation of new chemotherapeutic agents in treatment of multiple myeloma: IV. L-phenylalanine mustard (NSC-8806). Cancer Chemother. Rep. 21:87, 1962.
27. Brook, J., Bateman, J. R. and Steinfeld, J. L.: Evaluation of melphalan (NSC-8806) in treatment of multiple myeloma. Cancer Chemother. Rep. 36:25, 1964.
28. Brosdky, I., Kahn, S. B. and Brady, L. W.: Polycythaemia vera: Differential diagnosis by ferrokinetic studies and treatment with busulphan (Myleran). Brit. J. Haemat. 14: 351, 1968.
29. Council on Drugs, Subscommittee on Breast and Genital Cancer, Committee on Research, A.M.A.: Androgens and estrogens in the treatment of disseminated mammary carcinoma: Retrospective study of 944 patients. J.A.M.A. 172:1271, 1960.
30. Bloom, H. J. G.: Hormone treatment of renal tumours: Experimental and clinical observations. *In* Riches, E. (Ed.): Tumours of the Kidney and Ureter. Baltimore: Williams and Wilkins, 1964, p. 311.
31. Gardner, F. H. and Pringle, J. C., Jr.: Androgens and erythropoiesis. I. Preliminary clinical observations. Arch. Intern. Med. 107:846, 1961.
32. Kennedy, B. J.: Androgenic hormone therapy in lymphatic leukemia. J.A.M.A. 190:1130, 1964.
33. West, W. O.: Treatment of bone marrow failure with massive androgen therapy. Ohio Med. J. 61:347, 1965.
34. Wettstein-Frey, M. and Craddock, C. G.: Testosterone-induced depletion of thymus and marrow lymphocytes as related to lymphopoiesis and hematopoiesis. Blood 25:257, 1970.
35. Yoffey, J. M.: The lymphocyte. Ann. Rev. Med. 15:125, 1964.
36. Brodsky, I., Ross, E. M., Kahn, S. B. and Braverman, S. D.: The effect of cortisol on Rauscher virus infection. Cancer Res. 28:297, 1968.
37. Dimitrov, N. V. and Brodsky, I.: Asparagine metabolism in some lymphoproliferative disorders. Cancer Res. 30:1338, 1970.
38. Morley, A. and Stohlman, F.: Cyclophosphamide induced cyclical neutropenia. New Eng. J. Med. 282:643, 1970.
39. Gardner, F. H. and Nathan, D. G.: Androgens and erythropoiesis. III. Further evaluation of testosterone treatment of myelofibrosis. New Eng. J. Med. 274:420, 1966.
40. Wolk, H., Wilde, R. C., Carabasi, R. A. and Bisel, H. F.: Antitumor efficacy of norandrolone phenpropionate compared with testosterone propionate in advanced breast cancer. Cancer 18:651, 1965.
41. Johnston, I. D. A. and Burn, J. I.: Effect of nandrolone (Durabolin) on the white cell counts of rats treated with chlorambucil. *In* Value of Cytotoxic Agents and Anabolic Steroids in the Treatment of Advanced Malignant Disease; Sheffield Symposium. London: Parcener, 1966, pp. 45–55.

IV. HEMATOLOGIC NEOPLASMS

Chemotherapy of Acute Leukemia

By EMIL FREI, III, M.D.

THE SUBSTANTIAL AND CONTINUING PROGRESS in the chemotherapy of childhood acute leukemia is summarized in Figures 1 to 3. In Figure 1, the median survival of children with acute leukemia from 1946 to 1963 is plotted. Prior to the introduction of the folic acid antagonists, the first agents capable of producing complete remission in childhood leukemia,[1] the median survival was two months. With the successive introduction of the folic acid antagonists, the corticosteroids, and the thiopurines, there was a progressive increase in median survival to 10 months by 1953.[2] From 1953 to the early 1960s, the median survival did not change appreciably. In the early 1960s, a number of clinical and basic concepts were applied, with a resultant resurgence of progress in the chemotherapy of acute leukemia (Fig. 2). These represent data from various studies performed by the Acute Leukemia Group B (ALGB).[3]

From 1960 to 1967, the median survival increased from 12 months to 30 months and, for one of the treatment programs introduced 3 years ago, almost 80 per cent of patients were alive and in complete remission at 24 months (see Fig. 2). This extrapolates to a median survival of 3 to 4 years and a 5-year survival rate of 20 to 30 per cent.

The prognosis of patients surviving beyond the fifth year is illustrated in Figure 3,

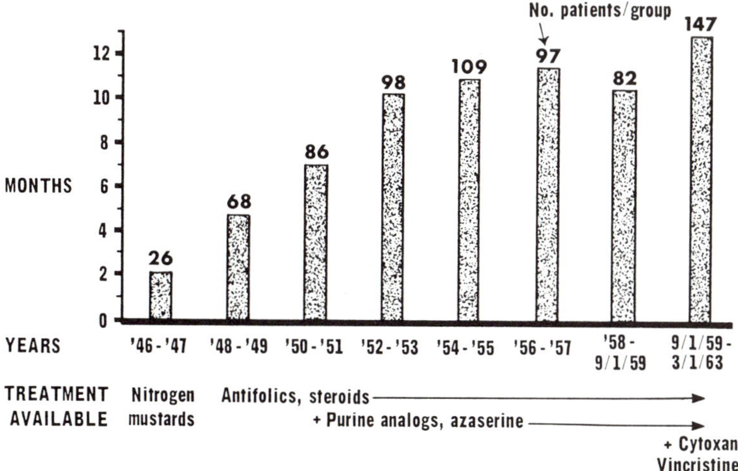

FIG. 1.—Survival of children with acute leukemia from 1946 to 1963. Data from Memorial Hospital for Cancer and Allied Diseases, New York, N. Y. (Statistics through courtesy of Joseph H. Burchenal, M.D.)

From the University of Texas M. D. Anderson Hospital and Tumor Institute at Houston, Houston, Texas.

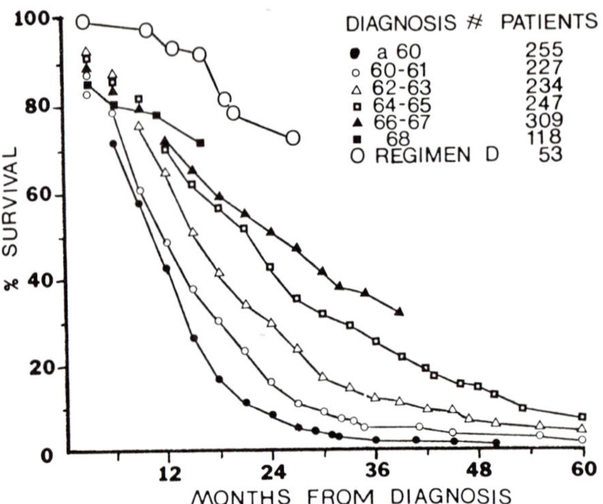

FIG. 2.—Survival of 1390 patients with acute lymphocytic leukemia under age 20. From data of Acute Leukemia Group B (ALGB), cited in Holland,[3] with permission.

where the risk of relapse or fatality per year beyond the fifth year is plotted.[4] The risk of relapse decreases sharply from the fifth to the eighth or ninth year, after which the risk of recurrent disease is minimal. Thus, approximately 25 per cent of patients surviving beyond the fifth year will experience continued long-term leukemia-free survival. Assuming a 20 per cent survival at 5 years, 5 per cent of currently treated patients are destined for long-term leukemia-free survival. It would appear that we are in process of moving beyond the palliative era in the treatment of childhood acute leukemia.[3]

Factors responsible for this marked increase and effective survival in childhood acute leukemia include the introduction of agents capable of producing complete

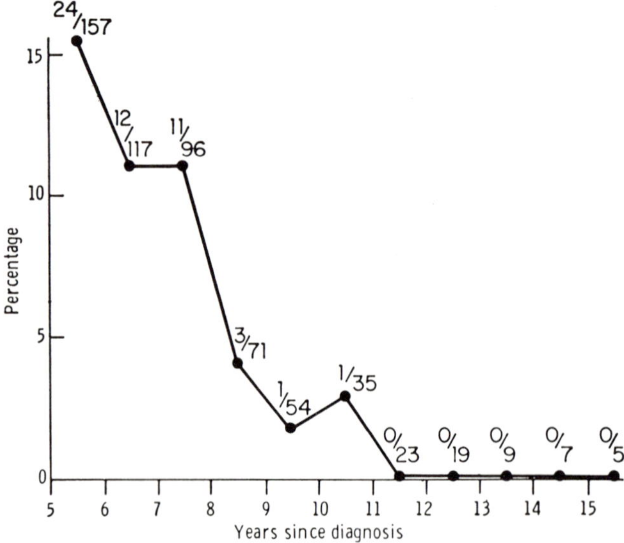

FIG. 3.—Percentage of population at risk dying of acute leukemia, for each year after the fifth year. From Burchenal,[4] with permission.

remission; concepts and application of combination chemotherapy which have resulted in complete remission rates of greater than 90 per cent; recognizing the significance of the complete remission state and its analysis by quantitative studies on the duration of unmaintained and maintained remissions; and the increase in the duration of complete remission by intensive treatment, optimized dose schedules, combination chemotherapy, cyclic therapy, and intermittent reinduction during remission.[1,2,5-11] In parallel with the above, there has been a substantial increase in the effectiveness of supportive care. This has included platelet transfusions for the prophylaxis and treatment of thrombocytopenic hemorrhage and better antibiotic regimens for treating infections.[12,13] Finally, and perhaps most important in the long run, has been the increasingly close and effective interaction of clinical scientists with basic scientists in disciplines relating to therapeutics. This relates particularly to experimental tumor biology, pharmacology, cell population kinetics (cytokinetics), and molecular biology. Experimental tumor biologists and cytokineticists particularly are responsible for a number of newer therapeutic concepts and rationales for clinical trials.[14-16]

The treatment of adult acute leukemia, which is predominantly acute myelocytic leukemia (AML), has progressed much slower than the treatment of childhood leukemia. In the treatment of adult leukemia, we are still at the level of attempting to devise therapeutic regimens which will produce complete remissions in most patients. The rest of this chapter will deal with this objective since it involves the application of many of the concepts listed above.

Within the past several years, two new agents have been found effective in the induction of complete remissions in adults with leukemia. These are arabinosylcytosine (ara-C) and daunarubicin.[17-18] A number of additional agents, such as L-asparaginase, 6-methylmercaptopurine ribonucleoside (MMPR), and dimethylaminoimidazole carboxamide triazeno, have been evaluated and have been found to produce remission rates of less than 15 per cent.

Four major treatment programs which we have used for adult AML are presented in Tables 1 and 2. All the programs involved intensive courses of treatment at 2- to 3-week intervals. This is based on the observation in both the laboratory and

TABLE 1.—*Treatment Programs and Rationale in Acute Myelogenous Leukemia of Adults*

Treatment programs	*Dosage and route*	*Rationale*
MP	90 mg/M^2/day orally	Activity in S 180
MP + *MMPR*	MP 300 mg/M^2/day × 5 intravenously MMPR 100 mg/M^2/day × 5 intravenously 5-day courses every 2 weeks	No cross reference and synergism in L1210 and Ehrlich
Ara-C	200 mg/M^2/day by continuous infusion: 5-day courses every 2 weeks.	Intermittent courses more active in L1210
Ara-C + *Cyclo.*	Ara-C and cyclo. 150 mg/M^2/day for 4 days (given intravenously every 8 hours). 4-day courses every 2 weeks.	Synergism between alkylating agents and ara-C in experimental systems
COAP	Cytoxan and ara-C as above plus prednisone and Oncovin (vincristine).	See text

Abbreviations: MP = 6-mercaptopurine; MMPR = 6-methylmercaptopurine ribonucleoside; ara-C = arabinosylcytosine; cyclo = cyclophosphamide (Cytoxan); COAP = a combination of cyclophosphamide, Oncovin (vincristine), ara-C and prednisone.

TABLE 2.—*Acute Myelocytic Leukemia in Adults: Induction of Remission by Treatment Program*

Patient categories	*MP*[5]	*MP + MMPR*	*ara-C*	*ara-C + Cyclophos.*	*COAP*
Time of study	'58–'60	'66–'67	'66–'67	'67–'68	'68–
Total entered	31	34	36	40	51
Adequate trial*	14	18	24	34	40
Adequate trial / Total entered	45%	53%	67%	83%	79%
Complete remission	3	8	9	16	23
Complete remission / Adequate trial	21%	44%	38%	47%	57%
Complete remission / Total entered	9%	24%	25%	40%	45%

Abbreviations: See Table 1.
* Adequate trial = 6 weeks or more of treatment.

the clinic that intensive, spaced courses of treatment tend to be superior to sustained daily treatment for rapidly proliferating tumors.[11,19,20] The cytokinetic basis for this is discussed below.

MMPR is an adenosine analogue which is converted to the nucleotide, the active intermediate for inhibition of purine biosynthesis, by the enzyme adenosine kinase.[21] Since this enzyme is not deleted in experimental tumors resistant to 6-mercaptopurine (MP), MMPR maintains its activity against MP-resistant L1210 leukemia and Ehrlich ascites carcinoma.[21,22] This was not true for man, however, in that MMPR was not found to be active in inducing remission in patients with acute leukemia initially or in patients who had received and were refractory to MP.[23] In experimental systems, MP and MMPR are synergistic.[22,24] This is perhaps related to the fact that they have separate allosteric sites for feedback inhibition of PRPP* amidotransferase, the first enzymatic step in purine biosynthesis. The combination of MP and MMPR produced a 24 per cent complete remission rate in adults with acute myelogenous leukemia as compared with a 9 per cent complete remission rate for MP alone (see Table 2) and a complete remission rate of zero for MMPR used alone. There are substantial pharmacologic differences between MMPR and MP. Thus, the plasma half-time and urinary excretion of MMPR are prolonged and delayed compared with those of MP. In addition, MMPR concentrates markedly within cells.[25,26] Because of this, a variety of schedules and drug ratios for this combination were studied in experimental systems and in man, but none proved superior to that listed in Table 1. The MP in Table 2 is a historical control,[5] and it remains possible that MP used alone with an intermittent dose schedule in a setting of modern supportive care would produce a complete remission rate comparable to that of MP plus MMPR. However, since other therapeutic leads were more compelling, we have discontinued studies of MP plus MMPR in the treatment of AML.

A demonstration of the application of cytokinetic information to experimental chemotherapy is summarized in Table 3.[27] Ara-C is a cell-cycle-specific agent affecting cells only during the S-phase (DNA synthesis phase) of the mitotic cycle. When ara-C is given by daily schedule to mice bearing L1210 leukemia, a substantial antileukemic

*Phosphoribosyl pyrophosphate.

TABLE 3.—*Combined Therapy with ara-C and Alkylating Agents in L1210 Mouse Leukemia*

Agent(s)	*Schedule*	*Dose* (*Fraction of* LD_{10})	*Response* *Increase in life span* (*median*) (%)	*"Cures"*
	Daily	1	200	0
Ara-C	Every 3 hours × 8 every 4 days	1	450	0
	Single dose	1	200	0
Nitrosourea (CCNU)*	Every 3 hours × 8 every 4 days	1	80	0
Ara-C + CCNU*	Every 3 hours × 8 every 4 days	0.5 0.5	900	90%

Treatment started 48 hours before deaths of controls, i.e., at time when animals have 6 to 7×10^8 cells.
* CCNU = cyclohexylnitrosourea.

effect is achieved, as evidenced by a 200 per cent or three-fold increase in median life span. To affect all the cells at least once during the S-phase, ara-C had to be given continuously over twice the generation time, i.e. over a 24-hour period. The plasma half-time of ara-C in mice is relatively long, so that treatment every three hours constitutes an approximation of continuous treatment.

It has been demonstrated by Bruce[16] that 24 hours of continuous treatment with a cell-cycle-specific agent is not lethal to mice since 20 per cent of bone marrow stem cells are in the nonproliferating pool and reenter the proliferating pool following treatment. Three 24-hour courses of treatment were given every 4 days. It was determined both cytokinetically and in toxicology studies that such an interval allows for complete recovery of the bone marrow and gastrointestinal stem cells.[27-29] Thus, toxicity for such a program was not cumulative and maximal safe doses of 24-hour courses of treatment could be repeated every four days.

This treatment program, at the same cost in host toxicity, produced a much greater antileukemic effect than daily treatment[27] (see Table 3). This treatment program was extrapolated to man (Tables 1, 2 and 4). Ara-C given by 24-hour infusion every 4 days produced a marked increase in cumulative toxicity in man, indicating that the human bone marrow stem cells do not recover in the short interval (3 days) required in the mouse.[30] Cytokinetic and clinical studies showed that 8 to 9 days are required for such recovery in man.[31,32] The generation time of acute myelogenous leukemic cells in man is 2 to 4 days, in contrast to 12 hours for L1210 leukemia cells in the mouse.[33] Accordingly, 5-day courses of ara-C by continuous infusion were given every 2 weeks. The complete remission rate for daily treatment was 13 to 16 per cent, whereas, for the 5-day courses of infusion, the complete remission rate was 30 per cent[17,18,34] (see Table 4).

An important cytokinetic difference between L1210 mouse leukemia and human leukemia is the fact that a substantial proportion of human leukemia cells is in the nonproliferating pool, whereas in L1210 mouse leukemia almost all the cells are

TABLE 4.—*Ara-C and Cyclophosphamide in Acute Myelogenous Leukemia in Man*

Agent(s)	Dosage	Total entered	Complete remission No.	Complete remission %	Source and ref.*
	Daily	8	1	13	MDA
		98	16	16	ALGB
Ara-C	5-day courses of	16	5	31	MDA
	continuous infusion				
	every 2 weeks	79	25	32	SWCCSG
Cyclophosphamide	Daily or weekly			<10	ALGB
Ara-C + cyclo-	4-day courses every				
phosphamide	2 weeks	32	14	44	MDA

* Abbreviations: MDA = M. D. Anderson Hospital; ALGB = Acute Leukemia Group B; SWCCSG = Southwest Cancer Chemotherapy Study Group.

in the proliferating pool.[35] Nonproliferating cells would not be sensitive to a cell-cycle-specific agent such as ara-C. However, the alkylating agents, and particularly the nitrosourea class of alkylating agents, have substantial activity against nonproliferating cells as well as proliferating cells. For these and other reasons, the nitrosourea derivative cyclohexylnitrosourea (CCNU) was studied in combination with ara-C in the treatment of L1210 mouse leukemia.[36] Nitrosourea alone has moderate activity in L1210 mouse leukemia. However, neither ara-C nor nitrosourea at any dosage produced "cures" in this transplanted leukemia. When ara-C and cyclohexylnitrosourea were combined at the optimal dosage, a cure rate was achieved (see Table 2).[36] Thus, in experimental systems, this combination of agents is highly synergistic.

Accordingly, ara-C and an alkylating agent were studied in combination in man. Cyclophosphamide was chosen rather than a nitrosourea because cyclophosphamide has some activity in acute leukemia and does not produce the delayed toxicity that complicates the use of the nitrosoureas in man. This combination produced a complete remission rate of 40 per cent [37](see Tables 2 and 4).

The efficacy of vincristine and prednisone in acute myelogenous leukemia has been controversial. However, remission rates as high as 20 per cent have been observed with prednisone alone, and recently vincristine has been found to produce objective remissions in the acute phase of chronic myelogenous leukemia. Moreover, prednisone and vincristine have produced an additive and perhaps synergistic increase in the response rate in patients with acute lymphocytic leukemia.[7] Prednisone and vincristine do not depress the bone marrow. Because of this, it was possible to add the prednisone and vincristine to the regimen of ara-C plus cyclophosphamide and not produce a significant increase in toxicity (Tables 1 and 5). The resulting program (COAP) has produced an overall complete remission rate of 45 per cent (see Table 2). This program is concurrently being compared with a program using ara-C alone in a multi-institutional study.

Infections and hemorrhage are a major cause of morbidity and mortality in adults with acute leukemia. Indeed, the risk of fatal hemorrhage per month of active acute leukemia approaches 50 per cent. In addition, these complications may markedly compromise the application of appropriate chemotherapy which in itself is myelosuppressive. Consequently, clinical research has focused on techniques for the

TABLE 5.—*Adequate Trial in Acute Leukemia*

$$\text{Adequate trials/Total entered} \sim \frac{\dfrac{\text{Patient selection}}{\text{(youth, low WBC, etc.)}} \times \text{Supportive care}}{\text{toxicity}}$$

Treatment	*MP*	*MP + MMPR*	*ara-C*	*ara-C + cyclo.*	*COAP*
Years	'58–'60	'66–'67	'66–'67	'67–'68	'68–
Patient's age (median)	—	56	42	51	55
Toxicology*: marrow	2+	3+	4+	4+	4+
gastrointestinal	2+	3+	1+	1+	1+
Supportive care	Platelets →	→	→	→	→
		Life Island →	→	→	→
			Laminar air →	→	→
				Carbenicillin →	→

Abbreviations: See Table 1.
* Toxicity = 0–4+ scale.

prevention and treatment of such hemorrhage and infection, and the efficacy of chemotherapeutic programs must be interpreted against the background of this supportive care. We propose that a good measure of the adequacy of supportive care is the proportion of patients receiving an adequate trial, which is defined as a minimum of 6 weeks of remission induction chemotherapy at full dose. Inadequate trials almost invariably result from the threat or presence of hemorrhage and infection or death therefrom, that is, they result from inadequate supportive care. The concept of an adequate trial and its relation to the chemotherapeutic programs discussed in this chapter are illustrated in Tables 2 and 5. Patient factors, particularly youth, correlate positively with the percentage of adequate trials, and supportive care should increase the proportion of patients having an adequate trial. On the other hand, the more toxic the treatment program the less likely is the patient to tolerate an adequate trial (see Table 5). The median age for the patients on the therapeutic programs described in this study was reasonably comparable. The marrow toxicity in terms of severity of thrombocytopenia and granulocytopenia was greater for the more recent programs than for the earlier programs. In contrast, the gastrointestinal toxicity was less severe with the more recent programs as compared with the MP and MP plus MMPR programs. Supportive care techniques were relatively limited in the era of the 6-MP control (1958 to 1960) and have been increasingly introduced since that time (see Table 5).

The interrelation of supportive care to chemotherapy is illustrated in Table 2. With regard to 6-MP, in a trial conducted from 1958 to 1960, only 45 per cent of the patients in the study received 6 weeks of adequate dose treatment, that is, only 45 per cent of patients had an adequate trial.[5] With the successive introduction of such techniques as platelet transfusions, protected environment and prophylactic antibiotic programs, and new antibiotics such as carbenicillin for the treatment of *Pseudomonas* infections, there has occurred a progressive increase in the proportion of patients receiving an adequate trial. Since the start of 1967, approximately 80 per cent of patients have achieved an adequate trial (see Table 2). This is true despite the fact that the more recent treatment programs are more myelosuppressive; this, if anything, should decrease the chances of an adequate trial (see Table 5). The chemotherapeutic specificity is perhaps best expressed by the proportion of patients achieving a complete remission divided by the proportion of patients who have had adequate treatment with the specified remission induction program. As evidenced from Table 2, this has increased progressively from 21 per cent for the original MP program to 60 per cent for the COAP program. Thus, the effectiveness of supportive care has progressively increased during the past 5 years, as has the chemotherapeutic specificity of the treatment programs.

The sum of these efforts, that is, supportive care plus chemotherapy, is presented in the bottom line of Table 2. With each successive program there has been an increment of about 10 per cent in the remission rate, so that with the last program (COAP), almost 50 per cent of all patients achieved complete remission. It should be emphasized that the very important progress which occurred in acute childhood leukemia was made possible by the development of remission induction programs that were effective with most patients. It is reasonable to hope that we are on the threshold of such an attainment in acute myelogenous leukemia in adults.

For the above treatment programs, the same treatment employed for remission induction was continued (with increasing intervals between courses) during remission. The median duration for complete remissions is indicated in Table 6. For the COAP program the median duration of complete remission is 10 months. The ultimate criterion for evaluating treatment is effective survival. It has been demonstrated that the increased survival of children with acute leukemia is a function of time spent in complete remission. Since such patients are asymptomatic and active, the improved survival is "effective" survival. This has also been demonstrated for adults. However, because of the above, the median or 50 per cent survival is not likely to be affected in a significant way by complete remission rates of less than 50 per cent. The effectiveness of the improved treatment programs in terms of remission induction and remission maintenance is evidenced, nevertheless, by the 25 per cent survival rate, that is, the median time from start of treatment to the point in time when 25 per cent of patients are surviving. As is shown in Table 6, this period has increased from 5 to 12 months.

TABLE 6.—*Acute Myelocytic Leukemia in Adults: Remission Maintenance*

*Treatment program**	*Year*	*Complete remission* Rate (%)	Duration *(median in months)*	*Survival after treatment* 50%	25%
MP	'58–'60	9	5	2	5
MP + MMPR	'66–'67	24	7	3	—
Ara-C	'66–'68	25	10	3	9
Ara-C + Cytoxan	'67–'68	40	6	4	12
COAP	'68–	45	10	4	12

* Abbreviations: See Table 1.

REFERENCES

1. Farber, S., Diamond, L. K., Mercer, R. D., Sylvester, R. F. and Wolff, V. A.: Temporary remission in acute leukemia in children produced by folic antagonist amethopteroylglutamic acid (aminopterin). New Eng. J. Med. 238:787, 1948.

2. Burchenal, J. H., Murphy, M. L., Ellison, R. R., Sykes, M. P., Tan, T. C., et al.: Clinical evaluation of a new antimetabolite, 6-mercaptopurine, in the treatment of leukemia and allied disease. Blood 8:965, 1953.

3. Holland, J. F.: Who should treat acute leukemia? J.A.M.A. 209:1511, 1969.
4. Burchenal, J. H.: Long-term survivors in acute leukemia. Cancer 21:595, 1968.
5. Frei, E., III, et al.: Studies of sequential and combination antimetabolite therapy of acute leukemia: 6-Mercaptopurine and methotrexate. Blood 18:431, 1961.
6. Freireich, E. J, Karon, M. and Frei, E., III: Combined chemotherapy (VAMP) in the treatment of acute leukemia in children. Proc. Amer. Ass. Cancer Res. 5:20, 1964.
7. Frei, E., III and Freireich, E. J: Progress and perspectives in the chemotherapy of acute leukemia. *In* Goldin, A., Hawking, F. and Schnitzer, R. J. (Eds.): Advances in Chemotherapy, Vol. 2. New York: Academic Press, 1965, pp. 269–298.
8. Selawry, O.: Acute Leukemia Group B. New treatment schedule with improved survival in childhood leukemia: Intermittent parenteral versus daily oral administration of methotrexate for maintenance of induced remission. J.A.M.A. 194:75, 1965.
9. Chevalier, L. and Glidewell, O.: Schedule of mercaptopurine and effect of inducer drugs in prolongation of remission maintenance of acute leukemia. Proc. Amer. Ass. Cancer Res. 8:10, 1967.
10. Zuelzer, W. W.: Implications of long-term survival in acute stem cell leukemia of childhood treated with composite cyclic therapy. Blood 24:477, 1964.
11. Skipper, H. E., Schabel, F. M. and Wilcox, W. S.: Experimental evaluation of potential anticancer agents. XIII. On the criteria and kinetics associated with "curability" of experimental leukemia. Cancer Chemother. Rep. 35:3, 1964.
12. Freireich, E. J: Effectiveness of platelet transfusion in leukemia and aplastic anemia. Transfusion 6:50, 1966.
13. Bodey, G. P., Rodriguez, V. and Stuart, B.: Clinical pharmacologic studies of carbenicillin. Amer. J. Med. Sci. 257:185, 1969.
14. Goldin, A., Vendetti, J. M., Humphreys, S. R. and Mantel, N.: Influence of the concentration of leukemic inoculum on the effectiveness of treatment. Science 123:840, 1956.
15. Skipper, H. E., Schabel, F. M. and Wilcox, W. S.: Experimental evaluation of potential anticancer agents. XIII. On the criteria and kinetics associated with "curability" of experimental leukemia. Cancer Chemother. Rep. 35:1, 1964.
16. Bruce, W. R., Meeker, B. E. and Valeriote, F. A.: Comparison of the sensitivity of normal hematopoietic and transplanted lymphoma colony-forming cells to chemotherapeutic agents administered *in vivo*. J. Nat. Cancer Inst. 37:233, 1966.
17. Ellison, R. R., et al.: Arabinosylcytosine: A useful agent in the treatment of acute leukemia in adults. Blood 32:507, 1968.
18. Bodey, G. P., Freireich, E. J, Monto, R. W. and Hewlett, J. S.: Cytosine arabinoside (NSC-63878) therapy for acute leukemia in adults. Cancer Chemother. Rep. 53:59, 1969.
19. Burkitt, D., Hutt, M. S. R. and Wright, D. H.: The African lymphoma: Preliminary observations on response to therapy. Cancer 18:399, 1965.
20. Hertz, R., Bergenstal, D. M., Lipsett, M. B., Price, E. B. and Hilbish, T. F.: Chemotherapy of choriocarcinoma and related trophoblastic tumors in women. J.A.M.A. 168:845, 1958.
21. Bennett, L. L., Jr. et al.: Activity and mechanism of action of 6-methylthiopurine ribonucleoside in cancer cells resistant to 6-mercaptopurine. Nature 205:1276, 1965.
22. Wang, M. C., Simpson, A. I. and Paterson, A. R. P.: Combinations of 6-mercaptopurine and 6-methylmercaptopurine ribonucleoside in therapy of Ehrlich ascites carcinoma. Cancer Chemother. Rep. 51:101, 1967.
23. Luce, J. K., Frenkel, E. P., Uletti, T. J., Isassi, A. A., Hernandez, K. W. and Howard, J. P.: Clinical studies of 6-methylmercaptopurine riboside in acute leukemia. Cancer Chemother. Rep. 51:535, 1967.
24. Schabel, F. M., Laster, W. R. and Skipper, H. E.: Chemotherapy of leukemia L1210 by 6-mercaptopurine in combination with 6-methylthiopurine ribonucleoside. Cancer Chemother. Rep. 51:111, 1967.
25. Loo, T. L., Luce, J. K., Sullivan, M. P. and Frei, E., III: Clinical pharmacologic observations on 6-mercaptopurine and 6-methylthiopurine ribonucleoside. Clin. Pharmacol. Ther. 9:180, 1968.
26. Loo, T. L., Ho, D. H. W., Blossom, D. R., Shepard, B. J. and Frei, E., III: In vitro cellular uptake of purine antimetabolites. I. Uptake of 6-methylthiopurine ribonucleoside by human erythrocytes. Biochem. Pharmacol. 18:1711, 1969.
27. Skipper, H. E., Schabel, F. M. and Wilcox, W. S.: Experimental evaluation of potential anticancer agents. XXI. Scheduling of

arabinosylcytosine to take advantage of its S-phase specificity against leukemic cells. Cancer Chemother. Rep. 51:125, 1967.
28. DeVita, V. T., Denham, C. and Perry, S.: Relationship of normal CDF mouse leukocyte kinetics to growth characteristics of leukemia L1210. Cancer Res. 29:1067, 1969.
29. Leach, W. B., Laster, W. R., Mayo, J. G., Griswold, D. P. and Schabel, F. M.: Toxicity studies in mice treated with arabinofuranosylcytosine. Cancer Res. 29:529, 1969.
30. Frei, E., III, Luce, J. K. and Bonnet, J.: Further dose schedule studies of arabinosylcytosine in man. Cancer Chemother. Rep. (In press.)
31. Perry, S., Moxley, J. H., Weiss, G. H. and Zelen, M.: Studies of leukocyte kinetics by liquid scintillation counting in normal individuals and in patients with chronic myelocytic leukemia. J. Clin. Invest. 45:1388, 1966.
32. Frei, E., III, Bickers, J. N., Hewlett, J. S., Lane, M., Leary, W. V. and Talley, R. W.: Dose schedule and antitumor studies of arabinosylcytosine (NSC 63878). Cancer Res. 29:1325, 1969.
33. Clarkson, B. T., Ohkita, R. T., Ota, K. and Fried, J.: Studies of cellular proliferation in human leukemia. I. Estimation of growth rates of leukemic and normal hematopoietic cells in 2 adults with acute leukemia given a single injection of tritiated thymidine. J. Clin. Invest. 46:506, 1967.
34. Bickers, J. and Freireich, E. J (Southwest Cancer Chemotherapy Study Group): Phase II protocol, cytosine arabinoside (NSC-63878) in acute leukemia in adults.
35. Mauer, A. M. and Fisher, V.: Characteristics of cell proliferation in four patients with untreated acute leukemia. Blood 28:428, 1966.
36. Schabel, F. M., Jr.: *In vivo* leukemic cell kill kinetics and "curability" in experimental systems in the proliferation and spread of neoplastic cells. Baltimore: Williams & Wilkins, 1968, p. 379.
37. Bodey, G. P., Rodriguez, V., Hart, J. and Freireich, E. J: Therapy of acute leukemia with the combination of arabinosylcytosine and cyclophosphamide. Cancer Chemother. Rep. 54:225, 1970.

Editors' Note

The current emphasis on the therapy of acute myelocytic leukemia (AML) in adults is encouraging for patients afflicted with this dread malady. As bright as this star seems to be, an even brighter one appears to be the result of therapy of acute lymphoblastic leukemia of childhood. As a result of the pioneering efforts of Farber,[1] Frei,[2] and others, recent studies estimate that 50 per cent or more of these patients may survive for more than 5 years, even without maintenance chemotherapy.[3] Present-day therapy involves intensive combination chemotherapy coupled with CNS irradiation given at a dosage of 2400 R to the entire cerebrospinal axis.[3] Treatment begins by inducing a remission with vincristine and prednisone, usually requiring several weeks. Cytotoxic therapy is then given, utilizing three drugs, such as 6-mercaptopurine, methotrexate and cyclophosphamide. This requires about one week, after which CNS irradiation is administered. Once the bone marrow has recovered, maintenance therapy is continued with the three cytotoxic agents. At periodic intervals, reinduction courses of vincristine and prednisone are given.[3]

It is clear from these data that the therapy of acute lymphoblastic leukemia is now at a point where cure may be expected in a sizeable number of patients. Management of these patients is most appropriate in a center where various supportive and therapeutic modalities are available.

A final note of caution seems advisable, despite the current enthusiasm regarding cure of this disease. In lower animals, lymphoma and leukemia are caused by viruses.[4] However, rigid proof of the viral causation of leukemia in human beings is suggested but still uncertain. Thus, although cytotoxic chemotherapy aims at eradicating every last tumor cell, these drugs are not effective in eradicating the virus (at least in animal systems).[5] It is disturbing to read reports that, in children with acute leukemia treated with total body irradiation and then transplanted with marrow from another person, the disease *recurs in the transplant.*[6]

These data, while overtly discouraging, should not invalidate the rather high survivals being currently reported. Perhaps by reduction of the tumor cell population to low levels, the immune system can then eradicate both the disease and its cause. Continued efforts to develop newer, more effective agents may eventually result in cure of leukemia in most patients, even before the causative agent is discovered and despite the inability of chemotherapy to eradicate the virus per se.

References to Editors' Note

1. Farber, S., Diamond, L. K., Mercer, R. D., Sylvester, R. F., Jr. and Wolff, J. A.: Temporary remission in acute leukemia in children produced by folic acid antagonist 4-aminopteroyl glutamic acid (aminopterin). New Eng. J. Med. 238:787, 1948.
2. Frei, E., III: Chemotherapy of acute leukemia. *In* Brodsky, I. and Kahn, S. B. (Eds.): Cancer Chemotherapy. New York: Grune & Stratton, 1967, p. 185.
3. Pinkel, D.: Five year follow up of total therapy of childhood lymphocytic leukemia. J.A.M.A. 216:648, 1971.
4. Borron, M., Levy, J. P. and Peries, J.: *In vitro* investigations on murine leukemia viruses. Progr. Med. Virol. 9:341, 1967.
5. Brodsky, I., Ross, E. M., Kahn, S. B. and Braverman, S. D.: Effect of cortisol on Rauscher virus infection. Cancer Res. 28:297, 1968.
6. Fialkow, P. J., Thomas, E. D. and Bryant, J. I.: Leukaemic transformation of engrafted human marrow cells *in vivo*. Lancet 1:251, 1971.

Immunotherapy of Leukemia

By Edward S. Henderson, M.D. and Brigid G. Leventhal, M.D.

ALTHOUGH IMMUNOTHERAPY OF CANCER is older in concept and practice than chemotherapy, the major advances in medical control of disseminated neoplasms have been attributable largely to the introduction of effective chemical agents. A prominent factor in the resurgence of interest in immunotherapy has been the identification of tumor-specific antigens in animals and man during the last two decades, during which chemotherapy has frequently palliated but infrequently cured neoplastic disease. Drug therapy for acute leukemia has resulted in improved average survival of childhood acute leukemia[1] and has been followed by apparent cures in a small fraction of cases in both adults and children.[2] However, the improving initial efficacy of drugs and drug combinations, while increasing the frequency or duration of remission, has not as yet proved curative in most cases.[3,4]

A series of therapeutic trials at the National Cancer Institute illustrates this point. Between 1962 and 1964, two intensive combination programs—VAMP (vincristine, amethopterin, mercaptopurine and prednisone) and BIKE (bi-cycle)—were administered to 33 children with previously untreated acute lymphoblastic leukemia.[5] The median duration of remission after termination of drug treatment was 140 days, and the median survival of the group was exactly 2 years. Ten patients lived 4 years or longer; one patient has been in continuous complete remission for 7 years, while a second experienced a local relapse (ovary) 4 years ago, but has remained in otherwise perfect health for 7 years after initial treatment.

After these initial attempts at eradicating disease, a longer and more intensive course with a four-drug combination—prednisolone, Oncovin (vincristine), methotrexate and Purinethol (POMP)—was started for 35 children with the same disorder.[4,6] The 240-day median duration of unmaintained remission was nearly double that of the earlier studies, and the median survival increased to 34 months. Nevertheless, the 4-year survival rate (8 of 35) and long-term continuous remission rate (2 of 35) were not superior to those of the earlier regimens.

Analysis of the relapses from these several studies revealed no significant difference in the mode of leukemia recurrence, the rate of marrow repopulation by lymphoblasts, or the responsiveness of the disease to subsequent attempts at remission induction. Estimates of the degree of leukemia cell reduction based on average tumor doubling times and duration of unmaintained remission suggested that the rapidly replicating component of the leukemic population had been eliminated in most patients by the POMP protocol. Nevertheless, there were fatal recurrences in the vast majority of these patients.[4]

Four frequently advanced explanations for late recurrences are (1) the existence of pharmacologic sanctuaries for residual tumor cells, e.g., within the central nervous system, into which most antileukemic drugs penetrate to a degree inadequate for cytolysis; (2) induction of a new leukemia cell line by the same factor which caused the initial illness; (3) the selection of residual cells resistant to additional drug therapy

---

From the Leukemia Service, Medicine Branch, National Cancer Institute, National Institutes of Health, Bethesda, Maryland.

through alterations in cell metabolism; and (4) the selection of cells resistant to chemotherapy by virtue of preexistent or induced kinetics of growth. Pharmacologic sanctuaries alone could not account for late relapses, since, if the usual kinetics of growth persisted, evidence of recurrent disease should appear at the same rate as that usually observed, if not earlier. Acute leukemia is not characterized by a characteristic karyotypic abnormality such as the Ph^1 chromosome of chronic myelocytic leukemia. However, specific karyotypic markers, when seen, regularly recur at relapse, including late relapse,[7-9] an extremely improbable phenomenon if reinduction were responsible for recurrence. The almost uniform response of patients at their first relapses to the identical chemotherapy used for initial remission induction argues against rapid development of a significant degree of biochemical resistance.[5,6] Persistence, despite intensive therapy, of nondividing or slowly dividing leukemic cells, protected from the effects of most antileukemic therapy by their replicative dormancy, is entirely consistent, on the other hand, with the results observed by the National Cancer Institute and elsewhere.[3,4]

Therapy directed against a population of kinetically inactive leukemic "stem cells" would require either a greater degree of specificity than that demonstrated by current chemotherapy or, alternatively, the provision of extensive protection during the phase of obligate toxicity, or replenishment of normal stem cells by grafting. Because of the specificity inherent in most immunologic mechanisms, immunotherapy is a most attractive consideration for the elimination of theoretic leukemia stem cells.

With forms of acute leukemia less responsive to chemotherapy, e.g., acute myelocytic leukemia or the blastic phase of chronic myelocytic leukemia, the need for greater therapeutic specificity is immediately apparent. Severe marrow hypoplasia is a necessary prelude to remission with all currently effective remission induction therapies,[1,10-12] and remissions, when obtained, are usually of brief duration despite continued drug maintenance.[1]

Pharmacologic sanctuaries would probably not be eliminated by immunologic reactions since antibody and cellular access to the central nervous system is limited. Intracerebral or other extramedullary sites of recurrence have complicated otherwise suggestively successful immunotherapy attempts.[13-15] On the other hand, both biochemically resistant cells and oncogenic viruses might prove attractive targets for immunotherapy.

Requisites for Immunotherapy

The obvious primary requisite for any immunologic attack on leukemia is the existence of either a specific tumor antigen or a heightened susceptibility of leukemic tissue to immune reactions. Secondarily, one must be concerned with the ability to develop and administer suitable immunization, antisera, or immunocytes with safety to all concerned (patient and, where apropos, donor). Finally, the limits of the antileukemic effects of immunologic reactions must be determined and the patient prepared appropriately so as to benefit maximally from application of immune therapy.

In animals tumor-specific antigens have been documented in a variety of virus-induced[16-19] and chemically induced tumors[20-22] and in spontaneous neoplasms.[22] Evidence for such antigens in man had until recently been only surmised from the occurrence of spontaneous remissions in melanoma,[23,24] Burkitt's tumor,[25] choriocarcinoma,[26] and leukemia[27,28]; from the observation that neoplasia occurred more frequently in patients with hereditary,[29] spontaneously acquired,[30,31] and iatro-

TABLE 1.—*Tumor-Specific Antigens in Human Solid Neoplasms*

Tumor	*Test for detection*	*Reference*	*Comments*
Burkitt's tumor	1) Membrane immunofluorescence	Klein et al.[42]	
		Henle and Henle[43]	
	2) Humoral cytotoxicity	Herberman and Fahey[44]	
	3) Delayed hypersensitivity	Fass et al.[36]	
Melanoma	1) Cytoplasmic immunofluorescence	Muna et al.[45]	
	2) Humoral cytotoxicity	Lewis et al.[39]	Cross-reactive
	3) Delayed hypersensitivity	Fass et al.[46]	
	4) Membrane immunofluorescence	Morton et al.[47]	
Sarcoma	1) Membrane immunofluorescence	Morton et al.[48]	Cross-reactive
	2) Complement fixation	Eilber and Morton[49]	
Colon	1) Immunologic tolerance	Gold and Freedman[50]	
	2) Immune absorption		
Neuroblastoma	1) Cell and plasma mediated tumor-colony inhibition	Hellstrom et al.[51]	
Breast carcinoma	1) Cell mediated tumor-colony inhibition	Pierce et al.[52]	
Hodgkin's disease	2) Delayed hypersensitivity	Hughes and Lytton[53]	
Lung carcinoma		Stewart[54]	
		Herberman and Oren[55]	
Stomach carcinoma	3) In vitro inhibition of leukocyte migration	Andersen et al.[56]	Breast only

genic[32-35] immunologic deficiencies; and from observations correlating a favorable response to therapy with the demonstration of general immune competence[24,35-40] or histologic evidence of immunologic activity at the site of the tumor.[41] Within the last 6 years tumor antigens, distinct from histocompatibility antigens identified on normal cells of the tumor-bearing patient, have been identified by a number of techniques (Table 1). Most such antigens have been unique to the individual patient's tumor, whereas others, notably that of osteogenic sarcoma,[48] have been tumor-specific and cross-reactive from patient to patient. Cross reactivity has been claimed[39] but not confirmed[46] for melanoma.

Tumor-specific antigens have been detected in acute leukemia by similar techniques (Table 2). Fink and coworkers noted cytoplasmic immunofluorescence occurring with certain human leukemic cell lines exposed to fluorescein-labelled antisera prepared in rabbits against human leukemia virus or Rauscher virus, or both.[57] Although this observation has been confirmed by others,[58,59] the significance of such an intracellularly situated antigen in control of the disease is questionable. Doré et al.[60] noted, in addition to immunofluorescence reactions, an occasional incidence of cytotoxic and complement fixing antibodies directed against autochthonous leukemia. Cross reactivity against allogeneic leukemic cells was not investigated. Delayed hypersensitivity reactions against intradermally administered leukemic cell extracts have been reported by Herberman and Oren.[55] Using cell extracts containing less than 0.33 mg of protein per 0.1 ml of interadermal injection, they observed positive delayed reactions in 2 of 6 patients with acute lymphocytic leukemia, 3 of 8 with chronic lymphocytic leukemia, 7 of 10 with acute myelocytic leukemia and 4 of 10 with chronic myelocytic leukemia, as compared with positive reactions in 3 of 28 normal volunteers. In two patients with acute lymphoblastic leukemia, positive reactions were observed in remission status but were not detectable in relapse, similar

TABLE 2.—*Tumor-Specific Antigens in Human Leukemia*

Assay used	*Type of leukemia* and results*	*Authors (Ref.)*
1. Cytoplasmic immunofluorescence with rabbit anti-Rauscher virus serum	AML and ALL: 11/14 relapse marrows and 2/8 remission marrows positive; 5/5 positive tests in erythroleukemia	Fink et al.[57]
2. Cytoplasmic immunofluorescence with rabbit anti-Rauscher virus serum	Positive tests in 11/11 ALL, 5/11 AML, 4/5 CLL, 0/1 CML, at relapse	Ioannides et al.[58]
3. Cytoplasmic immunofluorescence with rabbit anti-Rauscher virus serum	Positive tests in 3/3 AML, 2/2 ASCL, 6/6 CML, 1/1 ALL, 3/3 CLL, in relapse	Bates et al.[59]
4. Cytotoxicity, immunofluorescence, complement fixation, immune adherence	Occasional positives in ALL, AML, and CLL; 4 CML patients negative in all assays	Doré et al.[60]
5. Mixed leukocyte culture; membrane immunofluorescence	6/9 positive ALL, 0/1 AML, 1/10 sera-positive; no cross reactivity	Fridman and Kourilsky[61]
6. Mixed leukocyte culture	3 positives/5 cases (ALL, AML, CML)	Viza et al.[62]
7. Delayed skin hypersensitivity to leukemia cell extracts (< 0.33 mg protein/0.1 ml intradermal test dose)	2/6 ALL, 3/8 CLL, 7/10 AML, 4/10 CML positive; 0/3 positives in patients in long-term remission	Herberman and Oren[55]

* ALL = Acute lymphocytic leukemia; AML = acute myelocytic leukemia; ASCL = acute stem cell leukemia; CML = chronic myelocytic leukemia; CLL = chronic lymphocytic leukemia.

to the findings in Fass et al. in Burkitt's tumor.[36] Fridman and Kourilsky, employing cultures of mitomycin-treated lymphoblasts acquired at relapse, stored and frozen at $-180°C$, plus mature lymphocytes obtained from the same patient during remission, showed three-fold stimulation of ^3H-thymidine incorporation in 6 of 9 patients with acute lymphocytic leukemia.[61] Only the serum from one of these patients contained a weak antibody against autochthonous lymphoblasts demonstrable by membrane immunofluorescence techniques. This antibody was not cross-reactive with leukemic cells from the other patients. Viza and coworkers also used the mixed leukocyte culture in a similar study to demonstrate apparent tumor specific antigens on leukemia cells from 3 of 5 patients.[62]

Such studies suggest that tumor specific antigens do exist on leukemic cells from at least some patients, and encourage attempts at exploitation of this phenomenon.

Given a target, albeit elusive, for immunotherapy, a number of questions, some general and others unique to clinical medicine, must be answered before therapy can be securely and rationally initiated. Are all leukemia antigens identical? Does a finite number of antigens exist, as in virus-induced animal tumors, or is each patient's leukemia antigen unique? Does a state of permanent tolerance exist within a patient to the antigenic differences of his tumor, or is the lack of effective immunologic control at relapse a matter of "enhancing" antibodies which protect cells from immunologic destruction, excess antigen which overwhelms the immune system, or some other potentially reversible immunologic defect? In what host, and by what means, should antileukemia immunity be elicited? Should one actively immunize the patient himself, or can and must one induce immunity in another individual, man or animal, and transfer this protection to the patient by infusion or engraftment? And finally, what are the limitations of even the most potent immunologic attack in terms of the size, anatomic distribution, proliferative capacity, and mutability of the malignant tissue target?

The specificity of the observed leukemia antigens requires more extensive testing. Cross reactivity has not been evaluated systematically, and clinical trials which in part test the hypothesis of a common antigen have been suggestive but inconclusive.[63] Prospective studies of the relation of immunization to the clinical state have only recently been undertaken, the results of Fridman and Kourilsky,[61] Viza et al.,[62] and Herberman and Oren[55] being provocative but preliminary. These questions should soon be resolved by clinical studies now in progress.

The mode of inducing or transferring antileukemia immunity is a more complex and difficult problem.

Passive transfer of tumor specific antibody or sensitized immunocytes, although demonstrably effective in animals,[17,64–67] is compromised by the short duration of effect of each infusion,[68] the potential risks and discomfort attendant upon immunizing human donors with leukemic tissue or extracts, and the problems of sensitization to heterologous proteins when animals are used as a source of antibody or immunocytes. Adoptive immunotherapy, requiring engraftment of immunocompetent cells, entails the additional risks of immunosuppression of the patient recipient and severe graft-versus-host disease. Except in the rare case of leukemia occurring in one member of a monozygous multiple birth, isogeneic adoptive or passive transfer is impossible, and the high incidence of leukemia in the "normal" identical sibling, together with the absence of normal histocompatibility barriers, interdicts immunization of the genetically identical sibling with leukemia cells or extracts. To date, transfusion or transplantation of normal isologous plasma and bone marrow from donors not intentionally immunized against tumor-specific antigens has had no demonstrable effect upon animal or human neoplasms, including leukemias.[69–74] The observation of Law[17] that positive transfer of isologous sera can reconstitute (as opposed to induce) native resistance of $BC3HF_1$ mice to XM-131 after immunosuppression with X-irradiation, is a special case not in conflict with this thesis.

Xenogeneic antisera have been used in animal systems and against human tumor. Miller et al.[75] were able to prolong the survival of BDF_1 mice inoculated with leukemia L1210 by pretreatment with L1210 antisera prepared in rabbits or goats, and Reif and Kim[76] demonstrated a similar effect in the case of leukemia L1210 in isogeneic DBS/26 mice. Hill et al.,[77] in another syngeneic tumor/host combination (BW5147) in AKR/J mice, were able to extend survival by rabbit or horse antisera administration. Old and coworkers[68] developed an antiserum specific for Gross virus-induced tumors in rats and used this antiserum to successfully treat the Gross virus-induced G+ leukemia in mice. This technique obviated hyperimmunization of the donor against normal xenogeneic transplantation antigens. In humans, however, the technique could be applicable only for tumors induced by a virus which could be cultivated or to which animals were naturally exposed.

Xenogeneic antisera have been used against human leukemia and solid tumors since the nineteenth century with marginal, uninterpretable or unreproducible results (see review of Southam[78]). However, one probable response has been reported[79] in which a gestational choriocarcinoma remitted after administration of rabbit antiserum prepared against the leukocytes and gamma globulin of the patient's husband.

Allogeneic immune sera, from patients exhibiting spontaneous remissions of melanoma have occasionally induced documented remissions in other patients with melanoma.[23,80] Similar results in Burkitt's lymphoma, using late remission sera, have been reported by Ngu[13] and Burkitt,[81] but have not been confirmed by others,[82] despite the use of plasma with documented high titers of antibody cytotoxic to Burkitt cells in vitro.

Cellular transfer of immunocytes from sensitized isogeneic[66,67,83–85] or unstimulated[86,87] allogeneic donors has been reported therapeutic in studies with animal tumors. Boranic has shown that allogeneic marrow transplantation, causing short-term graft-versus-host disease reversed by ablative chemotherapy, prolonged survival of tumor bearing mice.[88] Using cross immunization and passive leukocyte transfer techniques, Nadler and Moore have observed responses in some human solid tumors (melanoma, breast, colon and sarcoma).[89]

Perhaps the most interesting form of passive transfer of immunity involves RNA from lymphocytes sensitized to tumor antigens. Inhibition in the growth or transplantability of isogeneic tumors has been observed in animals receiving injections of either "immune" RNA[90,91] or spleen cells previously exposed to "immune" RNA in vitro.[92] The resultant immunologic responses were specific to the tumor employed. In two experiments,[90,92] RNA was obtained from lymph node or splenic lymphocytes from xenogeneic donors (sheep or guinea pig) immunized with the tumor. Such procedures had little, if any, effect on the normal tissues of the recipient tumor-bearing animals, and, if they could be adapted to man, might provide a safe form of passive immunization.

Despite these partial successes, the most direct and least hazardous method of immunization remains active immunization. Studies in animals suggest that nonspecific, as well as specific, active immunization can be effective in retarding or preventing tumor growth[93–105] (Table 3). Since frequently it may be impossible to obtain adequate amounts of tumor in clinical situations, nonspecific immunization has great appeal. A variety of bacterial antigens,[95,98–103] mitogens[104] and polynucleotides[105] have been successfully used in animal or in vitro models, and clinical responses have occasionally been reported. These substances have been given intravenously, subcutaneously, intradermally or directly into the tumor.[24,100] Since in the last-mentioned approach, regression usually has been limited to the local neoplasm, it may have scant applicability to leukemia. To date there has been no clear evidence of increase in tumor growth when any of the above approaches have been used clinically, although such a phenomenon has been observed occasionally in animal tumors.[101,105–108]

Limits of Immunotherapy

There is considerable evidence to suggest that even an optimal immunologic response to specific tumor antigens would not in all cases eradicate established tumors. Many studies of transplantable animal tumors have indicated that both humoral and cellular immune reactions to tumors follow zero order kinetics, i.e., a specified number of immune competent cells or tumor antibodies are required for the lysis of each tumor cell.[95,97,98,109,110] Several independent investigations have suggested that the upper limit of immunologic control in rodents is reached when a tumor reaches the order of 10^3–10^6 cells.[17,95,97,98,109] The correlation of limited extent of disease to curability in melanoma[39,89] and Burkitt's tumor[25,36] and the occasional regression of metastases in Wilms' tumor and neuroblastoma following resection of the primary tumor are consistent with, though in no way confirmatory of, this postulate.

TABLE 3.—*Active Immunization in Animal Tumors*

	Authors	*Immunizing agent*	*Target cells*	*Comment*
Specific	Oettgen et al.[93]	Tumor homogenates	Chemically induced sarcomas, guinea pig	Prophylaxis
	Zbar et al.[94]	Living tumor cells	Chemically induced hepatomas, guinea pig	Prophylaxis
	Mathé[95]	Irradiated tumor cells	Murine leukemia L1210	Therapy
	Kronman et al.[96]	Living tumor cells	Chemically induced hepatoma, guinea pig	Therapy
	Parr *in* [97]	Living tumor cells	Chemically induced sarcoma, rats	Therapy
	Alexander and Hall[97]	Living tumor cells	Chemically induced sarcoma, rats	Therapy
Nonspecific	Amiel[98]	Bacille Calmette-Guérin (BCG)	Murine viral leukemia	Prophylaxis
	Old et al.[99]	BCG	Chemically induced murine tumors	Prophylaxis
	Mathé[95]	BCG	Murine leukemia L1210	Therapy
	Zbar[100]	BCG	Chemically induced guinea pig hepatoma	Local therapy
	Weiss et al.[101]	BCG fraction	Virus-induced murine sarcomas, carcinomas, leukemia	Prophylaxis
	Wissler et al.[102]	*Bordetella pertussis; Corynebacterium parvum*	Spontaneous carcinoma and chemically induced sarcoma in mice	Prophylaxis
	Holm and Perlman[104]	Phytohemagglutinin	Chang cells	In vitro with lymphocytes
	Levy et al.[105]	Polyinosinic-polycytidylic acid	Murine sarcomas and leukemias	Therapy

Estimates of residual leukemia, based on observed doubling times at relapse and the duration of unmaintained remission, have been applied to human acute lymphoblastic leukemia by Zelen,[111] Frei and Freireich,[112] and others.[1,113] These approximations suggest that, to insure the reduction of leukemic blasts to 10^5–10^6, initial therapy should be such that relapse occurs no less than three months after the cessation of treatment. This degree of leukemia suppression has been achieved in childhood acute leukemia utilizing intensive combination chemotherapy.[3–5,113] Although the above discussion is woven from assumption, it would seem reasonable to attempt maximal tumor cell reduction before institution of immunotherapy, provided such cytolytic treatment did not seriously impair the patient's response to subsequent immunization.

Differences in the expression of humoral and cellular immunity in different anatomic locations must also be taken into account. For example, it would be vital to take great care to eradicate central nervous system leukemia, which might be expected to resist immunotherapy,[14,15] by radiation therapy or local chemotherapy.

With few exceptions, when multiple remissions are achieved in a patient, they tend to be of successively shorter duration, despite the administration of maintenance regimens of theoretically equivalent efficacy.[1] Among the leading candidate causes for this phenomenon is a progressive reduction in native host resistance to the

TABLE 4.—*Immunotherapy Trials in Human Leukemia*

Type	*Antigen or other substance used*	*Purpose of therapy*	*Results*	*Reference*
Active, specific	—	—	—	—
Active, nonspecific	Allogeneic leukemic cells ± BCG	Remission maintenance—ALL	7/20 long-term remissions	Mathé et al.[63]
	Allogeneic leukemic cells	Remission induction—ALL	1 complete remission on immunization alone	Skurkovich et al.[115]
	BCG	Remission maintenance—ALL	No effect demonstrable to date	BMRC[116]
	Bordetella pertussis	Remission maintenance	Increased median duration of remission in ALL	Guyer and Crowther[14]
	Multiple viruses	Remission induction—AML	Reduction in node, spleen and marrow infiltration by leukemic myeloblasts	Wheelock and Dingle[118]
	Poly I-poly C	Remission induction—ALL, AML	5/15 complete remissions of ALL in early relapse	Mathé et al.[117]
Passive, xenogeneic	Rabbit anti-human-leukemia sera	Remission induction—CML	Complete remission in 4/10	Lindstrom[122]
	Rabbit anti-human-leukemia sera	Remission induction—CML	Decreased spleen size, increased WBC	Hueper and Russell[121]
	Sheep anti-human-leukemia sera	Remission induction—CML, ASCL	Transient reduction in WBC in 1/10 CML, 1/1 ASCL	Izawa et al.[123]
Passive, allogeneic	Normal human antileukemia plasma	Remission induction—CML, ASCL	Transient fall in WBC and % blasts in 3/3 CML, 1/1 ASCL	Izawa et al.[123]
	Plasma and cells from multiply transfused patient with thalassemia	Remission induction—ALL, AUL	Transient decrease in circulating leukemic cells	Djerassi[127]
	Normal human antileukemia plasma	Remission induction—CML	No definite response (1 case)	Brittingham and Chaplin[124]

	Normal plasma, unrelated donor, normal plasma, related donor	Remission maintenance—ALL	No response (112 cases)	Albo et al.[128]
	Normal plasma and lymphocytes from specifically immunized donors	Remission maintenance—ALL	No definite effect (2 cases)	Andrews et al.[125]
	Plasma from multiply transfused normal donors	Remission induction—CLL, CML	Decreased WBC, spleen and lymph node size (CLL), no effect on blastic phase of CML	Lazlo et al.[126]
Passive, isogeneic	Remission cells and plasma	Remission maintenance—ALL	Marked increase in long-term remissions	Skurkovich et al.[15]
Adoptive, syngeneic	Normal twin bone marrow	Remission maintenance—ALL, AML	No definite effect, grafts in 80%	Thomas and Epstein[70] Pegg[71] National Cancer Institute[69]
Adoptive, allogeneic	Bone marrow(s) from normal relatives	Remission induction and maintenance—ALL and AML	Grafts in 17/24, long remissions in 3/24 with death from graft-vs.-host disease (GvH)	Mathé[129]
	HL-A matched normal sibling bone marrows	Remission induction and maintenance—ALL	Grafts in 7/8. No definite antileukemic effect. Death from GvH 2/8	Graw et al.[132]
	CML leukocytes	Induction maintenance—AML	Graft with ? related 70-day remission	Freireich et al.[130]
	CML leukocytes	Induction—ALL, AML	Grafts, GvH, and short remission in 9/21	Schwarzenberg et al.[131]

Abbreviations: BCG = bacille Calmette-Guérin; BMRC = British Medical Research Council; Poly I-poly C = polyinosinic-polycytidylic acid; ALL = acute lymphocytic leukemia; AML = acute myelocytic leukemia; CML = chronic myelocytic leukemia; ASCL = acute stem cell leukemia; CLL = chronic lymphocytic leukemia; AUL = acute undifferentiated leukemia.

leukemia. Since immune reactivity against other antigenic stimuli is usually not lost during the course of the illness (except during periods of intense immunosuppressive treatment), resistance most probably develops through the continual selection of hypoantigenic variants of the tumor cell population. Accordingly, immunotherapy should be initiated and sustained early in the course of the disease (or as soon as the tumor size is suitably reduced) to minimize the development of leukemic cell variants under the pressures of multiple chemotherapies and native immune reaction.

Immunotherapeutic Trials in Leukemia

Despite the inherent difficulties of clinical immunotherapy, a growing number of attempts to simulate encouraging laboratory models have been reported (Table 4). Most of these trials have been preliminary and uncontrolled, concerned more with determining risks and feasibility than with documenting therapeutic gain. Since they have not been always so interpreted, most careful scrutiny is required.

Active specific therapy using autochthonous leukemia cells or their derivatives as antigen has not been reported during the last decade. Previous attempts, reviewed by Southam in 1961, were inconclusive,[114] and although Mathé et al. consider the allogeneic leukemic inoculations included in their immunotherapy protocols to be specific,[63] immunologic cross reactivity has not been proved for human leukemia.

Mathé et al.[63] and Skurkovich et al.[115] have attempted to immunize acute leukemia patients with allogeneic acute leukemia cells. Skurkovich et al. treated six pairs of children, all but one pair at their first presentation with acute lymphocytic, myelocytic or undifferentiated leukemia. The authors state that "not all the patients received cytostatic therapy" and that prednisolone was not given during the period of immunization.

In each pair, cross immunization was attempted by inoculating live leukemic cells from one patient to the other. Peripheral blood cells 5×10^6 to 4×10^9 in 50 to 70 ml donor plasma were given intravenously, and 3×10^7 to 1×10^9 cells in 5 to 7 ml plasma intramuscularly, at intervals of 2 to 4 days for a total of 2 to 5 injections. Five of the patients also received 8 to 145×10^6 bone marrow cells intramuscularly on up to four occasions. At least some patients developed delayed hypersensitivity reactions to the immunizing cells. Eight to 15 days after immunization, plasma was exchanged 2 to 3 times between the immunized pairs at doses of 50 to 70 ml of plasma containing 6 to 40×10^7 lymphocytes at 1- to 4-day intervals.

Three complete and 5 partial hematologic remissions were observed during the active immunization phase. All complete remissions had received both allogeneic leukemic peripheral blood and bone marrow. Two of the complete and 5 of the partial remissions received steroid and cytostatic therapy as well, but one complete remission was achieved with immunotherapy alone, and was maintained for longer than 6 months with semiweekly intramuscular injections of 10^9 cells. Improvement in bone marrow differentials was usually most marked within the first 4 weeks.

In Skurkovich's approach, patients were immunized at the time of extensive leukemia. Mathé and coworkers, on the other hand, prepared their patients for immunotherapy by inducing complete remission and administering multiple-drug cytotoxic chemotherapy for a period varying between 7 and 24 months.[63,114] Thirty patients, aged 3 to 50, with acute lymphocytic leukemia, who had remained in remission throughout the period of chemotherapy, were allocated to 4 groups: 10 controls received no further therapy; 8 patients were treated every fourth day for the first month and once weekly thereafter with 2 ml (75 mg) of Pasteur Institute bacille Calmette-Guérin (BCG) applied to 20 epidermal scratches 5 cm long; 5 patients received 4×10^7 pooled formalinized or irradiated allogeneic acute lymphocytic leukemia cells by subcutaneous injection once weekly; and 7 patients received simultaneous BCG and allogeneic leukemia cells at the above doses and schedules. All control patients had relapsed within 130 days after chemotherapy was completed. The median time to relapse for the controls was only 74 days, indicative of an estimated drug induced reduction to 10^6 to 10^7 residual leukemic cells. Patients receiving BCG or leukemia cell injections, or both, relapsed at a rate comparable to that of the controls for the first month, after which the rate of recurrence was dramatically reduced. Only 9 of the 20 had relapsed by day 130, and 7 remained in remission more than 28 months after the last drug administration. This study provides the most striking exhibition of control of residual leukemia by nonchemotherapeutic means yet reported. The biphasic curve apparent in plotting the rate of the immunotherapy group relapses implies that immunotherapy was effective only for those patients whose tumor cell populations were most significantly reduced and/or most slowly regrowing. The inflection point occurred at 30 days, consistent with a reduction of leukemia of less than 3 logs (to 10^8 to 10^9). Therefore, this experiment and that of Skurkovich et al. suggest that human host-defense mechanisms have a greater capacity for cell control than the 10^5 cell threshold observed in rodents (see above). By the same reasoning, the "cytoreductive" therapy employed by Mathé in preparation for immunotherapy was clearly less effective than other reported drug regimens,[3,4] so that the possibility exists that more vigorous preparatory chemotherapy resulting in greater leukemia cell reduction might yield still better results.

The above reports have stimulated a number of attempts to confirm and extend these observations. Guyer and Crowther[14] used *Bordetella pertussis* vaccine as the nonspecific immunizing agent, based on the findings of Wissler et al. in transplantable murine tumors.[102] Sixteen patients with acute leukemia were divided into two groups matched for age, sex, and the duration of leukemia. Remission induction with prednisone plus either mercaptopurine or vincristine, and a 3-month period of combination chemotherapy in remission preceded the immunotherapy trial. *B. pertussis* vaccine was given to 8 patients, 0.5 ml once or twice per week intramuscularly, with a median remission period of 186 days on the vaccination alone. The longest remission in this group was 455 days. The median post-chemotherapy remission for the control group was 112 days. One of these was still in remission at over 2 years.

The early reports of a large collaborative immunotherapy trial conducted by the British Medical Research Council have recently been published.[116] This program was based directly on Mathé's study using early remission drug therapy (16 weeks of mercaptopurine, vincristine intermittently, and prednisone daily), followed by 6 weeks of combined asparaginase and intramuscular and intrathecal methotrexate. Patients were then randomized to weekly BCG, intermittent methotrexate, or no further treatment. The BCG regimen differed from Mathé's, the antigen being obtained from Glaxo and administered by means of a Heath gun rather than by linear scarifications. Seventy-one patients completed initial chemotherapy. Ten of 18 controls and 18 of the 35 BCG-treated patients have thus far relapsed, with a median remission duration of 130 to 160 days. In contrast, there have been only 3 relapses (all with meningeal leukemia) in patients receiving methotrexate. Although continued drug therapy was clearly the superior treatment at the point of randomization 5½ months into remission, and although there has not yet been a difference between the BCG and control groups, it is still possible that a difference in the number of long-term remissions in the latter two groups will become manifest, particularly in light of the apparent all-or-nothing response to BCG seen in Mathé's series.

Obviously, since the techniques of antigen administration differed, and since there is no established direct assay of enhancement of antileukemia immunity, the two studies may be no more than superficially comparable.

Two other reports of nonspecific immunization deserve mention. Several polynucleotides have been shown to induce interferon, enhance immunologic reactions, and exert antitumor activity in mice. A recent report of Mathé and coworkers[117] notes 5 complete remissions in 15 patients treated at the point of early and/or partial relapse with polyinosinic-polycytidylic acid. No effect was seen in patients in whom leukemic marrow infiltration was greater than 50 per cent. The role of such compounds, and the mechanism(s) of their action, remain to be elucidated. A recent report of the antitumor activity of interferon against isogeneic murine leukemia suggests that at least part of the polynucleotide effect is through this pathway, rather than the strictly immunologic route.[118]

The observation of remissions occurring in patients suffering spontaneous viral illnesses prompted Wheelock and Dingle to advertently infect a patient with acute myelocytic leukemia no longer responsive to drugs with repetitive challenges of a variety of viruses.[119] Repeated reduction of peripheral blast levels, spleen, and lymph node size were observed, and at autopsy a marked reduction in bone marrow blasts was observed. The possibility that coincident virus infection, in this case infectious mononucleosis, during remission, may increase the duration of remission and survival has recently been raised by Stevens et al.[120]

Passive Immunotherapy

Since Hueper and Russell's[121] and Lindstrom's[122] articles on the treatment of myelocytic leukemia with rabbit anti-human-leukemia sera, only one attempt to passively immunize with xenogeneic plasma or cells has been reported. Izawa and colleagues[123] achieved transient depression of peripheral blood leukocyte counts in 1 of 10 patients with chronic myelocytic leukemia and in the only patient with acute leukemia receiving sheep anti-human-leukemia sera. Passive immunization with allogeneic plasma or serum has been attempted more frequently. Brittingham and Chaplin[124] attempted to influence the course of chronic myelocytic leukemia with sera obtained from immunized normal human donors. Andrews et al. treated acute leukemic children with thoracic duct lymphocytes from parents immunized with killed lymphoblasts.[125] Laszlo et al.[126] and Djerassi[127] treated chronic lymphocytic leukemia and acute lymphocytic leukemia with plasma and leukocytes, respectively, obtained from patients or volunteers sensitized to normal transplantation isoantigens through multiple transfusions. Skurkovich et al., as part of the experiment detailed above,[115] transfused putative specific immune plasma to half of his patients previously actively immunized. In all cases results were never dramatic, being limited in most instances to a reduction in peripheral blast counts or slight regression in the size of lymph nodes. In the only large-scale study of serotherapy in leukemia, Children's Cancer Group A compared plasma infusions (4 ml per kilogram of body weight each week) plus 6-mercaptopurine versus the antipurine alone as maintenance treatment for 112 children with acute lymphocytic leukemia.[128] One group received plasma obtained from unrelated donors, and a second plasma from parents or other relatives dwelling with the child and thus possibly immunized to a theoretical leukemogen. Remission durations were comparable in the plasma and control groups.

Skurkovich and coworkers reinfused stored autologous plasma, and intramuscularly injected stored leukocytes, at 1- or 2-week intervals as an adjunct to drug maintenance with 6-mercaptopurine in 9 children in their first complete remission from acute leukemia.[15] Nine comparable patients received only 6-mercaptopurine. At the time of their report, 6 of the 9 "passively autoimmunized" patients had continued in remission 11 to 48 months, while 8 of the 9 controls had relapsed by 8½ months. All 3 immunized patients who relapsed did so initially at extramedullary sites, one each in the skin, central nervous system, and testes.

Adoptive Immunotherapy

Transplantation of bone marrow and peripheral blood has been pursued with renewed interest with the partial identification and systematization of human transplantation (HL-A) isoantigens. Mathé et al. reported unexpectedly prolonged remission after marrow allografting in a few patients whose tumor had become refractory to drug therapy.[129] Freireich et al.[130] and Schwarzenberg et al.[131] noted transient remissions after transfusions of chronic myelocytic leukemia cells. In contrast, the transplantation of normal syngeneic bone marrow has not been associated with any apparent antileukemic effect.[68,72] Mathé, Schwarzenberg and their colleagues have suggested that the effectiveness of stem cell grafts is proportional to the degree of histocompatibility differences, the therapeutic limit being the toxicity of graft-versus-host reactions (GvH),[118] a position consonant with Boranic's grafting experiments in mice.[88]

Despite occasional successes, stem cell grafting remains a hazardous experiment. Matching of donor and recipient by HL-A typing and mixed lymphocyte culture has improved the rate of engraftment but has not eliminated the risk of fatal graft-versus-host reactions.[132-134] Mathé has reported that pretreatment of the graft recipient with antilymphocyte serum minimizes the threat of GvH but simultaneously negates the therapeutic effect of the allograft.[135] Up to the present time, because of the hazards involved, allogeneic marrow grafting has been undertaken only in late-stage or poor-risk patients, so that optimal reduction of leukemia cell populations have not been achieved prior to grafting.

Discussion

The immunotherapy of leukemia, although generally ineffective in the past, has received a modicum of scientific support and achieved a few tentative successes. As with other forms of tumor therapy, objective measures of tumor specificity and potency are urgently required. As blood and tissue levels are important to chemotherapy, so is the measurement of immunologic activities necessary for rational immunotherapy. A screening program with appropriate in vitro and animal models will probably be necessary to evaluate candidate adjuvants and nonspecific immunogens.

Furthermore, one must recall another lesson from chemotherapy and be wary of discarding a therapy as valueless on the basis of trials centering on only a single arbitrary regimen. Immunologic reactions can provide a more specific cytotoxic effect than any other known therapy. In combination with appropriate modalities of greater potency but less specificity, the full value of both approaches may be finally appreciated.

References

1. Henderson, E. S.: The treatment of acute leukemia. Seminars Hemat. 6:271, 1969.
2. Burchenal, J. H.: Formal discussion: Long-term survival in Burkitt's tumor and in acute leukemia. Cancer Res. 27:2616, 1967.
3. Holland, J. F.: Therapy of acute leukemia. XIII International Congress of Hematology. Munich: J. F. Lehmanns, 1970, pp. 58–65.
4. Henderson, E. S. and Samaha, R. J.: Evidence that drugs in multiple combinations have materially advanced the treatment of human malignancies. Cancer Res. 29:2272, 1969.
5. Freireich, E. J, Henderson, E. S., Karon, M. R. and Frei, E., III: The treatment of acute leukemia considered with respect to cell population kinetics. *In* The Proliferation and Spread of Neoplastic Cells. Baltimore: Williams & Wilkins, 1968, pp. 441–452.
6. Henderson, E. S.: Combination chemotherapy of acute lymphoblastic leukemia of childhood. Cancer Res. 27:2570, 1967.
7. Whang-Peng, J., Henderson, E. S., Knutsen, T., Freireich, E. J, and Gart, J. J.: Cytogenetic studies in acute myelocytic leukemia with special emphasis on the occurrence of Ph^1 chromosome. Blood 36:448, 1970.
8. Zuelzer, W. W. and Cox, D. E.: Genetic aspects of leukemia. Seminars Hemat. 6:228, 1969.
9. Whang-Peng, J., Freireich, E. J, Oppenheim, J. J., Frei, E., III and Tjio, J. H.: Cytogenetic studies in 45 patients with acute lymphocytic leukemia. J. Nat. Cancer Inst. 42:881, 1969.
10. Boiron, M., Weil, M. and Jacquillat, C.: Daunorubicin in the treatment of acute myelocytic leukaemia. Lancet 1:330, 1969.
11. Ellison, R. R. et al. (Acute Leukemia Cooperative Group B): Arabinosyl cytosine: A useful agent in the treatment of acute leukemia in adults. Blood 32:507, 1968.
12. Freireich, E. J, Bodey, G. P., Harris, J. E. and Hart, J. S.: Therapy for acute granulocytic leukemia. Cancer Res. 27: 2573, 1967.
13. Ngu, V. A.: Host defenses to Burkitt's tumour. Brit. Med. J. 1:345, 1967.
14. Guyer, R. J. and Crowther, D.: Active immunotherapy in treatment of acute leukemia. Brit. Med. J. 4:406, 1969.
15. Skurkovich, S. V., Makhonova, L. A., Reznichenko, F. M. and Chervonskii, G. I.: Treatment of children suffering from acute leukemia by passive cyclic immunization with autoplasma and autoleukocytes obtained during remission. Probl. Gemat. 12:18, 1967.
16. Old, L. J. and Boyse, E. A.: Antigens of tumors and leukemias induced by viruses. Fed. Proc. 24:1009, 1965.
17. Law, L. J.: Studies of the significance of tumor antigens in induction and repression of neoplastic disease. Cancer Res. 29:1, 1969.
18. Gilden, R. V., Beddow, T. G. and Huebner, R. J.: Production of high titer antibody in serum and ascitic fluid of hamsters for a variety of virus-induced tumor antigens. Appl. Microbiol. 15:657, 1967.
19. Kalnins, V. I., Stich, H. F., Gregory, C. and Yohn, D. S.: Localization of tumor antigens in adenovirus-12-induced tumor cells and in adenovirus-12-infected human and hamster cells by ferritin-labeled antibodies. Cancer Res. 27:1874, 1967.
20. Prehn, R. T. and Main, J. M.: Immunity to methylcholanthrene-induced sarcomas. J. Nat. Cancer Inst. 18:769, 1957.
21. Churchill, W. H., Jr., Rapp, H. J., Kronman, B. S. and Borsos, T.: Detection of antigens of a new diethylnitrosamine-induced transplantable hepatoma by delayed hypersensitivity. J. Nat. Cancer Inst. 41:13, 1968.
22. Riggins, R. S. and Pilch, Y. H.: Immunity to spontaneous and methylcholanthrene induced tumors in inbred mice. Cancer Res. 24:1994, 1964.
23. Sumner, W. C. and Foraker, A. C.: Spontaneous regression of human melanoma: Clinical and experimental study. Cancer 13:79, 1960.
24. Morton, D. L., Eilber, F. R., Malmgren, R. A. and Wood, W. C.: Immunological factors which influence response to immunotherapy of malignant melanoma. Surgery 68:158, 1970.

25. Burkitt, D. P. and Kyalwazi, S. K.: Spontaneous remission of African lymphoma. Brit. J. Cancer 21:14, 1967.
26. Bardawil, W. A. and Toy, B. L.: The natural history of choriocarcinoma: Problems of immunity and spontaneous regression. Ann. N.Y. Acad. Sci. 80:197, 1959.
27. Southam, C. M., Craver, L. F., Dargeon, W. and Burchenal, J. H.: A study of the natural history of acute leukemia. Cancer 4:39, 1951.
28. Burkett, L. L., Fields, M. L. and Diggs, L. W.: A possible immune reaction producing spontaneous remission in leukemia. Blood 25:541, 1965.
29. Fraumeni, J. F., Jr. and Miller, R. W.: Epidemiology of human leukemia: Recent observations. J. Nat. Cancer Inst. 38:593, 1967.
30. Medical Research Council: Hypogammaglobulinaemia in the United Kingdom. Lancet 1:163, 1969.
31. Leventhal, B. G., Waldorf, D. S. and Talal, N.: Impaired lymphocyte transformation and delayed hypersensitivity in Sjogrens syndrome. J. Clin. Invest. 46:1338, 1967.
32. Wilson, R. E., Hager, E. B., Hampers, C. L., Corson, J. M., Merrill, J. P. and Murray, J. E.: Immunologic rejection of human cancer transplanted with a renal allograft. New Eng. J. Med. 278:479, 1968.
33. Calne, R. Y.: Immunosuppression and cancer. Lancet 1:625, 1969.
34. McKhann, C. F.: Primary malignancy in patients undergoing immunosuppression for renal transplantation. Transplantation 8:209, 1969.
35. Zukoski, C. F., Killen, D. A., Ginn, E., Matter, B., Lucas, D. O. and Seigler, H. F.: Transplanted carcinoma in an immunosuppressed patient. Transplantation 9:71, 1970.
36. Fass, L., Herberman, R. B. and Ziegler, J.: Cutaneous hypersensitivity to extracts of Burkitt's lymphoma cells. New Eng. J. Med. 282:776, 1970.
37. Sokol, J. E. and Aungst, C. W.: Response to BCG vaccination and survival in advanced Hodgkin's disease. Cancer 24: 128, 1969.
38. Brown, R. S., Haynes, H. A., Foley, H. T., Godwin, H. A., Berard, C. W. and Carbone, P. P.: Hodgkin's disease: Immunologic, clinical and histologic features of 50 untreated patients. Ann. Intern. Med. 67:291, 1967.
39. Lewis, M. G., Ikonopisov, R. L., Nairn, R. C., Phillips, T. M., Hamilton Fairley, G. et al.: Tumour-specific antibodies in human malignant melanoma and their relationship to the extent of the disease. Brit. Med. J. 3:547, 1969.
40. Crowther, D., Fairley, G. H. and Sewell, R. L.: Significance of the changes in the circulating lymphoid cells in Hodgkin's disease. Brit. Med. J. 2:473, 1969.
41. Stewart, T. H. M.: The immunologic reactivity of patients with cancer: A preliminary report. Canad. Med. Ass. J. 99:342, 1968.
42. Klein, G., Klein, E. and Clifford, P.: Search for host defenses in Burkitt's lymphoma. Membrane immunofluorescence tests on biopsies and tissue culture lines. Cancer Res. 27:2510, 1967.
43. Henle, G. and Henle, W.: Immunofluorescence in cells derived from Burkitt's lymphoma. J. Bact. 91:1248, 1966.
44. Herberman, R. B. and Fahey, J. L.: Cytotoxic antibody in Burkitt's tumor and normal human serum reactive with cultures of lymphoid cells. Proc. Soc. Exp. Biol. Med. 127:938, 1968.
45. Muna, N. M., Marcus, S. and Smart, C.: Detection by immunofluorescence of antibodies specific for human malignant melanoma cells. Cancer 23:88, 1969.
46. Fass, L., Herberman, R. B., Ziegler, J. L. and Kiryabwire, J. W. M.: Cutaneous hypersensitivity to autologous extracts of malignant melanoma cells. Lancet 1:116, 1970.
47. Morton, D. L., Malmgren, R. A., Holmes, E. C. and Ketcham, A. S.: Demonstration of antibodies against human malignant melanomas by immunofluorescence. Surgery 64:233, 1968.
48. Morton, D. L., Malmgren, R. A., Hall, W. T. and Schidlovsky, G.: Immunologic and virus studies with human sarcomas. Surgery 66:152, 1969.
49. Eilber, F. R. and Morton, D. L.: Demonstration in sarcoma patients of anti-tumour antibodies which fix only human complement. Nature 225:1137, 1970.
50. Gold, P. and Freedman, S. O.: Specific carcinoembryonic antigens of the human digestive system. J. Exp. Med. 122:467, 1965.
51. Hellstrom, I., Hellstrom, K. E., Pierce, G. E., and Bill, A. H.: Demonstration of cell-bound and humoral immunity against neuroblastoma cells. Proc. Nat. Acad. Sci. 60:1231, 1968.

52. Pierce, G. E., Hellstrom, I. E., Hellstrom, K. E. and Yang, J. P. S.: Demonstration of cellular immunity against human tumors. Surg. Forum 20:112, 1969.
53. Hughes, L. E. and Lytton, B.: Antigen properties of human tumours. Delayed cutaneous hypersensitivity reactions. Brit. Med. J. 1:209, 1964.
54. Stewart, T. H.: The presence of delayed hypersensitivity reactions in patients toward cellular extracts of their malignant tumors. I. The role of tissue antigen, nonspecific reactions of nuclear material, and bacterial antigen as a cause for this phenomenon. Cancer 23:1368, 1969.
55. Herberman, R. B. and Oren, M.: Delayed cutaneous hypersensitivity reactions to membrane extracts of human tumor cells. Clin. Res. 17:403, 1969.
56. Andersen, V., Bendixen, G. and Schiodt, T.: An *in vitro* demonstration of cellular immunity against autologous mammary carcinoma in man. Acta Med. Scand. 186:101, 1969.
57. Fink, M. A., Karon, M., Rauscher, F. J., Malmgren, R. A. and Orr, H. C.: Further observations on the immunofluorescence of cells in human leukemia. Cancer 18:1317, 1965.
58. Ionnaides, A. K., Rosner, F., Brenner, M. and Lee, S. L.: Immunofluorescent studies of human leukemic cells with antiserum to a murine leukemia virus (Rauscher strain). Blood 31:381, 1968.
59. Bates, H. A., Bankole, R. O. and Swaim, W. R.: Immunofluorescence studies in human leukemia. Blood 34:430, 1969.
60. Doré, J. F., Motta, R., Marholev, L., Hrsak, I., Colas de la Noue, H., et al.: New antigens in human leukemic cells and antibody in the serum of leukemic patients. Lancet 2:1396, 1967.
61. Fridman, W. H. and Kourilsky, F. M.: Stimulation of lymphocytes by autologous leukemic cells in acute leukemia. Nature 224:277, 1969.
62. Viza, D. C., Bernard-Degani, O., Bernard, C. and Harris, R.: Leukemia antigens. Lancet 2:493, 1969.
63. Mathé, G., Amiel, J. L., Schwarzenberg, L., Schneider, M., Cattan, A., et al.: Active immunotherapy for acute lymphoblastic leukemia. Lancet 1:697, 1969.
64. Gorer, P. and Amos, D. B.: Passive immunity in mice against C57Bl leukosis E.L. 4 by means of iso-immune serum. Cancer Res. 16:338, 1956.
65. Alexander, P., Cornell, D. I. and McKulska, Z. B.: Treatment of a murine leukemia with spleen cells or sera from allogeneic mice immunized against the tumor. Cancer Res. 26:1508, 1966.
66. Delorme, E. J. and Alexander, P.: Treatment of primary fibrosarcoma in the rat with immune lymphocytes. Lancet 2:117, 1964.
67. Fefer, A.: Immunotherapy and chemotherapy of Moloney sarcoma virus-induced tumors in mice. Cancer Res. 29:2177, 1969.
68. Old, L. J., Stockert, E., Boyse, E. A. and Geering, G.: A study of passive immunization against a transplanted G+ leukemia with specific antiserum. Proc. Soc. Exp. Biol. Med. 124:63, 1967.
69. Freireich, E. J, Karon, M. and Henderson, E. S.: Unpublished observations.
70. Thomas, E. D. and Epstein, R. B.: Bone marrow transplantation in acute leukemia. Cancer Res. 25:1521, 1965.
71. Pegg, D. E.: Bone marrow transplantation. Chicago: Year Book Medical Publishers, 1966.
72. Bortin, M. M.: A compendium of reported human bone marrow transplants. Transplantation 9:571, 1970.
73. Klein, G., Sjogren, H. O., Klein, E. and Hellstrom, K. E.: Demonstration of resistance against methylcholanthrene induce sarcomas in the primary autochthonous host. Cancer Res. 20:1561, 1960.
74. Henderson, E. S.: Unpublished observations.
75. Miller, D. G., Moldovanu, G., Kaplan, A. and Tocci, S.: Antilymphocyte leukemia serum and chemotherapy on the treatment of murine leukemia. Cancer 22:1192, 1968.
76. Reif, A. E. and Kim, C.-A. H.: Therapy of transplantable mouse leukemias with anti-leukemia sera. Nature 223:1377, 1969.
77. Hill, G. J., II, Atkins, R. C., Parks, S., Littlejohn, K. and Eiseman, B.: Immunotherapeutic effect of sensitized leukocytes and anti-serum on mouse leukemia. Surg. Forum 20:122, 1969.
78. Southam, C. M.: Applications of immunology to clinical cancer. Cancer Res. 21:1302, 1961.
79. Cinader, B., Hayley, M. A., Rider, W. D. and Warwick, O. H.: Acquired tolerance, autoantibodies, and cancer. Canad. Med. Ass. J. 84:306, 1961.
80. Teimourin, B. and McCune, W. S.: Surgical management of malignant melanoma. Amer. Surg. 29:515, 1963.

81. Burkitt, D.: Clinical evidence suggesting the development of an immunological response against African lymphoma. Conference on the Chemotherapy of Burkitt's Tumor, Kumpala, Uganda, 1966; Treatment of Burkitt's Tumor (UICC Monograph Series, Vol. 8, 1967, p. 197). Berlin: Springer Verlag, 1967.
82. Fass, L., Herberman, R. B., Ziegler, J. and Morrow, R. H.: Evaluation of the effect of remission plasma on untreated patients with Burkitt's lymphoma. J. Nat. Cancer Inst. 44:145, 1970.
83. Glynn, J. P., Halpern, A. and Fefer, A.: An immunochemotherapeutic system for the treatment of a transplanted Moloney virus-induced lymphoma in mice. Cancer Res. 29:515, 1969.
84. Wepsic, H. T., Kronman, B. S., Zbar, B., Borsos, T. and Rapp, H. J.: Immunotherapy of an intramuscular tumor in strain-2 guinea pigs: Prevention of growth by intradermal immunization and by systemic transfer of tumor immunity. J. Nat. Cancer Inst. 45:377, 1970.
85. Fisher, J. C. and Hammond, W. G.: Inhibition of tumor growth by syngeneic spleen cell transfer. Surg. Forum 17:102, 1966.
86. Woodruff, M. F. A. and Nolan, B.: Preliminary observations on treatment of advanced cancer by injection of allogeneic spleen cells. Lancet 2:426, 1963.
87. Symes, M. O.: The use of immunologically competent cells in the treatment of cancer. Brit. J. Cancer 21:178, 1967.
88. Boranic, M.: The time-pattern of the antileukaemic effect of the graft-versus-host reaction. Transplant. Proc. 3:394, 1971.
89. Nadler, S. H. and Moore, G. E.: Immunotherapy of malignant disease. Arch. Surg. 99:376, 1969.
90. Alexander, P., Delorme, E. J., Hamilton, L. D. G. and Hall, J. G.: Effect of nucleic acids from immune lymphocytes on rat sarcomata. Nature 213:569, 1967.
91. Londner, M. V., Morini, J. C., Font, M. T. and Rabasa, S. L.: RNA-induced immunity against a rat sarcoma. Experientia 24:598, 1968.
92. Pilch, Y. H. and Ramming, K. P.: Transfer of tumor immunity with ribonucleic acid. Cancer 26:630, 1970.
93. Oettgen, H. F., Old, L. J., McLean, E. P. and Carswell, E. A.: Delayed hypersensitivity and transplantation immunity elicited by soluble antigens of chemically induced tumors in inbred guinea pigs. Nature 220:295, 1968.
94. Zbar, B., Wepsic, H. T., Rapp, H. J., Borsos, T., Kronman, B. S. and Churchill, W. H., Jr.: Antigenic specificity of hepatomas induced in strain-2 guinea pigs by diethylnitrosamine. J. Nat. Cancer Inst. 43:833, 1969.
95. Mathé, G.: Immunothérapie active de la leucémie L1210 appliquée après la greffe tumorale. Rev. Franc. Etud. Clin. Biol. 13:881, 1968.
96. Kronman, B. S., Wepsic, H. T., Churchill, W. H., Jr., Zbar, B., Borsos, T. and Rapp, H. J.: Immunotherapy of cancer: An experimental model in syngeneic guinea pigs. Science 168:257, 1970.
97. Alexander, P. and Hall, J. G.: The role of immunoblasts in host resistance and immunotherapy of primary sarcomata. Advances Cancer Res. 13:1, 1970.
98. Amiel, J.-L.: Immunothérapie active non-spécifique par le B.C.G. de la leucémie virale E [male] G2 chez des receveurs isogeniques. Rev. Franc. Etud. Clin. Biol. 12:912, 1967.
99. Old, L. J., Benacerraf, B., Clarke, D. A., Carswell, E. A. and Stockert, E.: The role of the reticuloendothelial system in the host reaction to neoplasia. Cancer Res. 21:1281, 1961.
100. Zbar, B. Personal communication.
101. Weiss, D. W., Bonhag, R. S. and Leslie, P.: Studies on the heterologous immunogenicity of a methanol-insoluble fraction of attenuated tubercle bacilli (BCG). II. Protection against tumor isografts. J. Exp. Med. 124:1039, 1966.
102. Wissler, R. W., Craft, K., Kesden, D., Polisky, B. and Dzoga, K.: Inhibition of the growth of the Morris hepatoma (5123) in buffalo rats using a mixture of pertussis vaccine and irradiated tumor. *In* Dausset, J. (Ed.): Advance in Transplantation. Baltimore: Williams and Wilkins, 1968, p. 539.
103. Woodruff, M. F. A. and Boak, J. L.: Inhibitory effect of injection of *Corynebacterium parvum* on the growth of tumor transplants in isogenic hosts. Brit. J. Cancer 20:345, 1966.
104. Holm, G. and Perlman, P.: Cytotoxic potential of stimulated human lymphocytes. J. Exp. Med. 125:721, 1967.
105. Levy, H. B., Law, L. W. and Rabson, A. S.: Inhibition of tumor growth by polyinosinic-polycytidylic acid. Proc. Nat. Acad. Sci. 62:357, 1969.
106. Gorer, P. A.: The antigen structure of tumours. Advances Immun. 1:345, 1961.

107. Hellström, I., Hellström, K. E., Evans, C. A., Heppner, G. H., Pierce, C. E. and Yang, J. P. S.: Serum-mediated protection of neoplastic cells from inhibition by lymphocytes immune to their tumor specific antigens. Proc. Nat. Acad. Sci. 62:362, 1969.
108. Kaliss, H. and Bryant, B. F.: Factors determining homograft destruction and immunological enhancement in mice receiving successive tumor inocula. J. Nat. Cancer Inst. 20: 691, 1958.
109. Wilson, D. B.: Quantitative studies on the behavior of sensitized lymphocytes *in vitro*. I. Relationship of the degree of destruction of homologous target cells to the number of lymphocytes and the time of contact in culture and consideration of the effects of isoimmune serum. J. Exp. Med. 122:143, 1965.
110. Borsos, T., Colten, H. R., Spalter, J. S., Rogentine, N. and Rapp, H. J.: The C′1a fixation and transfer test: Examples of its applicability to the detection and enumeration of antigens and antibodies at cell surfaces. J. Immun. 101:392, 1968.
111. Zelen, M.: Leukemia models: Mice and men. In The Proliferation and Spread of Neoplastic Cells. Baltimore: Williams & Wilkins, 1968, pp. 463–477.
112. Frei, E., III and Freireich, E. J: Progress and perspectives in the chemotherapy of acute leukemias. Advances Chemother. 2:269, 1965.
113. Holland, J. F.: Clinical studies of unmaintained remissions in acute lymphocytic leukemia. *In* The Proliferation and Spread of Neoplastic Cells. Baltimore: Williams & Wilkins, 1968, pp. 453–462.
114. Mathé, G., Schwarzenberg, L., Amiel, J. L., Schneider, M., Cattan, A. and Schlumberger, J. R.: The role of immunology in the treatment of leukemias and hematosarcomas. Cancer Res. 27:2542, 1967.
115. Skurkovich, S. V. Kisljak, N. S., Machonova, L. A. and Begunenko, S. A.: Active immunization of children suffering from acute leukemia in acute phase with "live" allogenic leukaemic cells. Nature 223:509, 1969.
116. Fairley, G. H.: Immunotherapy of acute lymphoblastic leukemia. XIII International Congress of Hematology. Munich: J. H. Lehmanns, 1970, p. 278.
117. Mathé, G., Amiel, J.-L., Schwarzenberg, M., Schneider, M., Hayat, M., et al.: Remission induction with poly IC in patients with acute lymphoblastic leukemia. Eurp. J. Clin. Biol. Res. 15:671, 1970.
118. Graff, S., Kassel, R. and Kastner, O.: Interferon. Trans. N.Y. Acad. Sci. 32:545, 1970.
119. Wheelock, E. F. and Dingle, J. H.: Observations on the repeated administration of viruses to a patient with acute leukemia. A preliminary report. New Eng. J. Med. 271:645, 1964.
120. Stevens, D. A., Levine, P. H., Lee, S. K., Sonely, M. J. and Waggoner, D. E.: Concurrent infectious mononucleosis and acute leukemia. Amer. J. Med. 50:208, 1971.
121. Hueper, W. C. and Russell, M.: Some immunologic aspects of leukemia. Arch. Intern. Med. 49:113, 1932.
122. Lindstrom, G. A.: Myelotoxic sera in myeloid leukemia. Acta Med. Scand. J. Suppl. 22:1, 1927.
123. Izawa, T., Sakurai, M., Atsuta, Y. and Yoshizumi, T.: Antigenicity of leukemia and antiserum therapy. Ann. Paediat. Jap. 12:346, 1966.
124. Brittingham, T. E. and Chaplin, H.: Production of human "antileukemic leukocyte" serum and its therapeutic trial. Cancer 13:412, 1960.
125. Andrews, G. A., Congdon, C. C., Edwards, C. L., Gengozian, N., Nelson, B. and Vodopick, H.: Preliminary trials of clinical immunotherapy. Cancer Res. 27:2535, 1967.
126. Laszlo, J., Buckley, C. E., III and Amos, D. B.: Infusion of isologous immune plasma in chronic lymphocytic leukemia. Blood 31:104, 1968.
127. Djerassi, I.: Transfusion of lymphocyte antibodies and lymphocytes from multitransfused donors: A possible immunologic approach to the reduction of leukemic cell mass in children. Clin. Pediat. 7:272, 1968.
128. Albo, V., Krivit, W. and Hartman, J.: Fresh plasma as an adjuvant to the chemotherapy of acute lymphatic leukemia in children. Proc. Amer. Ass. Cancer Res. 9:2, 1968.
129. Mathé, G., Amiel, J. L., Schwarzenberg, L., Schneider, M., Cattan, A., et al.: Bone marrow transplantation in man. Transplant. Proc. 1:16, 1969.
130. Freireich, E. J., Levin, R. H., Whang, J., Carbone, P. P., Bronson, W. and Morse, E. E.: The function and fate of transfused leukocytes from donors with chronic myelocytic leukemia in leukopenic recipients. Ann. N.Y. Acad. Sci. 113:1081, 1964.

131. Schwarzenberg, L., Mathé, G., Amiel, J. L., Cattan, A., Schneider, M. and Schlumberger, J. R.: Study of factors determining the usefulness and complications of leukocyte transfusions. Amer. J. Med. 43:206, 1967.

132. Graw, R. G., Jr., Leventhal, B. G., Yankee, R. A., Rogentine, G. N., Whang-Peng, J., et al.: HL-A and mixed leucocyte culture matched allogeneic bone marrow transplantation in patients with acute leukemia. Transplant. Proc. 3:405, 1971.

133. deKoning, J. and Dooren, L. J.: Bone marrow transplantation in an immune deficient infant: 1½ year follow up. XIII International Congress of Hematology. Munich: J. H. Lehmanns, 1970, p. 169.

134. Santos, G. W., Sensenbrenner, L. L., Burke, P. J., Colvin, O. M., Owens, A. H., et al.: Marrow transplantation in man following cyclophosphamide. Transplant. Proc. 3:400, 1971.

135. Mathé, G.: Personal communication.

Therapy of Myeloproliferative Disorders

By S. Benham Kahn, M.D. and Isadore Brodsky, M.D.

THE MYELOPROLIFERATIVE DISORDERS originate in the bone marrow or potential bone marrow sites; they have no known cause, are malignancies, and are characterized by an overgrowth of hematopoietic stem cells which give rise to erythrocytes, leukocytes, platelets, and fibroblastic reticulum.[1] Their classification is given in Table 1. Clinically and hematologically, all but the most acute are easily distinguished from the lymphoproliferative disorders.

Dameshek's hypothesis that these disorders are related etiologically to each other was prompted by their morphologic similarities. However, despite apparent similarities among entities,[2] workers have recently challenged the idea that these disorders share common causes or that they are transformed from one to another.[3] This fact must be kept in mind when eventually specific cures for these diseases are found. Therapy is still noncurative and nonspecific in that the cytotoxic agents used suppress normal tissue as well as malignant tissue. Because of the nonspecificity of therapy, we urge adherence to the concept of myeloproliferative disease since this approach still remains most useful in directing the physician towards proper diagnosis and treatment of patients with disorders which do not fit into single-disease categories.

In this chapter we shall consider therapy of the chronic disorders, since the acute syndromes are covered in a chapter dealing with therapy of acute leukemia.

Table 1.—*Types of Myeloproliferative Disorders**

Chronic myeloproliferative disorders
Polycythemia vera (PV)
Myelofibrosis, myelosclerosis with myeloid metaplasia (MMM)
Hemorrhagic thrombocytosis (HT)
Chronic myelogenous leukemia (CML)
Acute myeloproliferative disorders
Di Guglielmo's syndrome and variants
Acute myelogenous leukemia (AML)

*After Dameshek.[1]

Polycythemia Vera

The prototype of these disorders is polycythemia vera (PV). This disease is a panmyelopathy, resulting at various times in its course in elevation of red blood cell (RBC) count, white blood cell (WBC) count, platelet count, or all three.[4,5] The principal complication of this disorder is hemorrhage or thrombosis, or both.[6] The pathogenesis of these complications is related to the increase in blood viscosity and to thrombocytosis, particularly when associated with increased platelet turnover and abnormalities in platelet function.[7]

Treatment is aimed at reducing the blood volume and suppressing marrow activity.

From the Division of Hematology and Medical Oncology, Department of Medicine, Hahnemann Medical College and Hospital, Philadelphia, Pennsylvania.

Phlebotomy will reduce the blood volume rapidly but must be considered adjunctive therapy in most patients, since it does not alter the fundamental abnormality of the disease.[8] Only in the most benign cases does it produce anything more than transient improvement. Repeated phlebotomy seems to become less efficacious in time and may lead to symptoms of its own by producing severe iron deficiency. Phlebotomy is useful in the following situations: (1) when rapid reduction of the blood volume is necessary, as in acute heart failure or before emergency surgery; (2) before therapy with ^{32}P, since this suppressive agent requires four to six weeks before effects are seen; (3) in the later stages of the disease when chemotherapy is used to suppress the WBC count or platelet count; and (4) when the only manifestation of the disease is an elevated RBC mass unassociated with other symptoms. Hemolytic drugs, such as phenylhydrazine, cannot be recommended in present-day management. The same is true for iron-restricted diets. Actually, diets high in protein and minerals are suggested to prevent severe deficiency states, particularly in patients requiring frequent phlebotomy.

The myelosuppressive therapy of this disorder is now in a state of evolution, with more emphasis being placed on chemotherapy and less on radiophosphorus treatment. There is no consensus as to the best method. Indeed, all treatments are palliative and, while long symptom-free remissions may ensue, the disease may eventually cause death. Indications for myelosuppressive therapy in PV include thrombocytosis, leukocytosis, symptomatic splenomegaly (hypersplenism, infarcts, pressure and bowel symptoms), hyperuricemia with gout or renal stones, and symptoms such as pruritus, weight loss, gastrointestinal distress and headaches.[9] Erythrocytosis unassociated with any of the above is unusual; but when such a pattern is seen, phlebotomy alone may control the situation for a period of time.

Radiophosphorus (^{32}P)

Lawrence and his group introduced this form of therapy in the late 1930s. Experience since then has indicated that ^{32}P is an extremely effective form of therapy for this disease.[4,10–14] The rationale behind its use resides in the fact that actively dividing tissues have a high requirement for phosphorus, since this element is a key constituent of DNA and RNA. Radiophosphorus is a pure beta emitter of high intensity. In effect, radiation is delivered to the marrow and selectively to the nucleus of the dividing cell, and ^{32}P is advantageous because it is relatively inexpensive, can be given in a single dose, and does not create a radiation hazard to others.[4,12] The material is administered as sodium phosphate, preferably intravenously. It can be given orally, but about 25 per cent of the dose may not be absorbed if it is given in this fashion.[4] There is inadequate knowledge of the dosimetry of ^{32}P, and methods of estimating the therapeutic dose are empirical. Dosages based on body weight, height of RBC count, amount of RBC mass, or combinations of these factors have been advocated. The generally administered single dose is 3 to 7 millicuries (mc), depending on the above factors.[12–14] In one series of patients,[13] the average dose per course was 7.7 mc, with a mean of 10 mc. Generally venesection is performed before administration of ^{32}P although it is not necessary unless circulatory overload or other acute symptoms are present. Urinary loss of injected ^{32}P has been estimated at about 10 per cent in 48 hours, with a range of 3 to 31 per cent.[12] The physical half-life of ^{32}P is 14.3 days. The biologic half-life of the material is about 8 days. Therefore, significant radiation effects may exist for 4 to 6 weeks.

The first effect of radiophosphorus is on the platelets, and this is usually maximal in 3 to 4 weeks. In 6 to 12 weeks, depression of the RBC count is found. The effect on the WBC count generally, but not always, follows that of the platelet count. The apparent delayed effect of ^{32}P on erythropoiesis is due to the long life span of the RBC. Therefore, another dose of ^{32}P should never be given until at least four months have passed. Ferrokinetic study is useful in estimating the degree of marrow activity when repeat courses of ^{32}P are being considered.[5,15] The patient should be followed up at monthly intervals until remission occurs. If the RBC mass rises during the first 4 months after therapy, phlebotomy should be used for control of symptoms. Chemotherapeutic drugs should not be given during this time, as they are additive to the effects of ^{32}P. Full remission can be expected in about 80 per cent of cases and partial remission in 15 per cent more.[12] Thus, only a small number of patients fail on ^{32}P therapy. About two-thirds of the responders do so after one injection and the remainder on two injections. Rarely are three injections required.[12] The vast majority of patients have a complete remission in 6 months, and remissions will usually last 1 to 2 years. In one series the average length of remission was 22.3 months.[12] When relapse occurs, retreatment with ^{32}P is indicated. In one series of 107 patients,[13] followed up for 18 years, the highest total dose of ^{32}P given to any one patient was 42 mc.

Radiophosphorus has the following disadvantages:

(1) Suppression of leukocytosis and thrombocytosis is not as long-lasting as is suppression of erythrocytosis.[16]

(2) A radiation therapist is required to administer the material. In addition, because of its short physical half-life, the material must be ordered in advance, since storage is not possible.

(3) There is a danger of overestimating the dose, which may result in leukopenia, thrombocytopenia, and anemia.[4]

(4) A 10 per cent incidence of acute leukemia as a late complication of therapy has been shown to occur.[17] However, statistics indicate that this complication does not appear to shorten over-all life span when patients treated with ^{32}P are compared with those not treated with ^{32}P.[11,18] This increased incidence of acute leukemia, although debated by some workers,[19,20] is generally accepted as a valid criticism[21] of the use of ^{32}P. The entire issue of ^{32}P-induced leukemogenesis may have a factor of genetic susceptibility superimposed upon it, making final resolution of this debate even more difficult.[16,22]

Although we agree that radiophosphorus therapy will decrease the thrombotic and hemorrhagic complications of this disorder to some extent, it is our current practice to avoid its use and to administer chemotherapeutic agents when we believe myelosuppressive therapy is indicated. Exceptions to this rule of practice include the elderly, in whom the advanced age of the patient makes the risk of leukemia an acceptable one, and in those patients who, for one reason or another, cannot or will not take chemotherapy and in whom suppression of their disease is mandatory.

Chemotherapy of Polycythemia Vera

Although in the last 6 years increased interest has been shown in the use of chemotherapy, workers in the United Kingdom[16] had previously suggested that chemotherapy would induce remissions equivalent to those with ^{32}P. However, their data indicated that chemotherapy was more troublesome to administer than was ^{32}P,

TABLE 2.—*Myelosuppressive Drugs Useful in the Therapy of the Myeloproliferative Disorders*

Generic name	*Brand name*
Polycythemia Vera	
Busulfan	Myleran
Melphalan	Alkeran
Chlorambucil	Leukeran
Pipobroman	Vercyte
Cyclophosphamide	Cytoxan
Chronic Myelocytic Leukemia	
Busulfan	Myleran
Melphalan	Alkeran
Hydroxyurea	Hydrea
Demecolcine	Colcemid
Dibromomannitol	—

but this disadvantage was counterbalanced by a low incidence of leukemia in the patient treated with chemotherapy. More recent studies in the United States have demonstrated that control of the proliferative aspects of PV can be accomplished by proper use of alkylating agents.[5,9,15]

The drugs useful in the chemotherapy of this disorder are listed in Table 2. As with ^{32}P, the suppressive effects of therapy on the RBC mass are delayed, whereas the suppressive effects on WBC and platelet production are noted early. These drugs have cumulative effects, and the total dose administered should be carefully monitored. Unlike the situation with antimetabolites, the total dose administered is more important than the daily dose rate. Alkylating agents are more effective in the therapy of PV than are antimetabolites because in PV the proliferative cell is not much different from the normal cell.[23] Under these circumstances a noncycle-active agent would produce more even control of cellular growth since the malignant and normal cell proliferative rates are nearly the same.

Busulfan. This alkylating agent has been used extensively in the therapy of polycythemia vera.[5,9,15,16] In our experience this agent has proved to be the best and least expensive mode of treatment for this disorder.[5,9] Our studies in the therapy of PV over a period of 6 years are summarized in Table 3.

We have studied 21 patients in that time, and for some the diagnosis had been made before they came under our care. All patients achieved remission. For the most part therapy was begun with no more than 4 mg daily, often with 2 mg, or one tablet, daily. These low daily doses are different from our approach in chronic myelogenous leukemia (CML), where higher initial doses are used. In PV we recommend low daily doses, since higher daily doses would mandate frequent checks of the blood count because total dosage would accumulate rapidly.

Most patients can be seen every 2 to 3 weeks during therapy; if personal visits are not practical, the blood count should be checked in the laboratory and a follow-up phone call made. When remission occurs or if the platelet count drops to 300,000/cu mm or less, therapy is stopped. Even after cessation of therapy, a downward drift in the count will occur. This is especially true of the platelet count.

The median dose to response ranges between 150 mg and 200 mg.[5,15] The usual length of time to induce remission is in the range of 35 to 90 days. Phlebotomy is not necessary unless the initial RBC mass is very high and the patient symptomatic.

TABLE 3.—*Polycythemia Vera: Summary of Hematologic and Therapeutic Data on Busulfan-Treated Patients*

Total number of patients:			21
	Before therapy:	Median	16.1
		Range	(5.2–35.9)
WBC		% Leukopenic	0
(thousands/mm³)	After therapy:	Median	6.7
		Range	(2.1–30.2)
		% Leukopenic	14
	Before therapy:	Median	648
		Range	(126–2900)
Platelets		% Thrombocytopenic	0
(thousands/mm³)	After therapy	Median	202
		Range	(48–512)
		% Thrombocytopenic	14
Dose to remission (mg):		Median	186
		Range	(112–1080)
Duration of therapy (days):		Median	62
		Range	(34–370)

It should be kept in mind that the peripheral hemoglobin concentration and hematocrit are poor measures of RBC mass, since in the later phases of the disease plasma volume rises as rapidly as does the RBC mass.[5,15] In these instances measurement of the total RBC mass usually indicates severe hypervolemia, while hemoglobin concentration and hematocrit values suggest that the RBC mass is well controlled.[5]

We do not recommend maintenance chemotherapy for most patients with PV, since in our experience remissions of 18 to 24 months are commonplace after a single course of busulfan. This experience is similar to that of others.[9,16]

Adherence to this schedule has led to little toxicity. Platelet counts of less than 100,000/cu mm and WBC counts less than 5,000/cu mm occurred in 14 per cent of our patients. Wasserman and Gilbert found thrombocytopenia in 27 per cent of their patients treated with busulfan.[9] However, they used busulfan on a more continuous basis and gave higher total doses. Other toxic effects of busulfan are distinctly unusual.

Relapse is indicated by the occurrence of symptoms (pruritus, weight loss, sweating, etc.), splenomegaly, or a rising WBC or platelet count. Repeat therapy is then indicated. A rising RBC mass in the absence of the above symptoms can usually be controlled by phlebotomy alone.

Several of our patients have died of leukemia, but all except one had been treated with ^{32}P before we saw them. However, one of our patients, never treated with any agent other than busulfan, died some months ago of acute leukemia. Her overall survival was 18 years. Whether her terminal leukemia was a result of chemotherapy or a natural consequence of the disease cannot be determined.

Chlorambucil. This agent, which is more frequently used in the therapy of lymphoproliferative disease than in other diseases, has also been found to be effective in the therapy of PV.[9] Wasserman and Gilbert recommend that therapy be started with 6 to 8 mg daily; a total dose in the range of 800 mg is required to control the symptoms and signs of the disease.[9] However, unlike the situation with busulfan, relapse is likely in about 6 months if maintenance therapy is not used. For this reason a "4 weeks on and 4 weeks off" program has been recommended for smooth control.[9] A 10 to 15 per cent incidence of thrombocytopenia has been reported, as well as a small percentage of instances of alopecia. Both chlorambucil and busulfan are supplied in 2 mg tablets and their costs are similar. Thus, chlorambucil has the disadvantage of increased expense to the patient, since three to four tablets are used daily, as contrasted with a one- to two-tablet dose of busulfan. In addition, the continued use of this drug increases the likelihood of other side effects, such as skin rash, urticaria, and alopecia.

Pipobroman. This recently developed, clinically available alkylating agent is used in a daily dose of 1 to 1.5 mg/kg. Therapy is continued until a therapeutic response is obtained or toxicity is seen. Maintenance therapy at 0.1 mg/kg may then be used. Few side effects have been noted with this drug. More experience is necessary before its usefulness can be determined.

Cyclophosphamide. Wasserman and Gilbert[9] report that this drug, given in daily doses of 100 to 150 mg, will produce prompt organ shrinkage and a rapid drop in hematocrit. A total dose in the range of 9 gm is necessary for remission. Again, unmaintained patients have short remissions and the cost to the patient is high. Distressing side effects of this drug are alopecia and cystitis, both of which are proportional to the amount of drug given and the length of time administered. As with chlorambucil, maintenance therapy is necessary.

Melphalan (L-phenylalanine mustard). This agent seems to be very similar to busulfan. Although recent reports[24] suggest that therapy be begun with 10 mg daily, we recommend doses of 4 mg daily to start. A total dose of 1.5 to 3 mg/kg is needed for control. Thrombocytopenia and leukopenia are the most deleterious side effects. By careful follow-up (and, in our opinion, by reduced doses) these side effects can be avoided. This drug is probably the best alternative to the use of busulfan, since it does not share any of the other nonhematopoietic side effects of busulfan. However, maintenance therapy with melphalan is recommended; this is not so with busulfan.

Other Agents. Although the mainstay of therapy has been the alkylating agents, other drugs have been tried in the therapy of PV with some success. Over 10 years ago a folic acid antagonist, pyrimethamine, was shown to produce subjective and objective improvement in some patients.[25] Recently therapy with azauridine intravenously or azaribine orally, both cycle-active drugs (as is pyrimethamine) was found to produce rapid shrinkage of organs and prompt suppression of erythropoiesis. However, the data demonstrate rapid recovery of marrow function following use of these agents, making more continuous therapy mandatory.[26] It is likely that in proper circumstances almost any cancer chemotherapeutic drug might produce enough hematopoietic suppression to be deemed somewhat useful in the therapy of PV. Whether any of these agents, or any newer ones of the same type that will be developed, offer any advantages over currently tested agents will require further study.

We conclude from these data that busulfan is the best agent for control of this disease. Melphalan follows closely behind. The remissions induced by these agents are quantitatively and qualitatively similar to those obtained by ^{32}P therapy[5,9] and the incidence of hematologic side effects no worse than with ^{32}P. The incidence of leukemic transformation seems to be less than with ^{32}P.[17] Thorough follow-up over the next decade will prove or disprove this latter contention.

CHRONIC MYELOCYTIC LEUKEMIA (CML)

This disorder is the most malignant of the chronic myeloproliferative diseases in that survival is relatively short and terminally the patient develops a hematologic picture very similar to that in acute leukemia.[1,11,27,28] Although treatment in CML may or may not prolong life, once the diagnosis is established therapy should be begun even though the patient feels fairly well. The reason for this is that the disease, once it produces symptoms, is relentlessly progressive and therapy is highly successful in inducing remission.

Therapy is directed toward suppression of the myeloid hyperplasia. Unlike therapy of acute lymphoblastic leukemia, therapy of CML reduces the abnormal population of cells but does not eradicate it.[29] However, since the malignant cells behave almost normally, merely reducing their number to normal levels controls symptoms and signs of the disease. The therapeutic modalities used include chemotherapy, splenic irradiation, and radiophosphorus.

Chemotherapy of Chronic Myelocytic Leukemia (CML)

Busulfan. In many clinics, including ours, busulfan is the therapy of choice in CML.[29,30] The principles of therapy are similar to those outlined for PV.

A daily dose of 4 to 8 mg of busulfan is used to induce remission. Experience with this drug indicates that with a daily dose ranging from 4 to 8 mg a total dose of 125 to 250 mg will produce remission in most patients initially so treated. However, wide ranges in the total amount of drug required for remission have been reported. Several investigators have reported a total dose to remission in 40 separate courses of 84 to 849 mg.[31,32] Huguley et al. (the Southeastern Cancer Chemotherapy Cooperative Study Group)[33] found that for WBC counts in excess of 100,000/cu mm, 47 days and 204 mg of drug were required for control; for WBC counts between 50,000 and 100,000/cu mm, 32 days and 178 mg of drug were required; and for WBC counts below 50,000/cu mm, 26 days and 128 mg of drug were necessary for control.

Once therapy is begun, the condition of the patient should be checked weekly. Little change may be noted by the patient for a week to 10 days. During this period, there may be a transient rise in the total WBC count. Subsequently, the WBC count begins to fall, with the younger cells disappearing before the more mature cells.[29] Subjective improvement occurs. The spleen will then begin to decrease in size and the hemoglobin concentration will rise as the WBC count falls. The rate of fall of the WBC count at times appears to be an exponential function of the number of leukocytes per cubic millimeter at the start of treatment.[29,34] This rate of fall is independent of the daily dose rate of the drug and tends to remain constant during repeated courses. Some workers, therefore, suggest that each time the WBC count halves, the daily dose of busulfan should also be halved.[1] On the other hand, at daily dose rates of 4 to 8 mg, it is probably best to reduce the drug dose when the total WBC count reaches 15,000/cu mm.[29] Subsequently, an attempt is made to maintain the WBC count at 10,000/cu mm or below by adjustment of the dose. Usually, a daily dose of 2 mg is required, although doses of 2 mg twice a week are, at times, all that is necessary. In most patients the platelet count remains above 200,000/cu mm during this time. Should the platelet count fall to below 200,000/cu mm during the induction or maintenance phase, then therapy should be stopped until recovery occurs.

It is possible with busulfan therapy to control the disease in 90 per cent of patients initially treated.[27,33] Haut et al.[34] report only one failure out of 31 patients so treated. Even patients becoming resistant to splenic irradiation may respond to the drug.[35] However, eventually, all patients become resistant to busulfan's effects and die of the disease.[29]

On the basis of data reported in the literature, patients with CML treated with supportive therapy alone have a 31-month median survival,[36] and ^{32}P or X-ray therapy does not improve survival times appreciably.[37] Data from the United Kingdom reveal a median survival of 156 weeks in patients treated with irradiation, whereas treatment with busulfan resulted in a 188-week median survival.[28] This study also demonstrated busulfan's superiority over irradiation therapy in that patients treated with chemotherapy had significantly higher hemoglobin concentrations during and after treatment, and splenic enlargement was better controlled by busulfan than by X-ray therapy.[28,29] Indeed, in the later phases of the disease, when splenic enlargement was common, busulfan-resistant patients often responded to other drugs but rarely to radiation therapy.[29]

There is no doubt that maintenance therapy is superior to intermittent busulfan therapy in the management of this disease.[29] Hemoglobin concentrations are higher in patients treated with continuous busulfan therapy as opposed to intermittently treated patients. The case for increased survival is less clear but suggestive.[28] However, in our experience, regardless of continuous or intermittent therapy, those patients in whom mild leukopenia develops without a fall in platelet count below 100,000/cu mm have long survivals.

Toxicity and Side Effects of Busulfan. The most important toxic effect of busulfan is excessive bone marrow depression. The patient taking busulfan should have blood counts checked weekly initially and more frequently, if necessary, at the time the WBC count is approaching 10,000/cu mm. It is vital to follow up the platelet count at this point because severe thrombocytopenia may occur before or at the same time that the WBC count falls to normal.

Thrombocytopenia is the chief limiting factor in continuous busulfan therapy; once it occurs, it may persist for several months.[29,34] The patient may even manifest leukocytosis and reactivation of the leukemic process during busulfan-induced thrombocytopenia. Indeed, patients may enter the blastic phase as the marrow recovers. More frequently, recovery of the megakaryocytes is accompanied by recovery of the leukemic granulocytes.[29] In our experience and that of others,[29] complete aplasia of the marrow may be induced by injudicious use of busulfan. In one of our patients, myelopoiesis and thrombopoiesis recovered three months before erythropoiesis. In some instances the blast crisis occurs during the aplastic phase.[38] By frequent observation and careful adjustment of the dose during therapy, excessive bone marrow depression may be avoided. It must be emphasized that marrow suppression in busulfan-treated patients is a serious problem and one which can be insidious.[29]

It should also be noted that this agent, like most alkylating agents, has cumulative effects and severe downward drift in the blood count can be seen for weeks after cessation of therapy. We and others have produced the typical aplastic anemia syndrome[29,38] by overdoses of this drug. The survival of these patients, who often recover following testosterone therapy,[39] is no longer than that of other patients who do not become aplastic.[29] Indeed, some of the longest remissions on record have occurred in patients who did not show severe hypoplasia.[40] For this reason we do not recommend "pushing" chemotherapy to the extreme of aplasia.[29]

Other toxic side effects of busulfan include the development occasionally of interstitial pulmonary fibrosis[41] and hyperpigmentation of the skin.[34,42] Also rare is a syndrome resembling adrenal insufficiency, characterized by brownish pigmentation of the skin, debility, anorexia, and weight loss.[43] Unlike that in Addison's disease, the discoloration does not affect the mucous membranes or palmar creases. Steroid production by the adrenal glands is normal. The syndrome may persist for months after the drug is discontinued, and death may occur if treatment is not interrupted. All these toxic effects have been described in patients who have taken the drug for more than 24 months. There is no relation between these toxic manifestations and the leukemic process per se.[1,41,43]

Other side effects include sterility, cataract formation, and amenorrhea.[1] In some patients amenorrhea may persist even after therapy is stopped. One should not ascribe amenorrhea to drug therapy unless the possibility of pregnancy has been excluded. The occurrence of pregnancy during therapy with busulfan has been reported; normal infants have been delivered.[44] However, it is best to withhold therapy during early gestation.

Hydroxyurea (*Hydrea*). This clinically available agent is not an alkylating agent.[45] It can be administered orally and will control some busulfan-resistant patients.[46] The usual initial dose is 40 to 50 mg/kg/day in divided doses. Therapy is continued until the WBC becomes normal. If the patient is truly busulfan-resistant and not entering the blast crisis, rapid control of leukocytosis and associated thrombocytosis will be seen. The spleen will also regress. Maintenance therapy is necessary in doses of about 30 mg/kg daily.[29,45,46]

Hydroxyurea has an advantage: Unwanted excessive marrow suppression is easily corrected, since the WBC and platelet counts rise rapidly following cessation of treatment.[45,46] However, side effects such as anorexia, nausea, vomiting, alopecia and skin rash have been reported. The number of tablets prescribed for daily use is high, and thus expense to the patient is a disadvantageous factor. The need for divided doses is also disadvantageous. This drug is an important addition to our armamentarium, but it is not to be recommended unless busulfan has failed or cannot be used.

Melphalan. Over 6 years ago the Southeastern Cancer Chemotherapy Cooperative Study Group began evaluating this drug in the therapy of CML. In the first volume of this symposium series it was suggested that this agent might be as useful as busulfan. Studies reported in the future will probably indicate that melphalan (L-phenylalanine mustard) is very useful in the therapy of CML.[47] The principles of therapy with melphalan have been discussed in the above section dealing with PV.

Other Chemotherapeutic Agents. Demecolcine[48] and dibromomannitol,[49] pipobroman[50] and mercaptopurine[33] have each been tried in this disease with some success. None offers an advantage over busulfan, melphalan, or hydroxyurea. In general, they require continuous therapy and are not useful in controlling the blast crisis.

Radiation Therapy

There seems to be no doubt that splenic irradiation or ^{32}P therapy is no longer considered optimal therapy for this disorder. Overall survival seems lower and hemoglobin concentration not as well maintained in comparison with that of patients treated with busulfan.[28]

In the patient resistant to busulfan who is not yet in the blast crisis, small doses of X-ray to the spleen (200 to 400 rads over 4 to 6 elapsed days) may result in clinical improvement. This type of treatment may find its greatest use in the unusual patient who, early in the course of the disease, presents with thrombocytopenia. In this instance, busulfan treatment would be dangerous. However, in view of our expanded chemotherapeutic potentialities, most likely this patient's disease would be better controlled with a drug such as hydroxyurea or small doses of melphalan, rather than by splenic X-ray or ^{32}P.

Resistance to Therapy

A few patients are resistant to all forms of therapy from the onset. However, it is unusual to find this situation in classic cases of CML.[33,34] Krauss et al.[51] reported a group of patients whose disease resembled CML, except that the Philadelphia chromosome was absent. These patients had rapidly deteriorating courses despite treatment. An analysis of survival rates indicated that the longest survivals occurred in those patients who were Ph-positive. Hardisty et al.[52] reported that in children with the juvenile form of granulocytic leukemia, chromosome analysis did not reveal the Ph chromosome. These patients have a short survival and fail to respond to busulfan therapy. Therefore, the Ph chromosome may serve not only as a diagnostic marker of leukemia, but also as a prognostic marker in regard to response to chemotherapy.

When patients with CML become resistant to therapy, there is usually a rise in the blast count.[29] The so-called blast cell crisis occurs more commonly in CML than in any of the other myeloproliferative syndromes. Its manifestations are variable, and it is not necessarily a rapidly occurring phenomenon. It may happen in the first 12 months following therapy. In some instances, the increase in blast count may occur over a period of months. There does not appear to be any increased incidence of this phenomenon in those patients treated with busulfan versus those treated with ^{32}P. There is no currently available agent that prevents the blast crisis.[29] Interestingly, as the blast crisis occurs, other chromosomal changes besides that relating to the Ph chromosome may be noted, indicating that CML may be characterized by a genetically unstable population in which therapy is acting as one of the selective factors.[11] Some patients in the terminal phases of CML have fever, weight loss, and pancytopenia without an increase in the blast count. Bone marrow examination reveals hypoplasia and fibrosis. These patients are refractory to all forms of chemotherapy and usually succumb to infection.[1] Recent work suggests that chemotherapy of the blast crisis with drugs used in the therapy of acute leukemia might result in some improvement (see the chapter by Frei, this volume).

Myelofibrosis with Myeloid Metaplasia (MMM)

Therapy of this disease depends upon the degree of marrow function and the role of the spleen in blood production and destruction. The main problem is usually anemia. Pharmacologic doses of testosterone have been used with some success to stimulate erythropoiesis.[53,54] This agent should be tried initially in patients with this disorder, since for the most part leukocytosis and thrombocytosis are not as distressing as is the anemia. If a response occurs, then the high WBC and platelet counts can be controlled by busulfan or melphalan. Patients with MMM are extremely sensitive to the effects of chemotherapy, and no more than 2 mg of busulfan or melphalan should be started.[8] The blood count should be checked weekly.

Splenectomy is of use in those patients in whom hypersplenism develops.[55] Hypersplenism would be suggested by a fall in blood count or by a rising need for transfusion. Since marrow failure is a usual occurrence in MMM, it is important to show shortened survival of the formed elements before attempting splenectomy. We have recently demonstrated the usefulness of ^{75}Se-selenomethionine platelet survival in predicting the effectiveness of splenectomy in the disease. The importance of this procedure will become more apparent as experience is gained.[7]

Hemorrhagic Thrombocytosis

This is an unusual form of myeloproliferative disease in which there is a severe anemia secondary to chronic hemorrhage related to the presence of marked thrombocytosis. The predominant therapeutic effort should be toward reduction of the platelet count. This is best accomplished by the use of busulfan or melphalan.[56] The anemia responds to iron therapy once the bleeding stops. As in cases of PV with thrombocytosis, but without anemia, these patients are poor surgical risks because frequently hemorrhage occurs, even after trivial procedures. Once the platelet count is reduced to normal, surgery may be safely performed.[57]

Hyperuricemia in the Myeloproliferative Disorders

The myeloproliferative disorders are characterized by hyperuricemia due to excessive production of uric acid by proliferating cells. Renal excretion of urates is increased, and urate stones or uric acid deposition in the kidneys may complicate the disease or occur as a result of therapy. Acute gouty arthritis may also occur. A xanthine oxidase inhibitor, allopurinol, has been shown to be effective in reducing serum urate concentration in patients with myeloproliferative disorders.[58] Patients who have renal stones or gout due to myeloproliferative disease should be treated with high fluid intake, alkalinization of the urine with sodium bicarbonate, and allopurinol, 200 to 600 mg per day.

References

1. Dameshek, W. and Gunz, F.: Leukemia. 2nd ed. New York: Grune & Stratton, 1964.
2. Silverstein, M. N.: Myeloproliferative diseases: Their shifting spectrum. Postgrad. Med. 43:167, 1968.
3. Glasser, R. M. and Walker, R. I.: Transitions among the myeloproliferative disorders. Ann. Intern. Med. 71:285, 1969.
4. Pike, G. M.: Polycythemia vera. New Eng. J. Med. 258:1250, 1958.
5. Brodsky, I., Kahn, S. B. and Brady, L. W.: Polycythemia vera: Differential diagnosis by ferrokinetic studies and treatment with busulfan (Myleran). Brit. J. Haemat. 14:351, 1968.
6. Wasserman, L. R. and Gilbert, H.: Complications of polycythemia vera. Seminars Hemat. 3:199, 1966.
7. Brodsky, I., Ross, E. M., Petkov, G. and Kahn, S. B.: Platelet and fibrinogen kinetics with (^{75}Se) selenomethionine in patients with myeloproliferative disorders. Brit. J. Haemat. (in press).
8. Gurney, C. W.: Polycythemia vera and some possible pathogenic mechanisms. Ann. Rev. Med. 16:169, 1965.
9. Wasserman, L. R. and Gilbert, A. S.: The treatment of polycythemia vera. Med. Clin. N. Amer. 50:1501, 1966.
10. Lawrence, J. H.: Polycythemia: Physiology, diagnosis and treatment based on 303 cases. New York: Grune & Stratton, 1955, p. 136.
11. Galton, D. A. G.: Problems in the management of the myeloproliferative states. Ser. Haemat. 1:37, 1965.

12. Szur, L., Lewis, S. M. and Goolden, A. W. G.: Polycythaemia vera and its treatment with radioactive phosphorus. Quart. J. Med. 28:397, 1959.
13. Halnan, K. E. and Russell, M. H.: Polycythaemia vera: Comparison of survival and causes of death in patients managed with and without radiotherapy. Lancet 2:760, 1965.
14. Gardner, F. H.: Treatment of polycythemia vera. Seminars Hemat. 3:220, 1966.
15. Brodsky, I.: The use of ferrokinetics in the evaluation of busulfan therapy in polycythemia vera. Brit. J. Haemat. 10:291, 1964.
16. Perkins, J., Israels, M. C. G. and Wilkinson, J. F.: Polycythemia vera: Clinical studies on a series of 127 patients managed without radiation therapy. Quart J. Med. 33:499, 1964.
17. Modan, B. and Lilienfeld, A. M.: Polycythemia vera and leukemia: The role of radiation treatment. Medicine 44:305, 1965.
18. Modan, B.: Computing length of survival in long term disease. J.A.M.A. 192:609, 1965.
19. Osgood, E. E.: Polycythemia vera: Age relationships and survival. Blood 26:143, 1965.
20. Osgood, E. E.: Contrasting incidence of acute monocytic and granulocytic leukemias in P^{32}-treated patients with polycythemia vera and chronic lymphocytic leukemia. J. Lab. Clin. Med. 64:560, 1964.
21. Dameshek, W.: Comments on the therapy of polycythemia vera. Seminars Hemat. 3:226, 1966.
22. Nathan, D. G.: Comments on treatment of polycythemia vera leukemia as a complication of polycythemia vera. Seminars Hemat. 3:230, 1966.
23. Stohlman, F.: Pathogenesis of erythrocytosis. Seminars Hemat. 3:181, 1966.
24. Logue, G. L., Gutterman, J. U., McGinn, T. G., Laszlo, J. and Rundles, R. W.: Melphalan, therapy of polycythemia vera. Blood 36:70, 1970.
25. Frost, J., Jones, R. and Jonsson, W.: Pyrimethamine in the treatment of polycythemia vera. Southern Med. J. 51:1260, 1958.
26. DeConti, R. D. and Calabresi, P.: Treatment of polycythemia vera with azauridine and azaribine. Ann. Intern. Med. 73:575, 1970.
27. Wintrobe, M. M.: Clinical Hematology. 5th ed. Philadelphia: Lea and Febiger, 1961.
28. Medical Research Council, Working Party for Therapeutic Trials in Leukaemia: Chronic granulocytic leukaemia: Comparison of radiotherapy and busulphan therapy. Brit. Med. J. 1:201, 1968.
29. Galton, D. A. G.: Chemotherapy of chronic myelocytic leukemia. Seminars Hemat. 6:323, 1969.
30. Krakoff, I. H.: Management of the chronic myeloproliferative disorders. Med. Clin. N. Amer. 50:803, 1966.
31. Haut, A. and Altman, S. J.: Chemotherapy of leukemia, Hodgkin's disease and related disorders. Ann. Intern. Med. 41:447, 1954.
32. Wintrobe, M. M.: The use of Myleran in the treatment of chronic myelocytic leukemia. Arch. Intern. Med. 96:451, 1955.
33. Huguley, C. M., Jr. et al. (Southeastern Cancer Chemotherapy Cooperative Study Group): Comparison of 6-mercaptopurine and busulfan in chronic granulocytic leukemia. Blood 21:89, 1963.
34. Haut, A., Abbott, W. S., Wintrobe, M. M. and Cartwright, G. E.: Busulfan in the treatment of chronic myelocytic leukemia: The effect of long term intermittent therapy. Blood 17:1, 1961.
35. Galton, D. A. G. and Till, M.: Myleran in chronic myeloid leukaemia. Lancet 1:425, 1955.
36. Minot, G. R., Backman, T. E. and Isaacs, R.: Chronic myelogenous leukemia: Age, incidence, duration, and benefit derived from irradiation. J.A.M.A. 82:1489, 1924.
37. Tivey, H.: The prognosis for survival in chronic granulocytic and lymphocytic leukemia. Amer. J. Roentgen. 72:68, 1954.
38. Weatherall, D. J., Galton, D. A. G. and Kay, H. E. M.: Letter to the editor. Brit. Med. J. 1:638, 1969.
39. Kahn, S. B. and Brodsky, I.: Personal observation.
40. Djaldetti, M., Pinkhas, J., Padeh, B. and deVries, A.: Prolonged remission in chronic myeloid leukaemia after a single course of Myleran. Israel J. Med. Sci. 1:827, 1965.
41. Oliver, H., Schwartz, R., Rubio, F., Jr. and Dameshek, W.: Interstitial pulmonary fibrosis following busulfan therapy. Amer. J. Med. 31:134, 1961.
42. Galton, D. A. G.: Chronic myeloid leukaemia. Brit. J. Radiol. 26:285, 1953.
43. Dameshek, W.: A syndrome resembling adrenal cortical insufficiency associated with long-term busulfan therapy. Blood 18:497, 1961.
44. Dennis, L. H. and Stein, S.: Busulfan in pregnancy: Report of a case. J.A.M.A. 192:715, 1965.

45. Fishbein, W. N., Carbone, P. P., Freireich, E. J., Misra, D. and Frei, E.: Clinical trials of hydroxyurea in patients with cancer and leukemia. Clin. Pharmacol. Ther. 5:574, 1964.
46. Kennedy, B. J. and Yarbro, J. W.: Metabolic and therapeutic effects of hydroxyurea in chronic myeloid leukemia. J.A.M.A. 195:1038, 1966.
47. Rundles, R. W. and Logue, G. L.: Melphalan therapy of chronic granulocytic leukemia. (In preparation.)
48. Lessmann, E. M. and Sokal, J. E.: A colchicine derivative in therapy of chronic myelocytic leukemia. J.A.M.A. 175:741, 1961.
49. Eckhardt, S., Sellei, C., Horvath, I. P. and Institoris, L.: Effect of 1,6 dibromo 1,6-dideoxy-D-mannitol on chronic granulocytic leukemia. Cancer Chemother. Rep. 33:57, 1963.
50. Evaluation of two antineoplastic agents, pipobroman (Vercyte) and thioguanine. J.A.M.A. 200:619, 1967.
51. Krauss, S., Sokal, M. E. and Sandberg, A. A.: Comparison of Philadelphia chromosome-positive and -negative patients with chronic myelocytic leukemia. Ann. Intern. Med. 61:625, 1964.
52. Hardisty, R. M., Speed, D. E. and Till, M.: Granulocytic leukaemia in childhood. Brit. J. Haemat. 10:551, 1964.
53. Gardner, F. H. and Pringle, J. C.: Androgens and erythropoiesis. II. Treatment of myeloid metaplasia. New Eng. J. Med. 264:103, 1961.
54. Gardner, F. H. and Nathan, D. G.: Androgens and erythropoiesis. III. Further evaluation of testosterone treatment of myelofibrosis. New Eng. J. Med. 274:420, 1966.
55. Amorosi, E. L.: Hypersplenism. Seminars Hemat. 2:249, 1965.
56. Bensinger, T. A., Logue, G. L. and Rundles, R. W.: Hemorrhagic thrombocythemia: Control of postsplenectomy thrombocytosis with melphalan. Blood 36:70, 1970.
57. Wasserman, L. R. and Gilbert, H. S.: Surgical bleeding in polycythemia vera. Ann. N. Y. Acad. Sci. 15:122, 1964.
58. Yu, T. F. and Gutman, A. B.: Effect of allopurinol (4-hydroxypyrazolo[3,4-*d*]pyrimidine) on serum and urinary uric acid in primary and secondary gout. Amer. J. Med. 37:885, 1964.

Treatment of Lymphoproliferative Disease

By FRANK H. GARDNER, M.D.

LYMPHOPROLIFERATIVE DISEASE as an inclusive term has nosologic value to emphasize the similarity between lymphocytic leukemia and a variety of malignant disorders manifested by lymph node and organ enlargement. The schematic classification of Custer is useful to appreciate the variations in tumor histology that may be seen in individual lymph nodes (Fig. 1).[1] While we may initially use one histologic classification, we need to recognize that clinic experience has taught us to expect transitions from one type to another. This is most notable in the patient with lymphosarcoma. During wide dissemination, the tumor may have a blood-borne phase that may not be distinguishable from that in chronic lymphocytic leukemia (CLL).

In our experience, the most common lymphoproliferative disease is chronic lymphocytic leukemia. We are aware of the remarkable character of the illness, which, generally speaking, occurs in the later decades of life, chiefly in men (Fig. 2).[2] Some series will have a male/female ratio of 3 to 1 or 4 to 1; there is no

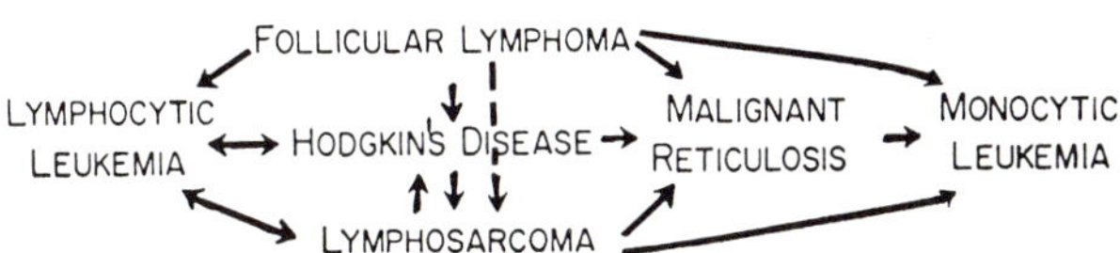

FIG. 1.—Schematic outline to emphasize the transitional morphologic relations of lymphoproliferative disease. Diagram derived from data of Custer.[1]

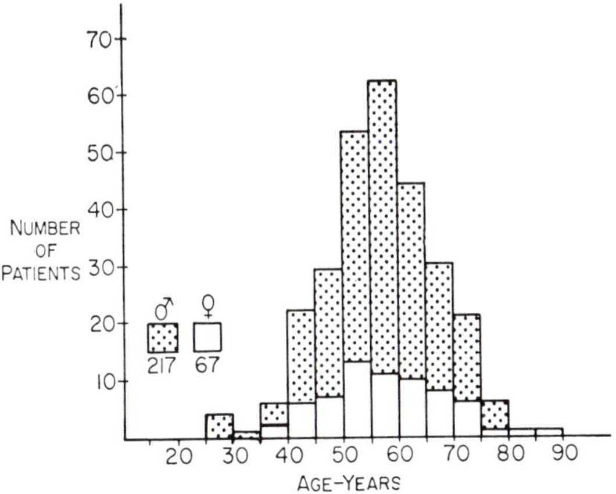

FIG. 2.—Incidence of chronic lymphocytic leukemia. The peak level of disease is observed in the sixth and seventh decades of life, with a high percentage of males. Redrawn from Boutis et al.[2]

From the Hematology Research Laboratory and Department of Medicine, Presbyterian-University of Pennsylvania Medical Center, and the Department of Medicine, University of Pennsylvania School of Medicine, Philadelphia, Pennsylvania.

Supported in part by grants AM11188-03 and AM11188-04 from the USPHS and by a grant from the John A. Hartford Foundation, Inc.

adequate explanation for this sex predominance. In recent years, the increased opportunity for medical observation among elderly patients has made all physicians aware that CLL can exist for years without symptoms.[3,4] During the past decade, more emphasis has been oriented towards the concept of CLL as a mutant proliferating lymphocyte clone that has no recognition for control by the stem cell pool of lymphocytes. It has been proposed that the normal lymphocyte will develop a mutant clone that does not respond to antigenic stimuli.[5]

In the early phase of such a mutation, these abnormal clone lymphocytes will be considered as abnormal cells, and the residual normal lymphocytes' response will lead to their destruction. However, as more abnormal lymphocytes are formed from the abnormal clone, there is an inadequate number of normal lymphocytes available to recognize and destroy the abnormal (CLL) lymphocyte.[6] The aberrant clone continues to replicate, and this type of abnormal lymphocyte replaces the majority, if not all, of the circulating lymphocyte pool (Fig. 3). Lymphocytes derived from this abnormal clone have lost their ability to react to antigenic stimuli as measured by specific protein antigens and phytohemagglutinin material (PHA).[7,8] With an inadequate response to antigens, there is less opportunity for these cells to be destroyed, and they continue to accumulate slowly in the circulation with a lifespan of 50 to 60 days.[9] Such lymphocytes retain the capacity for mitogenesis and protein synthesis but at a slower rate. They may produce abnormal globulins and have decreased synthesis of the normal immunoglobulins.[10]

The patient with the slow proliferation but progressive accumulation of mature, abnormal lymphocytes has in most instances no symptoms from the lymphocytosis for prolonged intervals. The careful histologic studies of Wasi and Block have demonstrated that the bone marrow may have intensive invasion by mature lymphocytes without evidence of anemia or thrombocytopenia.[11] It is important for the clinician to appreciate that the bone marrow may be almost totally replaced by

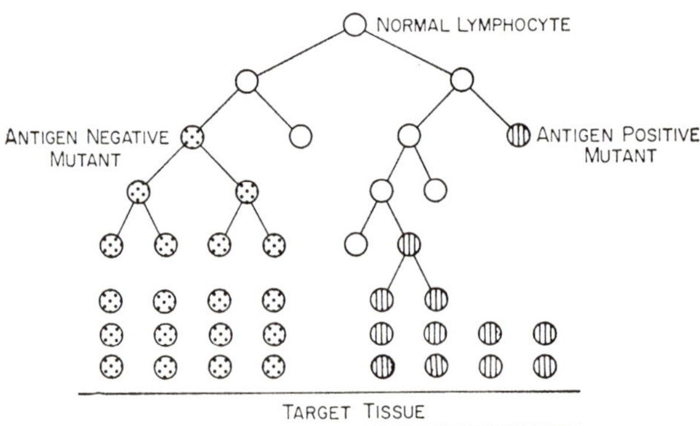

FIG. 3.—Schematic outline for proliferation of abnormal lymphocytes. The initial formation of an antigen positive mutant that could produce abnormal protein is destroyed in the initial phase by normal lymphocytes. However, as additional lymphocytes are formed without such reactivity (antigen negative mutants), there are inadequate normal lymphocytes available to destroy the antigen positive mutant. The circulating lymphocytes in chronic lymphocytic leukemia (CLL) can be considered to be for the most part antigen negative mutants, their primary function being to invade and replace the target tissue, i.e., lymph nodes and bone marrow. Antigen positive mutant lymphocytes form abnormal proteins that bind to the target tissue (red cells and platelets) to allow increased destruction by the reticuloendothelial tissue. Redrawn from Fudenberg.[6]

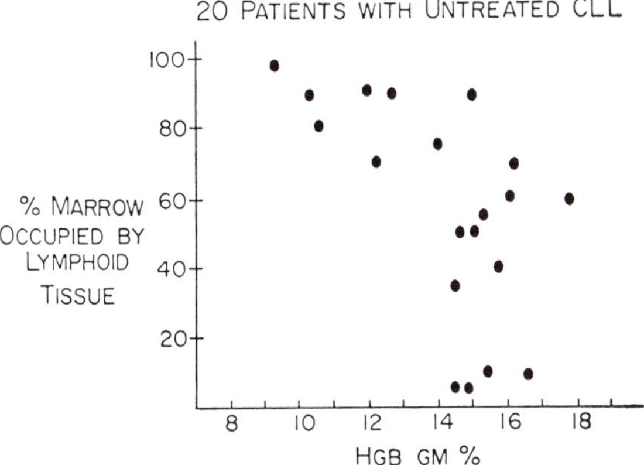

FIG. 4.—Correlation of bone marrow lymphocytosis with peripheral hemoglobin levels observed in 20 patients with untreated chronic lymphocytic leukemia (CLL). Most of the bone marrow may be replaced with lymphocytes (80 per cent) without significant anemia. Redrawn from Wasi and Block.[11]

diffuse lymphocytosis or hyperplastic nodules of lymphocytes without classical symptoms (Fig. 4). There is a relatively stable marrow replacement (50 to 60 per cent) until the peripheral lymphocytosis exceeds 100,000/cu mm. Thereafter, the marrow replacement has no correlation with peripheral blood measurements (Fig. 5). However, the capacity of the marrow compartment to expand erythroid production prevents any accurate assessment of the total body burden of abnormal lymphocytes. As a general consideration, the clinician can expect up to 80 to 90 per cent of marrow replacement before the onset of anemia.

Should the patient with CLL who has no symptoms from anemia or discomfort from lymphoid masses be treated? From the current information, I am not certain that we can say that we have the facts at hand to know when to treat such a patient. In view of the benign course of the disease that may be observed for years, I am

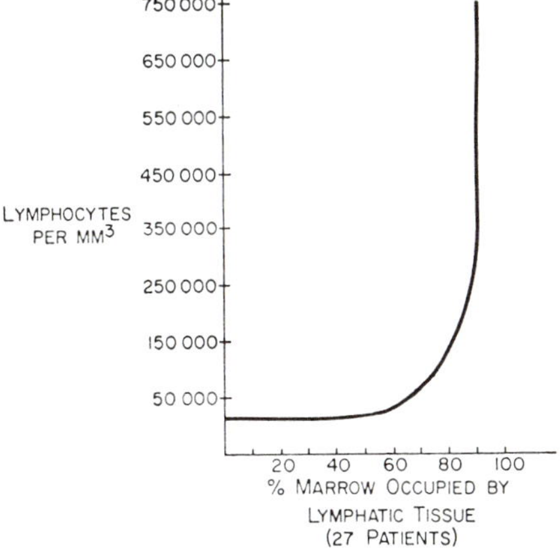

FIG. 5.—Schematic relation of peripheral blood lymphocyte count to bone marrow replacement by lymphatic invasion. With peripheral blood measurements above 150,000/cu mm, one can predict that the marrow will have more than 80 per cent of the cellularity replaced with lymphocytes. However, such measurements do not permit prediction of onset of anemia. Redrawn from Wasi and Block.[11]

hesitant to add the risk of chemotherapy or irradiation.[4] Certainly the physician should not treat the peripheral blood lymphocyte count per se.[12] If the disease is followed by casual diagnosis from incidental laboratory measurements, one may expect little or no clinical complications for years (Fig. 6). From the series observed by Boggs et al., physical findings or symptoms imply a more advanced collection of abnormal lymphocytes, with shortened survival.[13] The practical conclusion from the benign course in curve A, Figure 6[13] would imply careful observation without therapy. I am not convinced that we should treat this phase of lymphocyte accumulation. Although adequate data do not exist, I would suspect that such patients represent the minimal invasion associated with modest lymphocytosis. For those patients whose disease becomes symptomatic, whether preceded by a prolonged period free of symptoms or not, treatment is related to control of one or more of five chief problems: (1) localized nodes or organ enlargements that threaten normal physiologic functions; (2) "metabolic" symptoms (fever, sweating, weight loss) related to total proliferating lymphoid tissue mass; (3) anemia; (4) thrombocytopenia and granulocytopenia; and (5) infections. Glands in neck and axillae may be reduced in size by irradiation. However, the use of irradiation may initiate lympholysis and progressive activity of the disease, or severe hemolytic anemia or thrombocytopenia.[14] "Metabolic" symptoms are rarely observed without anemia.

Although nitrogen mustard and triethylene melamine (TEM) have historical interest, the oral alkylating agents chlorambucil and cyclophosphamide are the favored drugs in use today.[15,16] The response rate is similar for these two latter drugs, but the complications of hemorrhagic cystitis and alopecia have made cyclophosphamide less desirable as the initial drug of choice.[17] During the last 10 years, more clinicians have used chlorambucil, and most laboratory groups have accepted an initial daily dosage of 0.1 to 0.2 mg/kg orally as a safe schedule. Usually the total dose should not be above 10 to 12 mg per day. In most instances, there is no critical haste to reduce the white blood count rapidly. In the initial period of 2 to 3 weeks after therapy has begun, the lymphocytosis may increase. One should expect to achieve normal values in a 2- to 3-month interval. As a general rule, the dosage should be decreased by 50 per cent when the leukocyte count is halved. When a

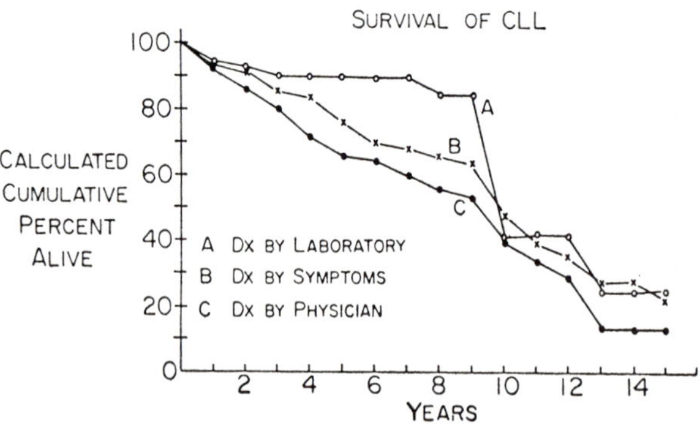

FIG. 6.—Survival curves in chronic lymphocytic leukemia (CLL). The incidental diagnosis (dx) of CLL by laboratory measurements usually shows a more benign course (curve A). Diagnosis on the basis of symptomatic complaint or by the physician indicates a similar pattern of survival. The abrupt alteration in curve A may suggest that the mutant clone has a common proliferation pattern that is moderated in a selected group of patients. Redrawn from data by Boggs et al.[13]

leukocyte count in the range of 10,000 to 20,000/cu mm is achieved, the dosage may be reduced to 2 mg daily or even to 2 mg three times a week. Many clinics will then stop medication and may resume when a definite leukocytosis has been observed. As a personal preference, I will maintain the patient on medication indefinitely, for there are adequate data to indicate that we can expect a better survival rate with continuous alkylating treatment.[18] For reasons not well understood, a patient resistant to chlorambucil after a period of treatment may respond to cyclophosphamide. If the latter agent is used, one may follow a daily program of 3 to 4 mg/kg orally. If administration of cyclophosphamide is initiated after an impaired response to chlorambucil, the physician need be aware that there may be less myeloid reserve with additional chemotherapy.

The anemia associated with a marked lymphoid invasion of the marrow initially has some response to chemotherapy. Also, as the leukocytosis declines, usually the peripheral blood differential count continues to manifest a high percentage of mature lymphocytes. Hence there can be a white count of 10,000/cu mm with 60 to 80 per cent mature lymphocytes. Since androgens have stimulated erythropoiesis nonspecifically in a variety of malignancies, for the past 10 years clinicians have used pharmacologic doses of testosterone in patients with CLL when there have been granulocytopenia and anemia.[19-21] The anemia may respond to androgens alone without chemotherapy, but the opportunity to obtain a more normal peripheral blood film differential is more easily achieved with the combination therapy. There is no experimental evidence to demonstrate a possible lympholytic effect of androgens in human leukemia. However, rodent lymphocytic leukemia can be suppressed with pharmacologic doses of testosterone.[22] Androgens enhance erythropoiesis in elderly male subjects, and this response may have special merit when applied to CLL, a disease with a sharply peaked incidence in the later decades[23] (see Fig. 2). When possible, administration of androgens should be started in the patient with CLL 4 to 6 weeks prior to the use of chlorambucil. With testosterone therapy, we have been able to maintain higher hematocrit levels. If anemia is present, sodium restriction is started prophylactically in this age group because of the higher incidence of cardiovascular complications and the marked sodium-retaining potential of androgens. With androgen therapy in myeloproliferative disorders, a marked nonspecific myeloid response is observed; indeed, granulocyte counts may be increased to 50,000/cu mm. This is a valuable adjunct to therapy to have granulocytes available for combating infection (Fig. 7).

The oral androgen fluoxymesterone has been used predominantly at a dose of 1 mg/kg daily during the initial treatment until a normal white blood count is observed. Thereafter, a dosage of 20 mg daily can be used indefinitely. In parenteral therapy testosterone enanthate or testosterone cypionate has been used in the induction phase at a dosage of 600 mg weekly. While the disease is in remission, 600 mg should be used at monthly intervals. Since most patients are males, there is minimal concern regarding side effects of virilization.

Many patients with CLL may have marked thrombocytopenia as well as anemia and granulocytopenia when the diagnosis is made or symptoms develop. As noted above, granulocytopenia and thrombocytopenia almost always are associated with marrow replacement by the lymphocytic tumor. The extent of the marrow invasion should be assessed by marrow trephine core biopsy. In such patients, the safest initial therapy is massive corticoid therapy, usually prednisone, 80 to 100 mg daily.[24,25]

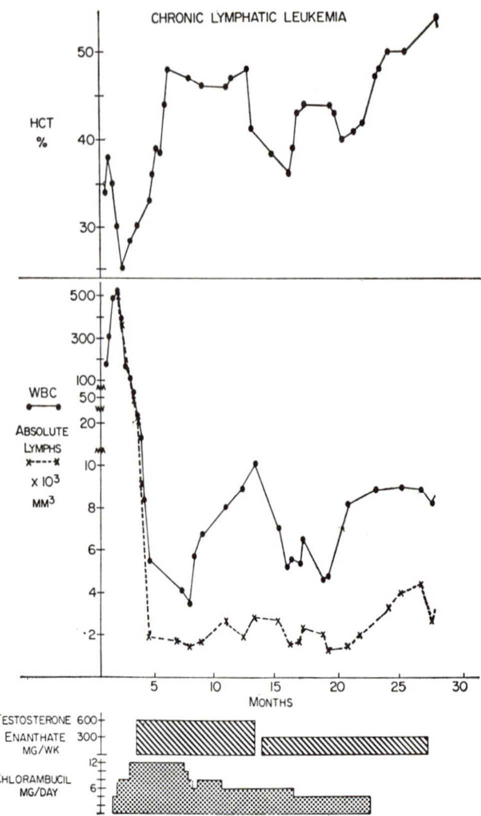

FIG. 7.—Treatment of chronic lymphocytic leukemia (CLL) in a 62-year-old man by means of chlorambucil and androgens. Note the nearly normal absolute lymphocyte count with the combined therapy.

This therapy has two objectives: first, to achieve lympholysis and to permit some repopulation of the marrow with megakaryocytes and myeloid elements; and second, to suppress possible peripheral blood destruction (hemolysis) that may be related to reticuloendothelial function. This dosage may be continued for 6 to 10 weeks, and if no response is seen in that time, the medication should be stopped. As the leukocytosis declines, one may wish to add chlorambucil (2 mg/day) along with small doses of prednisone (20 mg/day). The prolonged use of corticoids is related to increased frequency of infections, and chlorambucil treatment should be substituted if possible. Patients with osteoporosis, usually elderly women, may fracture the dorsolumbar vertebrae if they receive corticoids for a period of more than 3 to 4 months. One should try to induce fluorosis in these patients by the use of fluoride and calcium salts.[26]

When corticosteroids and chemotherapy fail to reverse thrombocytopenia or granulocytopenia, splenic irradiation should be considered. It should be recognized that neither splenic irradiation nor splenectomy is as effective in myelophthisic CLL as they would be in localized lymphosarcoma of the spleen, where the megakaryocytic and myeloid series may be hyperactive and the peripheral destructive component more obvious. Without doubt, the onset of fulminating hemolytic anemia or thrombocytopenia, or both, threatens to be a serious and possibly life-threatening response in lymphoproliferative disease. Here, we may suspect that abnormal lymphoid cells are producing IgG proteins with binding sites to the red cells. In most instances, these patients will demonstrate isotope localization of red cells in the spleen by surface scanning. The abnormal protein may be derived from destruction of the abnormal lymphocytes and hemolysis may be induced by lympholysis from chemotherapy, irradiation or corticoids.[27] If corticoid therapy does not control the hemolysis or thrombocytopenia, splenic irradiation should be used (Fig. 8). In the presence of tuberculosis or peptic ulcer, splenic irradiation should be instituted initially. If splenic irradiation and corticoids have proved ineffective, splenectomy should be done. It should also be reemphasized here that "idiopathic" hemolytic anemia may be due to CLL, in which case the disease is "unmasked" by the histologic examination of the spleen after a latent period of months or years.

With any treatment program in CLL, there should be careful attention to control and prevention of infection by adjunctive measures. Whenever prolonged corticoid therapy is used, isonicotinic acid hydrazide (INH) therapy should be employed as prophylaxis for possible activation of tuberculosis. The skin should be cleansed by daily baths with hexachlorophene soap. Elective surgical treatment of teeth or hemorrhoids, for example, should be avoided until a remission is achieved. However, during a remission, the physician should be energetic to be certain that he has eliminated any potential source of infection which could overwhelm the patient during relapse. Infections, especially of the urinary tract and lungs, are more frequent in the terminal stages of CLL.[28] Onset of fever warrants treatment with antibiotics while the source of infection is sought. The high incidence of urinary tract infections in the male may suggest combinations of cephalothin, kanamycin, and colistin until cultures have defined bacterial sensitivity. Infections are more frequent with hypogammaglobulinemia; prophylactic injections of gamma globulin may be used intramuscularly and injections repeated when the serum electrophoresis levels of IgG are below 40 mg %.

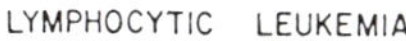

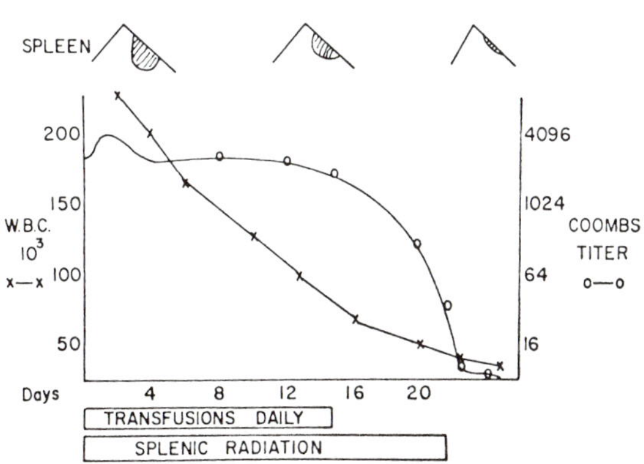

FIG. 8.—Acquired hemolytic anemia in chronic lymphocytic leukemia (CLL) of a 67-year-old man, Rapid improvement in the hemolysis was obtained by splenic irradiation, tabulated here by the disappearance of the abnormal red cell coating globulin (Coombs' test). The peripheral lymphocytosis was well controlled by the irradiation (850 rads).

Although alkylating therapy has been used for more than a decade, it has rarely resulted in complete hematologic remission. Such remissions are defined as absence of physical findings of lymphoid disease (adenopathy, splenomegaly or hepatomegaly), normal hemogram, and a bone marrow with less than 30 per cent lymphoid infiltration.[29] Previous reports of complete remission primarily have been associated with X-ray therapy. In a series of 144 patients with CLL, 2 remissions were achieved with chlorambucil and 4 with splenic irradiation.[30] Whole-body irradiation has been equally successful. In a series of 17 previously untreated patients with CLL, 8 achieved remission with total-body irradiation, for durations similar to those obtained with chlorambucil.[31] In this series, 4 patients in remission had a normal mitogenic lymphocyte response to PHA stimulation. This report suggests that a clone of normal lymphocytes survives during the massive invasion of the marrow by mutant cells, and these residual lymphocytes have the capacity to regenerate with normal antigenic response when the myelophthisic infiltration is destroyed by irradiation. Huguley has reported that the Southeastern Cancer Chemotherapy Group demonstrated a 10 per cent complete remission rate among 111 patients with CLL treated daily with chlorambucil. The duration of remissions in all these series has varied from 1 to 10 years. Although the response appears to be more effective with irradiation therapy, the use of high-dose intermittent chemotherapy with chlorambucil has not had adequate trial for a fair evaluation. Such data should encourage clinicians to consider new programs in the years ahead with chemotherapeutic agents.[18]

Lymphosarcoma

What is there about this lymph node disorder that makes the mature lymphocyte response different from that in CLL? The age pattern of patients is similar to the grouping noted with CLL. However, until late in the course of the disease, the abnormal lymphocyte does not circulate. Indeed, the maturation pattern may be different, with morphologic alterations that lead some hematologists to define the lymphocyte in the peripheral blood as a "lymphosarcoma" type cell.[32,33] As the abnormal lymphocytes proliferate, they remain in and efface the architecture of lymph nodes. In contrast to CLL with the slow expansion of the abnormal lymphocyte, most of the cells remain outside the vascular tree; this suggests that a membrane receptor has been lost to allow transit into lymph channels.[34] Later in the course of the illness, with sheets of lymphocytes replacing the nodule structure, we can then expect to see this lymphoid cell escape into the circulation. When the white count is elevated, the term leukosarcoma has been used to define a leukemic phase of a previous lymphosarcoma. At present, the diagnosis of lymphosarcoma must be made by node biopsy. Lymphoid cells derived from such nodes have similar characteristics to those in CLL in that they have poor response to antigenic (PHA) stimulation and impaired immunoglobulin production.[35]

When the histologic diagnosis is made, the physician should consider carefully whether the disease is unicentric, for such a classification may warrant irradiation in a "curative" dose schedule, as proposed for Hodgkin's disease. At the present time, I do not believe we have data to consider laparotomy for assessing splenic involvement. Unfortunately, as evidenced by careful bone marrow biopsies and lymphangiograms, the disease almost always has widespread distribution. In recent years, I have only found one patient who could qualify for intensive "mantle" irradiation. At the time of the diagnosis by biopsy, if no other disease has been found, the localized nodes, as well as proximal draining regions, should be irradiated. Effort should be made to achieve an initial tumor dose of 3,500 rads utilizing medium voltage or megavoltage therapy.[36] It should be emphasized that the asymptomatic patient should have intravenous urograms done annually so that the physician can be alerted to early obstructive uropathy. Such a prophylactic program will allow irradiation to be done safely to prevent risk of hydronephrosis. Whenever large nodes are observed to impinge on lymphatic or venous drainage, nitrogen mustard treatment remains valuable for acute resolution, usually in a dosage of 0.2 mg/kg for 2 consecutive days. With the phenothiazine drugs available, this drug is well tolerated by the ambulatory patient.

Systemic lymphosarcoma with toxic symptoms of weight loss, fever and malaise can be treated in a similar fashion to CLL with primary reliance on a combination of chlorambucil and androgens. In all instances of small lymphocyte destruction, an associated destruction of platelets and red cells may be noted concurrently. For this reason, some physicians would propose that corticoids be given during the initial phase of lympholysis by irradiation or alkylating drugs. As a general rule, I would doubt if such programs are necessary, recognizing that sudden hemolysis can be treated by the addition of corticoids if necessary.

I would emphasize again that cyclophosphamide is equally effective if an alternative to chlorambucil is needed for gastrointestinal tolerance. In contrast to CLL, these patients more frequently have pancytopenia initially when the diagnosis is made. This response is related to massive expansion of the bone marrow lymphoid nodules similar to the process noted with the late stage of CLL. Initial therapy in the face of pancytopenia should be intensive corticoid therapy, 60 to 80 mg, or prednisone daily, for 4 to 6 weeks. The effects sometimes are salutary, even in the presence of extensive organ and node involvement (Fig. 9). Thereafter, the corticoid program should be discontinued and alkylating therapy with chlorambucil used in a dose of 6 mg daily.

For the most part, combination with the *Vinca* alkaloids has not had wide use. It should be recognized that a lack of response to chlorambucil does justify the physician to initiate a trial with *Vinca* alkaloids.[37] Despite the clinical benefits of irradiation for localized disease and the improvements noted with chemotherapy, survival spans have not improved markedly. As noted with CLL, total-body irradiation (TBI) also has been used in the treatment of lymphosarcoma.[38] The response to fractionated TBI does appear encouraging. Further evaluation is needed to determine whether intermittent TBI can be supplemented with androgen therapy to prevent severe bone marrow depression and allow additional specific nodal irradiation.[19]

The value of splenectomy in lymphosarcoma has been generally overlooked. Splenectomy should be considered more frequently as a means for treatment if corticoids are not successful in reversing pancytopenia or if the spleen appears to be enlarging over a few months of observation. Unlike CLL, where marrow infiltration and replacement are the rule in association with moderate to great enlargement of the spleen, in lymphosarcoma the spleen may be massively enlarged with minimal marrow invasion. The marrow, in fact, may be normal or may show hyperplasia of the parent series in association with thrombocytopenia, granulocytopenia, or anemia. Usually, lymphosarcoma-type lymphocytes can be found in a careful examination of the buffy coat.[33] Irradiation of the massive lymphosarcomatous spleen should be

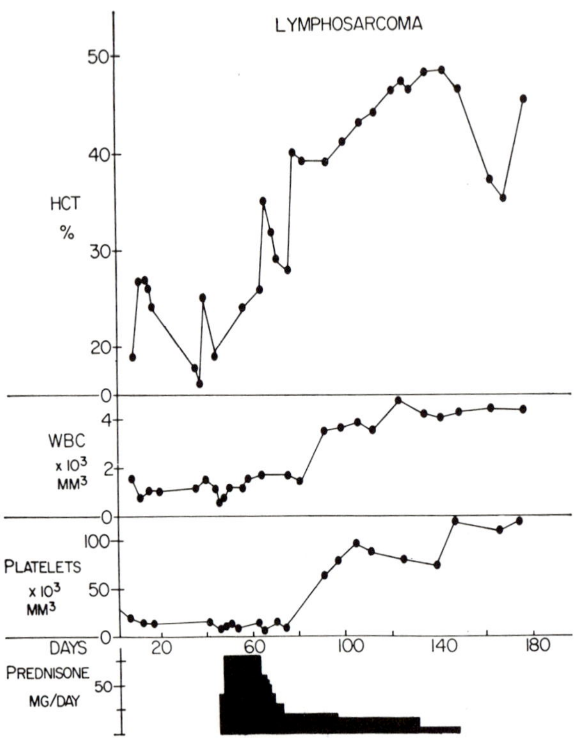

FIG. 9.—Treatment of small cell type lymphosarcoma in a 54-year-old man with pancytopenia. The lympholysis of a "packed bone marrow" by prednisone (80 mg/day) improved the anemia and hemorrhagic complications from severe thrombocytopenia.

tried, but if some regression of spleen size is not apparent after 500 rads have been given, then splenectomy should be considered. Corticosteroids may help to prepare the patient for surgery by raising platelet and granulocyte counts to protective levels. The courses of these patients demonstrate that large localized tumor masses can be removed, with great comfort to the patient. Splenectomy in small and large cell types of lymphosarcoma does not potentiate transformation into a leukemic phase (leukosarcoma). Hickling has emphasized the possibility of prolonged remission or cure in giant follicle lymphoma or lymphosarcoma by splenectomy when the spleen is the main site of tumor proliferation.[39]

Reticulum Cell Sarcoma (Malignant Reticulosis)

The neoplastic proliferation of primitive mesenchymal or reticulum cells represents a classification of malignant lymphoma in which most therapies have had limited success. Indeed, the tumor often is confused with anaplastic carcinoma and the sarcoma type of Hodgkin's disease. One can appreciate immediately how therapeutic evaluation might well be misinterpreted since the error in classification may misdirect treatment. Usually, one can expect to observe multicentric areas of malignancy that can be clinically similar to lymphosarcoma. I have not assumed that staging for intensive irradiation should be done. Careful evaluation of retroperitoneal adenopathy is advisable to assess any tumor encroachment on the kidney. From our current

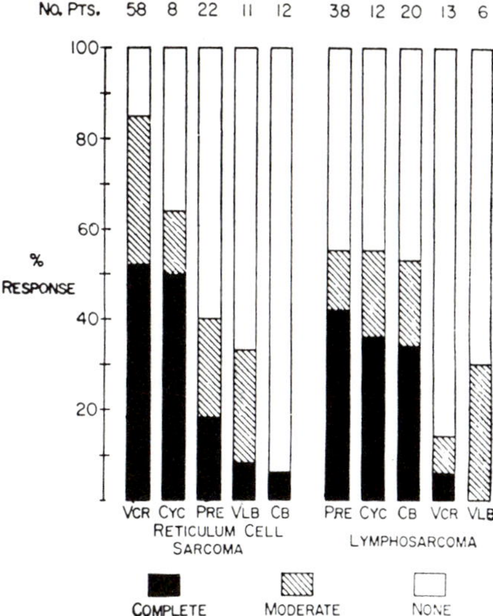

FIG. 10.—Response to treatment with chemotherapeutic agents in reticulum cell sarcoma compared with the response in lymphosarcoma. The response rate with vincristine is similar to that with cyclophosphamide, but does offer an additional medication in this disease. Response rate for lymphosarcoma (LS) is tabulated for comparison for this particular clinic. VCR = vincristine; Cyc = cyclophosphamide; pre = prednisone; Vlb = vinblastine; CB = chlorambucil. Reference 41 gives the exact definition of clinical response. Data modified from Desai et al.[41]

experience, we need to have cautious interpretation for all treatments. Increased survival percentages beyond 6 to 9 months would be encouraging data for any treatment program. However, any evidence of localized disease continues to warrant intensive irradiation (3,500 rads) to the involved nodes and the contiguous area as noted previously for lymphosarcoma.[36]

Disseminated disease should be treated with chemotherapy, preferably cyclophosphamide.[40] The drug has been used orally without a "loading" dose at a daily dose of 2 mg/kg. For marrow protection, androgens have been prescribed with the oral medication. Evidence of relapse or poor response after 6 weeks of therapy should prompt a change of treatment to vincristine.[41] For short-time remission of 1 or 2 months, dosage of 1 to 2 mg at 2- or 3-week intervals may be helpful. Alteration of therapy with previous chemotherapy already in use carries a high risk of further bone marrow suppression to limit the total dose that can be achieved. The resultant neuromuscular toxicity and gastrointestinal atony have limited the duration of therapy with vincristine. Nevertheless, several acceptable therapies are now available to the physician and offer a better opportunity for treating this disorder (Fig. 10). Corticoid therapy has had limited value, and should be considered only when there is pancytopenia, as noted also in the treatment of lymphosarcoma.[25]

ACKNOWLEDGMENT

The author is indebted to Dr. E. C. Reifenstein, Jr., Squibb Institute for Medical Research, New Brunswick, New Jersey, who kindly supplied testosterone enanthate (Delatestryl) and fluoxymesterone (Ora-Testryl).

References

1. Custer, R. P.: The changing pattern of lymphocytic malignancies. *In* Rebuck, J. W. (Ed.): The Lymphocyte and Lymphocytic Tissue. New York: Paul B. Hoeber, 1960.
2. Boutis, L., Obrecht, P., Musshoff, K. and Jochmann, P.: Zur Prognose der chronischen lymphatischen Leukämie. Deutsch. Med. Wschr. 44:2111, 1968.
3. Galton, D. A. G.: The pathogenesis of chronic lymphocytic leukemia. Canad. Med. Ass. J. 94:1005, 1966.
4. Han, T.: Benign chronic lymphocytic leukemia: Clinical and immunologic studies in 16 patients. Clin. Res. 17:406, 1970.
5. Dameshek, W.: Chronic lymphocytic leukemia: An accumulative disease of immunologically incompetent lymphocytes. Blood 29:566, 1967.
6. Fudenberg, H.: Are autoimmune diseases immunologic deficiency states? Hosp. Pract. 3:43, 1968.
7. Rubin, A. D., Havemann, K. and Dameshek, W.: Studies in chronic lymphocytic leukemia: Further studies of the proliferative abnormality of the blood lymphocyte. Blood 33:313, 1969.
8. Schrek, R.: Effect of phytohemagglutinin on lymphocytes from patients with chronic lymphocytic leukemia. Arch. Path. 83:58, 1967.
9. Zimmerman, T. S., Godwin, H. A. and Perry, S.: Studies of leukocyte kinetics in chronic lymphocytic leukemia. Blood 31:277, 1968.
10. Miller, D. G., Budinger, J. M. and Karnofsky, D. A.: A clinical and pathological study of resistance to infection in chronic lymphatic leukemia. Cancer 15:307, 1962.
11. Wasi, P. and Block, M.: The mechanism of the development of anemia in untreated chronic lymphatic leukemia. Blood 17:597, 1961.
12. Pisciotta, A. V. and Hirschboeck, J. S.: Therapeutic considerations in chronic lymphocytic leukemia: Special reference to the natural course of the disease. Arch. Intern. Med. 99:334, 1957.
13. Boggs, D. R., Sofferman, S. A., Wintrobe, M. M. and Cartwright, G. E.: Factors influencing the duration of survival of patients with chronic lymphocytic leukemia. Amer. J. Med. 40:243, 1966.
14. Djaldetti, M., DeVries, A., Levie, B. and Tikva, P.: Hemolytic anemia in lymphocytic leukemia: Treatment by irradiation of the spleen. Arch. Intern. Med. 110:449, 1962.
15. Silver, R. T.: The treatment of chronic lymphocytic leukemia. Seminars Hemat. 6:344, 1969.
16. Ultmann, J. E. and Nixon, D. D.: The therapy of lymphoma. Seminars Hemat. 6:376, 1969.
17. Goldman, R. L. and Warner, N. E.: Hemorrhagic cystitis and cytomegalic inclusions in the bladder associated with cyclophosphamide therapy. Cancer 25:7, 1970.
18. Huguley, C. M.: Survey of current therapy and of problems in chronic leukemia. *In* Leukemia-Lymphoma (a collection of papers presented at the Fourteenth Annual Clinical Conference on Cancer, 1969, at The University of Texas M. D. Anderson Hospital and Tumor Institute at Houston, Houston, Texas). Chicago: Year Book Medical Publishers, 1970, p. 317.
19. Gardner, F. H. and Pringle, J. C.: Androgens and erythropoiesis. I. Preliminary clinical observations. Arch. Intern. Med. 107:846, 1961.
20. Gardner, F. H.: Non-nutritional agents associated with nonspecific stimulation of erythropoiesis in man. *In* Jacobson, L. O. and Doyle, M. (Eds.): Erythropoiesis. New York: Grune & Stratton, 1962, p. 263.
21. Kennedy, B. J.: Androgenic hormone therapy in lymphatic leukemia. J.A.M.A. 190:1130, 1964.
22. Kirschbaum, A., Liebelt, A. G. and Falls, N. G.: Influence of gonadectomy and androgenic hormone on the induction of leukemia by methylcholanthrene in DBA/2 mice. Cancer Res. 15:685, 1955.
23. West, W. O.: The treatment of bone marrow failure with massive androgen therapy. Ohio Med. J. 61:347, 1965.
24. Freymann, J. G., Vander, J. B., Marler, E. A. and Meyer, D. G.: Prolonged corticosteroid therapy of chronic lymphocytic leukaemia and the closely allied malignant lymphomas. Brit. J. Haemat. 6:303, 1960.
25. Ezdinli, E. Z., Stutzman, L., Aungst, C. W. and Firat, D.: Corticosteroid therapy for lymphomas and chronic lymphocytic leukemia. Cancer 23:900, 1969.
26. Gardner, F. H. and Cohen, P.: The function of androgens and fluoride salts in the treatment of multiple myeloma. Trans. Amer. Clin. Climat. Ass. 77:226, 1965.

27. Lewis, F. B., Schwartz, R. S. and Dameshek, W.: X-radiation and alkylating agents as possible trigger mechanisms in the autoimmune complications of malignant lymphoproliferative disease. Clin. Exp. Immun. 1:3, 1966.
28. Shan, R. K., Szwed, C., Boggs, D. R., Fahey, J. L., Frer, E., et al.: Infection and immunity in chronic lymphocytic leukemia. Arch. Intern. Med. 106:467, 1960.
29. Rundles, R. W., Grizzle, J., Bell, W., Corley, C., Frommeyer, W., et al.: Myleran in chronic lymphocytic and granulocytic leukemia. Amer. J. Med. 27:424, 1959.
30. Han, T., Ezdinli, E. Z. and Sokal, J. E.: Complete remission in chronic lymphocytic leukemia and leukolymphosarcoma. Cancer 20:243, 1967.
31. Johnson, R. E.: Total body irradiation of chronic lymphocytic leukemia: Incidence and duration of remission. Cancer 25:523, 1970.
32. Zacharski, L. R. and Linman, J. W.: Chronic lymphocytic leukemia versus chronic lymphosarcoma cell leukemia. Amer. J. Med. 47:47, 1969.
33. Bierman, H. R., Marshall, J. and Winer, M. L.: The prediagnostic state of lymphoma. J.A.M.A. 86:185, 1963.
34. Vincent, P. C. and Gunz, F. W.: Control of lymphocyte level in the blood. Lancet 2:342, 1970.
35. Papac, R. J.: Lymphocyte transformation in malignant lymphomas. Cancer 26:279, 1970.
36. Lipton, A. and Lee, B. J.: Prognosis of Stage I lymphosarcoma and reticulum cell sarcoma. New Eng. J. Med. 284:230, 1970.
37. Carbone, P. P. and Spurr, C.: Management of patients with malignant lymphoma: A comparative study with cyclophosphamide and *Vinca* alkaloids. Cancer Res. 28:811, 1968.
38. Johnson, R. E., O'Conor, G. T. and Levin, D.: Primary management of advanced lymphosarcoma with radiotherapy. Cancer 25:787, 1970.
39. Hickling, R. A.: Giant follicle lymphoma of the spleen. Brit. Med. J. 2:787, 1964.
40. Stutzman, L., Ezdinli, E. Z. and Stutzman, M. A.: Vinblastine sulfate vs. cyclophosphamide in the therapy for lymphoma. J.A.M.A. 195:173, 1966.
41. Desai, D. V., Ezdinli, E. Z. and Stutzman, L.: Vincristine therapy of lymphomas and chronic lymphocytic leukemia. Cancer 26:352, 1970.

Extracorporeal Irradiation of Blood in Therapy of Leukemia

By Eugene P. Cronkite, M.D., Arjun D. Chanana, M.D., and Kanti R. Rai, M.D.

INTENSIVE EFFORTS of many investigators throughout the world have resulted only in modest control of leukemia and improvement in the allotransplantation of tissues. All too frequently, the chemotherapeutic and radiotherapeutic maneuvers that aid in the control of malignant cell proliferation and immunologic processes have serious widespread destructive effects upon normal tissues. The sequelae of these destructive effects upon the bone marrow or the bowel often result in the death of the patient. It is now known that immunologically competent cells are ceaselessly migrating from extravascular sites of production into and through the blood, and it is conceivable that leukemic cells act in a similar manner. In view of this continuous traffic through the blood stream, it can be hypothesized that immunity could be depressed and the leukemic process favorably influenced if one could destroy the immunologically competent cells on the one hand and the leukemic cells on the other hand by diverting a portion of the cardiac output extracorporeally through a shunt in a radiation field. With the possible exception of injury to circulating stem cells, the desired result might be accomplished without injury to the radiosensitive formative blood organs.

The notion of perturbing homeostasis by physical treatment of the blood through an extracorporeal shunt was initiated by Heymans[1] in 1921. Our group has perfected the technique of extracorporeal irradiation of the blood in man and animals. To date, we have described the production of a pronounced lymphopenia with a prolonged recovery time,[2] the induction of lymphocytosis by intravenously administered heparin,[3] the mathematical considerations of the dose distribution to the blood,[4] the combined effect of thoracic duct cannulation with drainage and extracorporeal irradiation upon the concentration of lymphocytes in the blood and the lymph,[5] the histologic picture of lymphoreticular tissues after prolonged extracorporeal irradiation,[6] observations on the effect of varying transit doses,[7] the effect of extracorporeal irradiation of the blood on erythrocyte survival in man,[8] the effect on circulating platelets in man,[9] experience with arteriovenous shunts in leukemic patients,[10] the effect of extracorporeal irradiation of the blood in the treatment of acute myelocytic leukemia,[11] the effect on chronic lymphocytic leukemia,[12] and the radiation sensitivity of chronic lymphocytic leukemia lymphocytes.[13]

The rationale for attempting to treat leukemia with extracorporeal irradiation of the blood (ECIB) is based on analogy among the behavior of leukemic cells, the behavior of normal lymphocytes, kinetic observations on the behavior of cells in the diverse types of leukemia, and theoretical considerations. Lajtha and colleagues[14] have assumed that the leukemic process was perpetuated by leukemic stem cells and that these cells are exchanging in both directions between marrow and blood. If this in reality occurs, there is a probability that all stem cells could be killed provided there is adequate exchange between marrow and blood and provided a fatal dose of

---

From the Medical Department, Brookhaven National Laboratory, Upton, New York.
Supported by the U. S. Atomic Energy Commission.

radiation can be delivered to the leukemic stem cell. The mathematical treatment of this problem has been expanded by Oliver and Shepstone.[15] In their analysis of the problem they assumed a blast cell doubling time of 10 days, continuous ECIB for periods up to 7 days, a blood blast turnover time of 16.7 hours, and as mentioned before, a two-way exchange between blood and marrow. There is also little to be gained by increasing the transit dose to the leukemic cells above 150 rads if leukemic and normal cells have about the same radiosensitivity. They conclude that there is a possibility of temporary remissions if long treatment times are possible. They do not consider intermittent ECIB for several months. Kinetic studies on leukemia suggest that their simple model of a two-way exchange between blood and tissues of the leukemic stem cells is probably an oversimplification of the problem. We have treated calves with chronic lymphocytic leukemia (CLL)[16] and have obtained results suggesting that the leukemia was being influenced favorably. Thomas and associates[17] applied intermittent ECIB in the treatment of CLL and in one patient with acute lymphocytic leukemia. Some patients with chronic lymphocytic leukemia responded very favorably, with decreasing blood lymphocyte counts, reticulocytosis, increasing platelet counts and improved general condition even though they had become refractory to chemotherapy.

Storb et al.[18] have extended these initial studies, and the results are similar to ours.[12,19] Our program has involved experimental therapy of several types of human leukemia[19] and the study of the effect of radiation upon the red cell and platelet of man.[8,9] The influence of ECIB can be discussed reasonably in the context of knowledge concerning the kinetics of leukemic cell proliferation.

The Effects of Extracorporeal Irradiation of the Blood (ECIB) upon the Human Red Cell

The radiation sensitivity of the human red cell has been studied.[8] Autologous erythrocytes were irradiated at doses of 35,000 to 200,000 rads, chromated, and the red cell survival studied. The 24-hour loss of labeled cells and the subsequent apparent erythrocyte survival times were functions of the radiation dose. Studies on several patients with leukemia undergoing ECIB demonstrated a mild red cell hemolysis during the course of therapy. It is believed that ECIB would be safe and would not produce acute hemolytic anemias if the accumulated dose was kept below 30,000 rads. A computer program (Sangrad II) makes it possible from given flow rates, blood volume and transit doses to calculate the accumulated dose to various fractions of the total blood volume for any given treatment schedule.

The *radiation resistance* of platelets has been studied.[9] In 5 leukemic patients receiving ECIB the platelets were labeled with ^{51}Cr. No effect was observed in the life span of the platelets, their ability to take up ^{51}Cr, or their ability to circulate shortly after autotransfusions. Platelets from a normal patient were similarly resistant to radiation up to 75,000 rads given in vitro, chromated and autotransfused. Clinical observation on platelet levels in all our patients suggests a lack of radiation damage. The doses of radiation delivered to platelets by extracorporeal irradiation of the blood in the treatment of leukemia do not seem to be a limiting factor to this form of treatment.

Another source of potential concern is the insertion of arteriovenous shunts in individuals with leukemia in light of their susceptibility to hemorrhage and infection. Thirty-three leukemic patients in whom shunts were placed have been studied.[10]

Postoperative wound bleeding was a frequent problem since most of the patients had striking thrombocytopenia. Pressure dressings, elevation of the cannulated arm and fresh blood transfusions controlled the bleeding in all cases except one. Infection occurred in 6 patients. In 4 patients the wound infection was controlled by systemic or local antibiotic treatment, or both. In two patients the wound infection was associated with irreversible clotting, and the shunts had to be removed. In two patients with acute myeloblastic leukemia, leukemic infiltrations developed at the shunt site simultaneously with the development of generalized subcutaneous infiltrations. Other minor complications are described by Chanana et al.[10]

Chronic Granulocytic Leukemia

Current notions on proliferation of cells and their exchange between blood and tissues are based primarily on the observations of Perry et al.[20] Cell proliferation in the marrow goes on in a manner analogous to normal granulocytopoiesis, the cells proliferating and flowing from the blast to the promyelocytic to myelocytic levels of maturation. Proliferation ceases at the myelocyte. Maturation continues through the metamyelocyte, band form, and segmented neutrophil. Normally, cells emerge from the marrow as segmented neutrophils, rarely as bands. In chronic granulocytic leukemia, cells leak into the blood at all levels of maturation and set up foci of proliferation predominantly in the spleen. All granulocytic cell types in the spleen exchange with the blood. There appears to be a free exchange between the blood, spleen and bone marrow of all types of leukemic cells. Six patients with chronic granulocytic leukemia have been treated with ECIB. Approximately 5 blood volumes per day were diverted through the irradiator, receiving a transit dose of 150 to 500 rads. Some patients had become drug resistant; others had not had prior treatment. ECIB reduced the blood count for varying periods in all patients. In the early stage of treatment, before the blood count started to fall, the spleen usually became larger and later substantially shrank. Hyperuricemia was prevented by allopurinol. Complete remissions were not obtained in any case. Decreasing blood counts accompanied by an increase in the size of the spleen suggest that the spleen is removing the radiation-damaged cells. The subsequent decrease in the size of the spleen supports the notion of Perry and associates that there is a free exchange between blood, spleen and bone marrow. Theoretically at least, in this model, one should be able to sterilize the body of all leukemic stem cells as suggested.[14,15] To date it has not been feasible to do so. Whether this is because of inadequate blood-bone marrow-spleen exchange rates, insufficient transit dose, or inadequate treatment time remains to be seen. However, since the probability of a chemotherapeutic cure is greater the smaller the mass of leukemic cells, it would be worthwhile to treat individuals with ECIB and then follow up with heavy chemotherapy.

Acute Myeloblastic Leukemia

A concept of acute myeloblastic leukemia based upon the work of many individuals has been published.[21] The marrow population consists of a leukemic stem cell population that may be identical with or lost among the obvious dividing leukemic cells. The ratio of dividing to apparent nondividing leukemic blast cells varies from 50:1 to 3:1 in the marrow. Later studies by Saunders and Mauer[22] suggest that the small apparent nondividing cells can reenter cycle. After thymidine labeling there is a difference between rate of entry of labeled cells into the blood and the loss of labeled cells from the blood. This difference could be interpreted as meaning that about 3 to 6 "nondividing cells" are entering the blood for each dividing cell. There is no direct evidence for return of leukemic cells to the marrow. However, a return of a small fraction of stem cells would not be detected by techniques currently available. In addition, there is a loss of leukemic stem cells from blood to tissue since tumor masses may develop subcutaneously. Rate of return is not known, and may not exist. In view of the apparent predominantly unidirectional flow from marrow to blood or the sluggish exchange of the dividing population, one would not expect to be able to kill the stem leukemic cell population in any reasonable length of single or repetitive treatment schedule. However, if the entrance rate into the blood were to increase with the diminished blood counts or if the proliferation rate were to be suppressed by peripheral killing of the leukemic cells through some negative feedback loop, one might anticipate a partial remission with some benefit to patients, particularly those who become refractory to chemotherapy. Another possibility to consider has been brought up by the studies of Chan et al.[23] These investigators have evidence suggesting that ECIB increases the mitotic and labeling index, possibly synchronizing the proliferative compartment in the marrow and thus perhaps making it more susceptible to chemotherapy aimed at specific stages of the cell cycle.

In our studies 14 adults with acute myelocytic leukemia received 16 courses of extracorporeal irradiation of the blood. The median survival time was 8 months. If the variable factors are taken into consideration, it was as good as, if not better than, studies previously reported despite the absence of hematologic remissions. Although no significant bone marrow changes were noted, there was a marked decrease in the peripheral leukemic cells in 75 per cent of the patients. There appears to be a correlation of increased survival time with a transit dose of ECIB over 340 rads. At the present time, the usefulness of this mode of treatment in the overall management of acute myelocytic leukemia is uncertain. It appeared to be of value in one patient to control leukostasis. It was also used in one patient with leukemia to carry her through pregnancy. These may be two definite indications. On the basis of the studies of Chan et al. and our data suggesting an increased survival time with higher transit doses, further studies on the use of ECIB in treatment and preparation of patients for chemotherapy are clearly indicated.

Chronic Lymphocytic Leukemia

Chronic lymphocytic leukemia (CLL) constitutes a spectrum of related disorders with many similarities but great differences in clinical aggressiveness. There is a benign, slowly advancing form of the disease for which treatment may not be required for many years, and a more aggressive type characterized by rapid clinical progression, with development of huge lymphocytic masses, resistance to standard therapy, hemolytic and infectious complications, and a rather short survival time. Between these extremes there is a group of syndromes which respond reasonably well to chemotherapy or internal or external radiation, or both. The median survival time is approximately 5 years.[12] It is not possible to distinguish among the various forms of CLL cytologically. There is great variability in the rate of increase of the lymphocyte count in the blood among patients. Without treatment, the counts may have doubling times from a few weeks to several years; in rare instances, the count may actually diminish with time or remain constant, implying a steady-state or near steady-state equilibrium between production and destruction of lymphocytes entering the blood.[12] A functional model of lymphocyte compartments in chronic lymphocytic leukemia has been devised by Schiffer.[12] This can be simplified by considering the blood lymphocyte compartment to comprise two subcompartments, one of which is rapidly exchanging with the other, making it possible to measure the size of this pool by dilution of labeled leukemic lymphocytes within it. These pools are exchanging with spleen and lymph nodes at relatively slow rates. There is an input into the blood from the bone marrow, and the mass of the lymphocytic tissue in the bone marrow, spleen and lymph nodes is perpetuated by a stem cell compartment that cannot be cytologically identified. This simplified model has been described earlier.[24] In such a model, where there is a sluggish exchange between the formative tissues and the blood, it is reasonable to expect that the blood compartment could be rapidly depleted by ECIB, which would equilibrate rapidly with the easily exchangeable pool of lymphocytes and slowly deplete the extravascular pools of lymphocytes in lymph nodes, spleen and bone marrow depending upon the exchange rates between the two. It could be hypothesized that with the sluggish exchanges with blood, a cure would be highly unlikely by ECIB.

To date 18 patients with CLL have been treated with ECIB. Some were refractory to chemotherapy and were anemic, thrombocytopenic and granulocytopenic. Some had had no previous therapy. In all cases, the blood lymphocyte pool was decreased in size by therapy. The rate at which lymphopenia developed was inversely related to ribonucleic acid turnover in the leukemic cells.[13] In some patients there was a decrease in lymph node and splenic size. Reticulocytosis and increased platelet counts were seen also in some patients. In one patient an apparent increase in marrow erythropoiesis was observed. In all cases there was a striking increase in uric acid excretion unless prevented by the administration of allopurinol. In no case was complete hematologic remission observed. Of the 18 patients treated, 6 are still alive. Rai et al.[25] have retrospectively surveyed the entire experience with chronic lymphocytic leukemia and its management at Brookhaven. To better evaluate the spontaneous survival and the influence of therapy, the disease was staged in a manner comparable to that for Hodgkin's disease:

Stage 0: Lymphocytosis of the blood and marrow exclusively.
Stage I: Lymphocytosis of blood and marrow plus enlarged lymph nodes.
Stage II: Stage I plus an enlarged spleen or liver, or both.
Stage III: Stage II plus anemia.
Stage IV: Stage III plus thrombocytopenia.*

In 12 years we observed 53 patients with chronic lymphocytic leukemia. In Table 1, the distribution of the living and dead patients among treatment groups is shown.

In Table 2, the survival time from diagnosis to death of patients treated conventionally for each stage of the disease is shown. An apparent good correlation is shown for survival and stage of disease at diagnosis. There are not sufficient data as yet to perform any meaningful statistics.

Table 3 shows the period of survival after diagnosis for those patients treated conventionally who were alive in September 1970. In Tables 2 and 3 it is noteworthy

* Lymphocytosis lymphocyte count greater than 15,000/mm^3; marrow lymphocytosis greater than 25 per cent in the bone marrow; anemia hemoglobin level of 11 gm% or less; and thrombocytopenia platelet count of less than 100,000/cu mm. For stages II, III and IV the last-noted criterion is used as decisive.

TABLE 1.—*Comparison of Patients with Chronic Lymphocytic Leukemia, Living or Dead, by Type of Treatment*

Treatment	Number of patients Alive	Dead	Total
Conventional only	12	24	36
Conventional and ECIB	4	11	15
ECIB only	2	0	2
	—	—	—
	18	35	53

TABLE 2.—*Survival Times Between Diagnosis and Death of Patients with CLL Who Did Not Receive ECIB*

Number of patients	Stage of disease at diagnosis	Survival after diagnosis (years) Mean	Range
7	IV	1.28	0.5–2.25
8	III	1.31	0.2–3.0
5	II	10.35	5.75–17.0
2	I	9.0	8–10
2	0	7.25	7–7.5

TABLE 3.—*Survival Times of Patients with CLL Who Received Only Conventional Therapy and Who Were Alive in September 1970*

Number of patients	Stage of disease at diagnosis	Survival after diagnosis (years)
2	II	1.0, 2.75
3	I	2.5, 3.0, 4.0
7	0	7.7 (mean); 1–20.0 (range)

TABLE 4.—*Survival Times, from Diagnosis to Death, of Patients with CLL Who Received Both ECIB and Conventional Therapy*

Number of patients	Stage of disease at diagnosis	Survival after diagnosis (years)
2	IV	1.3, 3.5
2	III	4.5, 8.0
2	II	2.5, 5.0
3	I	1.25, 3.0, 4.0
2	0	2.5, 5.5

that among the patients already dead, 15 of 24 (62 per cent) had been in stage III or IV at diagnosis, whereas among the patients who were still alive, none had been in these categories. However, 7 of 12 (58 per cent) had been in stage 0 at diagnosis.

In Table 4, the survival time from diagnosis to death is shown for those patients who received ECIB in addition to conventional therapy.

In Table 5, survival data after diagnosis are shown for patients treated with ECIB and conventional therapy who were alive in September 1970.

TABLE 5.—*Survival Data after Diagnosis on Patients Treated with ECIB and Conventional Therapy Who Were Alive in September 1970*

Number of patients	*Stage of disease at diagnosis*	*Survival after diagnosis (years)*
1	II	2.0
2*	I	1.5, 10.0
3*	0	4.0, 4.5, 6.3

* One patient treated with ECIB only.

In comparing the survival times of the patients who were treated with conventional therapy and who died (see Table 2) and those treated with conventional therapy plus ECIB (see Table 4), it is seen that the maximal survival in stage IV with conventional therapy is 2.25 years and that in stage IV with conventional therapy plus ECIB, maximal survival is 3.5 years. With conventional therapy in stage III, the maximal survival was 3 years, and for the 2 patients with ECIB combined with conventional therapy, survival was 4.5 and 8 years. For stages II, I and 0, the survival times in the group with conventional therapy combined with ECIB suggests that ECIB was not beneficial. It may be noted, however, that all these patients, irrespective of the stage of disease at diagnosis, were in stage III or IV at the time of ECIB. Clearly, no conclusions can be drawn at this stage and more data are required. In addition, meaningful comparisons among the groups treated with ECIB, with ECIB and conventional therapy, and with conventional therapy only cannot be made until after the deaths of the patients.

So far most patients who have been treated have had long-established disease; many were refractory to chemotherapy or had clinical indications for therapy (anemia, thrombocytopenia, or marked organomegaly, or a combination of these). Although clinically one gets the impression that several of these patients benefited from ECIB, conclusions cannot be drawn from anecdotal observations.

One wonders if CLL should be treated by ECIB early in the disease before there are extensive organomegaly and its sequelae. Whereas a cure is unlikely in principle, it may be possible to prevent organomegaly by intermittent depletion of the blood and of the rapidly exchanging lymphocytic pools. It is conceivable that this could be accomplished by a vein-to-vein ECIB using a pump rather than by inserting arteriovenous shunts.

A possible virtue of using ECIB in treating chronic lymphocytic leukemia is simply that there are no general toxic effects such as those encountered with chemotherapy and with general radiation therapy. There is also no local damage such as renal injury seen after extensive splenic irradiation.

REFERENCES

1. Heymans, J.-F.: Iso-hyper et hypothermisation des mammifères par calorification et frigorification du sang de la circulation carotido-jugulaire anastomosée. Arch. Int. Pharmacodyn. 25:1, 1921.
2. Cronkite, E. P., Jansen, C. R., Mather, G. C., Nielsen, N. O., Usenik, E. A., et al.: Studies on lymphocytes. I. Lymphopenia produced by prolonged extracorporeal irradiation of blood. Blood 20:203, 1962.
3. Jansen, C. R., Cronkite, E. P., Mather, G. C., Nielsen, N. O., Rai, K. R., et al.: Studies on lymphocytes. II. Production of lymphocytosis by intravenous heparin in calves. Blood 20:443, 1962.
4. Slatkin, D. N., Jansen, C. R., Cronkite, E. P. and Robertson, J. S.: Extracorporeal irradiation of the blood: Calculations and radiation dose. Radiat. Res. 19:409, 1963.

5. Cronkite, E. P., Jansen, C. R., Cottier, H., Rai, K. R. and Sipe, C. R.: Lymphocyte production measured by extracorporeal irradiation, cannulation and labeling technique. Ann. N.Y. Acad. Sci. 113:566, 1964.
6. Cottier, H., Cronkite, E. P., Jansen, C. R., Rai, K. R. and Singer, S.: Studies on lymphocytes. III. Effects of extracorporeal irradiation of the circulating blood upon the lymphoreticular organs in the calf. Blood 24:241, 1964.
7. Sipe, C. R., Chanana, A. D., Cronkite, E. P., Joel, D. D. and Schnappauf, Hp.: The influence of varying dose and repetitive short sessions of extracorporeal irradiation of the blood on the production of lymphopenia. Radiat. Res. 25:684, 1965.
8. Schiffer, L. M., Atkins, H. L., Chanana, A. D., Cronkite, E. P., Greenberg, M. L., et al.: Extracorporeal irradiation of the blood in humans: Effects upon erythrocyte survival. Blood 27:831, 1966.
9. Greenberg, M. L., Chanana, A. D., Cronkite, E. P., Schiffer, L. M. and Stryckmans, P. A.: Extracorporeal irradiation of blood in man: Radiation resistance of circulating platelets. Radiat. Res. 35:147, 1968.
10. Chanana, A. D., Cronkite, E. P., Greenberg, M. L., Rai, K. R., Schiffer, L. M., et al.: Experience with arteriovenous shunts in leukemic patients. Arch. Surg. 97:154, 1968.
11. Schiffer, L. M., Atkins, H. L., Chanana, A. D., Cronkite, E. P., Greenberg, M. L. and Stryckmans, P. A.: Extracorporeal irradiation of blood (ECIB) in man. II. Treatment of acute myelocytic leukemia. Blood 31:17, 1968.
12. Schiffer, L. M.: Kinetics of chronic lymphocytic leukemia. Series Haemat. 1:3, 1968.
13. Stryckmans, P. A., Chanana, A. D., Cronkite, E. P., Greenberg, M. L. and Schiffer, L. M.: Studies on lymphocytes. X. Influence of extracorporeal irradiation of the blood on lymphocytes in chronic lymphocytic leukemia: Apparent correlation with RNA turnover. Radiat. Res. 37:118, 1969.
14. Lajtha, L. G., Lewis, C. L., Gunning, A. J., Sharp, A. A. and Callender, S.: Extracorporeal irradiation of the blood. A possible therapeutic measure. Lancet 1:353, 1962.
15. Oliver, R. and Shepstone, D. J.: Extracorporeal irradiation of the blood: The mathematical problem of dosimetry. Brit. J. Haemat. 10:181, 1964.
16. Cronkite, E. P., Chanana, A. D., Schnappauf, Hp.: Extracorporeal irradiation of blood and lymph in animals: Its effects on homografts and on lymphoma. New Eng. J. Med. 272:456, 1965.
17. Thomas, E. D., Epstein, R. B., Eschbach, J. W., Jr., Prager, D., Buchner, C. D. and Marsaglia, G.: Treatment of leukemia by extracorporeal irradiation. New Eng. J. Med. 273:6, 1965.
18. Storb, R., Epstein, R. B., Buckner, C. D. and Thomas, E. D.: Treatment of chronic lymphocytic leukemia by extracorporeal irradiation. Blood 31:490, 1968.
19. Schiffer, L. M., Chanana, A. D., Cronkite, E. P., Greenberg, M. L., Joel, D. D., et al.: Extracorporeal irradiation of the blood. Seminars Hemat. 3:154, 1966.
20. Perry, S., Moxley, J. H., Weiss, G. H. and Zelen, M.: Studies on leukocyte kinetics by liquid scintillation counting in normal individuals and in patients with chronic myelocytic leukemia. J. Clin. Invest. 45:1383, 1966.
21. Cronkite, E. P.: Kinetics of leukemic cell proliferation. *In* Perspectives in Leukemia (Symposium of the Leukemia Society, 1966). New York: Grune & Stratton, 1968.
22. Saunders, E. F. and Mauer, A. M.: Reentry of nondividing leukemic cells into a proliferative phase in acute childhood leukemia. J. Clin. Invest. 48:1299, 1969.
23. Chan, B. W. B., Hayhoe, F. G. J. and Bullimore, J. A.: Effect of extracorporeal irradiation of blood on bone marrow activity in acute leukemia. Nature 221:972, 1969.
24. Cronkite, E. P.: Extracorporeal irradiation of the blood and lymph in the treatment of leukemia and for immunosuppression. Ann. Intern. Med. 67:415, 1967.
25. Rai, K. R., Chanana, A. D. and Cronkite, E. P.: Unpublished studies.

Therapy of Multiple Myeloma

By Ralph Wayne Rundles, Ph.D., M.D. and Harvey J. Cohen, M.D.

During the period since the first of this series of symposia on the chemotherapy of neoplastic disease was held, biologic, biochemical and clinical investigations have produced a flood of new and interesting information relating to plasma cell myeloma. The sheer mass of information which has accrued makes it difficult to carry out our present assignment, to summarize and present a fair consensus of the more relevant data pertaining to the causation, pathogenesis and treatment of plasma cell myeloma in man.

Myeloma began to be recognized as a relatively common clinical entity about 25 years ago. When a few responses to systemic chemotherapy were observed, widespread interest developed in the array of clinical and hematologic manifestations of the disease, the relation of the abnormal serum to urinary proteins and to plasma cell proliferation, the pathogenesis of the renal disease, etc. Attention began to be directed also to the study of experimental counterparts, plasma cell tumors in animals. These rare malignancies were first discovered to arise spontaneously in old mice, in a lymph node near the base of the cecum.[1] Later, Potter, Dunn and others found that plasma cell tumors could be induced experimentally with great frequency in one strain of inbred mice, BALB/c, by the intraperitoneal injection of mineral oil or adjuvants containing mineral oil, or by the intraperitoneal implantation of solid plastic materials, such as lucite.[2-4] Both types of agents produce a chronic granulomatous reaction in the submesothelial connective tissues around the root of the mesentery which become infiltrated by a variety of reticulum cells, lymphocytes, and plasma cells. After 6 to 14 months, or about one-third the mean life span of a mouse, plasma cell tumors begin to develop in these granulomas and then metastasize to involve proximal lymph nodes.[5] It was significant that the growth of plasma cells in the bone marrow of the mice was not affected by these experimental manipulations and that tumors arising from the submesenteric tissues synthesized predominantly immunoglobulins of the intestinal IgA type. These tumors can be transplanted from animal to animal indefinitely. The concentration of homogeneous Ig in the plasma is directly proportional to the weight of the tumor.[5]

Speculations regarding the causation of myeloma in man parallel to some extent the experimental findings in the mouse. Suspicion has been directed particularly to (1) prolonged abnormal immunologic stimuli, (2) genetic factors, and (3) age. Anomalous serum protein components and, eventually, plasma cell myeloma develop in a few individuals with chronic infections of the biliary tract or intestine,[6,7] The importance of genetic factors in the causation of plasma cell myeloma in man is illustrated by reports of several families in which two siblings or other first-degree relatives have had the disease.[8,9] Even though this incidence has been much lower than the impressively increased incidence of chronic lymphocytic leukemia among relatives of patients with this disease, plasma cell and lymphocytic proliferative

From the Division of Hematology and Oncology, Department of Medicine, Duke University School of Medicine, Durham, North Carolina.

Supported in part by USPHS Training Grant No. CA 05042 and Grant No. CA 03177 from the National Cancer Institute, National Institutes of Health.

abnormalities have developed concurrently in a few families. The inherited trait seems to be an unstable regulation of immunologic responses generally, since both high and low levels of immunoglobulin have been observed, as well as an increased incidence of autoimmune and hypersensitivity diseases. The possibility that inherited immunologic abnormalities may increase an individual's susceptibility to oncogenic viruses is relevant to the pathogenesis of myeloma, as it is to certain forms of leukemia.

Plasma cell tumors develop in old mice, and myelomatosis is a disease of the elderly in man. In recent years, as new series of patients have been reported, individuals in whom plasma cell myeloma develops seem to be older. The age of maximal incidence of the disease in New York and London, two to three decades ago, was between 50 and 60 years. In Copenhagen, the age of maximal incidence is now between 60 and 70 years and in Malmö, between 70 and 80 years.[10] It has been well demonstrated that immunologic competence decreases with age, and reduction in the effectiveness of surveillance mechanisms may be important.

It is more blessed, of course, for physicians to prevent a disease than to treat an established one. To prevent myeloma, one should choose ancestors with normal immunologic apparatus, avoid chronic infections and hyperimmune reactions, and not grow old!

To take a panoramic view of plasma cell myeloma, the basic phenomenon is, of course, the malignant growth of plasma cells (Fig. 1). The normal habitat of these

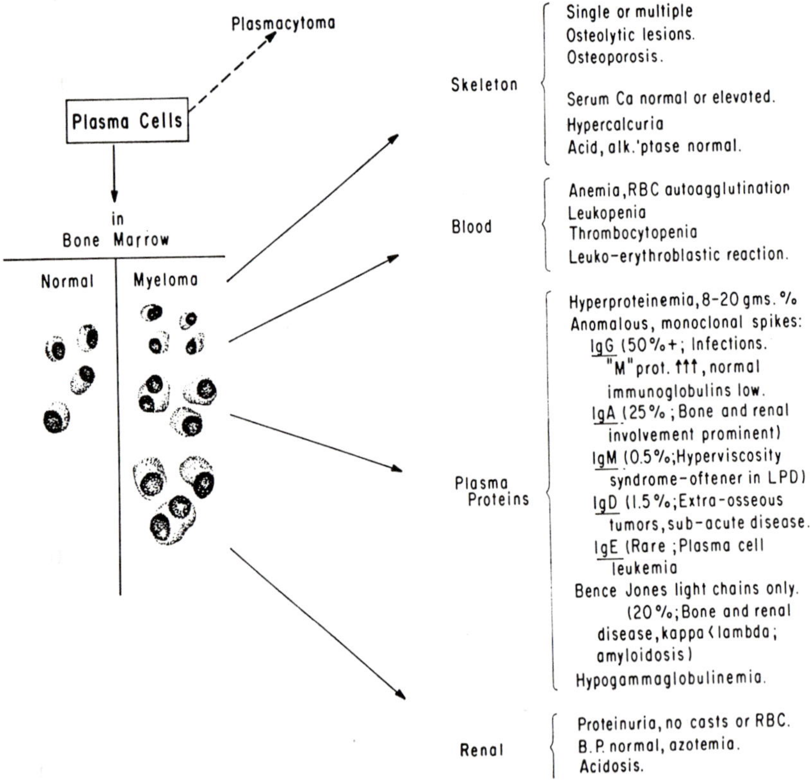

FIG. 1.—Pathogenesis of plasma cell myeloma.

cells in man is the red bone marrow housed in the short, flat bones of the skull, vertebrae, ribs, pelvis and the proximal portions of the long bones. These are the regions of the skeleton predominantly involved in plasma cell myeloma, but plasmacytomas occasionally develop elsewhere: in the tonsils, paranasal sinuses, epidural space, lymph nodes or distal long bones. The many manifestations of the disease relate for the most part to (1) the volume and bulk of the tumor, and (2) the consequences of perverted plasma cell function.

Bone marrow function is compromised to an important extent in nearly every patient by the overgrowth of abnormal plasma cells. Anemia or other cytopenias, or both, develop when half or more of the bone marrow tissue is replaced by plasma cells. For undefined reasons, bony trabeculae around foci of proliferating plasma cells are subject to dissolution. Perversions of plasma cell function associated with the malignant state are manifested by a variety of disturbances in the synthesis of immunoglobulin. Anomalous, homogeneous, monoclonal components occur with the approximate frequency shown in Figure 1. In some instances, H-chain moieties may be present in the plasma or excreted in the urine.[11] Isolated light chains of gamma globulin, Bence Jones proteins, are excreted in the urine, too, in amounts ranging from a few milligrams to many grams per 24 hours. There is considerable variation in the pattern of disease presentation, evolution and clinical complications, and in response to therapy. Some correlation between specific globulin abnormalities and the clinical features of the disease became apparent when a large group of patients was studied[12] (Table 1). This was particularly true with respect to the relation of reduced normal gamma globulin to infection and the association of light chain proteinuria with the development of myeloma renal disease, which accounts for the ultimate death of nearly half of all patients with this disease.

Plasma Cells

Plasma cell myeloma, like other varieties of leukemia, appears to originate from the mutation of a single stem cell. The morphologic identification of stem cells is somewhat uncertain, but neoplastic elements must have a survival advantage over

TABLE 1.—*Clinical Features of Myelomatosis Compared with Immunoglobulin Status*

	IgG	*IgA*	*BJ*
Number of patients	112	54	40
Myeloma protein in serum, mean concentration, gm%	4.3	2.8	±
Immunoglobulin <20% normal	68	30	19
Hospital admissions, infection, %	60	33	20
Osteolytic bone lesions, %	55	65	78
Hypercalcemia	33	59	62
Azotemia, urea above 79 mg%	16	17	33
Detected amyloidosis, %	0.5	7	10
Mean doubling time of myeloma protein (months)	10.1	6.3	3.4
Estimated duration of disease (years)	33	21	11

From data of Hobbs.[12]
BJ = Bence Jones protein.

normal cells. All plasma cells, wherever they are and whatever their functional commitment is destined to be, seem to be equally vulnerable to the mutagenic stimulus.

Differential Diagnosis

Plasmacytosis in the bone marrow, like leukocytosis appearing in the circulating blood, may follow chronic infection or be associated with hepatic or hypersensitivity disease. The differentiation of benign from malignant plasmacytosis is a critical matter which may be easy or exceedingly difficult. The number of plasma cells in the bone marrow and their morphology give the first clue. Benign or non-neoplastic diseases ordinarily produce at the maximum a plasmacytosis of 10 to 20 per cent, and the degree of plasma cell immaturity in the bone marrow is only modest. If 50 per cent or more of the marrow elements are plasma cells, or if sheets of these cells are present, the diagnosis of myeloma is virtually certain. There is no sharp morphologic distinction between reactive plasma cells and "myeloma" cells. The more abnormal the plasma cells are, however, the more certain is the diagnosis. The presence of large numbers of particularly bizarre plasma cells is generally associated, as noted below, with a poor prognosis.

The identification of anomalous serum and urine proteins is enormously helpful in the diagnosis of plasma cell myeloma, and in differentiating benign from malignant proliferation. The quantitation of abnormal proteins provides an indispensable guide to the management of therapy. The natural history of plasma cell myeloma is that of orderly and regular growth at first, but progression or exacerbation is frequent in late stages of the disease. When the abnormal plasma cell line is first established, the cells appear to divide and grow at a regular rate for many years. Symptoms may be produced by a few grams of plasma cells, if they erode a rib or produce a superficial tumor, but most patients with full-blown disease appear to have upwards of a kilogram of plasma cells distributed throughout their bone marrow and other tissues.[13] To produce this number of cells from a single mutant, as many as 39 cell doubling divisions are required, assuming the efficient survival of all cell descendants. The rate at which the untreated disease progresses has been measured in suitable patients, and this provides some indication of the probable duration of the occult, preclinical disease.[13] Extrapolation back from the observed rate at which the disease progresses, once it had been recognized clinically, indicated that the asymptomatic phase of the disease may range from 11 years for patients producing only light chains to 33 years for those producing IgG.

Population surveys have shown that the incidence of abnormal serum "M" components increases with age, and in elderly people may be upwards of 1 per cent.[14] The amount of abnormal protein in these individuals was usually low, only 300 to 600 mg%, and was sometimes present only transiently. Large amounts of protein occurred predominantly in individuals with myelomatosis. In a survey of patients with a variety of tumors, the incidence of abnormal components was about 1 per cent, too, apparently reflecting a random association.[15] "Myeloma" proteins must be differentiated from the anomalous components that occur in patients with lymphoma or lymphocytic leukemia, usually IgM, and in those with no evident primary disease. The quantity of protein, and its tendency to increase in amount, provide additional diagnostic clues.[16,17] In malignant proliferation of plasma cells, the amount of abnormal serum protein is usually 1 gm% or more, and Bence Jones light chain proteinuria is at least 10 to 20 mg per day. Progression is a basic characteristic of plasma cell myeloma, and increasing evidence of disease is nearly always found within a period of 2 or 3 years.

The diagnosis of "benign" monoclonal gammopathy should always be made tentatively. Patients who seem to have a nonprogressive, benign disease for some months or years may be found to have malignant plasma cell proliferation or some other lymphoproliferative disease only after a decade or more. Early in the course of this type of disease, the only diagnosis one can make is "potential malignancy."

An illustration of the course of myeloma, a rapid initial response to therapy followed by acute exacerbation a few months later, is shown in Figure 2. This 56-year-old man enjoyed excellent health until an unusual series of persistent respiratory, sinus and ear infections developed in the winter of 1963–64. In April 1964, his physician found that he had a mild degree of anemia and proteinuria. X-ray films of his skeleton, gall bladder and gastrointestinal tract, and pyelograms showed no relevant abnormalities. Survey blood chemical determinations were all normal except for a serum protein concentration of 11.2 gm%. Bone marrow aspirated from the sternum was moderately hypercellular, with about two-thirds of the cells being relatively mature plasma cells. Electrophoresis of the serum protein showed a large "spike" of gamma globulin amounting to 5.2 gm/100 ml. The urine protein was 1.1 gm per 24 hours and, on electrophoresis, was mostly a homogeneous globulin constituent.

Therapy with L-phenylalanine mustard (melphalan, Alkeran) was initiated. Ten mg was given in one dose before breakfast each morning for one week, and thereafter 10 mg once a week. His clinical status and laboratory abnormalities improved quickly, and for nearly one year he was well. At that time, however, protein reappeared in

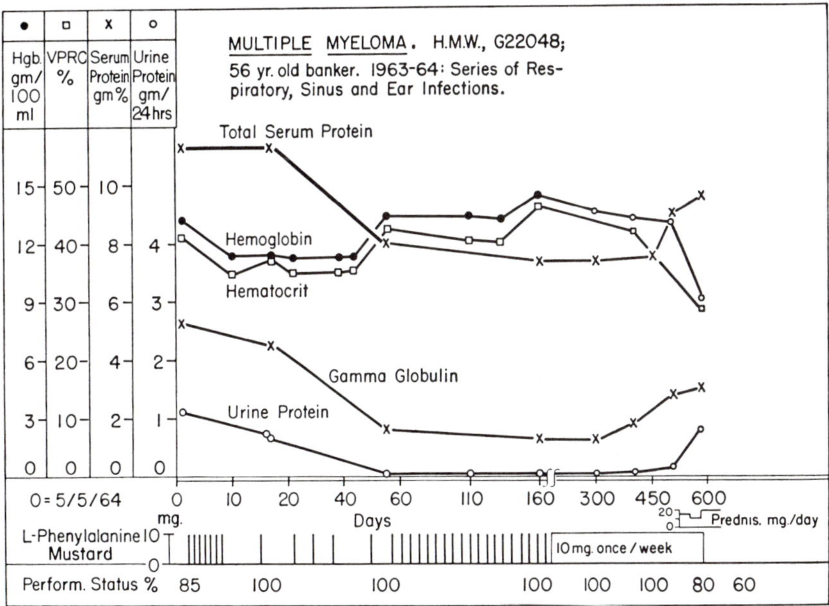

FIG. 2.—Rapid response to therapy in a patient with plasma cell myeloma, followed by acute exacerbation after 1 year.

his urine and the globulin component in his serum began to increase. Prednisone was added to his regimen, with some evidence of temporary improvement. Eighteen months after the beginning of therapy, he became anemic for the first time. Heavy proteinuria reappeared, and the abnormal serum component began to increase in concentration. He continued to get worse and evidence of renal insufficiency developed. The patient died 18 months after the diagnosis of myeloma had been established. At autopsy the main finding was acute necrosis of the renal tubules.

In this instance there was a quick response to what has become rather standard therapy, but a relatively acute, fatal exacerbation of the disease occurred one year later. Death resulted from renal insufficiency.

The exacerbation of plasma cell myeloma in late stages, or progression to plasma cell leukemia, has been recognized for some time. Concomitant with the use of more effective therapeutic measures to suppress plasma cell growth, transitions to other forms of myeloproliferative disease such as acute myelogenous or myelomonocytic leukemia, stem cell leukemia and erythroleukemia are now being reported.[18,19] There is no evidence that the therapeutic agents used are leukemogenic in these patients.

To make a prognosis in plasma cell myeloma is always difficult. A number of features, however, may be used to identify "high-risk" patients. The rapid onset of disease, impairment of renal function with azotemia, severe cytopenias with hypocellular bone marrow, the predominance of bizarre plasma cells in the bone marrow, etc., are all indicative of severe disease and a poor prognosis.

In a large cooperative group study, a significant correlation between the clinical features of myeloma and different types of immunoglobulin abnormalities was demonstrated[12] (see Table 1). The degree and rapidity with which patients responded to therapy were also important in predicting their survival. Individuals who did not respond to therapy and those in whom disease progressed despite therapy ordinarily lived only a few months. A slow and sustained response to therapy, moreover, was better than a rapid one. The 2-year survival of patients who responded quickly, in a matter of weeks, was 39 per cent as compared with a 78 per cent 2-year survival for those who improved slowly over a period of months.

The use and rationale of different therapeutic agents in plasma cell myeloma are outlined in Table 2. Two nitrogen mustard derivatives are the most effective agents presently available for the systemic suppression of plasma cell growth. In group studies, the overall therapeutic effectiveness of melphalan and cyclophosphamide is about equal.[20] A few of our patients, having responded poorly to phenylalanine mustard and prednisone, have shown a better response when cyclophosphamide was substituted for melphalan. Cyclophosphamide given by the intravenous route is sometimes more effective than when given orally.

Melphalan therapy has usually been initiated with the administration of the maximally tolerated dose, a total of approximately 1 mg per kilogram of body weight, given over a period of 1 to 3 weeks. Therapy is then suspended for 1 to 3 weeks to observe the degree to which bone marrow function is suppressed before maintenance therapy is begun. A variety of regimens for maintenance with melphalan have been used: 1 to 2 mg daily; 6 to 10 mg once a week; or 6 to 10 mg daily for 3 to 5 consecutive days, at intervals of 6 to 10 weeks.[21-23] Single doses of more than 10 to 12 mg produce nausea, vomiting, malaise and other symptoms which make the use of larger amounts impractical without inviting therapeutic rebellion. Many observers prefer to give melphalan intermittently for maintenance, allowing bone marrow

TABLE 2.—*Therapeutic Agents in Multiple Myeloma*

To suppress plasma cell growth:
Nitrogen mustard derivatives
Phenylalanine mustard (melphalan)
Cyclophosphamide
Adrenal corticosteroids, ACTH
Irradiation to local areas, tumors
To promote bone remineralization:
Physical therapy
Anabolic steroids
Androgens
Fluoride
To promote erythropoiesis:
Androgenic steroids
Testosterone
Fluoxymesterone
To relieve pain:
Physical therapy
Bed rest (acute)
Salicylates, etc.
X-ray

function to recover between doses, but whether the interval should be one week, two weeks or two months is difficult to say.

If patients have thrombocytopenia or severe neutropenia, cyclophosphamide is a better agent than phenylalanine mustard. Cyclophosphamide can be given intravenously or orally. If cytopenia is present before therapy is begun, the dose should be reduced to approximately half that tolerated by individuals with normal bone marrow function. The administration of 5 mg/kg intravenously daily, or every other day, for four to five doses initially is ordinarily safe in previously untreated patients. For long-term maintenance, cyclophosphamide can be given orally in doses of 50 to 100 mg daily. The total amount should be given in one dose before breakfast, with enough extra fluid to produce a morning polyuria to avert adverse effects on the bladder mucosa.

The adrenal corticoids are indispensable agents in the treatment of plasma cell myeloma. The use of prednisone in doses of 40 to 60 mg per day, or equivalent amounts of other corticosteroids, to treat acute hypercalcemia is well recognized. In addition, these compounds act to suppress the growth of plasma cells, stimulate bone marrow function, and appear to have a useful catabolic effect on abnormal myeloma proteins. Prednisone should never be used alone for prolonged therapy, however, but always in conjunction with a mustard compound. These two classes of compounds are synergistic, and their combined effect in the treatment of plasma cell myeloma is greater than that of either one alone.[23] The adrenal corticoids are given in many ways, and there are no conclusive data to indicate which regimen is most efficacious. Large doses should be avoided in the long-term therapy of patients with plasma cell myeloma, since they increase skeletal demineralization, susceptibility to infection and the likelihood of gastrointestinal bleeding. In those patients whose disease cannot be adequately controlled with one of the mustard agents alone, it is ordinarily safe to give 5 to 10 mg of prednisone every 12 hours for protracted periods. Some give an equivalent amount in one dose daily, others every other day, and still others during a two-week period every month or two.[23] There is no established rationale or adequate clinical study to show which regimen is superior.

Solitary plasma cell tumors or plasmacytomas are rare, but may be sensitive to radiation therapy. Plasmacytomas also develop in patients with generalized myeloma and may produce laryngeal obstruction, spinal cord compression or bone lesions of orthopedic significance. Local irradiation therapy in these instances may be used in conjunction with chemotherapy. Generalized skeletal demineralization is one of the most incapacitating complications of plasma cell myeloma. The irradiation of collapsed vertebrae may help relieve pain and increase bone healing, but the field should be limited to avoid further depression of bone marrow function. When bony involvement is widespread, irradiation becomes impractical. It is important to avoid immobilization whenever possible, and to encourage active physical therapy, even for patients confined to bed.

Androgenic steroids (fluoxymesterone, testosterone enanthate, testosterone cypionate) have a variety of effects when given in pharmacologic doses, which are valuable in the treatment of multiple myeloma. As plasma cell proliferation is being controlled by the mustard compounds and corticosteroids, the erythropoietic stimulus of androgens may be beneficial in alleviating anemia.[24] It has been suggested that androgens may protect the bone marrow to some extent from the adverse effects of mustard agents.[25] The protein anabolic effect of the androgens reduces bony demineralization in myeloma and counteracts the demineralizing effects of corticosteroids. Fluoxymesterone (Halotestin) can be given orally in doses of 10 to 40 mg a day, or long-acting testosterone compounds (testosterone enanthate, testosterone cypionate) can be administered intramuscularly, 100 to 200 mg per week. These agents are useful even though they have no demonstrable primary effect on plasma cell growth.

The effect of chronic fluoride ingestion on bone was described as early as 1891, but its clinical importance was not widely recognized until radiologic evidence of bony sclerosis following chronic industrial exposure was described in 1932.[26] The potential value of fluoride in the treatment of bone demineralization in multiple myeloma has been extensively studied since 1964.[27–29] Sodium fluoride is given orally in doses as tolerated, 50 to 150 mg a day. At least six months of therapy is required before there is a significant increase in radiologic density or histologic evidence of increased bone formation. This effect appears to result from the incorporation of fluoride into a more resistant hydroxyapatite structure and a positive calcium balance associated with decreased osteoclastic and increased osteoblastic activity. Pain relief has occurred in some patients, but there is no evidence that fluoride therapy increases the strength or stability of bone. Abnormal plasma cells may continue to grow in areas of fluoride-induced bone sclerosis.

Patients with plasma cell myeloma are particularly susceptible to bacterial infections, which require prompt and energetic therapy with the proper antimicrobial agents. Routine prophylactic treatment with gamma globulin, or gamma globulin supplementation during acute infections, has met with little success.[30] The catabolism of all gamma globulins is accelerated when a large amount of abnormal protein, especially IgG is present.[31] This reduces possible benefit from exogenously administered immune globulins. The administration of gamma globulin may be somewhat more valuable in patients with a low concentration of normal and myeloma immunoglobulins.

The hyperviscosity syndrome, recognized during the last 6 years, refers to circulatory and bleeding abnormalities associated with increased serum viscosity, tinnitus, CNS dysfunction, blurred vision, dilated retinal veins, retinal hemorrhages, mucous membrane bleeding and, occasionally, gastrointestinal bleeding.[32] Arterial hypertension, congestive heart failure and renal failure are less common, late manifestations. The syndrome most often occurs in patients with Waldenström's macroglobulinemia when the IgM concentration exceeds 2 gm% and the relative serum viscosity is increased to 6 to 8. A striking increase in plasma volume parallels the increased serum viscosity.[33] Impressive therapeutic benefits have resulted from plasmapheresis, probably related to the fact that almost all IgM produced stays in the intravascular space. In myeloma the hyperviscosity syndrome is rare but may develop in the presence of large quantities of IgG protein, circulating aggregates of IgG protein, or molecular configurations producing a high intrinsic viscosity.[34,35] Plasmapheresis may result in striking degrees of temporary benefit.[36]

The renal disease associated with plasma cell myeloma may be produced by a variety of causative factors, which include hypercalcemia, hyperuricemia, pyelonephritis, amyloid infiltration, plasma cell infiltration and tubular damage by anomalous proteins. Acute renal failure, a hazard in these patients, may be prevented by avoiding dehydration or procedures involving fluid restriction such as intravenous pyelograms, etc.[37] Cautious but prompt rehydration is advisable if dehydration does occur. Acute renal failure in multiple myeloma has been successfully treated by short-term renal dialysis in several instances, with return of good kidney function and prolonged survival with the concomitant control of plasma cell proliferation.[38] Chronic renal failure in myeloma has been more resistant to therapy. Slowly advancing azotemia frequently regresses with control of the underlying disease, but severe impairment of renal function with acidosis rarely improves. The exact pathogenesis of the "myeloma kidney" is not understood, but is currently believed to be related in some way to tubular damage produced by the excretion of low molecular weight Bence Jones protein.[39] Life can be prolonged somewhat by renal dialysis, but there is no evidence that the kidney lesion in chronic disease is reversible.

References

1. Dunn, T. B.: Normal and pathologic anatomy of the reticular tissue in laboratory mice, with a classification and discussion of neoplasms. J. Nat. Cancer Inst. 14:1281, 1954.
2. Merwin, R. M. and Algire, G. H.: Induction of plasma-cell neoplasms and fibrosarcomas in BALB/c mice carrying diffusion chambers. Proc. Soc. Exp. Biol. Med. 101:437, 1959.
3. Potter, M. and Robertson, C. L.: Development of plasma cell neoplasms in BALB/c mice after intraperitoneal injection of paraffin-oil adjuvant heat killed staphylococcus mixtures. J. Nat. Cancer Inst. 25:847, 1960.
4. Potter, M. and Boyce, C. R.: Induction of plasma cell neoplasms in strain BALB/c mice with mineral oil adjuvants. Nature 193:1086, 1962.
5. Potter, M.: The plasma cell tumors and myeloma proteins of mice. Meth. Cancer Res. 2:104, 1967.
6. Osserman, E. F. and Takatsuki, K.: Considerations regarding the pathogenesis of the plasmacytic dyscrasias. Series Haemat. 4:28-49, 1965.
7. Zawadzki, Z. A. and Edwards, G. A.: Dysimmunoglobulinemia associated with hepatobiliary disorders. Amer. J. Med. 48:196, 1970.
8. Herrell, W. E., Ruff, J. D. and Bayrd, E. D.: Multiple myeloma in siblings. J.A.M.A. 167:1485, 1958.
9. Leoncini, D. L. and Korngold, L.: Multiple myeloma in 2 sisters: An immunochemical study. Cancer 17:733, 1964.
10. Waldenström, J.: Diagnosis and Treatment of Multiple Myeloma. New York: Grune & Stratton, 1970.

11. Osserman, E. F. and Takatsuki, K.: Clinical and immunochemical studies on four cases of heavy (Hγ-2) chain disease. Amer. J. Med. 37:351, 1964.
12. Hobbs, J. R.: Immunochemical classes of myelomatosis: Including data from a therapeutic trial conducted by a Medical Research Council working party. Brit. J. Haemat. 16:599, 1969.
13. Hobbs, J. R.: Growth rates and responses to treatment in human myelomatosis. Brit. J. Haemat. 16:607, 1969.
14. Axelsson, U., Bachmann, R. and Hällén, J.: Frequency of pathological proteins (m-components) in 6995 sera from an adult population. Acta Med. Scand. 179:235, 1966.
15. Migliore, P. J. and Alexanian, R.: Monoclonal gammopathy in human neoplasia. Cancer 21:1127, 1968.
16. Waldenström, J. G.: Monoclonal and Polyclonal Hypergammaglobulinemia: Clinical and Biological Significance. Nashville, Tenn.: Vanderbilt University Press, 1968.
17. Hobbs, J. R.: Paraproteins, benign or malignant. Brit. Med. J. 3:699, 1967.
18. Anderson, E. and Videbaek, A.: Stem cell leukemia in myelomatosis. Scand. J. Haemat. 7:201, 1970.
19. Kyle, R. A., Pierre, R. V. and Bayrd, E. D.: Multiple myeloma and acute myelomonocytic leukemia. New Eng. J. Med. 283:1121, 1970.
20. Rivers, S. L. and Patno, M. E.: Cyclophosphamide vs. melphalan in treatment of plasma cell myeloma. J.A.M.A. 207:1328, 1969.
21. McArthur, J. R., Athens, J. W., Wintrobe, M. M. and Cartwright, G. E.: Melphalan and myeloma. Ann. Intern. Med. 72:665, 1970.
22. Hoogstraten, B., Costa, J., Cuttner, J., Forcier, J., Leone, L. A., et al.: Intermittent melphalan therapy in multiple myeloma. J.A.M.A. 209:251, 1969.
23. Alexanian, R., Haut, A., Khan, A. U., Lane, M., McKelvey, E. M., et al.: Treatment for multiple myeloma (combination chemotherapy with different melphalan dose regimens). J.A.M.A. 208:1680, 1969.
24. Gardner, F. H. and Pringle, J. C.: Androgens and erythropoiesis. I. Preliminary clinical observations. Arch. Intern. Med. 107:846, 1961.
25. Brodsky, I., Dennis, L. H., DeCastro, N. A., Brady, L. W. and Kahn, S. B.: Effect of testosterone enanthate and alkylating agents on multiple myeloma. J.A.M.A. 193:102, 1965.
26. Moller, P. F. and Gudjonsson, S. V.: Massive fluorosis of bone and ligaments. Acta Radiol. 13:269, 1932.
27. Cohen, P. and Gardner, F. H.: Induction of subacute skeletal fluorosis in a case of multiple myeloma. New Eng. J. Med. 271:1129, 1964.
28. Cohen, P., Nichols, G. L. and Banks, H. H.: Fluoride treatment of bone rarefaction in multiple myeloma and osteoporosis: A review. Clin. Orthop. 64:221, 1969.
29. Carbone, P. P., Zipkin, I., Sokoloff, L., Frazier, P., Cook, P. and Mullins, F.: Fluoride effect on bone in plasma cell myeloma. Arch. Intern. Med. 121:130, 1968.
30. Solomon, S. E., Somal, B. A., Hayes, D. M., Hosley, H., Miller, S. P. and Schilling, A.: Role of gamma globulin for immunoprophylaxis in multiple myeloma. New Eng. J. Med. 277:1336, 1967.
31. Solomon, A., Waldmann, T. A. and Fahey, J. L.: Metabolism of normal 6.6 S γ globulin in normal subjects and patients with macroglobulinemia and multiple myeloma. J. Lab. Clin. Med. 62:1, 1963.
32. Fahey, J. L., Barth, W. F. and Solomon, A.: Serum hyperviscosity syndrome. J.A.M.A. 192:120, 1965.
33. Mackenzie, M. R., Brown, E., Fudenberg, H. H. and Goodenday, L.: Waldenström's macroglobulinemia correlation between expanded plasma volume and increased serum viscosity. Blood 35:304, 1970.
34. Mackenzie, M. R., Fudenberg, H. H. and O'Reilly, R. A.: The hyperviscosity syndrome. I. In IgG myeloma. The role of protein concentration and shape. J. Clin. Invest. 49:15, 1970.
35. Smith, E., Kochwa, S. and Wassermann, L. R.: Aggregation of IgG globulin *in vivo*. I. The hyperviscosity syndrome in multiple myeloma. Amer. J. Med. 39:35, 1965.
36. Kopp, W. L., Bierne, G. J. and Burns, R. O.: Hyperviscosity syndrome in multiple myeloma. Amer. J. Med. 43:141, 1967.
37. Morgan, C. and Hammack, W. J.: Intravenous urography in multiple myeloma. New Eng. J. Med. 275:77, 1966.
38. Bryan, C. W. and Healy, J. K.: Acute renal failure in multiple myeloma. Amer. J. Med. 44:128, 1968.
39. Levi, D. F., Williams, R. C. and Lindstrom, F. D.: Immunofluorescent studies of the myeloma kidney with special reference to light chain disease. Amer. J. Med. 44:922, 1968.

Waldenström's Macroglobulinemia

By H. Hugh Fudenberg, M.D.

Waldenström's macroglobulinemia (WM) is a disease of unknown etiology, which clinically often mimics lymphoma and, in the laboratory, sometimes mimics multiple myeloma (MM). In WM, the immunocytes produce large quantities of monoclonal IgM (monoclonal: only one light chain type, κ or λ, never both on one protein). These proteins are of high molecular weight, i.e., 17 to 20 S (Svedberg) units, or about 800,000 to a million.[1] They are carbohydrate-rich (about 10 per cent of their total weight is carbohydrate). In normal serum, γ-macroglobulins represent only 0.1 gm % of the total protein.[2] The normal macroglobulin molecules are antibodies. They arise early in the normal immune response and contain, among other antibodies, the isoglutinins to the ABO blood groups, the cold agglutinins, etc.[3] WM is occasionally associated with a protein of tremendous titer of antibody activity, e.g., sera with cold agglutinin titers of a million represent sufficient macroglobulin to give the typical clinical and laboratory findings of WM.[4] Also, some patients with extremely high titers of rheumatoid factor, another 19 S antibody, have the clinical features of WM.

Patients with WM usually present complaints of fatigue, weakness, and weight loss, but other symptoms and signs differentiate these patients from those with multiple myeloma (Table 1). The statistics presented are on 48 patients studied during a 10-year period.[5] Forty per cent of the patients entered complaining of skin or mucous membrane bleeding, sometimes recurrent, or severe epistaxis, or both. Twenty-five per cent had various neurologic complaints, especially vertigo, and sometimes peripheral neuropathy. Ataxia may occur but is rare. Occasionally, there is a sudden

Table 1.—*Differential Diagnosis of Macroglobulinemia and Multiple Myeloma on Clinical Grounds in 48 Patients*

Clinical picture	*Macroglobulinemia*	*Multiple myeloma*
Recurrent infections	−	+
Bone pain	−	+
Mucous membrane bleeding	+	−
Hepatomegaly	+	−
Lymphadenopathy	+	−
Neuropathy	+	−
Sausage veins	+	−
Leukopenia	−	+
Thrombocytopenia	−	+
Hypercalcemia	−	+
Excretion of Bence Jones protein	−	+
Renal insufficiency	−	+
Lytic bone lesions	−	+
Hyperviscous serum	+	−

From the Section of Hematology and Immunology, Department of Medicine, University of California School of Medicine, San Francisco, California.

Supported by grants from the American Cancer Society (ET-13E) and Travenol Laboratories, Morton Grove, Illinois.

loss of consciousness. Less commonly, inguinal, axillary, or cervical lymphadenopathy leads the patient to consult a physician. Bone pain is almost never present.

Ecchymoses or purpura were among the predominant physical findings, as might be expected. In about 35 to 40 per cent of the patients, signs of hyperviscosity were present, as reflected in dilatation of the retinal veins on funduscopic examination. Hepatomegaly was present in about 60 per cent of the patients with WM, splenomegaly in about 35 per cent, and lymphadenopathy in about 45 per cent. Hence, upon encountering a patient with these findings, the first suspicion to enter the physician's mind is that this might be lymphoma.

The hemogram, however, is helpful. White cell counts and platelet counts are almost always normal, at least initially. There is usually a low hematocrit, and the cells are usually normocytic, normochromic. If there had been much blood loss, the red cells may be hypochromic. The "anemia" is more apparent than real because of greatly expanded plasma volume. The sedimentation rate is strikingly increased. Proteinuria is common, but only 10 per cent or less of the patients have Bence Jones protein. One sometimes sees a patient with macroglobulinemia who is referred from a thyroid clinic where the diagnosis of hypothyroidism has been made because of the patient's weakness. Some of these patients have a low serum protein-bound iodine or butanol-extractable iodine, or both, which would be compatible with the diagnosis of thyroid disease. These findings are due to the reduction in quantity of thyroxine-binding globulins which are synthesized. However, the serum cholesterol in WM is always less than 150 mg %, and in 50 per cent of the patients, it is less than 100 mg %. Although the total serum proteins range anywhere from 8 to 16, or 18 gm %, rarely do patients have total protein levels within the normal range. On serum electrophoresis, a characteristic narrow-based "spike" is present in the beta to gamma globulin region (Fig. 1). The presence of that spike does not differentiate myeloma

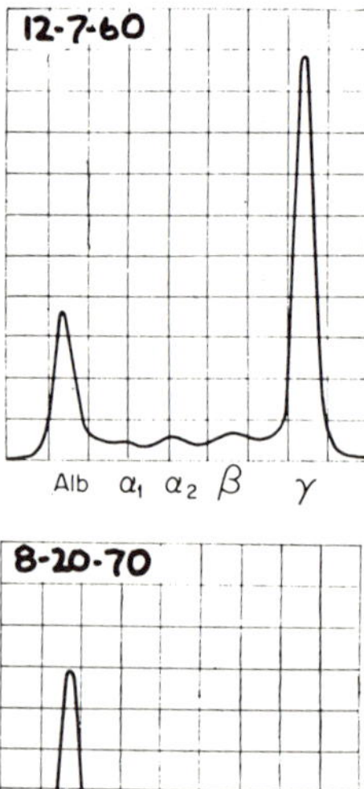

FIG. 1.—(Top) Electrophoretic pattern of WM serum before therapy. (Bottom) Electrophoretic pattern of the same patient after 10 years of plasmapheresis therapy.

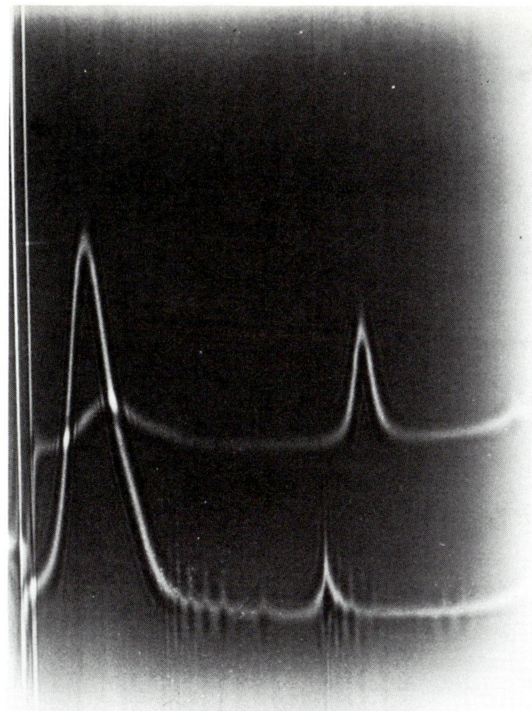

FIG. 2A.—Ultracentrifuge (UCF) patterns: (Top) WM serum diluted 1:20; 19S spike is to the left. (Bottom) Normal human serum diluted 1:5. Note decreased 7S protein in the WM serum and marked increase of 7S protein compared to 18S protein in the normal serum.

from macroglobulinemia. The mobility of the spike varies from one patient to another, but with time, whether the patient is treated or untreated, the mobility remains the same for the duration of the disease. In the untreated patient, usually the concentration of protein gradually rises.

Differentiation between myeloma and macroglobulinemia is essential because the natural histories of these disorders are quite different and the therapies are quite different. The laboratory diagnosis demands a combination of methods. Analytical ultracentrifugation (UCF) combined with immunoelectrophoresis (IEP)[6] can almost always help the clinician to definitively distinguish between WM and MM. Figure 2 shows a UCF pattern of an isolated WM protein at 16 minutes and at 40 minutes. The amount of macroglobulin in the serum was 20 times that which appears in normal serum.

In IEP, an antiserum to whole normal human serum is placed in a trough and is allowed to diffuse toward electrophoretically separated serum proteins. Figure 3 shows characteristic arcs, including the IgG arc and the IgA and IgM bands; the patterns obtained vary with the antisera. Many commercial antisera give widely differing results, even from batch to batch from the same company. I recommend that the antisera be made in the research laboratory, if possible.

Figure 4b represents a γG myeloma, with mobility in the mid-γ range. Figure 4c shows a protein of faster mobility; the patient was admitted with what was thought to be WM, because he had symptoms of hyperviscosity. Some myelomas, the rare ones,

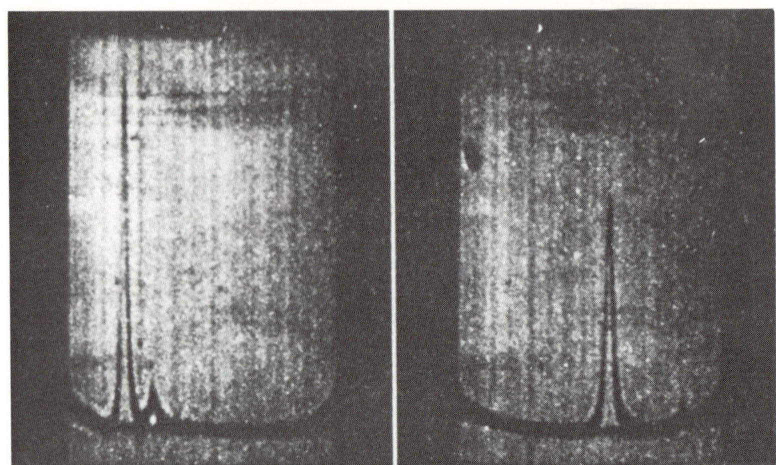

Fig. 2B.—Analytical ultracentrifuge pattern of a purified WM protein.

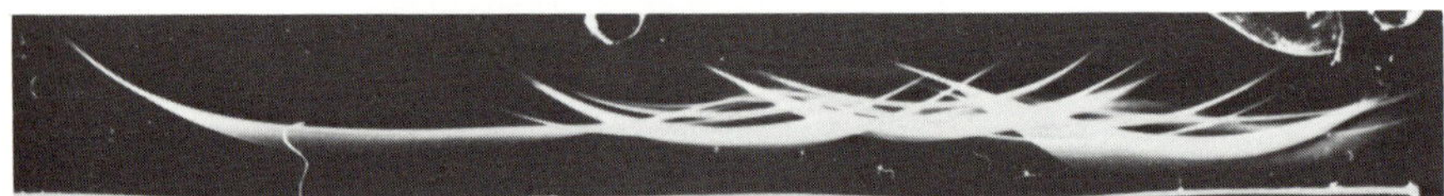

Fig. 3.—Normal serum in immunoelectrophoresis (IEP) versus antiserum to normal human serum.

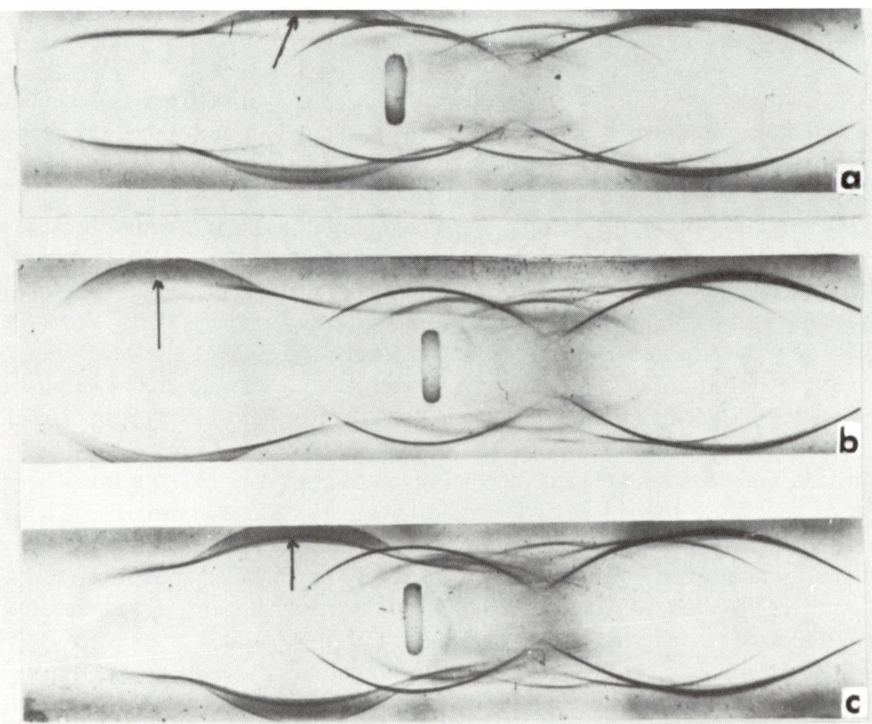

Fig. 4.—Record of immunoelectrophoresis of three myeloma serums. Arrows point to MM protein. (a) IgA: Note crossing of residual normal IgG over the IgA band. (b) IgG of mid-γ mobility. (c) IgG of fast γ mobility similar to mobility of IgA MM protein in (a).

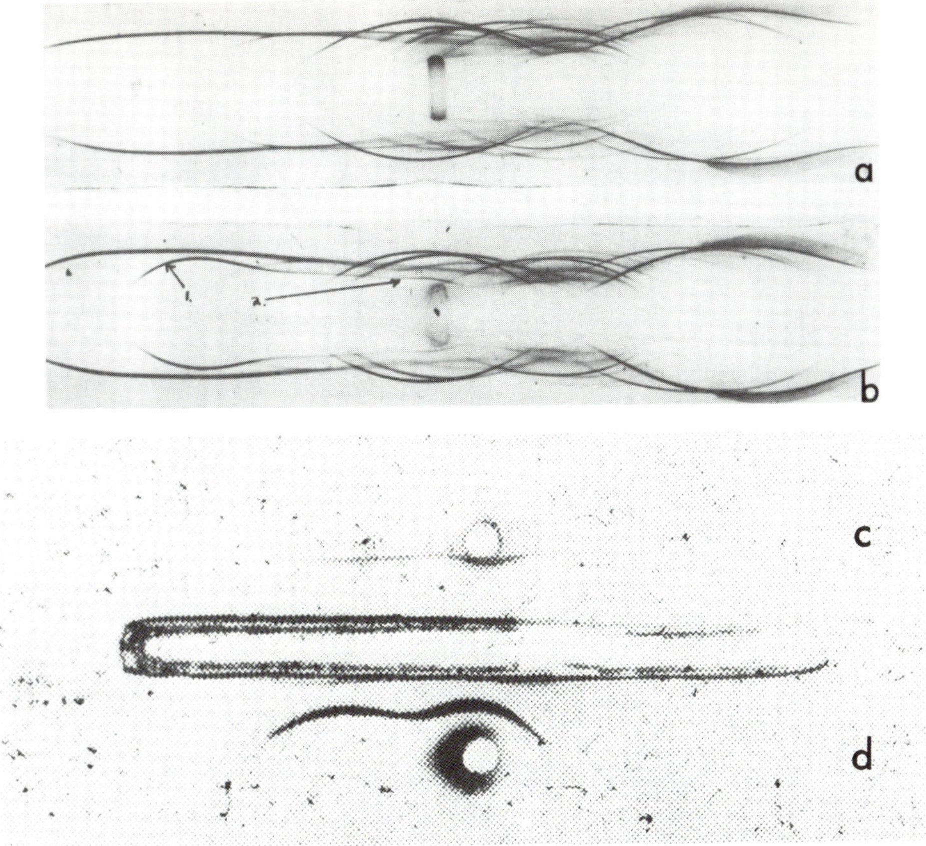

FIG. 5.—Immunoelectrophoresis using anti-normal human serum: (a) Normal human serum. Unfortunately, normal IgM band did not reproduce well. (b) WM serum. Arrow 1 points to pathologic WM; arrow 2 to residual normal IgM. Immunoelectrophoresis with antiserum to IgM: (c) Normal serum. (d) WM serum.

show hyperviscosity.[7] Figure 4a illustrates an IgA myeloma as shown by immunoelectrophoresis. Clinically, it does not resemble WM. (Note the residual normal IgG band in the IEP.)

Figure 5a shows the faint IgM of a normal serum. In contrast, Figure 5b shows the IgM of a patient with WM. (Note the residual IgG and also the marked increase in the IgM band.) Figure 5, c and d, shows the IEP when IgM antiserum, rather than normal antiserum, is used. When this particular IgM was run with anti-κ sera and anti-λ sera, it gave a line only with anti-κ. Normal macroglobulin gives lines with both anti-κ and anti-λ, but each WM protein, like each MM protein, has only one light chain type. There are pitfalls in IEP because some of the macroglobulins will precipitate out in solutions of about 0.05 ionic strength, which is the usual ionic strength used in IEP; if this occurs, an IgM arc is not seen. In the absence of an IgM precipitating arc, the clinical laboratory is likely to miss a macroglobulin protein because of its property of precipitating out in low ionic strength media. (Many laboratories still use the Sia test* as a screening test. A positive result is highly suggestive. A negative result is not particularly helpful.)

* This screening test is based on the insolubility of macroglobulins in distilled water; about 85 per cent are insoluble at this low ionic strength.

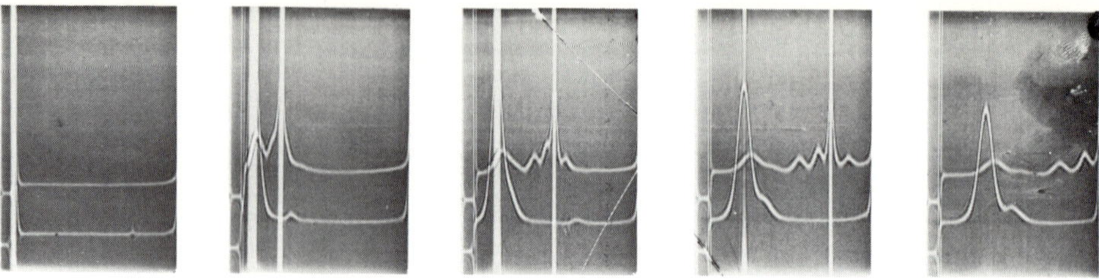

FIG. 6.—IgA polymer in analytical ultracentrifuge at 16-minute intervals. (Above) IgA MM polymer (serum diluted 1:10). (Below) Normal serum run simultaneously (diluted 1:5). Numerals alongside pictures represent time in minutes.

As stated earlier, most symptoms of macroglobulinemia are due to marked hyperviscosity. Any patient with the hyperviscosity syndrome merits study of his serum with both IEP and the analytical UCF. Sometimes the proteins responsible for these symptoms are polymers of IgA (Fig. 6). The size of these proteins can be anywhere from 7 S, 9 S, 11 S, up to 18 S. IgG myelomas only rarely produce the hyperviscosity syndrome.

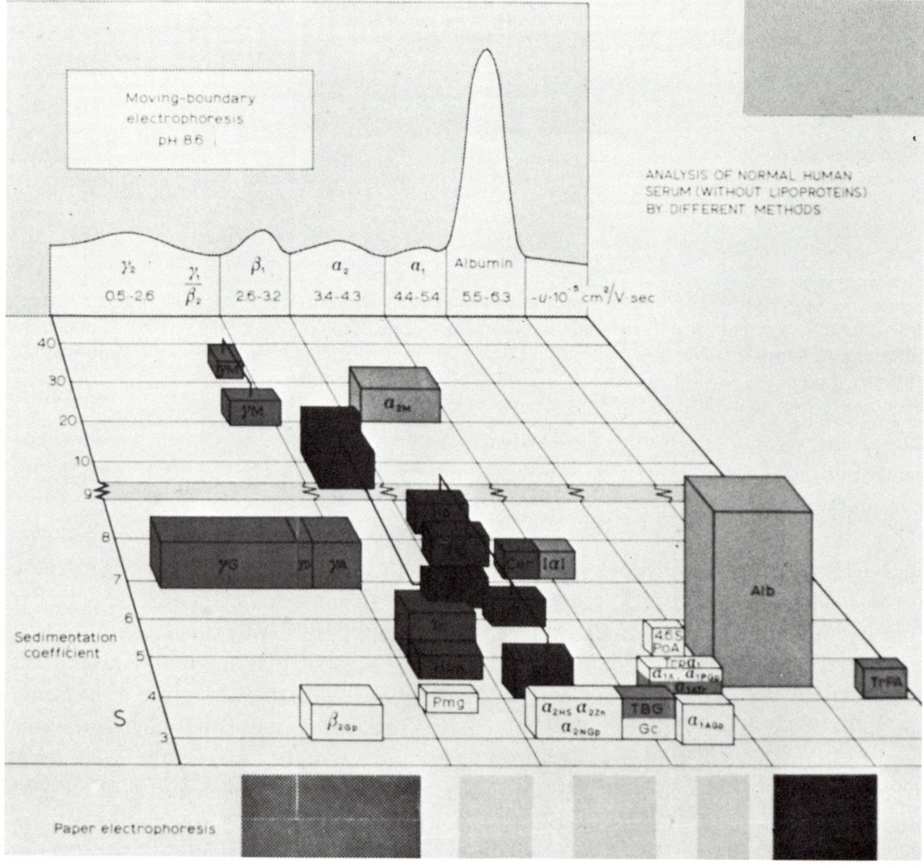

FIG. 7.—Three-dimensional plate of the plasma protein. From Schultze, H. E. and Heremans, J. F.: Molecular Biology of Human Proteins. Vol. 1, Nature and Metabolism of Extracellular Proteins. New York: Elsevier, 1966. With permission.

Indeed, several years ago we described a patient who had an 18 S spike and the hyperviscosity syndrome. It was thought initially that he had macroglobulinemia, but the 18 S protein, when isolated, turned out to be IgA; hence, the patient had myeloma, not macroglobulinemia.[8,9]

Again it should be emphasized that the natural histories and treatment of WM and MM are different. A few of the patients with hyperviscosity syndrome and myeloma of the IgG type have been reported; these are usually IgG aggregates. However, we have seen several patients who were initially thought to have had macroglobulinemia, because they came in with bleeding and distortion of the retinal veins, with enlarged liver and spleen. They actually had IgG hyperviscous myelomas, but the IgG was 7 S, not aggregated. To reiterate, most IgG myelomas associated with the hyperviscosity syndrome are polymers, i.e., 9, 11, or 13 S[10]; these are rare, but even rarer (and they do exist) are the 7 S hyperviscous myelomas.[11] Consequently, both IgG and IgA myelomas must be entertained under differential diagnosis of hyperviscosity syndrome.

It should be pointed out that finding an increased 17 to 20 S protein in the UCF does not establish a diagnosis of WM. Figure 7, a three-dimensional chart of the serum proteins, plots electrophoresis mobility on the x-axis, size on the y-axis, and concentration upward. The 18 to 20 S region contains two proteins, one IgM, the other α_2 globulin mobility. In normal serum, the IgM is about 100 mg %, and the α_2M, of the same molecular weight, is about 200 mg %. The α_2M can rise markedly in many chronic diseases[12]; indeed, cases of "macroglobulinemia" in 9-year-old children have been published, diagnosed solely on the basis of large amounts of 18 to 20 S protein seen in the UCF. Careful analysis shows that these patients always had chronic infections. Undoubtedly, they had an increase in α_2M, which showed up as increased 18 to 20 S material in the UCF; if so, these were not WM cases.

When one finds increased 18 to 20 S protein in the UCF, one good way to differentiate between the α_2M and IgM is through the technique of starch or acrylamide

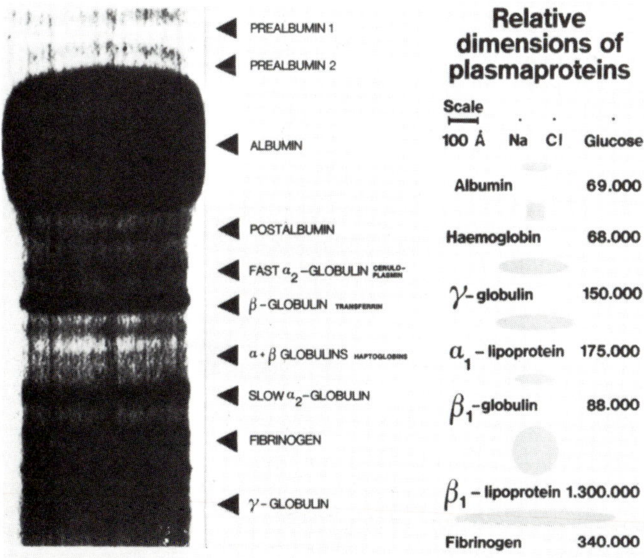

FIG. 8A.—Starch gel electrophoresis of normal serum.

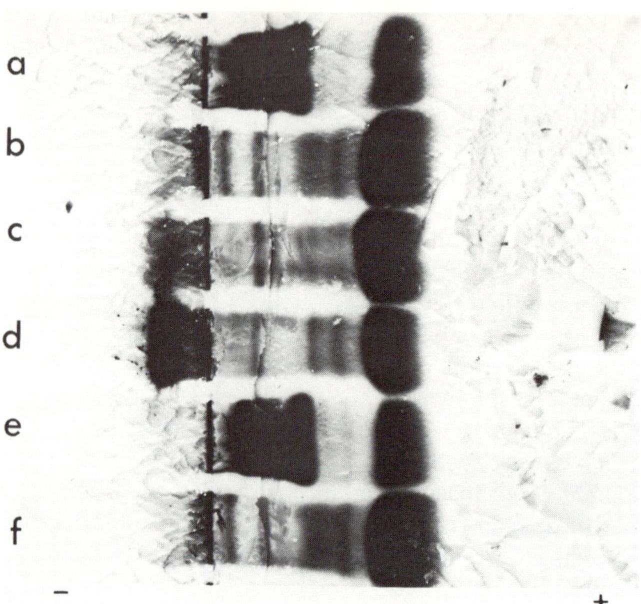

FIG. 8B.—Starch gel electrophoresis of sera containing the following: a = monoclonal IgA (both monomer and polymer form); b = monoclonal IgM; c = normal human serum; d = monoclonal IgG; e = monoclonal IgA (both monomer and polymer form); f = monoclonal IgM. Note that the IgM does not enter the gel but remains at the origin; also, the serum containing both monomer and polymer IgA gives at least two bands.

gel electrophoresis (Fig. 8); this technique separates proteins, not only on the basis of net electric charge, but also on the basis of size and shape. The α_2M molecule is oval. It enters the gel; it travels more slowly than most β-globulins, but it does enter the gel. The IgM molecule has a very peculiar configuration. It is somewhat like a spider,[13] or a ring with five arms sticking out, and it hangs up at the origin of the gel, and does not enter the gel. Thus, in a patient with WM, one finds a very sharp band right at the protein insertion slot. This is often a useful diagnostic technique. I think all three of these methods may be necessary when one has a patient in whom the diagnosis of WM is suspected. At least two must be done.*

It should be emphasized that many hematologists feel that they can always make the differential diagnosis between WM and MM by morphology. Plasma cells are characteristic in myeloma; cells intermediate between lymphocytes and plasma cells, called "lymphocytic plasmacytes" or "plasmacytic lymphocytes," are characteristic of WM.[14] It is true that most of the time the differential diagnosis can be made by morphologic study, but occasionally one sees a patient with WM with a marrow that looks like what most of us would call classical myeloma, e.g., Figure 9. One helpful morphologic indication is that the marrow from these patients often contains tissue mast cells; these are not seen in myeloma. In any event, morphology alone cannot be relied upon for differential diagnosis.[11]

As stated earlier, the cause of the symptoms in WM is the hyperviscosity. In a particular patient with myeloma, or a series of patients, the relative viscosity of the

* Rare cases of IgM monomer, differing clinically from WM,[15] have been described. Hence, UCF is mandatory.

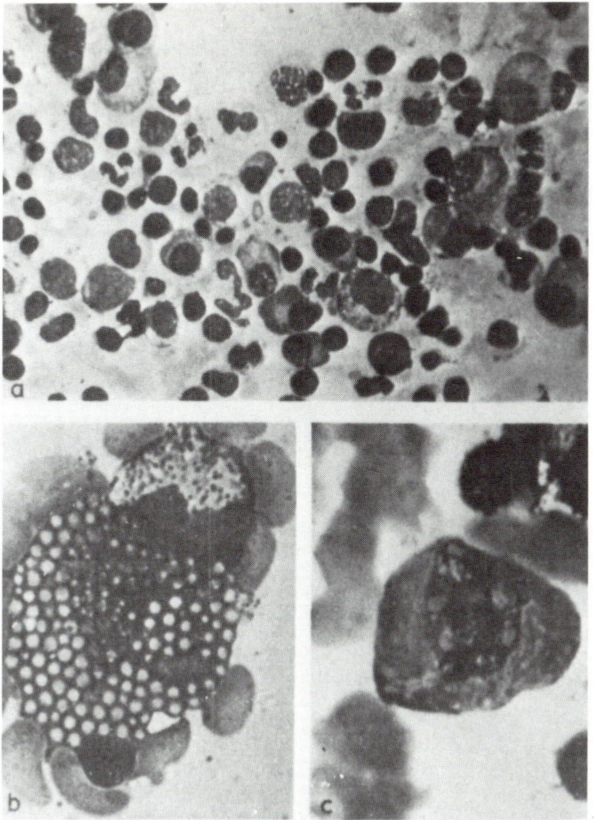

FIG. 9.—Bone marrow resembling myeloma from patient with WM.

serum changes very little as the IgG concentration rises. (Normal viscosity is 1.4 to 1.8. It is measured in an Ostwald viscometer.) However, with macroglobulinemia, after the paraprotein level reaches about 3 or 4 gm %, the viscosity starts climbing markedly. (Our arbitrary criterion for making the diagnosis of WM is a concentration of 1 gm %; increased viscosity is seen at about 2 gm %.) Normal serum takes about 1.4 to 1.8 times as long as water to traverse the Ostwald viscometer. With the ordinary myeloma, the relative viscosity is rarely above 3. With macroglobulinemia, it is anywhere from 4 to 20. Most patients remain symptomatic until the viscosity is above 6, but a particular patient will have symptoms at one given point, whether it is 4, 6, or 12. One can find that point and control the symptoms by maintaining the macroglobulin concentration and plasma volume at the given point, below which the viscosity does not cause symptoms. The plasma volume of most patients with WM is tremendously expanded when the relative serum viscosity is greater than 4,[16] being anywhere from 100 to 160 per cent greater than normal. In large part, this accounts for the spuriously low hematocrit, for the weakness, and probably for a number of other poorly understood symptoms. Further, plasmapheresis often reverses coagulation abnormalities.[17]

Our therapy for this disorder is based on the fact that WM occurs mainly in people 60 to 65 years of age. In patients studied in countries other than the United States, before the introduction of chemotherapeutic agents in 1957, the average life span after the onset was 40 months.[18] Most hematologists in the United States treat WM with chlorambucil or other cytotoxic agents. Our procedure is as follows: We bring the patients in to the hospital and perform plasmapheresis vigorously, i.e., 2 units a day for 5 to 7 days. Sometimes it takes 2 weeks. In most cases, this brings the viscosity down below the symptom threshold and reduces plasma volume to near-normal. It also often reverses coagulation abnormalities.[17] We then maintain the patients by plasmapheresis, once weekly on an outpatient basis, monitoring them by viscosity. If plasmapheresis becomes too time-consuming, we treat the patients with very small doses of chlorambucil. Usually, 2 mg per day is sufficient.

Currently, in our series of 48 patients, the average span of survival of those who have not already succumbed to complicating causes (i.e., coronary artery disease or malignant disease) is 5 years, and many are still alive (average age at the onset is 60 to 65 years). Two patients whom I have been treating since 1960, one by plasmapheresis alone and the other by plasmapheresis and 2 mg per day of chlorambucil thereafter, are now 80 years old, and both are doing well (see Fig. 1).

Immunosuppressive drugs used in renal transplantation have resulted in a high rate of malignant transformation[19]; so that with these agents, one runs the risk of converting a relatively "benign" disease in a person 65 to 70 years of age into something more malignant. Furthermore, macroglobulinemia is sometimes associated initially with lymphoma, although it may develop later. On rare occasions, protein production starts tapering off, and the patient winds up with reticulum cell sarcoma. It is, therefore, wise to avoid therapeutic agents that carry the possibility of inducing lymphoreticular malignancy[19] in patients already predisposed. I again emphasize that these patients have a much better prognosis than those with myeloma, at least in our hands. Consequently, we feel that chemotherapy should be given judiciously, if at all. Further, with conventional doses of chlorambucil or similar agents, aplastic anemia is likely to develop in many of these patients.[11] The aplasia in these patients lasted far longer than it did in others in whom aplastic anemia developed in association with the same drug, e.g., patients with lymphoma.[11] In WM, aplasia induced by chlorambucil may last up to 2 years.

Studies of these proteins and other monoclonal proteins have added immeasurably to our knowledge in many areas, i.e., immunochemistry, genetics, etc. Using these proteins, we have shown that 2 genes make 1 polypeptide chain,[20,21] in contrast to the "1 gene, 1 polypeptide chain" dogma stated in all textbooks.

Recommendation

WM is a disease of unknown origin, presumably due to an immunologic aberration, perhaps genetically determined. It arises mainly in elderly people, and the prognosis is generally favorable if it is managed cautiously. I urge the "ultra-dove" approach in its treatment.

References

1. Waldenström, J.: Incipient myelomatosis or "essential" hyperglobulinemia with fibrinogenopenia . . . a new syndrome? Acta Med. Scand. 117:216, 1944.
2. Stiehm, E. R. and Fudenberg, H. H.: Serum levels of immune globulins in health and disease: A survey. Pediatrics 37:715, 1966.
3. Fudenberg, H. H., Kunkel, H. G. and Franklin, E. C.: High molecular weight antibodies. Proc. 7th Cong. Int. Soc. Blood Trans., 1958, Rome, 1959, pp. 522–527.
4. Fudenberg, H. H. and Kunkel, H. G.: Physical properties of the red cell agglutinins in acquired hemolytic anemia. J. Exp. Med. 106:689, 1957.

5. MacKenzie, M. R. and Fudenberg, H. H.: Macroglobulinemia: An analysis of forty-eight cases. (In preparation.)
6. Heremans, J.: Les globulines sériques du système gamma. Paris: Masson, 1960.
7. MacKenzie, M. R., Fudenberg, H. H. and O'Reilly, R. A.: The hyperviscosity syndrome. I. In IgG myeloma, the role of protein concentration and molecular shape. J. Clin. Invest. 49:15, 1970.
8. Vaerman, J.-P., Johnson, L. B., Mandy, W. and Fudenberg, H. H.: Multiple myeloma with two paraprotein peaks: An instructive case. J. Lab. Clin. Med. 65:18, 1965.
9. Vaerman, J.-P., Fudenberg, H. H., Vaerman, C. and Mandy, W. J.: On the significance of the heterogeneity in molecular size of human serum γA-globulins. Immunochemistry 2:263, 1965.
10. Smith, E. G., Kochwa, S. and Wasserman, L. R.: Aggregation of IgG globulins *in vitro*. I. The hyperviscosity syndrome in multiple myeloma. Amer. J. Med. 39:35, 1958.
11. Fudenberg, H. H.: Unpublished observations.
12. Schultze, H. E. and Heremans, J. F.: Molecular Biology of the Serum Protein. Amsterdam: Elsevier, 1966.
13. Chesebro, B., Bloth, B. and Svehag, S. E.: The ultrastructure of normal and pathological IgM immunoglobulins. J. Exp. Med. 127:399, 1968.
14. Dutcher, T. F. and Fahey, J. L.: The histopathology of the macroglobulinemia of Waldenström. J. Nat. Cancer Inst. 22:887, 1959.
15. Solomon, A. and Kunkel, H. G.: A monoclonal type low molecular weight protein related to IgM macroglobulin. Amer. J. Med. 42:958, 1967.
16. MacKenzie, M. R., Brown, E., Fudenberg, H. H. and Goodenday, L.: Waldenström's macroglobulinemia: Correlation between expanded plasma volume and increased serum viscosity. Blood 35:394, 1970.
17. Perkins, H. A., MacKenzie, M. R. and Fudenberg, H. H.: Hemostatic defects in dysproteinemias. Blood 35:695, 1970.
18. Kappeler, R., Krebs, A. and Riva, G.: Klinik der Makroglobulinämie Waldenström Beschreibung von 21 Fällen und Übersicht der Literatur. Helv. Med. Acta 25:54, 1958.
19. Penn, I.: Malignant Tumors in Organ Transplant Recipients. New York: Springer-Verlag, 1970.
20. Wang, A. C., Pink, J. R. L., Fudenberg, H. H. and Ohms, J.: A variable region subclass of heavy chains common to immunoglobulins G, A, and M and characterized by an unblocked amino-terminal residue. Proc. Nat. Acad. Sci. USA 66:657, 1970.
21. Levin, A. S., Fudenberg, H. H., Hopper, J. E., Wilson, S. K. and Nisonoff, A.: Immunofluorescent evidence for control of synthesis of variable regions of light and heavy chains of IgG and IgM by the same gene. Proc. Nat. Acad. Sci. USA 68:169, 1971.

Radiation Therapy for Hodgkin's Disease

By LUTHER W. BRADY, M.D., DONALD S. FAUST, M.D., JOHN ANTONIADES, M.D., SRIPRAYOON PRASASVINICHAI, M.D. AND RICHARD J. TORPIE, M.D.

ALTHOUGH THE ORIGINAL DESCRIPTION of Hodgkin's disease by Thomas Hodgkin was made in 1832, the most important change in thinking about the disease has taken place within the last decade, when diverse interests converged to stimulate a more vigorous search for improvement in the treatment.[1,2] This has been brought about by the realization that frequently the disease can be, and has been, cured by the utilization of optimal radiation techniques. With the rapid evolution of ideas on the pathogenesis and primary treatment of Hodgkin's disease, it is difficult for the physician who sees only an occasional case to maintain a coherent view of the problems of management.[3]

The factors contributing to the main change in the attitudes toward treatment of Hodgkin's disease may be identified as follows:

(1) There have been optimistic reports of prolonged disease-free survivals in high percentages of patients treated aggressively with radiation techniques.

(2) At the beginning of this decade, megavoltage radiation therapy equipment such as the cobalt-60 teletherapy unit, the Van de Graaf generator, the linear accelerator, and the betatron became available for routine clinical application in more radiation therapy centers.

(3) The concentration on curative intent stimulated the need for a more precise definition of the extent of the disease, and the importance of lymphangiography as a vital contribution toward staging was apprecaited.

(4) There was an increasing awareness among internists, surgeons, and radiation therapists that a cooperative interdisciplinary approach to the management of patients with this disease might yield better results.

(5) There was growing disenchantment with retrospective studies as a prototype for clinical investigation. The concept of a well conceived prospective clinical trial was thought to be more productive in terms of information to be achieved.[4,5]

Fundamental to all attempts at curative treatment of Hodgkin's disease is the assumption that in a significant fraction of cases the process is localized at the time of diagnosis. Many reports now support this concept, more than 50 per cent of patients with localized disease surviving for 5 years or longer when treated by radiation techniques.[6-13] Peters' data[14-17] indicate that a substantial percentage alive at 5 years remained well 10, 15, and 20 years after radiation therapy. Easson[18] has shown that after the tenth year, the survival of irradiated patients with localized Hodgkin's disease approaches that of the normal population. Further support of the fundamental concept has been presented by Rosenberg and Kaplan,[19,20] who have demonstrated that new areas of involvement after radiation therapy of the localized

---

From the Department of Radiation Therapy and Nuclear Medicine, Hahnemann Medical College and Hospital, Philadelphia, Pennsylvania.

Supported by The Alexander and Margaret Stewart Trust; the Alperin Foundation; the Friends of the Radiation Therapy Center of the Hahnemann Medical College and Hospital; and by PHS Training Grants Nos. T01-CA05185-05 and T12-CA08024-05 from the National Cancer Institute.

form of Hodgkin's disease are immediately adjacent to the treated areas in more than 80 per cent of patients. This supports the fundamental premise that the spread is contiguous and predictable.

Even though the controversy as to the prognosis of Hodgkin's disease continues, there is little justification for such a pessimistic outlook. Considerable credit for the change in this point of view is due to three major developments leading to better diagnosis, definition and treatment. They are (1) Lower-extremity lymphangiography using radiopaque contrast medium; (2) megavoltage therapy for deep-seated lesions; and (3) renewed attack on the histopathology of the disease based on the Lukes system of classification.[21–25]

The goals of radiation therapy programs for the management of Hodgkin's disease should be directed toward the determination of whether intensive irradiation of lymph node regions immediately adjacent to those of proved involvement with Hodgkin's disease would increase the duration of remission or survival, the determination whether potentially curable doses of radiation given to all lymph node regions in patients with generalized disease might be more effective in increasing the duration of remission or survival than the repeated palliative doses given to regions of clinical involvement only, the accumulation of additional information on the natural history of Hodgkin's disease, and the evaluation of tolerance to irradiation in patients treated with extended fields in high doses.

It is obvious that the prognosis of Hodgkin's disease is influenced basically by histopathology, the clinical stage, and the presence or absence of systemic symptoms. The clinician must address himself to an analysis of each of these factors before the proper therapeutic measures are instituted.

Evaluation and Staging

The optimal treatment program for patients with Hodgkin's disease must be decided after determining the full extent of the disease, the histopathologic type, and the stage of disease of the patient.[26] To effectively stage a patient with newly diagnosed Hodgkin's disease, the following studies are pursued:

(1) The histopathologic interpretation by an experienced pathologist must be made. The classification is one of the most difficult problems in pathology (Table 1). In the past the disease was generally classified into three categories according to Jackson and Parker,[27] namely, Hodgkin's paragranuloma, Hodgkin's granuloma, and Hodgkin's sarcoma. Recently Lukes and other[21–25] have modified this pathologic description with an ability to correlate prognosis with pathology. The pathologic classification suggested by Lukes was lymphocytic predominance, which occurs in about 10 to 15 per cent of the cases, nodular sclerosis in 20 to 25 per cent, mixed cellularity in 20 to 40 per cent, and lymphocytic depletion, which comprises several histologic expressions of Hodgkin's disease that have in common lymphocytic depletion occurring in about 5 to 15 per cent of the cases.

(2) A careful clinical history with special attention to the characteristic symptoms of Hodgkin's disease must be obtained. The symptoms generally indicating more serious prognostic disease and indicative of systemic response are fever, night sweats, pruritus, and weight loss greater than 10 per cent of the normal body weight. Symptoms that are not necessarily thought to indicate systemic disease and not necessarily indicating Stage B are malaise, weakness, fatigue, anemia, leukocytosis, elevated sedimentation rate, cutaneous anergy, and pain associated with alcohol ingestion.

TABLE 1.—*Histopathologic Classification of Hodgkin's Disease*

Jackson and Parker[27]	*Rye, 1965*[2]	*Distinctive features*	*Relative frequency (%)*
Paragranuloma	Lymphocyte predominance	Abundant stroma of mature lymphocytes and/or histiocytes; no necrosis; Reed-Sternberg cells may be sparse.	10–15
	Nodular sclerosis	Nodules of lymphoid tissue, partially or completely separated by bands of doubly refractile collagen of variable width; atypical Reed-Sternberg cells in clear spaces ("lacunae") in the lymphoid nodules.	20–50
Granuloma	Mixed cellularity	Usually numerous Reed-Sternberg and atypical mononuclear cells with a pleomorphic admixture of plasma cells, eosinophils, lymphocytes, and fibroblasts; foci of necrosis commonly seen.	20–40
Sarcoma	Lymphocyte depletion	Reed-Sternberg and malignant mononuclear cells usually, though not always, numerous; marked paucity of lymphocytes; diffuse fibrosis and necrosis may be present.	5–15

(3) A physical examination must be done with extreme care, recording and describing all palpable lymph nodes in the cervical, supraclavicular, infraclavicular, axillary, brachial, epitrochlear, iliac, inguinal, femoral, and popliteal areas. Not all palpable lymphadenopathy in a patient with Hodgkin's disease is necessarily pathologic. Waldeyer's ring must be carefully examined, and abdominal examination must be directed toward identifying hepatic or splenic enlargement or abdominal masses.

(4) Radiologic studies of the chest should include tomography of the mediastinum and hila. To detect disease in the retroperitoneal space, lower extremity lymphangiography is indispensable.[28] The lymphogram has an accuracy of approximately 85 per cent, but there are 3 to 4 per cent false positives.[29]

False positive lymphograms may result from errors in interpretation, benign disease simulating lymphoma, or surgical removal of uninvolved nodes at the time of the abdominal exploration. False negative lymphograms may result from errors in interpretation, small unobservable defects in the nodes, or inadequate filling of the abdominal nodes by the contrast medium.

Since lymphangiography is a relatively benign procedure, its routine use is indicated in the initial evaluation of patients with Hodgkin's disease. It can be preceded by a gold-198 lymph scan as a screening procedure to choose those individuals for whom lymphangiography might be most valuable. At the present, lymphangiography is the most conclusive examination of the retroperitoneal area, which is not otherwise accessible to direct evaluation.[30]

Gallium-67 citrate for soft tissues and strontium-87 bone scans are also helpful in defining the extent of disease.

Palpable splenomegaly may cause error 40 per cent of the time in terms of involvement. The size of the spleen does not necessarily correlate with involvement. Occult disease in the abdomen is often confined to the spleen and splenic pedicle nodes.

Skeletal surveys are necessary for all patients with Hodgkin's disease or patients with pain that is suggestive of skeletal involvement. Barium studies of the stomach and bowel are indicated if organ involvement is suspected. An intravenous urogram is essential in all patients to establish that there are two kidneys and to identify any ureteral obstruction or displacement.

(5) Laboratory studies should include routine blood counts, liver function studies, and determinations of serum uric acid and renal function.

(6) It is important to search carefully for involvement of the bone marrow. The aspiration technique may demonstrate disease in some patients with Hodgkin's disease. Open biopsy or closed needle biopsy with the Westerman-Jensen needle or Stryker saw biopsy are more satisfactory techniques in evaluating bone marrow involvement. It is recommended that bone marrow biopsy be done on all patients with the diagnosis of Hodgkin's disease with at least one location and, in some instances, two different anatomical sites being tested.

(7) Frequently, liver biopsy may be necessary to attempt clarification of equivocal liver function tests. A normal result of needle biopsy of the liver, however, does not exclude involvement of the liver.

(8) Inferior vena cavography is extremely helpful in evaluating the nodes in the area of the cisterna chyli. This is a location not seen on intravenous urograms with any accuracy nor on lymphangiograms since nodes in this area are not generally filled by the contrast material.[31]

(9) The work-up on some patients will leave unanswered questions relative to the extent of the disease. Therefore, in these selected individuals exploratory laparotomy is a more satisfactory method for documenting the extent of involvement in the abdomen. It offers the opportunity to do biopsies of the retroperitoneal nodes, direct biopsies of the liver, and splenectomy for determining the presence or absence of splenic disease.[32]

TABLE 2.—*Clinical Staging in Hodgkin's Disease. Proposed Classification by Stanford University Medical Center, 1970*[11]

Stage I—Involvement of a single lymph node region (I) or of a single extralymphatic organ or site (I_{-E}).

Stage II—Involvement of two or more lymph node regions on the same side of the diaphragm (II) or solitary involvement of an extralymphatic organ or site and of one or more lymph node regions on the same side of the diaphragm (II_{-E}).

Stage III—Involvement of lymph node regions on both sides of the diaphragm (III), which may also be accompanied by involvement of the spleen (III_{-S}) or by solitary involvement of an extralymphatic organ or site (III_{-E}) or both (III_{-SE}).

Stage IV—Multiple or disseminated foci of involvement of one or more extralymphatic organs or tissue, with or without associated lymph node involvement.

In Hodgkin's disease denote also the absence (A) or presence (B) of systemic symptoms.

Comment: This proposed classification attempts to combine the best features of the Rye classification[2] and those of Peters et al., 1968, and Musshoff and Boutis, 1968[34]. It is intended for use not only in Hodgkin's disease but also in the non-Hodgkin's group of lymphomas.

(10) Studies on delayed hypersensitivity may offer information to predict response to treatment.[33]

When the diagnostic evaluation of the patient has been completed, the clinical classification can be made according to the international staging classification for Hodgkin's disease. The stages are based on the anatomic extent of the disease and are subclassified "A" or "B" depending on the absence or presence of systemic symptoms. The initial staging for Hodgkin's disease suggested by Peters[16] in 1950 has evolved into the present more practical staging (Table 2). Clinical staging has become more accurate when a complete, thorough diagnostic evaluation of the patient is carried out. Musshoff et al.,[34] Peters,[15] and Rosenberg and Kaplan[11] have suggested that Stage IV is often a dumping basket and therefore pointed out the need to separate the single extralymphatic lesions into separate groups.

Treatment

Once the patient has been categorized with respect to histopathology, clinical stage and symptomatology, a rational approach to therapy is possible. There are two separate but distinct goals in the management of Hodgkin's disease. The first is cure, a goal that can be achieved in a significant proportion of patients with the disorder. The concept of cure should be carried out within the framework of minimal complication from the treatment. The second goal in the management of Hodgkin's disease is the amelioration of symptoms which can be achieved with regularity but unfortunately may not be accompanied by significant prolongation of life. If the two goals are confused, the maximal therapeutic possibilities will not be realized. In localized Hodgkin's disease (Stage I and II) treatment should be directed toward cure, whereas in Stage IV, cure is usually impossible because the involved organs will not tolerate curative amounts of radiation. Stage III forms an intermediate group in which the possibility for cure has been neither proved nor ruled out.

Surgery

Radical dissection of lymph node disease has been used for localized Hodgkin's disease. The surgical procedure, however, is often followed by full courses of radiation therapy. In general, surgery is best restricted to diagnostic biopsy and to resection of certain rare lymphomas arising outside the lymphoid organs. Extensive surgical resection is not recommended for the treatment of Stage I Hodgkin's disease.[35]

Definitive Radiation Therapy

For localized Hodgkin's disease, radiation therapy with intent to cure is the treatment of choice. The possibility for cure of Hodgkin's disease with radiation techniques is based on two principles:

(1) If the tumor dose of radiation is raised to 4000 rads in 4 to 5 weeks, the local recurrence rate at the same site thus treated is less than 5 per cent; i.e., 95 per cent of the time an area of Hodgkin's disease can be sterilized with a high or radical dose of radiation.[9]

(2) Hodgkin's disease is unicentric in origin and tends to spread regionally first and to contiguous areas later. Therefore, the concept evolved in treatment of localized Hodgkin's disease is directed toward treatment not only of the primary known sites of disease but also contiguous, or apparently uninvolved, areas. This radical or extended field approach has proved rational and effective when applied in Stage I

and Stage II disease. The superiority of this technique over the palliative approach in this group of patients is absolutely beyond question.[36] Analysis of the data[6-13] indicates that control and possible cure at 5 years comprise 90 per cent of Stages IA and IIA. Similar, though slightly less impressive, results (75 per cent with no evidence of disease at 5 years) have been obtained in Stages IB and IIB, but the numbers of patients are few and the follow-up brief.

For Stage I and II Hodgkin's disease, radiation therapy can be effectively administered only with megavoltage equipment, and even some megavoltage units such as small cobalt units will not permit fields of sufficient size to ensure homogeneous distribution of the radiation dosage. Optimal therapy requires 3500 to 4000 rads over a period of 3.5 to 5 weeks. When the primary process is in the neck or axilla, there is little argument about treating the apparently uninvolved mediastinum, where detection of the early disease is difficult. In practice, a mantle port, including both cervical and axillary regions and the mediastinum treated in continuity, is the suitable treatment field for Hodgkin's disease localized above the diaphragm. The upper abdomen may be added as a treatment field if the hilar lymph nodes are involved.

For localized presentations in the groin, treatment should include at least a bilateral pelvic field and a periaortic field to the level of the diaphragm. In the latter situation, irradiation of the mediastinum may also be advisable when high periaortic nodes are diseased.

Waldeyer's ring should be treated when there is disease in the upper half of the neck. The value of this program in the management of Stage I and II Hodgkin's disease has been demonstrated by Peters,[14] Rosenberg and Kaplan,[11,37] Easson,[18] Smithers,[20] and others.[7-10,12,13]

There is no doubt that this form of treatment in Stage I and II Hodgkin's disease is a sophisticated and difficult undertaking. It requires not only adequate radiation therapy equipment but a radiation therapist with interest in the disorder, able to deal with the technically demanding problems of treatment and experience in the utilization of large treatment fields and high radiation dosage employed to treat the disease.

The proper treatment of Stage III Hodgkin's disease remains an open question. Information elicited from more cases treated aggressively with radiation techniques will be needed before it becomes clear that the extensive radiation therapy required in such disseminated cases is justified. Without such data at present, an attempt is being made in most radiation therapy centers to extend definitive radiation therapy to as many Stage III cases as possible including in particular, patients whose disease would have been classified as Stage I or II but for the finding of retroperitoneal lymph nodes on lymphangiography or patients who are found to have positive lymph node involvement on abdominal exploration. These cases are different from those with more advanced positive disease obvious on lymphangiographic examination. In the management of Stage III Hodgkin's disease, the program for treatment is far more complex than that required in Stage I or Stage II disease. The tumor is more widely disseminated, the fields of treatment and volumes being irradiated greater, and the complications of treatment more common. The most important information relative to the management of Stage III disease has developed from the program being pursued at the Stanford University Medical Center,[11] with the following goals:

(1) To determine whether intensive irradiation of lymph node regions immediately

adjacent to those of proved involvement with Hodgkin's disease would increase the duration of remission or survival;

(2) To determine whether potentially curative doses of radiation given to all lymph node regions in patients with generalized disease might be more effective in increasing the duration of remission or survival than repeated palliative doses given to regions of clinical involvement only;

(3) To accumulate additional information on the natural history of Hodgkin's disease;

(4) To evaluate tolerance to irradiation in patients treated with extended fields and high doses.

The Stanford study probably represents the most carefully controlled investigation relative to the most effective means of treatment in Stage III being carried out in the world. The results are difficult to interpret at present but do seem to be generally superior to those in cases managed with chemotherapy.[38-42] Thus far, the group reports a remarkably high long-term survival rate of 60 per cent for patients in Stage III.[11] Such patients had all been deemed incurable prior to 1962, when such intensive radiation therapy to all lymphoid areas was first initiated at Stanford. This high-dose, extended-field radiation is in wide use now in many radiation therapy centers. The problems[43] encountered with this treatment program are related to complications of radiation pneumonitis, pericarditis with effusion, necrotizing gastrointestinal lesions, and bone marrow depression. Shielding of critical areas such as lungs, heart and kidneys is a necessary protective device to avoid these difficulties. In 700 patients radically irradiated, the incidence is between 6 and 10 per cent.[11]

Chemotherapy, either by itself or preceded by radiation therapy, is an alternative approach in the treatment of Stage III disease, but radiation therapy should not be withheld if the known areas of disease can be encompassed with reasonable treatment fields.[44,45]

In Stage IV Hodgkin's disease there is seldom hope of cure because of widespread involvement of radiosensitive normal tissues. In such cases chemotherapy is usually the primary method of management, and the goal is relief of symptoms. Occasionally the anatomic involvement of parenchymal tissue is limited enough to justify an aggressive radiotherapeutic approach even in Stage IV disease. Likewise, an expeditious way to palliate a localized symptomatic area of adenopathy in Stage IV disease is often with radiation therapy, and this approach is often used in Hodgkin's disease of lung parenchyma or of bone.

Palliative Radiation Therapy

The intelligent management of Hodgkin's disease requires more mature clinical judgment and experience than other more standardized therapeutic programs of treatment.[46] Taking this into account, there are specific indications for radiation therapy in the treatment of advanced Hodgkin's disease.

Mediastinal compression leading to actual or anticipated mediastinal embarrassment requires prompt radiation therapy and may be associated with reasonably long life expectancy with prompt and dramatic response to the radiation therapy.[36] The effect is of longer duration than that achieved with chemotherapy alone. Treatment by radiation techniques may be indicated in patients with otherwise generalized disease along with chemotherapy. Spinal cord compression due to meningeal involvement is considered a clinical emergency. We have insisted upon immediate decompression surgically, followed by radiation therapy to a generous portion of the spinal cord. In this situation relief of compression by surgical techniques obviates permanent cord damage and permits time to achieve the maximal response from radiation techniques. Other authors have successfully used radiation treatment without decompression in patients in whom the neurologic symptoms were of a few days' duration. Nodes resistant to chemotherapy may require local radiation therapy depending on the situation and taking into account the location of these nodes, the symptomatology produced and the observed lack of sufficient regression with chemotherapy.

Radio-resistant nodes may occur in late stages of Hodgkin's disease but should not be confused with clinically ineffective irradiation used in the past or because the involvement is too widespread or too extensive to be reached by any local procedure. New and previously untreated involved lymph nodes can be as responsive in later stages as other nodes have proved to be in earlier stages. Recurrent nodes in areas previously irradiated seldom arise within our experience since our techniques of high-dose local treatment usually prevent recurrence. Where repeated treatment is necessary, retreatment will lead to fibrotic changes in the nodes and make radiation therapy less effective.

Visceral involvement can at times be effectively managed by radiation techniques, but indications and techniques are dependent on the evaluation of the individual situation. In advanced stages, involvement of the stomach or bowel by direct infiltration, or from contiguous retroperitoneal nodes, requires slow, low-dosage therapy to avoid lysis and perforation. Osseous involvement may require radiation therapy to the bony foci and critical areas such as weight bearing bones and vertebrae as it is indicated in the treatment of metastatic bone disease secondary to other neoplasms.

Discussion

The ability of the clinician to assess more precisely the prognosis in an individual case of Hodgkin's disease has been sharpened greatly by the refinements in histopathologic classification as well as techniques for locating all sites of disease. Nevertheless, difficulties in utilizing these criteria to make predictions do exist. Ultimately, the best prognostic indicator is the length of time a patient remains free of disease following initial therapy.[37] The greater the time interval between initial treatment and the first relapse, the better the prognosis. Those patients with Stage I and II who have continued free of disease for greater than 2 years after initial therapy have an excellent chance for cure.

The development of megavoltage equipment has significantly influenced the pattern of treatment, and these techniques are being accepted as the treatment of choice for Stage I and Stage II disease. The management of Stage IV disease is directed toward the utilization of chemotherapeutic techniques for systemic disease and local radiation therapy techniques for localized disease. The ideal treatment for Stage III Hodgkin's disease is not entirely clear. Enough data are not yet available, in terms of long-term survival following extended field or radical irradiation, to be certain that cure is possible. Using this modality in Stage III, nearly all major lymphatic areas are irradiated above and below the diaphragm, thus exposing a large amount of marrow to the suppressive effects of radiation.[47] If the patient has a remission of greater than one year, his marrow reserve may return to normal, and, should relapse occur later, chemotherapy frequently can be used without too much difficulty.[48] However, should there be a recurrence in less than 12 months, the use of highly effective chemotherapeutic agents may be curtailed. From the data being accumulated by the group at Stanford, a substantial number of patients with Stage III Hodgkin's disease are being cured by extended field treatment, and it thus seems that the sacrifice in marrow reserves is worthwhile.

One must stress that with respect to the interpretation of data presented in the treatment of Hodgkin's disease, the course is highly variable from case to case and is significantly influenced by the histopathology and stage of the disease. Therefore, a thoughtful practitioner in this field must proceed slowly in accepting innovations in therapy that must be classified as still experimental and accept them after they have withstood the test of time. Great damage is done in the irresponsible application of aggressive radiation therapy techniques in the treatment of Hodgkin's disease as well as by the utilization of aggressive chemotherapy techniques when they are not carried out within the environment of a careful, deliberate program of assessment of the multiple parameters of the disease process.

The primary management of Hodgkin's disease is a sophisticated and difficult undertaking. Both an internist and a radiation therapist with interest in this disorder should participate in the initial evaluation of the patient. Lymphangiography, which is essential for the assessment of early disease, is technically demanding and requires experience in interpretation. Furthermore, the large treatment fields and high radiation dosages employed make special demands upon the radiation therapist and his equipment.

Since Hodgkin's disease is a relatively uncommon disorder as well as one with many clinical peculiarities, there is much to be said for concentration of its initial management in a few centers of excellence. This is particularly true for young patients with Stage I and II disease, in whom some radiation therapists believe the chance of cure is as high as 80 per cent or greater and even advisable perhaps also for young people with Stage IIIA disease. With the realization that the hopeless prognosis of Hodgkin's disease still found in some textbooks is incorrect, haphazard radiation therapy can no longer be justified or tolerated. Procrastination, dilatory chemotherapy and irradiation to inadequate fields or in inadequate amounts can only jeopardize the chance for cure. High cure rates for Hodgkin's disease have been reported only from centers that practice careful, painstaking, sophisticated radiation therapy.

REFERENCES

1. Symposium: The clinical status of Hodgkin's disease. Cancer 26:1268, 1966.
2. Symposium: Obstacles to the control of Hodgkin's disease. Cancer Res. 26:1041, 1966.
3. Aisenberg, A. C.: Primary management of Hodgkin's disease. New Eng. J. Med. 278:93, 1968.
4. Bagshaw, M. A., Kaplan, H. S. and Rosenberg, S. A.: Extended-field radiation therapy in Hodgkin's disease: A progress report. Radiat. Clin. N. Amer. 6:63, 1968.
5. Nickson, J. J. and Hutchison, G. B.: Hodgkin's disease: Clinical trial. Sixth National Cancer Conference Proceedings, 1970, pp. 77–81.
6. Aisenberg, A. C.: Hodgkin's disease: Prognosis, treatment and etiologic and immunologic considerations. New Eng. J. Med. 270:508, 1964.
7. Chawla, P. I., Stutzman, L., Dubois, R. E., Kim, U. and Sokal, J. E.: Long survival in Hodgkin's disease. Amer. J. Med. 48:85, 1970.

8. Johnson, R. E., Thomas, L. B., Schneiderman, M., Glenn, D. W., Faw, F. and Hafermann, M.: Preliminary experience with total nodal irradiation in Hodgkin's disease. Radiology 96:603, 1970.
9. Kaplan, H. S.: The radical radiotherapy of regional Hodgkin's disease. Radiology 78:553, 1962.
10. Keller, A. R., Kaplan, H. S., Lukes, R. J. and Rappaport, H.: Correlation of histopathology with other prognostic indicators in Hodgkin's disease. Cancer 22:487, 1968.
11. Rosenberg, S. A. and Kaplan, H. S.: Hodgkin's disease and other malignant lymphomas. Calif. Med. 113:23, 1970.
12. Rubin, P.: Hodgkin's disease: Comment. J.A.M.A. 191:32, 1965.
13. Rubin, P.: Hodgkin's disease. J.A.M.A. 190:910, 1964.
14. Peters, M. V.: Hodgkin's disease: Radiation therapy. J.A.M.A. 191:28, 1965.
15. Peters, M. V.: The contribution of radiation therapy in the control of early lymphomas. Amer. J. Roentgen. 90:956, 1963.
16. Peters, M. V.: A study of survivals in Hodgkin's disease treated radiologically. Amer. J. Roentgen. 63:299, 1950.
17. Peters, M. V. and Middlemiss, K. C. H.: A study of Hodgkin's disease treated by irradiation. Amer. J. Roentgen. 79:114, 1958.
18. Easson, E. C. and Russell, M. H.: Cure of Hodgkin's disease. Brit. Med. J. 1:1704, 1963.
19. Rosenberg, S. A. and Kaplan, H. S.: Evidence for an orderly progression in the spread of Hodgkin's disease. Cancer Res. 26:1225, 1966.
20. Smithers, D. W.: Spread of Hodgkin's disease. Lancet 1:1262, 1970.
21. Lukes, R. J.: Hodgkin's disease: Prognosis and relationship of histologic features to clinical stage. J.A.M.A. 190:914, 1964.
22. Lukes, R. J., Butler, J. J. and Hicks, E. B.: Natural history of Hodgkin's disease as related to its pathologic picture. Cancer 19:317, 1966.
23. Lukes, R. J. and Butler, J. J.: The pathology and nomenclature of Hodgkin's disease. Cancer Res. 26:1063, 1966.
24. Lukes, R. J., Tindle, B. H. and Parker, J. W.: Reed-Sternberg-like cells in infectious mononucleosis. Lancet 1:1003, 1969.
25. Strum, S. B. and Rappaport, H.: Interrelations of the histologic types of Hodgkin's disease. Arch. Path. 91:127, 1971.
26. Brady, L. W. and Faust, D. S.: Radiation therapy in Hodgkin's disease and lymphoma. *In* Brodsky, I. and Kahn, S. B. (Eds.): Cancer Chemotherapy. New York: Grune & Stratton, 1967.
27. Jackson, H., Jr. and Parker, J., Jr.: Hodgkin's disease and allied disorders. New York: Oxford University Press, 1947.
28. Schwarz, G.: Hodgkin's disease: The role of lymphangiography. J.A.M.A. 190:912, 1964.
29. Wallace, S.: Personal communication.
30. Lee, B. J.: Correlation between lymphangiography and clinical status of patients with lymphoma. Cancer Chemother. Rep. 52:205, 1968.
31. Lee, B. J., Nelson, J. H. and Schwartz, G.: Evaluation of lymphangiography, inferior vena cavography and intravenous pyelography in the clinical staging and management of Hodgkin's disease and lymphosarcoma. New Eng. J. Med. 271:327, 1964.
32. Glatstein, E., Guernsey, J. M., Rosenberg. S. A. and Kaplan, H. S.: The value of laparotomy and splenectomy in the staging of Hodgkin's disease. Cancer 24:709, 1969.
33. Aisenberg, A. C.: Studies on delayed hypersensitivity in Hodgkin's disease. J. Clin. Invest. 41:1964, 1962.
34. Musshoff, K., Renemann, H., Boutis, L. et al.: Die extranoduläre Lymphogranulomatose (Hodgkin's disease). Fortschr. Roentgenstr. 109:776, 1968.
35. Slaughter, D. P.: Hodgkin's disease: Radical surgery. J.A.M.A. 191:26, 1965.
36. Landberg, T. and Forslo, H.: Radiosensitivity of mediastinal lymphomas in Hodgkin's disease treated with split-course radiotherapy. Acta Radiol. 9:177, 1970.
37. Kaplan, H. S.: Prognostic significance of the relapse: The interval after radiotherapy in Hodgkin's disease. Cancer 22:1131, 1968.
38. Gellhorn, A.: Hodgkin's disease: Management with chemotherapeutic agents. J.A.M.A. 191:315, 1965.
39. Karnofsky, D. A.: Hodgkin's disease chemotherapy. J.A.M.A. 191:30, 1965.
40. Lacher, M. J.: Chemotherapy of Hodgkin's disease. New York: Grune & Stratton, 1971.
41. Rubin, P.: Advanced Hodgkin's disease. J.A.M.A. 191:314, 1965.
42. Rubin, P.: Hodgkin's disease: Comment. J.A.M.A. 190:917, 1964.
43. Serpick, A.: Clinical case records in chemotherapy: Possible radiation pericarditis in Hodgkin's disease. Cancer Chemother. Rep. 54:199, 1970.

44. Anderson, A. P., Brincker, H. and Lass, F.: Prognosis in Hodgkin's disease with special reference to histologic types. Acta Radiol. 9:81, 1970.
45. Shimkin, M. B.: Hodgkin's disease: Effectiveness of treatment in control. J.A.M.A. 190:916, 1964.
46. Buschke, F.: Hodgkin's disease: Indications for radiation therapy. J.A.M.A. 1913:17, 1965.
47. Ellis, R. E.: The distribution of active bone marrow in the adult. Phys. Med. Biol. 5:255, 1960–61.
48. Curran, R. E. and Johnson, R. E.: Tolerance to chemotherapy after prior irradiation for Hodgkin's disease. Ann. Intern. Med. 72:505, 1970.

Chemotherapy of Hodgkin's Disease

By Mortimer J. Lacher, M.D.

ONE OF THE CHIEF OBSTACLES to the control of Hodgkin's disease is the fact that radiation therapy is not a curative form of therapy for most patients with this disorder.

Peters'[1] best data (applying only her selected group of 39 Stage I, 71 Stage IIA, 25 Stage IIB and 53 Stage III cases using high dose radiation of adjacent areas) reveal that 41 per cent of Stage I patients, 22 per cent of Stage IIA patients, and 92 per cent and 82 per cent of the Stage IIB and Stage III patients, respectively, were dead within 10 years after diagnosis.

Easson[2] has presented "statistically valid evidence that patients with Hodgkin's disease are potentially curable provided (a) that they are fortunate enough to have localized lymphadenopathy at the time of treatment, and (b) that they are treated by X-rays to an adequate volume of tissue and to an adequate level of dosage." Despite this, 43.5 per cent of his patients with localized Hodgkin's disease were dead by 5 years and 56.8 per cent were dead by 10 years. Among the "generalized" patients, 81.1 per cent were dead by 5 years and 88.7 per cent by 10 years. At the Memorial Sloan-Kettering Cancer Center,[3] although the 5-year survival rate appeared promising, 63 per cent of the Stage IA and IIA patients were dead by 10 years.

Considering the fact that the "generalized" patient group in Easson's report is double the size of the "localized" group and that in other balanced series the IA and IIA patients constitute only one-third or less of the total group, not too many patients are available for a tenth anniversary of survival. Since more than 75 per cent of all patients with Hodgkin's disease have died within 10 years of their initial therapy, much more emphasis must be placed on alternative methods of treatment, other than radiation therapy, if one is to achieve a "cure" for the majority of patients. Certainly some patients can be "cured" by radiation therapy (or is it just a peculiar feature of their natural history?) (Fig. 1). Despite this, the failure group remains inordinately large.

Another problem in evaluating the radiation therapy data is that these data are usually presented as if no interim therapy had been applied. This implies that the end results are all dependent upon the initial course of radiation therapy. This, of course, is not true. Considerable credit for lengthening survival must be given to chemotherapy.

Perhaps radical radiation therapy is superior to "ordinary" radiation therapy, but even Kaplan and Rosenberg[4] report that "in a series of 109 consecutive cases of Stage I and Stage II Hodgkin's disease treated with megavoltage radiotherapy, additional clinical manifestations of disease have appeared after the first course of treatment in 40 instances to date." Thirty-three of these 40 relapses occurred within two years of therapy. If this high relapse rate occurred in this selected group of potentially curable patients, what can one expect from radiation therapy of the Stage III and IV patients? The magnitude of the problem may be more fully appreciated by reviewing the findings at laparotomy after high dose (3000 to 4000 rads) and low dose (1500 rads) radiation therapy as presented by Glatstein et al.[5] (Table 1).

From the Memorial Hospital for Cancer and Allied Diseases, New York, New York.

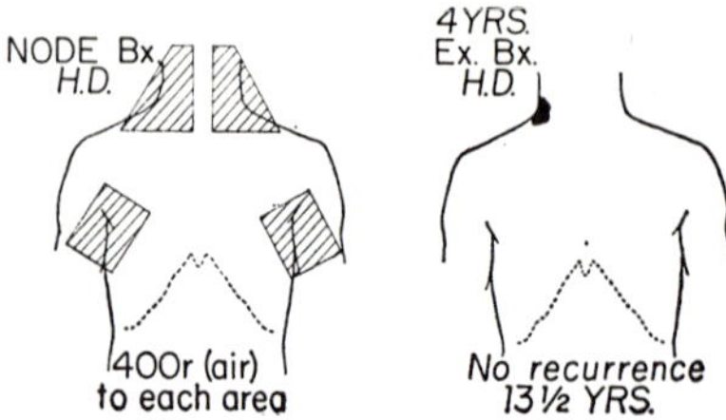

FIG. 1.—This patient achieved long survival after extraordinary minimal initial therapy. The first and only recurrence of pathologically reconfirmed tumor was treated by excisional biopsy only! This exceptional patient is an illustration of the fact that natural immunity cannot be completely ignored when reasons for long survival are considered.

Nine of these 12 patients received high radiation doses below the diaphragm, and despite this 7 of these 9 had persistent (or recurrent?) Hodgkin's tumor, confirmed by laparotomy, in nodes, liver or spleen. All three of the low dose group had residual or recurrent Hodgkin's disease below the diaphragm. This clearly demonstrates the failure of radiation therapy to eradicate the Hodgkin's tumor, especially when it is present below the diaphragm.

We therefore must remain concerned with the majority of patients, who have more widespread tumor, and with patients whose tumors recur despite high-dose, large-field and "prophylactic radiation" therapy. Besides, the destructive effects of high-dose radiation therapy are becoming more evident as its uses increase. Radiation pneumonitis, arteritis, myocarditis, pericarditis and myelitis are now more commonly encountered.

It is clear that a physical force such as radiation therapy has its physical limitations.

TABLE 1.—*Laparotomy in Hodgkin's Disease*

	Dose (rads)	*Area**	*Lapse*	*Histology* L	*Histology* S	*Histology* PA
I	1500	M, PA, S, P	2 months	+	+	+
II	1500	All Areas	1 year	+	+	NB
III	1500	M, PA, S, P	2 years	Neg.	+	Neg.
1	{4000	M, PA				
	{1500	S	8 months	+	+	+
2	4400	M, PA, S, P	7 months	+	+	NB
3	{1500	All Areas	3 years			
	{4000	All Areas	2 years	+	+	+
4	{3500	Neck, M	2 years			
	{4000	PA, Chemo	16 months	+	+	+
5	{4000	M, PA, P				
	{3200	S	2 years	NB	+	NB
6	4400	M, PA, S	18 months	Neg.	Neg.	+(iliac)
7	4000	M, PA	2 months	Neg.	Neg.	Neg.
8	{3000	M	18 months			
	{4000	PA, S, P	8 months	Neg.	Neg.	Neg.
9	4000	M, PA, P	2 years	+	+	+

Adapted from Glatstein, et al.[5]
* Abbreviations: M = mediastinum; PA = periaortic nodes; S = spleen; P = pelvic nodes; Chemo = chemotherapy.

With the increasing record of its failure to cure patients with widespread tumor, more emphasis must be placed on chemotherapeutic techniques as the eventual "cure" for most patients with Hodgkin's disease. The therapeutic priority given to radiation therapy, except in Stage IA and IIA patients, must be seriously questioned.

Extensive radiation therapy, especially when administered below the diaphragm, seriously compromises our ability to use chemotherapy. Data collected by Vogel et al.,[6] who used endotoxin and etiocholanolone stimulation of the bone marrow to measure "physiologic" marrow reserve, implied that full recovery of "marrow responsiveness" did occur within 5 months following intense radiation. In practice, unfortunately, this has not been the experience when the marrow is challenged by further chemotherapy.

Curran and Johnson[7] have recently reported that intensive radiation therapy "significantly reduces the bone marrow reserve." This results in an inability to apply adequate chemotherapy after extensive radiation therapy, which is then associated with "both failure to achieve drug-induced remissions and limited survival times."

They also observed that "the most distinct correlation existed when tolerance to chemotherapy was related to both the extent of bone marrow irradiated and the time interval after irradiation."[7] Tolerance to chemotherapy was reduced for nearly all patients with total nodal irradiation, whether they relapse early (less than 12 months after radiation therapy) or late. Patients with only 15 per cent to 30 per cent of irradiated marrow tolerated chemotherapy with little difficulty. Curran and Johnson had the impression that age was a factor and the bone marrow of older patients was more severely compromised after total nodal irradiation, an impression that many of us share. Their appeal to avoid fruitless irradiation of patients (for whatever reason) because "the resultant marked reduction of bone marrow reserve can only seriously hamper the clinically useful exploitation of modern chemotherapy" is a practical admonition long overdue.

We must, therefore, consider limiting high-dose radiation therapy to areas above the diaphragm and using radiation therapy in a restricted fashion below the diaphragm to prevent serious permanent marrow reserve suppression.

When nitrogen mustard was the only available chemotherapeutic agent, pessimism regarding long-term control of Hodgkin's disease was probably warranted. The Hodgkin's tumor, however, can be controlled with remarkable extended effectiveness by newer agents with little or no toxicity. Used in sequence, Hodgkin's patients can respond dramatically to many drugs; unfortunately, resistance to antitumor action finally appears and we are left without any more new agents to continue effective rotation. Maintenance chemotherapy alone, therefore, with currently available drugs is insufficient to achieve a "cure" (by any definition) for almost all patients. Combination therapy and rotational therapy are now being investigated but probably the final solution must await the development of still more effective drugs.

Up to now the dosage and timing of chemotherapy have been developed in an empirical manner and it remains in that unsatisfactory state at this time (Table 2).

We are, however, beginning to achieve a stricter definition of patient types through more detailed histologic analysis and intensive early work-up, which now includes splenectomy and periaortic node and liver biopsy.[8,9] With this new approach, we will be able to define more exactly who should have radiation therapy, who requires chemotherapy or who requires combinations of both modalities.

The hallmark of the next phase of attack against Hodgkin's disease will be the elucidation of the best treatment methods to suit each special category of patient. This will be characterized by modification of "radical" radiation therapy, a foray into the still untapped field of combination chemotherapy, and a persistent investigation for the best approach to sequential treatment.

Because of a fortunate absence of a nationwide or a worldwide monolithic structure of directed research, multiple groups of dedicated researchers and clinicians have been probing the empirical vastness of chemotherapeutic approaches to Hodgkin's disease, so that nitrogen mustard, thio-TEPA, chlorambucil, cyclophosphamide, vinblastine, vincristine, vinglycinate, procarbazine, indomethacin, prednisone and other agents have all been discovered, developed, condemned, praised, reevaluated and combined in myriad ways in an attempt to treat the patient with Hodgkin's disease.

The Plant Alkaloids

The plant alkaloids are perfect examples of empirical serendipity in both their discovery and application. Vinblastine sulfate and vincristine sulfate, intravenously administered, are now commercially available. Oral vinblastine, unfortunately, remains unavailable although its effectiveness has been clearly demonstrated.[10,11] Vinglycinate, another agent in the plant alkaloid series, has been withdrawn from experimental use although it was clearly demonstrated to be another extremely effective drug against the Hodgkin's tumor.[12]

Vinblastine sulfate is unusually effective against the Hodgkin's tumor. Sohier et al.[13] achieved clinically useful remissions in 22 of 35 cases of advanced Hodgkin's disease (Stage IIIB and IVB), of whom 33 were no longer responsive to the alkylating agents. "Despite the disadvantage of being secondary therapy, vinblastine appeared superior to the alkylating agents in quality and length of remission it produced." The responses with maintenance therapy lasted from 3 to 40 months, with one-third of the patients experiencing partial remissions of more than 1 year's duration.

Ezdinili and Stutzman[14] reported a 73 per cent objective response rate in patients with Stage III and IV Hodgkin's disease treated with vinblastine. In one of the very early trials of vinblastine, Armstrong et al.[15] reported that "it was of benefit in nine out of ten patients with Hodgkin's disease," and confirmed the work of Frei et al.,[16] Warwick et al.[17] and Whitelaw and Teasdale,[18] showing that vinblastine benefits some patients with this disease who have become refractory to radiation and alkylating agents. There is at least one instance of a seven year remission on maintenance vinblastine therapy in a patient with stage IIIB disease who had become refractory to both radiation therapy and the alkylating agents.

Bonadonna et al.[19] summarized 12 published reports of patients treated with vinblastine. Of the 300 patients reviewed, 37 had had no previous treatment, 14 were not specified and 249 patients had either radiation therapy previously or alkylating agents or both. The range of subjective and objective improvement greater than 1 month's duration varied from 33 per cent to 85 per cent in the different series. The average response rate was 62 per cent.

Bonadonna's series of 38 patients had all become refractory to radiation therapy and the alkylating agents. He showed a 65.7 per cent response rate, with a median duration of remission of 5 months.

The acceptance of vinblastine as a useful drug is now universal. How to use it and when to use it remain controversial.

The usual initial intravenous dose of vinblastine sulfate is 0.1 mg per kilogram of body weight. Higher initial doses do not appear to be more effective, but they produce more toxicity. Raising the dose may cause leukopenia but it will not enhance the antitumor effect. Armstrong et al.[15] stated that "in some of our patients remission from Hodgkin's disease . . . has been achieved with doses that did not produce leukopenia at any time." Warwick et al.[20] also noted "that there was no definite evidence of a correlation between the degree of leukopenia and the beneficial effect. Remissions in Hodgkin's disease have been observed in the absence of leukopenia following therapy."

It is not necessary to continue raising the dose of vinblastine by 50 per cent increments each week until toxicity occurs. The best maintenance technique is to apply the smallest dose increment once a week, once every 2 weeks, or for longer periods as long as a remission of the patient's symptoms and tumor masses is achieved.[21]

No one has determined whether or not it is better to maintain a "smooth" remission or to allow the patient to "escape" after each injection, with the development of fever or tumor growth prior to each injection. Sohier et al.[13] found it "very difficult to recover vinblastine remissions whose disease has exacerbated because administration has been too infrequent." Others have found this to be true for some patients but not for others. The critical feature separating these two types of patients is unclear. In general, the quest has been for "smooth" uninterrupted remissions. In each case, with rare exceptions, drug resistance finally develops, and raising the increment dose or shortening the interval between doses has no further antitumor effect.

Systemic toxicity to vinblastine depends on the dose and time interval between injections. From a practical view, leukopenia is the only significant hematologic reaction. Occasionally some nausea will occur after the injection but most often the effective antitumor doses are so low that no systemic toxicity occurs at all. In fact, this drug, as it is currently employed, is probably the least toxic agent in our armamentarium.

Local toxicity occurs if vinblastine is mistakenly injected subcutaneously. This results in a delayed reaction (3 to 24 hours) associated with local heat, redness, swelling, nodule formation, severe local pain, and peripherally and centrally radiating pain from the point of infiltration. Reaction is dose-dependent. The physician must watch his injection closely and stop at the first sign of a leak outside the vein. There is no apparent toxicity to the vein itself, and a truly intravenous injection has never resulted in phlebitis.

The pain associated with the inadvertent subcutaneous injection of vinblastine may be severe, especially when the dose injected exceeds 1 mg. The patient should be given a supply of an oral narcotic if subcutaneous injection does occur in anticipation of the need to sedate the patient for delayed pain reaction. When doses as large as 5 mg of vinblastine have been inadvertently administered subcutaneously, constant sedation with morphine sulfate for 24 to 36 hours has been required. Residual discomfort may persist for months as hyperesthesia and peripheral paresthesia. The subcutaneous nodule formation subsides slowly and eventually disappears.

Minute quantities of subcutaneous injections of vinblastine are annoying but are tolerated with minimal sedation by the average patient. When the infiltration is very superficial or even intradermal, vesicle formation may occur and a superficial ulceration may appear. This has been observed rarely. The skin integrity is usually maintained and slough does not usually ensue.

In patients with poor veins the alternative use of oral vinblastine has proved to be a blessing. One Stage IIIB patient who was originally started on intravenous vinblastine had to be switched to oral vinblastine 9 months later because of poor veins and frequent inadvertent subcutaneous injection. The patient has continued in remission on oral vinblastine for almost 6 years since that time. Since the oral vinblastine is generally unavailable, details of dosage may be obtained from references 10 and 11.

VINCRISTINE

Vincristine is also effective against the Hodgkin's tumor, but the remission rate is not as high as with vinblastine and the length of average remission is not as long.[22,23]

Systemic toxicity to vincristine is dependent upon the frequency and amount of the drug administered, but neurotoxicity usually occurs in doses necessary to achieve tumor control.

The mere loss of deep tendon reflexes, however, is not a sign to discontinue the medication. The loss of deep tendon reflexes may occur after the first few injections (1 to 3 mg given over a period of one to three weeks) but the patient may not have any further progression of neurotoxicity. Other patients, however, will manifest peripheral paresthesia and loss of muscle strength, inability to perform fine hand movements, loss of strength in the fingers and loss of proprioception. A slapping gait may be observed. These effects usually occur with prolonged administration of vincristine, but they are also dose-dependent and a single dose of sufficient quantity may cause the same effect.

When vincristine is used as part of a quadruple therapy regimen, the neurotoxic side effects may be quite prominent.

Other side effects include the development of isolated cranial nerve palsies and bowel ileus, and there may be partial or total loss of scalp hair. The unpleasant side effects are reversible after vincristine administration is stopped.

Hematologic toxicity to vincristine is fortunately minimal and is restricted for the most part to leukopenia.

VINGLYCINATE

Armstrong et al.[12] observed that "the oncolytic drugs which have been derived from *Vinca rosea*, the flowering periwinkle, are remarkable in that major differences in potency, toxicity and anti-tumor spectrum appear to depend on relatively minor differences in the side chains attached to the skeleton which they share in common." With these differences in mind "it appeared logical to produce more alkaloids of this series by chemically modifying some of the side chains." The lack of cross resistance among the active *Vinca* alkaloids was a further inducement to follow this line of research.

Vinglycinate was subsequently developed in the Lilly Research Laboratories. Significant objective evidence of beneficial response was demonstrated in patients with Hodgkin's disease. The dose limiting toxicity was leukopenia and, as with other *Vinca* alkaloids, no significant effects on the platelets or the red blood cells were encountered. The lack of cross resistance between vinglycinate and the other *Vinca* alkaloids was clearly demonstrated. Armstrong et al. concluded that "such biological and clinical findings as these encourage us to produce yet more derivatives of the *Vinca* alkaloids." Unfortunately, vinglycinate has never been made generally available.

Procarbazine

Procarbazine hydrochloride is a hydrazine derivative whose cytotoxic action has not been clearly defined. There is evidence that the drug causes inhibition of DNA synthesis.[24] No cross-resistance to other agents has been reported. It is probable that the cytostatic effect of the drug is dependent on a particular sensitivity of various tissues to the drug and not the concentration of the drug itself in the tissue.[25]

Procarbazine is currently available to us only in the oral form but it is rapidly absorbed from the intestine. Maximal plasma levels are found within 60 minutes of ingestion. The drug is then excreted in the urine (67 to 70 per cent is recovered in the first-day urine after oral administration) and it may concentrate in the liver.[25] Procarbazine therapy is usually started with a 50 mg dose and the dose is increased by 50 mg each day up to the desired total daily dose of 2 to 5 mg/kg of body weight. The purpose of this slow build-up is to minimize the frequently encountered nausea and vomiting that occur with the initiation of therapy. Generally, by the time the patient is ingesting 150 mg of procarbazine daily, tolerance has developed and no further gastrointestinal side effects occur. Some patients do have persistent nausea and some have such severe vomiting as to preclude further use of the drug by the oral route.

After 3 weeks of high dose administration a daily maintenance dose of 50 to 100 mg is usually adequate.[26] Bone marrow toxicity usually becomes evident, with a drop in white cell count and platelets, within 3 to 4 weeks. Increasing the total weekly dose of procarbazine "above 30 mg/kg body weight per week or prolonging the high dose phase of therapy beyond 3 weeks did not increase the response rate but did increase the severity of toxic manifestations."[27]

The total maintenance dose must be adjusted to suit the individual's blood count and clinical status, and effective maintenance doses vary from 50 mg every other day to 200 mg daily for a period of months. Rarely, patients have been maintained in complete remission on procarbazine for over 3 years after relapsing following temporary responses to radiation therapy, alkylating agents, vinblastine and vincristine.

When procarbazine is effective, a patient's anemia, leukopenia and thrombopenia will actually improve despite the known marrow depressing effect of the drug. For this reason, even in desperate situations, patients with pancytopenia may also be given a drug trial with procarbazine.

The response rate to procarbazine has varied from 14 of 14 with "objective improvement"[28] to 12 of 20 "useful responses," with significant regression of tumor masses and clinical improvement lasting at least one month.[27] These responses have occurred despite relapses following previous treatment with radiation therapy, alkylating agents, vinblastine or combinations of these.

In previously treated patients who have relapsed, the average length of remission after the use of procarbazine is about 4 to 6 months.[26–28] There is always the unusual individual who achieves an extended remission for a period of years, however. The value of procarbazine as initial therapy, prior to radiation therapy, has not been fully investigated.

The Alkylating Agents

The historically important nitrogen mustards may have a new role in combination therapy. Little can be added to the conclusions Rhoads made 24 years ago concerning these agents used singly: "The tumor regressions induced by these compounds [the nitrogen mustards], even with maximum dosages, are temporary, with maximal persistence rarely extending beyond several months." And in reference to the treatment of Hodgkin's disease, he stated, "improvement . . . continues only from two weeks to a few months and is followed by failure and rapid relapse. The relapses may respond to further therapy but the remissions induced are progressively shorter in duration."[29]

It is recommended that after nitrogen mustard is given, maintenance therapy with an oral alkylating agent such as chlorambucil be used to extend the useful remission that may be obtained.[30]

Attempts to compare the efficacy of nitrogen mustard with that of other chemotherapeutic agents against Hodgkin's disease have led to some peculiar conclusions. Ezdinili and Stutzman,[14] comparing vinblastine and nitrogen mustard, concluded that "both drugs are highly effective chemotherapeutic agents for the treatment of Hodgkin's disease and the superiority of one over the other could not be demonstrated."

In their study vinblastine therapy was arbitrarily stopped after six weekly injections. Nitrogen mustard was administered on two successive or four successive days until 0.4 mg/kg as a total dose was administered. Unmaintained median remission was 2.5 months with either drug from the time of maximal response. The initial objective response rate in the group of patients with Stage III and IV Hodgkin's disease was 80 per cent in the nitrogen mustard group compared to 73 per cent in the vinblastine group.

Repeated courses of nitrogen mustard are difficult to administer because of marrow toxicity, and resistance develops rapidly. In addition, vinblastine is not intended to be used only for a 6 weeks' course but is to be used as a maintenance drug. These factors did not enter into their study design and therefore an erroneous conclusion was reached regarding the equality of these two agents.

If the study had been conducted with patients who had completed an extensive and intensive course of radiation therapy and then had relapsed, would they still be able to conclude that "the superiority of one (HN2) over the other (VLB) could not be demonstrated"? After radiation-induced marrow toxicity, a full dose of nitrogen mustard could be dangerous, whereas maintenance therapy with vinblastine could be readily controlled and might be the only means to achieve remission.

BCNU, 1,3,BIS(β-CHLOROETHYL)-1-NITROSOUREA)

Lessner[31] reported "dramatic and rapid" responses to BCNU in 17 of 31 patients with Stage IIIB and IV Hodgkin's disease. The median duration of maintained remissions was over 120 days. Thirteen of 17 responders had received previous radiation therapy. All had previously received various combinations of alkylating agents, *Vinca* alkaloids and steroids. Lessner observed that when a response was not evident within two weeks of initial treatment, prolonged repeated treatment with BCNU was of no further value.

Nausea and vomiting may occur about 2 hours after administration in 50 per cent of the patients. The main limiting drawback, however, is the delayed hematologic toxicity, usually occurring in the third or fourth week after treatment. The recommended dose of 100 mg/m^2 daily for two consecutive days, therefore, cannot be repeated until the nadir of hematologic toxicity (pancytopenia) is passed. Experience has shown that this dose schedule must be drastically modified in patients with poor marrow reserve since the full dose might be fatal. BCNU may prove to be as effective in modest, less toxic doses (a single 50 mg dose repeated once every two to four weeks) as in the higher doses. This remains to be more adequately studied, however.

INDOMETHACIN

This drug has proved to be an extraordinary adjuvant agent in the management of the fever of Hodgkin's disease.[32] It has such an extraordinary ability to control fever and create a sense of well-being that occasionally one may have the eerie sensation that it also has some antitumor properties! This, of course, has not been established. The best technique is to give the drug in a "prophylactic" manner. The patient should be given one 25 mg capsule early in the morning, immediately on arising, and the dose should be repeated before lunch, supper and bedtime. Incredibly low rectal temperatures may be recorded (92°F), but the patient will remain unaware of this and will feel perfectly comfortable. If the temperature is allowed to rise, indo-

TABLE 2.—*Chemotherapy of Hodgkin's Disease*

Agent	*Route*	*Dose and schedule*	*Significant toxicity*
Alkylating			
HN2	IV	0.4 mg/kg traditional single dose or divided over 2 to 4 consecutive days	Nausea, vomiting, pancytopenia, skin vesication, phlebitis
Thio-TEPA	IV	0.8 mg/kg single dose	Pancytopenia
Chlorambucil	Oral	0.05 to 0.1 mg/kg daily single dose	Pancytopenia
Cyclophosphamide	Oral	2 mg/kg daily as a single or divided dose	Leukopenia (? platelet sparing), alopecia, hemorrhagic cystitis
	IV	14 mg/kg once a week; or various other schedules	
Plant alkaloids			
Vinblastine	IV	0.1 mg/kg every 1 to 3 weeks	Leukopenia; local reaction if given subcutaneously in error
Vincristine	IV	1 to 2 mg every 1 to 3 weeks	Neurotoxicity, alopecia
Other			
Procarbazine	Oral	1 to 5 mg/kg daily single or divided dose for 2 to 3 weeks, then reduced maintenance daily dose	Nausea, vomiting, pancytopenia, "Antabuse effect"
BCNU	IV	100 mg/m^2 2 days in a row; drastic modification if marrow reserve is low	Pancytopenia, liver toxicity
Bleomycin	IV		Skin rash, mucosal ulceration of gastrointestinal tract, lung fibrosis
Adjuvant drugs			
Indomethacin (for fever)	Oral	25 mg 4 times daily; start first dose 7 to 8 A.M. each day	
Allopurinol (for hyperuricemia)	Oral	100 to 200 mg 4 times daily	

methacin may effect an extremely rapid drop in temperature, with minimal sweating, but the value of keeping the temperature suppressed is lost. If infection supervenes, fever will occur despite the antipyretic effect of indomethacin. If the Hodgkin's tumor becomes totally resistant to any therapy, indomethacin will no longer suppress the fever.

Sequential Therapy

Nitrogen mustard and other alkylating agents (such as thio-TEPA, cyclophosphamide and chlorambucil), vinblastine, vincristine and procarbazine, and experimental agents such as vinglycinate, BCNU and bleomycin do suppress the Hodgkin's tumor. Therefore, "the judicious use of all of these drugs, provided they are adequately administered with a proper sequential schedule, by producing several consistent tumor regressions can keep the patient active, relatively asymptomatic and in good general condition for long periods of time."[19] The proper sequential schedule remains a mystery and a source of confusion.

At one center for Hodgkin's disease, patients not suitable for further radiation therapy receive nitrogen mustard followed by maintenance doses of chlorambucil. When the tumor becomes refractory to the alkylating agents, vinblastine is tried next, and then procarbazine. Further progression of the tumor is followed by the use of vincristine or cyclophosphamide.[19] Other investigators have used vinblastine first, followed by the combination of vinblastine plus chlorambucil, and then by procarbazine or vincristine, followed by available experimental agents such as BCNU or bleomycin.

Combination Therapy

Now, of course, most clinicians are involved in using multiple drugs as initial therapy for patients with Stage III and IV Hodgkin's disease. The anticipation, of course, is that a cure may be effected by combination chemotherapy.

Effective combinations of small doses of vinblastine and chlorambucil were reported in 1965.[33] Maintenance therapy was necessary to sustain remission in these patients. Two of the 16 patients in this study were still alive 7 years later. Both have received various interim courses of radiation therapy to local node groups. One patient (Stage IVB) continues on the vinblastine-chlorambucil combination and the other patient (Stage IIIB) is now on procarbazine maintenance therapy.

Skipper et al.,[34] using an experimental animal system, attempted to establish a scientific rationale for combination chemotherapy that would serve to back up the empirical quest for a drug "cure." Although they used a leukemia model and based their study on the concept that "cure" depended on the ability to "kill every leukemic cell," their work may be extended to other tumors. They realized that drug toxicity was a principal limiting factor in any system designed to kill every tumor cell. Thus, they concluded that "any modified therapeutic procedure which significantly increases the per cent kill of the host's total [leukemic] cell population without proportional increase in toxicity to the host may be considered as a gain."

In the L1210 leukemia system, there was little doubt that "the higher the single dose administered to the host (from the practical standpoint, up to the toxic or lethal dose) the greater the chance of killing all leukemic cells in the animal. . . . The potential of a single dose high level schedule is much superior to the chronic maximum daily schedule if one is seeking 'cures.' "[34]

Skipper[34] outlined three basic problems in attempting to "cure" leukemia: "(A) The relatively *low chemotherapeutic indices* of the available drugs. (B) The existence of *anatomical compartments* readily invaded by the tumor cells but not so readily by the anti-tumor agents. (C) Spontaneous or drug induced mutation to and drug selection of drug-resistant variants within a leukemic population . . . ." These problems are applicable to all tumors; therefore, "searches for optimal dosages and schedules as well as combinations (simultaneous or sequential) which might be additive or potentiating with regard to [leukemic] cell cytotoxicity but less than additive or potentiating in toxicity to the host are obviously important approaches."

DeVita et al.[35] have provided us with a very important and exciting contribution with regard to the potential "cure" of the Hodgkin's tumor using a quadruple drug regimen. They chose an empirical combination of nitrogen mustard (or cyclophosphamide), prednisone, vincristine and procarbazine and applied it to patients with Stage IVA and B and IIIA and B Hodgkin's disease (Fig. 2). Only patients who had not received previous therapy or only limited therapy were accepted into the study. "Demonstrated resistance to one or more of the agents to be used in the study was considered a significant reason for exclusion."

Of 43 patients studied between 1964 and July 1, 1967, 35 had complete remission following therapy, defined as a complete disappearance of all tumor and return to normal performance status. The median duration of response was not less than 29 and not more than 42 months at the time of the report. Fifteen of the 35 responders relapsed within 11 months. Of the 20 remaining patients, 17 still remain in remission and a few were in remission for almost 4 years at the time of this writing.

The most significant feature of this approach is the fact that long *unmaintained* remissions have been achieved following an intensive course of chemotherapy. Previous trials with single drug regimens or other multiple drug regimens have resulted in rapid relapse when maintenance therapy was stopped.

Even if one would quibble with DeVita's staging, because as a purist one might insist on laparotomy and biopsy of the retroperitoneal nodes or spleen for the ultimate in accurate staging, the results achieved are not detracted from in any way. Assuming that the long-term responders who have been in complete remission without maintenance therapy were all patients with Stage IA or IIA or IIB disease instead of IIIB or IVB, the results still mean that we have been brought a significant step closer to the possibility of "cure" of Hodgkin's disease through combination chemotherapy. With combination chemotherapy there is greater hope than ever before for the 75 per cent of patients with Hodgkin's disease seeking to achieve long survival. Besides, DeVita et al. have probably understated their case. Not only were there 17 survivors without

QUADRUPLE THERAPY OF HODGKIN'S DISEASE

	Days				
Drugs mg/m^2	1	2-7	8	9-14	28
VCR	1.4		1.4		
HN2	6.0		6.0		
Procarbazine	100.0	→	→	→	No therapy
Prednisone*	40.0	→	→	→	

* Cycles 1 and 4 only

FIG. 2.—Example of a single cycle of a 4-drug therapy scheme as proposed by De Vita et al.[35]

QUADRUPLE THERAPY OF HODGKIN'S DISEASE

Drugs	Days 1	2-7	8	9-13	14	42
VLB	10.0 mg		10.0 mg		10.0 mg	
HN2	6.0 mg/m²		6.0 mg			
Procarbazine	100.0 mg/m²	→	→	→	→	No therapy (4 weeks)
Prednisolone	40.0 mg/m²	→	→	→	→	

FIG. 3.—Example of a single cycle of a 4-drug therapy scheme as proposed by Nicholson et al.[36]

maintenance therapy, but there were also 11 survivors (ranging from 33 to 71 months, average survival 47 months) who continued in remission on repeated courses of therapy. The choice of chemotherapy in preference to radiation therapy as primary treatment for patients with Stage III and Stage IV disease is strongly supported by these results.

The fact that all the patients sensitized with dinitrochlorobenzene (DNCB) maintained their skin anergy after their "complete" clinical remission suggests, however, that the basic factors present when the Hodgkin's disease was active remain even though the patient appears to be in complete remission. Careful observation will be continued of all these patients during the period of follow-up.

DeVita et al. have attempted to use the various drugs in their study in "full doses" to enhance "cell kill" employing agents that they felt would increase the "cell kill" without proportional increase in toxicity. The rationale for this is based on the work of Skipper et al., as outlined previously. The current protocol, therefore, could be modified to combine other agents such as vinblastine in place of vincristine to attempt to achieve further enhancement of "cell kill."

Nicholson et al.[36] have adapted the NCI protocol and have substituted vinblastine for vincristine, with the significant advantage of avoiding the unpleasant neurotoxicity of vincristine (Fig. 3). Other modifications with regard to dose and timing of the injections were introduced. These results, too, indicate that "there is no doubt that combination chemotherapy produces a higher proportion of both complete and partial remissions than the use of single agents in generalized Hodgkin's disease." Further modifications will continue to be studied. As new agents (such as bleomycin) appear, they, too, will be substituted or added to these protocols. As long as the true mode of action of these drugs remains unclear, much empirical work remains to be done.

A single drug or a combination of drugs will eventually cure or permanently control the Hodgkin's disease patient. The exact combination of drugs has not yet been found.

REFERENCES

1. Peters, V. M.: Prophylactic treatment of adjacent areas in Hodgkin's disease. Cancer Res. 26:1232, 1966.
2. Easson, E. C.: Long-term results of radical radiotherapy in Hodgkin's disease. Cancer Res. 27:1244, 1966.
3. Lacher, M. J.: Long survival in Hodgkin's disease. Ann. Intern. Med. 70:7, 1969.
4. Kaplan, H. S. and Rosenberg, S. A.: Cure in Hodgkin's disease and other malignant lymphomas. Postgrad. Med. 43:146, 1968.
5. Glatstein, E., Guernsey, J. M., Rosenberg, S. A. and Kaplan, H. S.: The value of laparotomy and splenectomy in the staging of Hodgkin's disease. Cancer 24:709, 1969.

6. Vogel, J. M., Kimball, H. R., Foley, H. T., Wolff, S. M. and Perry, S.: Effect of extensive radiotherapy on the marrow granulocyte reserves of patients with Hodgkin's disease. Cancer 21:798, 1968.
7. Curran, R. E. and Johnson, R. E.: Tolerance to chemotherapy after prior irradiation for Hodgkin's disease. Ann. Intern. Med. 72:505, 1970.
8. Glatstein, E., Trueblood, H. W., Rosenberg, S. A. and Kaplan, H. S.: Surgical staging of abdominal involvement in unselected patients with Hodgkin's disease. Radiology 97:432, 1970.
9. Lowenbraun, S., Ramsey, H., Sutherland, J. and Serpick, A. A.: Diagnostic laparotomy and splenectomy for staging Hodgkin's disease. Ann. Intern. Med. 72:655, 1970.
10. MacDonald, C. A., Jr. and Lacher, M. J.: Oral vinblastine sulfate in Hodgkin's disease. Clin. Pharmacol. Ther. 7:534, 1966.
11. Wilson, H. E. and Louis, J.: The response of Hodgkin's disease to treatment with oral vinblastine sulfate. Ann. Intern. Med. 67:303, 1967.
12. Armstrong, J. G., Johnson, I. S. and Hargrove, W. W.: Some biological and clinical features of a chemically produced ester analog of vinblastine. *In* Burchenal, J. H. (Ed.): Treatment of Burkitt's Lymphoma. New York: Springer-Verlag, 1967.
13. Sohier, W. D., Jr., Wong, R. K. L. and Aisenberg, C. A.: Vinblastine in the treatment of advanced Hodgkin's disease. Cancer 22:467, 1968.
14. Ezdinili, E. Z. and Stutzman, L.: Vinblastine *vs.* nitrogen mustard therapy of Hodgkin's disease. Cancer 22:473, 1968.
15. Armstrong, J. G., Dyke, R. W., Fouts, P. J. and Gahimer, J. E.: Hodgkin's disease, carcinoma of the breast, and other tumors treated with vinblastine sulfate. Cancer Chemother. Rep. 18:49, 1962.
16. Frei, E., III, Franzino, A., Shnider, B., Costa, G., Colsky, J., et al.: Clinical studies of vinblastine. Cancer Chemother. Rep. 12:125, 1961.
17. Warwick, O. H., Darte, J. M. M. and Brown, T. C.: Some biological effects of vincaleukoblastine, an alkaloid, *Vinca rosea* Linn., in patients with malignant disease. Cancer Res. 20:1032, 1960.
18. Whitelaw, D. M. and Teasdale, J. M.: Vincaleukoblastine in treatment of malignant disease. Canad. Med. Ass. J. 85:584, 1961.
19. Bonadonna, G., Monfardini, S. and Oldini, C.: Comparative effects of vinblastine and procarbazine in advanced Hodgkin's disease. Europ. J. Cancer 5:393, 1969.
20. Warwick, O. H., Alison, R. E. and Darte, J. M. M.: Clinical experience with vinblastine sulfate. Canad. Med. Ass. J. 85:579, 1961.
21. Lacher, M. J.: Vinblastine sulfate in Hodgkin's disease. New York J. Med. 69:808, 1969.
22. Bohannon, R. A., Miller, D. G. and Diamond, H. D.: Vincristine in the treatment of lymphomas and leukemias. Cancer Res. 23:613, 1963.
23. Carbone, P. P., Bono, V., Frei, E., III and Brindley, C. O.: Clinical studies with vincristine. Blood 21:640, 1963.
24. Berneis, K., Kofler, M., Bollag, W., Kaiser, A. and Langemann, A.: The degradation of deoxyribonucleic acid by new tumor inhibiting compounds: The intermediate formation of hydrogen peroxide. Experientia 19:132, 1963.
25. Data on file. Hoffmann-La Roche, Inc., Nutley, New Jersey 07110.
26. Geller, W. and Lacher, M. J.: Hodgkin's disease. Med. Clin. N. Amer. 50:819, 1966.
27. Brunner, K. W. and Young, C. W.: A methylhydrazine derivative in Hodgkin's disease and other malignant neoplasms: Therapeutic and toxic effects studied in 51 patients. Ann. Intern. Med. 63:69, 1965.
28. Flatow, F. A., Ultmann, J. E., Hyman, G. A. and Muggia, F. M.: Treatment of advanced Hodgkin's disease with vinblastine (NSC-49842) or procarbazine (NSC-77213). Cancer Chemother. Rep. 53:39, 1969.
29. Rhoads, C. P.: Nitrogen mustards in the treatment of neoplastic disease. J.A.M.A. 131:656, 1946.
30. Scott, J. L.: The effect of nitrogen mustard and maintenance chlorambucil in the treatment of advanced Hodgkin's disease. Cancer Chemother. Rep. 27:27, 1963.
31. Lessner, H. E.: BCNU (1-3, bis(β-chloroethyl)-1-nitrosourea). Effects on advanced Hodgkin's disease and other neoplasia. Cancer 22:451, 1968.
32. Silberman, H. R., McGinn, T. G. and Kremer, W. B.: Control of fever in Hodgkin's disease by indomethacin. J.A.M.A. 194:127, 1965.
33. Lacher, M. J. and Durant, J. R.: Combined vinblastine and chlorambucil therapy in Hodgkin's disease. Ann. Intern. Med. 194:127, 1965.

34. Skipper, H. E., Schabel, F. N., Jr. and Wilcox W. S.: Experimental evaluation of potential anti-cancer agents. XIII. On the criteria and kinetics associated with "curability" of experimental leukemia. Cancer Chemother. Rep. 35:1, 1964.
35. DeVita, V. T., Jr., Serpick, A. A. and Carbone, P. P.: Combination chemotherapy in the treatment of advanced Hodgkin's disease. Ann. Intern. Med. 73:881, 1970.
36. Nicholson, W. M., Beard, M. E. J., Crowther, D., Stansfeld, A. G., Vartan, C. P., et al.: Combination chemotherapy in generalized Hodgkin's disease. Brit. Med. J. 3:7, 1970.

Lymphocyte Function in Hodgkin's Disease

By ALAN C. AISENBERG, M.D.

AMONG THE LYMPHOMAS, indeed among acquired human disorders, Hodgkin's disease stands out as an illustration of defective thymus-dependent immunity. The deficiency is characterized by a depression of cell-mediated immune reactions, i.e., tuberculin or bacterial allergy (delayed hypersensitivity), contact sensitivity and homograft rejection. Since cellular immunity is most conveniently studied in the skin, loss of this responsiveness is frequently termed "cutaneous anergy." Antibody-mediated (immediate) immune responses are, for the most part, preserved in Hodgkin's disease. The immune defect progresses with the disease and, in many patients with advanced disease, the frequent and bizarre infectious complications constitute as difficult a problem in management as the lymphoma itself.

LOSS OF PREEXISTING DELAYED HYPERSENSITIVITY

In the middle 1930s Parker et al.[1] and Steiner[2] observed that the percentage of Hodgkin's patients with positive tuberculin reactions was much lower than that of a comparable control population. The abnormal tuberculin status was thought by these workers to suggest a role of the tubercle bacillus in the pathogenesis of Hodgkin's disease, but with the investigations of Schier et al. in the middle 1950s[3] it became clear that this status reflected a defect in immunologic response to all cell-mediated antigens. Schier tested his patients with Hodgkin's disease with a group of delayed (cell-mediated) antigens. Fourteen per cent of these individuals reacted to mumps skin test antigen, whereas 90 per cent of controls reacted; 19 per cent of the patients with Hodgkin's disease reacted to *Candida albicans* extract, to which 92 per cent of controls reacted; 16 per cent reacted to *Trichophyton gypseum* extract, to which 68 per cent of controls reacted; and 23 per cent reacted to tuberculin PPD (purified protein derivative), to which 71 per cent of controls reacted. Schier's observations have been confirmed in other Hodgkin's disease clinics using the same[4] and other delayed allergens.[5]

LOSS OF ABILITY TO ACQUIRE NEW HYPERSENSITIVITIES

The evaluation of delayed hypersensitivity by testing for preexisting sensitivity has the disadvantage that in any particular instance anergy cannot be distinguished from the absence of exposure. This objection can be circumvented by active sensitization with a compound to which lack of prior exposure can be assumed, or can be established by preliminary testing. Induction of contact sensitivity with dinitrochlorobenzene (DNCB), a substance not present in the normal environment, has proved to be a satisfactory and simple method of evaluating delayed hypersensitivity. A very high percentage (more than 95 per cent) of normal controls will react to a low (0.1 per cent) concentration of DNCB three weeks after a small area of skin has been painted with a more concentrated solution (2 to 10 per cent) of the compound.

In an early study of 37 patients with Hodgkin's disease,[6] all 25 who had disease

From the John Collins Warren Laboratories of the Huntington Memorial Laboratory of Harvard University at the Massachusetts General Hospital, Boston, Massachusetts.

activity when tested were anergic, as indicated by their inability to acquire DNCB sensitivity. Patients who had passed more than 2 years without active Hodgkin's disease did acquire DNCB sensitivity, and those whose disease was inactive for lesser periods of time displayed either positive or negative reactions. Although in this early study it was clear that patients in good clinical condition with active disease were anergic, only a small number of individuals with active *localized* and untreated Hodgkin's disease were included; in these the localized character of the process was not verified by lymphangiographic examination of the retroperitoneal lymph nodes. Brown et al.[7] at the National Institutes of Health have also used DNCB, and they report a different picture in a carefully staged group of *untreated* Hodgkin's patients: 35 (70 per cent) of the 50 patients investigated became sensitive to DNCB, including some with advanced disease.

It has been found difficult[8] to immunize patients with Hodgkin's disease with diphtheria toxoid (0 of 9 immunized, compared with 9 of 14 controls), though in 10 of 12 Hodgkin's patients without systemic manifestations the tuberculin status was converted to positive with BCG.[4] (BCG may be acting as a secondary antigenic stimulus.)

The Homograft Reaction

There have been several small studies of skin homograft rejection involving a total of 29 Hodgkin's patients.[8–11] Of this total, in 17 (59 per cent) homograft rejection was delayed, as would be predicted from the defect in cellular immunity seen in Hodgkin's disease.

Antibody Formation

The ability of the patient with Hodgkin's disease to form antibody has been the subject of numerous studies (reviewed in reference 12) and considerable controversy. Nevertheless, certain conclusions appear reasonably established. First, the terminal patient loses the ability to form antibody, probably as a near agonal event,[13] a loss which is paralleled by the decrease in gamma globulin levels often seen in individuals with far-advanced disease.[14,15] Second, patients in good general condition with localized or moderately advanced disease retain the ability to form normal amounts of antibody to many antigenic stimuli[13,16,17] and have normal or slightly elevated gamma globulin levels[14,18] Finally, a minor defect in antibody formation in such favorably disposed patients with Hodgkin's disease is suggested by a depressed response to primary (as opposed to secondary) antigenic stimuli[19] and to certain weak antigenic stimuli, by a failure to retain antibody levels as long as normal controls do,[13,16] and by a selective reduction of IgM levels.[20] Thus, the proviso that there are suggestions of subtle alterations must be added to the generalization that antibody formation is intact in anergic Hodgkin's patients.

Lymphocyte Counts

Since several lines of evidence have now established the small lymphocyte as the cell which mediates delayed hypersensitivity,[21,22] it is evident that investigation of this cell is a logical approach to understanding the anergy of Hodgkin's disease. Tissue lymphocyte depletion was described in some detail by Rosenthal[23] in 1936, and the degree of such depletion linked to prognosis. All subsequent pathologic classifications of Hodgkin's disease, including those of Jackson and Parker[24] and Lukes and Butler,[25] have used the degree of this depletion as a major criterion and have found severe lymphocyte loss associated with poor prognosis. As early as the middle 1930s, Wiseman[26] found depression of the peripheral lymphocyte in 87 per cent of the 31 untreated patients with Hodgkin's disease in his series, a finding which he remarked to be consistent with the experience of most hematologists of the period.

In a more recent series of autopsies of Hodgkin's patients,[27] profound lymphopenia was regularly found in the final 6 months of life, whereas in the same group of individuals two-thirds were moderately to severely lymphopenic at the time the disease was diagnosed. However, in a more favorable series drawn from the outpatient department of the same institution, most patients had lymphocyte counts in the low normal range at the time of diagnosis.

Lymphocyte counts were also studied in 50 untreated patients at the National Institutes of Health.[7] Two-thirds of the group displayed normal lymphocyte counts, with lymphocytopenia being more prevalent with advanced stage (wider dissemination) and with a lymph node histology of lymphocyte depletion. Lack of reactivity to tuberculin and other delayed allergens and to DNCB correlated in general with lymphopenia, but individual anergic patients had normal lymphocyte counts and some lymphopenic patients were reactive.

Thus, it seems likely that the profound lymphopenia of advanced Hodgkin's disease contributes to the severe immunologic depression of this type of patient, but that the anergy observed early in the disease is not accounted for solely by an insufficient total level of circulating lymphocytes. However, it is plausible that the anergy of the early Hodgkin's patient is related to the lack of a particular population of small lymphocytes. Recent evidence in both experimental animals and man suggests that small lymphocytes, though morphologically indistinguishable, can be separated on functional grounds.[21]

Lymphocyte Function

The response of cultures of Hodgkin's lymphocytes to a variety of stimuli has been examined in several laboratories. In an early report,[28] lymphocytes from 6 of 10 patients with Hodgkin's disease failed to react to phytohemagglutinin (PHA) and mixed-cell culture (mitogenic stimuli to which normal lymphocytes react). Hersh and Oppenheim[29] studied the lymphocytes from 23 Hodgkin's patients in more detail, and found that 87 per cent showed a diminished response to in vitro stimulation with phytohemagglutinin and vaccinia virus. In their study, the phytohemagglutinin Hodgkin's cultures contained a median of 11 per cent transformed cells compared to 70 per cent in PHA controls, and the vaccinia-stimulated cultures 0 per cent as compared with 8 per cent in vaccinia controls. Advanced clinical stage and the presence of systemic manifestations were both more frequently associated with unreactive lymphocytes than were their contraries. It should be noted that others have not found as high a percentage of unreactive Hodgkin's patients; two-thirds of the 9 patients of Holm et al.[30] and half of the 8 patients of Trubowitz et al.[31] were unresponsive to phytohemagglutinin. Indeed, only one-third of a group of 44 untreated patients with Hodgkin's disease showed such impaired lymphocyte response to PHA in a recent study[7] in which in vitro unresponsiveness could be correlated with in vivo reactivity to tuberculin and other intradermal allergens and to dinitrochlorobenzene. Finally, an extension of tissue culture studies has demonstrated that Hodgkin's lymphocytes lack the cytotoxicity of normal lymphocytes towards cultured human liver cells.[30]

In summarizing the lymphocyte culture work it is clear that at least one-third, and possibly two-thirds, of patients with Hodgkin's disease possess lymphocytes which are normally responsive in vitro. The available data suggest that lymphocyte unreactivity as conventionally defined is not the determining factor in the observed anergy.

Lymphocyte Transfer Reaction

The lymphocyte from the patient with Hodgkin's disease can also be studied by observing its reaction when transferred to the skin of another individual, the so-called "lymphocyte transfer reaction." This reaction, the complete interpretation of which is complex, is in part a reaction of grafted lymphocytes against the recipient and so can be used to study the immune competence of the lymphocyte donor. In one recent study, that part of the reaction that was ascribed to graft-versus-host reactivity of the donor lymphocytes was consistently depressed when Hodgkin's lymphocytes were used,[32] confirming the cell culture work. However, other investigators[33] failed to observe this depression, perhaps because the lymphocytes obtained were from patients earlier in the course of their disease.

Transfer of Delayed Hypersensitivity to Patients with Hodgkin's Disease (Lawrence-Type Transfers)

Lawrence has shown that it is possible to transfer delayed hypersensitivity from a sensitive individual to a nonsensitive one by the intradermal injection of buffy coat prepared from a small (100 to 200 ml) volume of blood.[34] Three groups of investigators have tried to transfer tuberculin sensitivity from tuberculin-positive normals to Hodgkin's patients and failed.[8,35,36] However, it should be pointed out that Lawrence-type transfers can be performed equally well with cell-free material; indeed, the active principle is small enough to be dialyzable. Therefore, manipulations of this type involve the transfer of information about the antigen, to be sure not antigen itself, which then must be replicated and incorporated into the recipient's lymphocytes. Thus a Lawrence-type transfer is almost as demanding of the recipient's immunologic apparatus as immunization itself, and it is doubtful whether this type of experiment gives us further insight into the immunologic difficulties of the patient with Hodgkin's disease. There have been no reported attempts to transfer delayed hypersensitivity from such patients to normal controls, a very interesting but difficult experiment.

Phagocytic Function

Phagocytosis is an aspect of immunologic responsiveness which is intact in patients with Hodgkin's disease. A very careful study has shown that individuals with this disorder clear labeled particles from the blood more effectively than normal controls.[37] The enhanced phagocytic ability might be predicted from the reticulum cell hyperplasia which is often a prominent histologic feature of the Hodgkin's lymph node.

Infectious Complications

Secondary infection with a variety of esoteric and nonesoteric organisms is characteristic of the advanced stages of Hodgkin's disease.[10,24,38] Clearly, it is difficult to disentangle the contribution of treatment to this susceptibility to infection since each agent used to treat this disorder (X-irradiation, alkylating agents, periwinkle alkaloids and procarbazine) has been proved to be immunosuppressive. The characteristic opportunistic infections are those caused by fungi (*Candida*, *Torula*, *Aspergillus*, *Actinomyces* and *Histoplasma*); viruses of the herpes group (*herpes zoster* and cytomegalovirus), and certain protozoa (*Pneumocystis carinii* and *Toxoplasma*). With all these agents, resistance is thought to involve cellular immunity. Tuberculosis, which at one time was the most frequent infectious complication seen in Hodgkin's disease, has become much less common as the disease has declined in the general population. However, listeriosis is now being reported in lymphoma patients.

It is of interest that in Hodgkin's disease *herpes zoster* usually remains segmental, whereas in chronic lymphatic leukemia (another disorder in which *herpes* is frequently seen), a disease which primarily affects antibody formation, the infection more often disseminates.[39] This observation suggests that the defect in cellular immunity in Hodgkin's disease permits segmental infection but intact antibody formation usually limits dissemination. Indeed, it has been pointed out that *herpes zoster* in Hodgkin's disease is mainly a manifestation of active lymphoma at the appropriate level.[39]

Although the esoteric fungous and viral infections are the *characteristic* infections of Hodgkin's disease, the most *common* infections are the more mundane bacterial problems (pneumonia, skin infections and septicemia) with organisms such as *Staphylococcus aureus*, *Pseudomonas* and *Escherichia coli*.[10,38] It should be stressed that, in contrast to the antibody-deficiency syndromes, the infectious complications of Hodgkin's disease usually occur in the final stages of the disorder. It is a common experience to control serious complicating infection only to have the patient with Hodgkin's disease die from the underlying disease.

The frequency of infectious complications in Hodgkin's disease can be appreciated from the National Cancer Institute series of 51 cases which were recently reported by Casazza et al.[38] In this small group of patients, 86 separate infections were observed of which 56 were bacterial, 17 viral, 10 fungal, and 3 protozoal.

Anergy in Other Clinical Situations

Loss of delayed hypersensitivity has been described in the advanced stages of a variety of debilitating illnesses (e.g., cancer, leukemia, uremia and tuberculosis). Cancer patients have been investigated in most detail. It appears that individuals in good condition with localized neoplasms react normally to delayed allergens and DNCB,[5,40,41] but when metastatic disease appears, DNCB sensitization is frequently difficult to produce,[40,42] and preexisting sensitivities are often lost.[15,18] It remains to be proved that the depression of cellular immunity seen in metastatic carcinoma reflects more than debilitation in an aged population. Whereas anergy is seen in Hodgkin's disease when patients are in good condition, in other neoplasms it is usually observed in patients whose condition has deteriorated.[5]

Of considerable interest is the anergy which accompanies the acute stage of a variety of viral infections. In measles it has been shown that tuberculin anergy occurs during the incubation period, the first 4 days of the rash, and even during vaccination with live-virus vaccine.[43] This anergy is presumably related to virus invasion, with the intense disruption of lymphoid tissue which takes place during this disorder. Another infection in which anergy is documented is leprosy, particularly the lepromatous form,[44] where the progressive nature of the disorder has been linked to the immune defect.

Anergy is also seen in sarcoid, a generalized disease of unknown etiology which widely involves the lymphoid system. Skin tests to common antigens are depressed, sensitization to dinitrochlorobenzene is impaired, and lymphocyte response to phytohemagglutinin is abnormal.[45,46] Anergy in sarcoid appears to be less intense than that of Hodgkin's disease, but like the latter disorder the defect is associated with active disease. It is not clear that there are critical differences between the anergies of the two conditions.

Progression of Anergy During the Course of Hodgkin's Disease

The immune defect of Hodgkin's disease is a deficiency which evolves as the disease progresses (Table 1). Early in the condition the loss of delayed hypersensitivity is not complete, and a fraction of patients respond normally to new antigens (DNCB) and to skin testing with common delayed antigens.

At the present time published documentation is not complete concerning the frequency with which anergy occurs in lymphangiogram-verified *localized* (Stage I: disease in a single lymph node group; Stage II: disease in two or more lymph node groups either above or below the diaphragm) and *untreated* Hodgkin's disease. The best data available indicate that untreated patients with Stage I have normal reactivity, but that more than two-thirds of individuals with Stage II, Stage III (disease in lymph nodes above and below the diaphragm), or Stage IV (disease in lymph nodes and nonlymphoid organs) are unreactive either to DNCB or to a battery of intradermal allergens.[7] Thus, it appears that even at the onset of the disorder and before treatment, some evidence of anergy can be found in most patients with Hodgkin's disease. It seems likely that individuals with normal cellular immunity at the outset have: (1) a more localized process; or (2) a more favorable prognosis; or (3) a favorable histology such as lymphocyte predominance[25]; or (4) a combination of these; but this important point requires further investigation. It has been observed that the disorder follows a more favorable course in patients with sufficient cellular immunity to acquire tuberculin sensitivity after BCG vaccination than in those who remain

Table 1.—*Progression of Immune Defect in Hodgkin's Disease*

Normal immunity
1. Stage I disease—at onset, untreated.
2. 30 to 40% of Stage II, III and IV—at onset, untreated.*
3. Local disease in remission 2+ years after radiation.
4. Anergic Stage III and IV after quadruple chemotherapy.

Anergy (negative skin tests and/or response to DNCB)
1. 60 to 70% of Stage II, III and IV—at onset, untreated.*
2. Almost all patients under medical care with active and incurable disease.†

Profound immune depression (anergy, depressed humoral immunity, marked susceptibility to infectious agents)
1. Patients with far-advanced and near-terminal disease.

* Anergy is more frequent in the lymphocyte depletion variant than in mixed cellularity or nodular sclerosis. It seems likely, but is unproved, that anergy is associated with a less favorable prognosis.

† Anergy is progressive and the intensity related to prognosis. Patients who acquire tuberculin sensitivity after BCG survive longer than those who do not.

tuberculin-negative.[47] It has also been found that patients may recover responsiveness to DNCB[6,48] or to tuberculin[4,45] after radiation to a localized area of adenopathy. However, while normal immunity is observed in patients in prolonged remission (longer than 2 years) in whom the question of cure may be raised, it cannot be assumed that these same individuals were necessarily anergic when the disease began.

Certainly, depressed delayed hypersensitivity (as determined by failure to become sensitized with DNCB and unreactivity to common skin test antigens) is present in most patients with active Hodgkin's disease under medical observation. This includes patients in good clinical condition without debility or systemic manifestations, and individuals in whom most lymph node areas are free of clinical disease and have not been irradiated. However, even though lymph nodes away from the primary site of involvement are free of clinical and presumably overt pathological evidence of Hodgkin's disease, it is possible that they are functionally impaired by the early stages of the same process. Gamma globulin levels are usually normal or slightly elevated[14,18] in such anergic patients and gross antibody formation is intact.

The immunologic deficiency of the deteriorating patient with far-advanced Hodgkin's disease is more complex. In such individuals profound anergy (negative skin tests and DNCB sensitization) is often accompanied by defective antibody synthesis and low gamma globulin levels, and in such patients secondary infections become a severe problem. The nonspecific deficiency of debility is now added to the characteristic immunologic defect of Hodgkin's disease.

Except in the untreated patient, it is difficult to assess the contribution of treatment to the observed immunologic defect. Over the past decade, as radiation therapy and chemotherapy in Hodgkin's disease have become more aggressive, this assessment has become an increasing problem. Certainly, treatment must be a contributory factor in the far-advanced patient under essentially continuous immunosuppression. However, it is noteworthy that anergic patients with stage III and IV disease usually recover delayed hypersensitivity reactions after six months of intensive quadruple (nitrogen mustard, vincristine, procarbazine and prednisone) chemotherapy with a drug regimen that is itself immunosuppressive.[49]

Pathogenesis of the Immunologic Defect in Hodgkin's Disease

It should be clear from the preceding section that the anergy of Hodgkin's disease (excluding the far-advanced patient) is unrelated to debility or to obliteration of the lymphoid system by anatomically verifiable disease. A variety of evidence suggests that this anergy is mediated through the peripheral small lymphocyte. First is the evidence that this cell subserves that type of immunity which is defective in the Hodgkin's patient. Second, the observed profound depletion of blood and tissue lymphocytes undoubtedly contributes to the anergy of individuals with advanced disease. Third, direct evidence from lymphocyte culture and lymphocyte transfer experiments suggests that the Hodgkin's lymphocyte may be functionally impaired. Finally, recovery of responsiveness after treatment argues against a tolerance-like central mechanism. However, in the individual patient the qualitative methods available have so far been inadequate to relate anergy to lymphocyte function, and conclusive proof of the relationship awaits quantitative techniques.

The immunologic deficiency of Hodgkin's disease involves that function which in experimental animals has been shown to be thymus-dependent,[50] and many features

TABLE 2.—*Thymus-Dependent Immunity and Hodgkin's Disease*

	Thymectomized animal	*Hodgkin's disease patient*
A. Cellular immunity		
1. Homograft reaction	↓ or ↓↓	↓ or ↓↓
2. Graft-vs.-host reaction	↓↓	↓ (lymphocyte transfer reaction)
3. Delayed hypersensitivity		
a) Bacterial	↓↓ (rat)	N to ↓↓
b) Contact	?	N to ↓↓
4. Lymphocytes		
a) Number	↓↓ to about 40% normal, selective loss of long-lived cells	N to ↓↓↓
b) Transformation	?	N to ↓
B. Humoral immunity		
1. Immunoglobulin levels	N, ?↓ IgA (rat)	N or ↑, except late ↓ or ↓↓ (IgM > IgG)
2. Plasma cells	N	? N
3. Antibody formation	↓↓ to N	↓ to N
	a) BSA > ShC > Pneumo, Fer., Hemo.	a) Typhoid, Tet. > Pneumo.
	b) Primary > Secondary	b) Primary > Secondary
	c) IgG > IgM	
C. Infection	Wasting in newborn. Protection by germ-free environment. Susceptibility to hepatitis virus	Susceptibility to various viral, fungal, protozoal and bacterial agents, often of low pathogenicity: *Herpes* group (CMV, *H. zoster*), *Torula*, *Histoplasma*, *Candida*, *Nocardia*, *Pneumocystis*, *Listeria*, *etc.*

Abbreviations: N = normal; ↓, ↓↓, ↓↓↓ = slight, moderate or severe decrease or impairment; > = more impaired than; BSA = bovine serum albumin; ShC = sheep erythrocytes; Pneumo = pneumococcus polysaccharide; Fer. = ferritin; Hemo. = hemocyanin; Tet. = tetanus toxoid; CMV = cytomegalovirus.

of the Hodgkin's patient resemble (Table 2) those of the thymus-deficient animal.*[12,51,52] Thus, in both the patient with Hodgkin's disease and the thymectomized animal, the defect in cellular immunity is more severe than the antibody deficiency. In both there is marked depression of the homograft reaction and susceptibility to secondary infection, but immunoglobulin levels are well maintained. Both show depression of tissue and circulating lymphocytes. Even the details of the antibody deficiency in the two states are similar, insofar as data are available to establish a parallel: In both the antibody response to pneumococcus polysaccharide is preserved better than that to protein antigens; the 19S response is preserved better than the 7S; and the secondary response preserved better than the primary.[53]

However, it seems unlikely[54] that Thomson[55] was correct in ascribing the seat of Hodgkin's disease to the thymus, but likely rather that Hodgkin's disease involves

* A decade ago Kaplan and Smithers[56] pointed out the similarities between graft-versus-host reactions of experimental animals and human malignant lymphomas, and suggested that this reaction might play a role in the causation of Hodgkin's disease. More recently, Schwartz et al. have described malignant lymphomas (of host origin) in mice subject to chronic graft-versus-host reactions.[57] Although there are a number of superficial similarities between these two fatal wasting disorders of lymphoid tissue, most investigators believe that the disparate pathology of the two conditions makes it unlikely that the experimental disorder plays a role in the pathogenesis of the human disease.[51]

that immune system (the small lymphocyte) which is thymic in origin. Thus, the immunologic deficiency reveals the cellular site at which the etiologic agent of Hodgkin's disease is acting. It is plausible that in anergic patients this etiologic agent is acting on thymus-dependent lymphocytes throughout the lymphoid system although histologically recognizable Hodgkin's disease is present only in limited anatomic locations. Since known viruses have been associated with anergy, a viral causation of Hodgkin's disease offers a credible explanation for the observed immune defect.

References

1. Parker, F., Jr., Jackson, H., Jr., Fitzhugh, G. and Spies, T. D.: Studies of diseases of lymphoid and myeloid tissues. IV. Skin reactions to human and avian tuberculin. J. Immun. 22:277, 1932.
2. Steiner, P. E.: Etiology of Hodgkin's disease. II. Skin reaction to avian and human tuberculin proteins in Hodgkin's disease. Arch. Intern. Med. 54:11, 1934.
3. Schier, W. W., Roth, A., Ostroff, G. and Schrift, M. H.: Hodgkin's disease and immunity. Amer. J. Med. 20:94, 1956.
4. Sokal, J. E. and Primikirios, N.: The delayed skin test response in Hodgkin's disease and lymphosarcoma: Effect of disease activity. Cancer 14:597, 1961.
5. Lamb, D., Pilney, R., Kelly, W. D. and Good, R. A.: A comparative study of the incidence of anergy in patients with carcinoma, Hodgkin's disease and other lymphomas. J. Immun. 89:555, 1962.
6. Aisenberg, A. C.: Studies on delayed hypersensitivity in Hodgkin's disease. J. Clin. Invest. 41:1964, 1962.
7. Brown, R. S., Haynes, H. A., Foley, H. T., Godwin, H. A., Bernard, C. W. and Carbone, P. P.: Hodgkin's disease: Immunologic, clinical and histologic features of fifty untreated patients. Ann. Intern. Med. 67:291, 1967.
8. Kelly, W. D., Lamb, D. L., Varco, R. L. and Good, R. A.: An investigation of Hodgkin's disease with respect to the problem of homotransplantation. Ann. N.Y. Acad. Sci. 87:187, 1960.
9. Green, I., Inkelas, M. and Allen, L. B.: Hodgkin's disease: a maternal-to-fetal lymphocyte chimaera? Lancet 1:30, 1960.
10. Miller, D. G.: Patterns of immunological deficiency in lymphomas and leukemias. Ann. Intern. Med. 57:703, 1962.
11. Miller, D. G., Lizardo, J. B. and Snyderman, R.: Homologous and heterologous skin transplantation in lymphomatous disease. J. Nat. Cancer Inst. 26:569, 1961.
12. Aisenberg, A. C.: Hodgkin's disease: Prognosis, treatment and immunologic considerations. New Eng. J. Med. 270:508, 565, 617, 1964.
13. Aisenberg, A. C. and Leskowitz, S.: Antibody formation in Hodgkin's disease. New Eng. J. Med. 269:1269, 1963.
14. Arends, T., Coorad, C. V. and Rundles, R. W.: Serum proteins in Hodgkin's disease and malignant lymphoma. Amer. J. Med. 16:833, 1954.
15. Ultmann, J. E., Cunningham, J. K. and Gellhorn, A.: The clinical picture of Hodgkin's disease. Cancer Res. 26:1047, 1966.
16. Hoffmann, G. T. and Rottino, A.: Studies of immunologic reactions of patients with Hodgkin's disease: Antibody reaction to typhoid immunization. Arch. Intern. Med. 86:872, 1950.
17. Millian, S. J., Miller, D. G. and Schaeffer, M.: Viral complement-fixing antibody in patients with Hodgkin's disease, lymphosarcoma, reticulum cell sarcoma and chronic lymphatic leukemia. Cancer 18:674, 1965.
18. McKelvey, E. M. and Fahey, J. L.: Immunoglobulin changes in disease: Quantitation on the basis of heavy polypeptide chains, IgG (γ-G), IgA (γ-A), and IgM (γ-M), and light polypeptide chains, type K (I) and type L (II). J. Clin. Invest. 44:1778, 1965.
19. Barr, M. and Fairley, G. H.: Circulating antibodies in reticuloses. Lancet 1:1305, 1961.
20. Goldman, J. M. and Hobbs, J. R.: The immunoglobulins in Hodgkin's disease. Immunology 13:421, 1967.
21. Gowans, J. L.: Life-span recirculation and transformation of lymphocytes. Int. Rev. Exp. Path. 5:1, 1966.
22. Gowans, J. L. and McGregor, D. D.: The immunological activity of lymphocytes. Progr. Allerg. 9:1, 1965.
23. Rosenthal, S. R.: Significance of tissue lymphocytes in the prognosis of lymphogranulomatosis. Arch. Path. 21:628, 1936.

24. Jackson, H., Jr. and Parker, F., Jr.: Hodgkin's Disease and Allied Disorders. New York: Oxford University Press, 1947.
25. Lukes, R. J. and Butler, J. J.: The pathology and nomenclature of Hodgkin's disease. Cancer Res. 26:1063, 1966.
26. Wiseman, B. K.: The blood picture in the primary diseases of the lymphatic system. J.A.M.A. 107:2016, 1936.
27. Aisenberg, A. C.: Lymphopenia in Hodgkin's disease. Blood 25:1037, 1965.
28. Aisenberg, A. C.: Quantitative estimation of the reactivity of normal and Hodgkin's disease lymphocytes with thymidine-2-C^{14}. Nature 205:1233, 1965.
29. Hersh, E. M. and Oppenheim, J. J.: Impaired *in vitro* lymphocyte transformation in Hodgkin's disease. New Eng. J. Med. 273:1006, 1965.
30. Holm, G., Perlmann, P. and Johansson, B.: Impaired phytohaemagglutinin-induced cytotoxicity *in vitro* of lymphocytes from patients with Hodgkin's disease or chronic lymphocytic leukemia. Clin. Exp. Immun. 2:351, 1967.
31. Trubowitz, S., Masek, B. and del Rosario, A.: Lymphocyte response to phytohemagglutinin in Hodgkin's disease, lymphatic leukemia and lymphosarcoma. Cancer 19:2019, 1966.
32. Aisenberg, A. C.: Studies of lymphocyte transfer reactions in Hodgkin's disease. J. Clin. Invest. 44:555, 1965.
33. Levin, A. G., Miller, D. G. and Southam, C. M.: Lymphocyte transfer tests in cancer patients and healthy people. Cancer 22:500, 1968.
34. Lawrence, H. S.: Some biological and immunological properties of transfer factor. *In* Wolstenholme, G. E. W. and O'Connor, M. (Eds.): Ciba Foundation Symposium on Cellular Aspects of Immunity. Boston: Little, Brown, 1960.
35. Fazio, M. and Calciati, A.: Transfer of antibodies of the delayed tuberculin type in lymphogranuloma. Panminerva Med. 4:162, 1962.
36. Müftüoglu, A. U. and Balkuv, S.: Passive transfer of tuberculin sensitivity in Hodgkin's disease. New Eng. J. Med. 277:126, 1967.
37. Shaegren, J. W., Block, J. B. and Wolff, S. M.: Reticuloendothelial system function in patients with Hodgkin's disease. J. Clin. Invest. 46:855, 1967.
38. Casazza, A. R., Duvall, C. P. and Carbone, P. P.: Summary of infectious complications occurring in patients with Hodgkin's disease. Cancer Res. 26:1290, 1966.
39. Williams, H. W., Diamond, H. D., Craver, L. F. and Parsons, H.: Neurological Complications in Lymphomas and Leukemias. Springfield, Ill.: Charles C Thomas, 1959.
40. Gross, L.; Immunological defect in aged populations and its relation to cancer. Cancer 18:201, 1965.
41. Solowey, A. C. and Rapaport, F. T.: Immunologic responses in cancer patients. Surg. Gynec. Obstet. 121:756, 1965.
42. Levin, A. G., McDonough, E. F., Jr., Miller, D. G. and Southam, C. M.: Delayed hypersensitivity response to DNFB in sick and healthy persons. Ann. N.Y. Acad. Sci. 120:400, 1964.
43. Starr, S. and Berkovich, S.: Effect of measles, gamma globulin-modified measles and vaccine measles on the tuberculin test. New Eng. J. Med. 27:394, 1964.
44. Waldorf, D. S., Sheagren, J. N., Trautman, J. R. and Block, J. B.: Impaired delayed hypersensitivity in patients with lepromatous leprosy. Lancet 2:773, 1966.
45. Chase, M. W.: Delayed-type hypersensitivity and the immunology of Hodgkin's disease, with a parallel examination of sarcoidosis. Cancer Res. 26:1097, 1966.
46. Jones, J. V.: Development of sensitivity to dinitrochlorobenzene in patients with sarcoidosis. Clin. Exp. Immun. 2:477, 1967.
47. Sokal, J. E. and Aungst, C. W.: Response to BCG vaccination and survival in advanced Hodgkin's disease. Cancer 24:855, 1967.
48. Kaplan, H. S., Eltringham, J. R. and Rosenberg, S. A.: Delayed hypersensitivity to DNCB in patients with malignant lymphoma. Clin. Res. 15:132, 1967.
49. DeVita, V. T., Serpick, A. and Carbone, P. P.: Combination chemotherapy in advanced Hodgkin's disease: The NCI program, a progress report. Proc. Amer. Ass. Cancer Res. 10:19, 1969.
50. Miller, J. F. A. P.: The thymus and the development of immunologic responsiveness. Science 144:1544, 1964.
51. Aisenberg, A. C.: Immunologic status of Hodgkin's disease. Cancer 19:385, 1966.
52. Dent, P. B., Gabrielson, A. E., Cooper, M. D., Peterson, R. D. A. and Good, R. A.: The secondary immunologic deficiency diseases associated with lymphoproliferative disorders. *In* Miescher, P. A. and Muller-Eberhard, H. J. (Eds.): Textbook of Immunopathology, Vol. II. New York: Grune & Stratton, 1969, p. 406.

53. Taylor, R. B.: Cellular cooperation in the antibody response of mice to two serum albumins: Specific function of thymus cells. Transplant. Rev. 1:114, 1969.

54. Marshall, A. H. E. and Wood, C.: The involvement of the thymus in Hodgkin's disease. J. Path. Bact. 73:163, 1957.

55. Thomson, A. D.: The thymic origin of Hodgkin's disease. Brit. J. Cancer 9:37, 1955.

56. Kaplan, H. S. and Smithers, D. W.: Autoimmunity in man and homologous disease in mice in relation to malignant lymphomas. Lancet 2:1, 1959.

57. Schwartz, R. S., André-Schwartz, J., Armstrong, M. Y. K. and Beldotti, L.: Neoplastic sequelae of allogenic disease. I. Theoretical considerations and experimental design. Ann. N.Y. Acad. Sci. 129:804, 1966.

V. REGIONAL TECHNIQUES

Cancer Chemotherapy Using Isolation Perfusion

By JOSEPH G. STRAWITZ, M.D.

THE CONCEPT OF DELIVERING a chemotherapeutic agent directly into a tumor site was first introduced by Klopp et al.[1] These workers placed a cannula in a major artery supplying a tumor bearing area and administered nitrogen mustard (HN2) in single or fractionated doses. Bierman et al.[2] and Sullivan et al.[3] experimented with this method and reported that the cytotoxic effect of nitrogen mustard in particular appeared to be enhanced by its intra-arterial administration. These developments followed the initial observations of Gilman and Phillips,[4] who reported that the mustard compounds appeared to have a cytotoxic effect on certain experimental tumors. The findings were confirmed clinically by Jacobsen et al.,[5] who observed that while tumor growth was retarded, an injurious action on normal tissues, particularly the hematopoietic system, appeared to be the limiting factor in the use of the agent.

Following these developments, many workers, eager to test this new-found concept of chemotherapy in the treatment of neoplastic disease, were frustrated by the toxicity factor; long-term treatment results were rarely reported. Creech et al.[6] showed that it was anatomically feasible to isolate a tumor bearing area from the rest of the circulation and to perfuse it with otherwise lethal doses of tumoricidal agents with the aid of a pump oxygenator system. With this method they showed that it was possible to use large doses of chemotherapeutic drugs while avoiding the various severe toxic effects commonly seen with systemic therapy. Surgeons began to use the recently developed heart-lung equipment to isolate nearly every part of the human anatomy. The purpose of this chapter is to review the techniques which have been developed and to give a progress report on the experiences of a number of investigators who have had the broadest experience in the use of isolation perfusion.

THE TECHNIQUE OF ISOLATION PERFUSION

Almost any pump oxygenator system familiar to the operator can be used (Fig. 1). We have used two sigma-motor coronary sinus pumps with a Hymen Oxygenator (Pulmo-pak) (Abbott Laboratories, North Chicago, Ill.). With this type of equipment, tissue oxygen tension in an isolated area can be elevated above normal levels. A venous reservoir is used with a priming volume of 750 to 1000 cc of whole blood. The oxygenator column is connected to rubber tubing in the venous pump head, while the venous reservoir is connected directly to rubber tubing in the arterial pump head. The venous reservoir gravity drainage is placed between the patient and the venous pump. Citrated blood is used in the arterial reservoir, to which 3000 units of sodium heparin is added, and the circuit is primed through the venous pump. The oxygen flow into the oxygenator is at a level of 3 to 4 liters per minute. Priming

---

From the Departments of Surgery, American Oncologic Hospital and the University of Pennsylvania Medical School, Philadelphia, Pennsylvania.

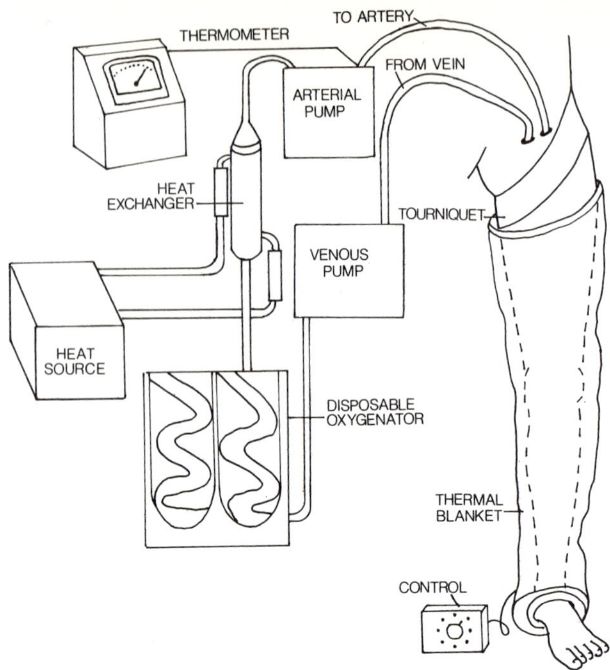

FIG. 1.—Diagram of apparatus for isolation perfusion.

blood is circulated through this system continuously until cannulations have been completed and the patient is prepared for perfusion. Before the artery and the vein are cannulated, the patient is heparinized with 150 units per kilogram of total body weight. In our experience, nitrogen mustard in an average dose level of 0.6 mg/kg has been administered with a syringe and needle into the tubing in the arterial pump head. The injection is given fractionally over a 60-minute perfusion period at approximately 10-minute intervals.

When hyperthermic perfusion is used, the blood is heated by a closed-circuit water-circulating unit connected to a heat exchanger with a temperature range of 45–150°F. The average temperature of the blood is kept at 115°F or 46°C. An increase in skin temperature can be produced by using a thermal blanket. The temperatures of the circulating blood, skin and muscle are monitored.

Upon completion of the perfusion, the pumps are shut off and the tourniquets released. The sites of cannulation in the artery and vein are repaired. Adequate blood flow in both the proximal and distal ends of the vessels is required before making the repair. After the repair is completed, protamine sulfate, a heparin antagonist, is administered systemically by the anesthesiologist in an amount equivalent to that of the heparin given prior to the perfusion.

Perfusion of the Lower Extremities

When lesions below the knee are being treated, the perfusion is carried out through the superficial femoral artery and vein in the mid-portion of the thigh (Fig. 2). A tourniquet is placed about the upper third of the thigh and inflated prior to the perfusion. These vessels are cannulated in a distal direction. The catheters used for venous drainage have two or three perforations near the tips and are usually size 16

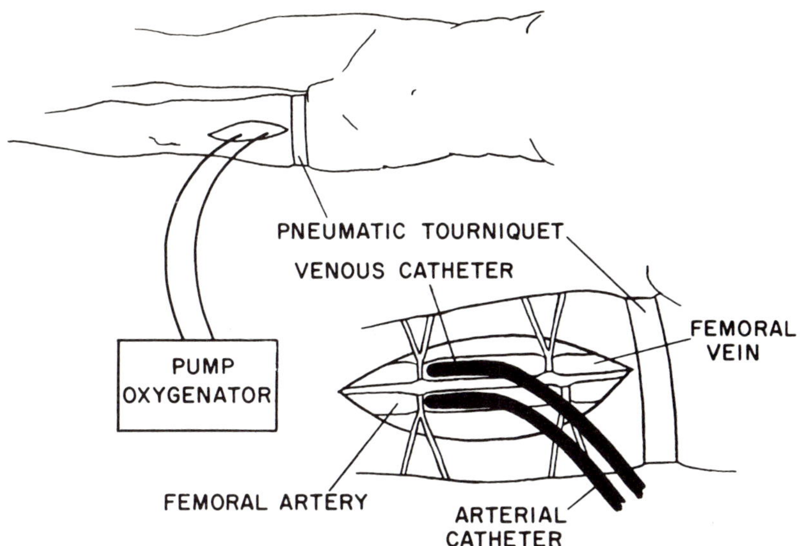

FIG. 2.—Perfusion of the lower extremities. From Strawitz,[15] with permission.

to 18 French, while the arterial catheters are size 10 to 12 French. A flow rate of 175 to 225 ml per minute is maintained provided the venous return remains constant. Venospasm occurs in many patients and requires a reduction in the flow rate. In perfusion of the upper leg, cannulation is carried out in a similar manner except that larger catheters are employed. In such a circumstance the tourniquet is passed over the iliac crest and is maintained in this position by towel forceps; if this poses a problem, a Steinmann pin thrust through the soft tissues below the iliac crest, coupled with an Esmarch bandage placed tightly about the limb and over the pin, is usually effective. Upper-extremity perfusion is carried out in a similar manner with cannulation of the brachial artery and vein. A pneumatic tourniquet is placed above the site of cannulation.

Perfusion of the Pelvis

With the patient under general anesthesia, pneumatic tourniquets are applied around the upper thighs (Fig. 3). Balloon catheters (Dotter-Lucas No. 2, American Instrument and Catheter Co., New York, N.Y.) are passed through the femoral artery and vein into the lower abdominal aorta and vena cava. These vessels are occluded by expanding balloons and perfused through separate cannulas inserted below the entrance of the balloon catheters in the artery and the vein. This method has been substituted for the initial cross-clamping of the aorta and vena cava, which requires an abdominal incision. The only disadvantage in connection with the use of ballon catheters pertains to rupture of the balloons when they are placed under pressure. Testing balloon catheters for strength prior to use is necessary to obviate this possible complication.

Perfusion of the Head and Neck

The external carotid artery is exposed on the tumor bearing side (Fig. 4). The internal jugular vein or common facial vein is cannulated and the blood passed

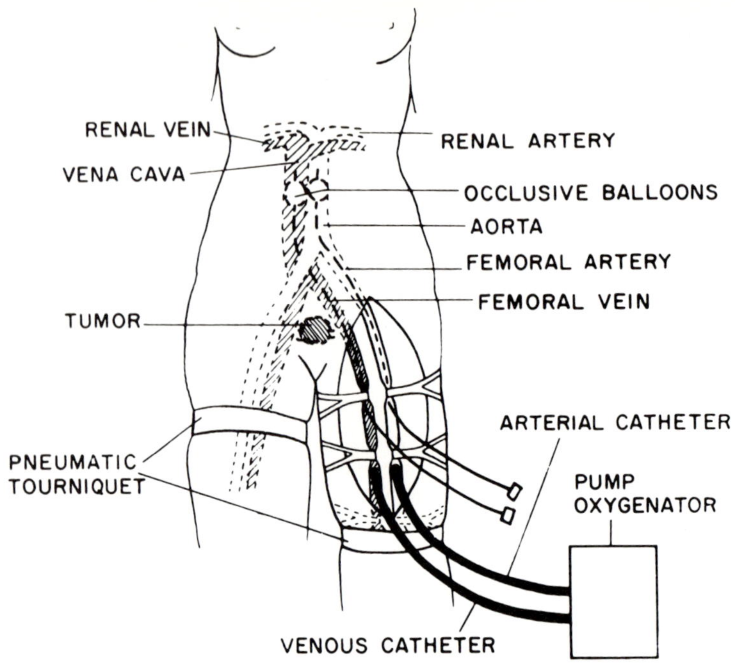

FIG. 3.—Perfusion of the pelvis using balloon catheters. From Strawitz,[15] with permission.

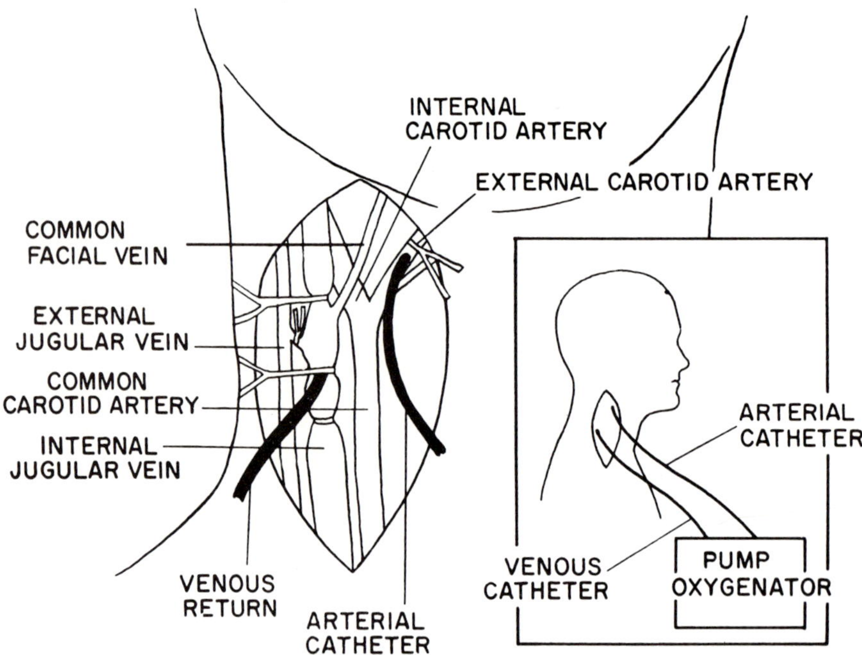

FIG. 4.—Perfusion of the head and neck. From Strawitz,[15] with permission.

through tubing into the pump oxygenator system. The blood, with the drug added, is pumped into the external carotid artery through a catheter inserted into it or through the superior thyroid artery, with the origin of the external carotid artery clamped or ligated. Gravity drainage or pump activated suction is used on the venous side. Low flow and pressure are necessary to avoid severe edema of the head, which has proved to be a serious complication, particularly in the elderly patient. Cerebrovascular spasm can also be a serious complication with perfusion and infusion techniques.

Perfusion of Intra-Abdominal Malignancy

In general, the more central the perfusion the less isolation is possible. Initially, investigators tended to isolate the liver and pancreas by cross-clamping the aorta and vena cava in the chest and introducing balloon catheters below, in a manner similar to the procedure described in pelvic perfusion. Martin[7] devised a tourniquet that could be applied at the time of laparotomy that effectively isolated the abdomen. Lawrence[8] and associates improved isolation in the abdomen by application of an external pneumatic tourniquet about the diaphragmatic region coupled with intra-arterial occlusions of the aorta and vena cava by balloon catheters. However, infusion techniques seem to be preferable to these procedures since the difficulties involved in the procedures are too great and the complication rate is high for palliative results.

Retroperitoneal and Posterior Mediastinal Perfusion of Lymphatics

The basic work in connection with this particular development is described by Strawitz et al.,[9] who showed that a substance with a molecular weight of 5000 or more remains within the lymphatic vessels and can have therapeutic value, particularly if the lymphatic system is not obstructed. The procedure (Fig. 5) involves the cannulation of a lymphatic vessel in the dorsum of the foot after the injection of approximately 3 cc of methylene blue subcutaneously in the first interdigital space. A small transverse incision is made in the dorsum of the foot, and a # 27 needle with

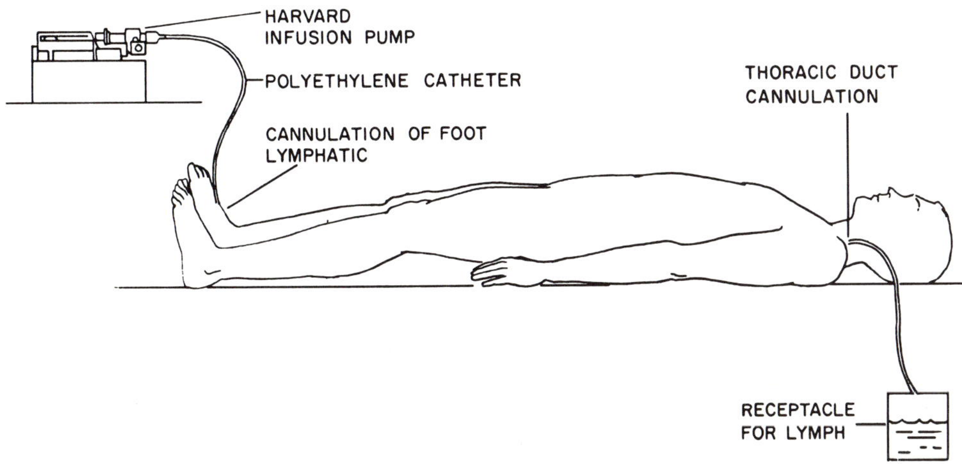

FIG. 5.—Retroperitoneal and posterior mediastinal perfusion of the lymphatics. From Strawitz,[15] with permission.

an attached polyethylene catheter is introduced into a lymphatic vessel, which is easily visualized since it contains the methylene blue previously injected.

The cannulation of the thoracic duct is done at the same time with the introduction of a polyethylene catheter from which drainage is recovered. Systemic blood volume is determined by the Evans blue method with 59 mc of ^{131}I (RISA) introduced through a foot lymphatic using a Harvard Infusion Pump (Harvard Apparatus Co., Cambridge, Mass.). Fifteen-minute samples are taken from the thoracic duct catheter simultaneously with blood samples from a systemic vein over 2 or 3 hours and counted immediately in a well-scintillation counter. The dose of chemotherapeutic agent is calculated from the extent of recovery of RISA from the thoracic duct so that the systemic leak does not exceed the recommended systemic dose.

Determination of Systemic Leak

Radioiodinated serum albumin ^{131}I (RISA) is added to the priming pump in the pump oxygenator system. The dose consists of 50 mc of ^{131}I during the period of recirculation prior to connecting the apparatus to the patient. In this way, thorough mixing of the indicator into the circulation is assured. Samples of blood are taken simultaneously from the extracorporeal circuit and the systemic vein prior to the perfusion and at 15-minute intervals thereafter until the treatment period is completed. Concentration of radioiodinated albumin is determined; the blood volume of the extracorporeal system is known, whereas the volume in the perfused and the systemic circulation is estimated. The percentage of systemic leak is determined from the amount of radioactivity found in the systemic blood samples as counted in the well-scintillation counter.

Choice of Chemotherapeutic Drugs

The agents used in isolation procedures by a number of investigators vary almost as much as those used systemically (Table 1). Nitrogen mustard has been employed most commonly, particularly for carcinomas, and has been the favorite for sarcomas such as liposarcoma and rhabdomyosarcoma as well as for melanoma. Melphalan (aminophenylalanine mustard) has been used frequently for sarcoma of the limbs and sometimes combined with triethylene thiophosphoramide (TSPA) for carcinoma of the breast and for melanoma. Numerous other agents have been used, including AB 100 for carcinoma of the pelvis. However, it has been the experience of most investigators that the antimetabolites appear to be more effective when given by

Table 1.—*Drug Dose Related to Area Perfused*

Region	*Drug*	*Dose (mg/kg of body weight)*
Head and neck		
One side	Nitrogen mustard	0.2
Both sides	Nitrogen mustard	0.3
Arm	Nitrogen mustard	0.4
	Phenylalanine mustard	0.6
	Actinomycin D	0.005
Pelvis	Nitrogen mustard	0.6
	Phenylalanine mustard	0.6
Leg	Nitrogen mustard	0.6
	Actinomycin D	0.005

intra-arterial infusion rather than by perfusion. Antibiotic agents have not commonly been used in perfusions described in the literature because of limited therapeutic responses and marked toxicity.

Results

Since the leak factor has been well controlled in the extremities, isolation perfusion has been applied extensively, and there are adequate data to assess its value in these locations. Krementz et al.[10] reported a study of 597 patients with advanced malignancy, and 690 instances of regional perfusion; 350 of this group had melanoma, 164 had carcinomas and 83 had sarcomas. Early regression of tumors was observed in approximately 70 per cent of the patients with melanoma and in about 60 per cent with carcinoma and sarcoma, but the responses were short. They cited a small series of patients with regional nodes or satellitosis or local recurrence in an extremity, 30 per cent of whom showed control for 5 years after perfusion. A small group of patients with primary melanoma confined to a limb had a 5-year survival rate of 90 per cent after conservative excision, node dissection and perfusion. Ten of 14 patients with soft-tissue sarcomas survived 5 years after perfusion. Stehlin[11] reported a $6\frac{1}{2}$-year study of 221 patients receiving perfusion for melanoma of an extremity. In this group the overall 5-year survival rate was 53.1 per cent for all stages, 72.7 per cent of 107 patients with Stage I melanoma surviving for the same period. These results appear to be improved over those reported using standard surgical methods without perfusion as adjunctive therapy.

In another series Stehlin[12] indicated that greater benefits in terms of survival, particularly in treating melanomas, can be obtained when hyperthermia is added to the perfusion system. This method evolved subsequent to the finding of Cavaliere et al.[13] of irreversible damage to the respiration of Novikoff hepatoma cells incubated at 42° and 44°C. However, complications consisting of swollen and painful limbs postoperatively, local burns and bleeding from incision sites are frequent. Two deaths in a group of 50 patients have been reported by Stehlin as the result of hemolysis, with secondary effects on the kidney and the cardiovascular system.

In other parts of the anatomy, the results after perfusion are less encouraging, with systemic leak being the limiting factor. For example, in the head and neck area the leak factor from the isolation circuit is above 50 per cent; however, relief of pain appeared to be a significant additional benefit of perfusion, as reported by Golomb.[14] Cerebrovascular spasm and cerebral edema were found to be serious complications, particularly in elderly patients. Despite the sizeable leak factor in pelvic perfusions, Strawitz and coworkers[15] and others have reported remarkable results after perfusion. Several patients manifested sloughing of pelvic tumors, and relief of pain was found to be a common benefit. However, the complication rate was excessive, with postoperative vaginal bleeding and sloughing of irradiated skin. Long-term survivors after pelvic perfusion have not been reported in any series so far as we are aware. The perfusion of intra-abdominal malignancy has not been reported often in the literature. Again, the main problem in dealing with these tumors is the large leak factor and the extensive operative procedures which must be used for palliation.

Discussion

Isolation perfusion has been used extensively during the past 10 years in the treatment of advanced malignant tumors of the extremities and other parts of the human body. At this time it appears that the technique has its greatest value in the treatment of tumors of the extremities, particularly malignant melanoma. The high leak factor in the head and neck, pelvis and abdominal viscera has reduced its value in these locations; the use of infusion techniques would seem more appropriate. Hyperthermia is a relatively new development and apparently enhances the effectiveness of perfusion. However, the complications associated with this additional technique are not to be underestimated. The limiting factor in perfusion as well as systemic therapy still relates to the lack of drug specificity and the absence of appropriate sensitivity tests.

Relief of pain appears to be a common additional benefit in patients who are perfused with nitrogen mustard. The explanation for this observation is based on the selective affinity that nitrogen mustard has for peripheral nervous tissue. Systemic leak appears to be crucial in determining whether the technique of isolation should be used in a particular location. In our opinion, lesions of the extremity appear to offer the best opportunity for treatment because of the very small leak factor. Infusion techniques are better used in the other locations since the dosage of drug delivered is almost equivalent to that in isolation perfusion. The perfusion of retroperitoneal and posterior mediastinal metastases and lymphoma has not progressed since our previous report, because chemotherapeutic agents of large enough molecular size have not yet been developed. Our studies have indicated that a molecular size of no less than 5000 would be necessary to maintain an adequate drug level within the lymphatic system.

The successful use of isolation perfusion systems depends upon the availability of special equipment and knowledgeability in vascular surgery and solid tumor chemotherapy. Consequently, this method cannot be recommended for general use but should remain in the hands of those who have these qualifications and who regard it as being in a phase of development.

References

1. Klopp, C. T., Alford, T. C., Bateman, J., Berry, G. M. and Winship, T.: Fractionated intra-arterial cancer chemotherapy with methyl - bis - amine hydrochloride: Preliminary report. Ann. Surg. 132:811, 1950.
2. Bierman, H. R., Kelley, K. H., Byron, R. L., Dod, K. S. and Shimkin, M. B.: Studies on the blood supply of tumors in man: Intra-arterial nitrogen mustard therapy of cutaneous lesions. J. Nat. Cancer Inst. 11:891, 1951.
3. Sullivan, R. D., Jones, R., Jr., Schnabel, T. G., Jr. and Shorey, J. M.: Treatment of human cancer with intra-arterial nitrogen mustard utilizing simplified catheter technique. Cancer 6:121, 1953.
4. Gilman, A. and Philips, F. S.: Biologic actions and therapeutic applications of β-chloroethyl amines and sulfides. Science 103:409, 1946.
5. Jacobsen, L. O., Spurr, C. L., Barron, E. S. G., Smith, T., Lushbough, C. and Dick, G. F.: Nitrogen mustard therapy: Studies on the effect of methyl-bis(beta-chlorethyl)-amine hydrochloride on neoplastic disease and allied disorders of the hematopoietic system. J.A.M.A. 132:263, 1946.
6. Creech, O., Jr., Krementz, E. T., Ryan, R. F. and Winblad, J. N.: Chemotherapy of cancer: Regional perfusion utilizing an extracorporeal circuit. Ann. Surg. 148:616, 1958.
7. Martin, D. S., Hobbs, J. C., II, White, H. M., Jr. and Pickens, J.: Experience with a pelvic tourniquet in man. Surg. Forum 12:434, 1961.
8. Lawrence, W., Jr., Clarkson, B., Kim, M., Clapp, P. and Randall, H. T.: Regional perfusion of pelvis and abdomen by an indirect technique. Cancer 16:567, 1963.
9. Strawitz, J. G., Eto, K., Kitsuoha, H., Olney, C., Parient, F. and Howard, J. M.: Molecular weight dependence of lymphatic permeability: The concept of regional cancer chemotherapy by lymphatic perfusion. J. Microvasc. Res. 1:58, 1968.

10. Krementz, E. T., Creech, O., Jr. and Ryan, R. F.: Evaluation of chemotherapy of cancer by regional perfusion. Cancer 20:834, 1967.
11. Stehlin, J. S., Jr.: Perfusion for melanoma of the extremities: 6½ years' experience with 221 cases. Proc. Nat. Cancer Conf. 5:525, 1964.
12. Stehlin, J. S., Jr.: Hyperthermic perfusion with chemotherapy for cancers of the extremities. Surg. Gynec. Obstet. 129:305, 1969.
13. Cavaliere, R., Ciocatto, E. C., Giovanella, B. C., Heidelberger, C., Johnson, R. O., et al.: Selective heat sensitivity of cancer cells. Cancer 20:1351, 1967.
14. Golomb, F. M.: Perfusion and infusion chemotherapy for cancer of the head and neck. Proc. Nat. Cancer Conf. 5:561, 1964.
15. Strawitz, J. G.: Cancer chemotherapy using isolation perfusion. *In* Brodsky, I. and Kahn, S. B. (Eds.): Cancer Chemotherapy: Basic and Clinical Applications. New York, Grune & Stratton, 1967.

Arterial Infusion Cancer Chemotherapy for Solid Tumors

By Robert D. Sullivan, M.D. and Chester J. Semel, M.D.

EXTENSIVE CLINICOPHARMACOLOGIC PROGRAMS designed to develop chemical agents for the treatment of various forms of advanced cancer in man have been under investigation for more than a decade. Despite the prodigious efforts of preclinical and clinical programs, progress has been slow, and except for methotrexate in choriocarcinoma, no chemical agents capable of a general curative effect on disseminated forms of cancer are presently available. Nevertheless, definite progress has been made in recent years in the introduction of new chemical compounds and special techniques of their administration.

Several techniques of regional cancer chemotherapy have been developed in an effort to enhance the antitumor effects of compounds that are in clinical use for patients with locally confined cancer. One method of regional cancer chemotherapy which we introduced in 1959 is *protracted arterial infusion cancer chemotherapy.*[1] This method of administration consists of the continuous, 24-hour infusion of a drug through a catheter inserted into the arterial blood supply of tumors. An infusion pump of the small, ambulatory, portable type impels the drug through the infusion catheter. Continuous, around-the-clock infusion is accomplished in multiple courses of treatment of three to six weeks each. Sterile water is infused between courses of active drug treatment.

We have previously reported techniques of catheter insertion in various arterial sites,[1-3] methods of maintenance of high- and low-volume infusion,[4] and the results of treatment in head and neck cancer,[5,6] pelvic cancer,[7] tumors of the trunk and extremities, and primary and secondary brain tumors.[8] Our preliminary experiences with the effects of this form of treatment on liver neoplasms and tumors of the biliary system have been the subject of earlier reports.[9,10] In this chapter we shall describe our expanded experience with the use of protracted ambulatory arterial infusion in patients with locally confined cancer, with special emphasis on advanced cancer of the liver and biliary system.

Rationale of Therapy

Certain forms of cancer, although incurable, often remain localized throughout a greater part of their evolution, and produce symptoms and death as a result of their relatively localized but uncontrolled growth. This is particularly true of primary and metastatic cancer of the liver, gall bladder, and bile ducts. Since the nutrient blood supply of these forms of cancer is accessible, higher concentrations of antimetabolite result from the arterial route of administration.

Our rationale for prolonged drug administration is predicated on the concept that prolonged and continuous exposure of tumor cells to certain antimetabolites is necessary if all cells of the given tumor population are to be exposed to the agent as they randomly enter their vulnerable metabolic phase.[1,5] Most antimetabolites produce their antitumor effect by interfering with the de novo synthesis of nucleic acids, the substances necessary for cell growth and multiplication. Cancer cells are

From Los Angeles, California.

TABLE 1.—*Dosages of Drugs Used in Arterial Infusion Therapy*

Drug	*Dosage*
5-Fluorouracil (FU)	5.0–7.5 mg/kg/24 hrs.
5-Fluoro-2′-deoxyuridine (FUDR)	0.1–0.3 mg/kg/24 hrs.
Methotrexate (MTX)	5 mg/24 hrs.
Methotrexate	50 mg/24 hrs.
and leucovorin (intramuscularly) (antidote)	6 mg every 6 hrs.

most active in the production of these essential metabolites and, hence, are most vulnerable to antimetabolite compounds just before cell division. Studies of cancer growth rates in humans suggest that in most cases greater than three months is required for tumor doubling.[11] In a small series, we estimated similar doubling time of individual patients with metastatic colonic and rectal cancer from calculations derived from measurements of the mean diameter of pulmonary metastases. Thus, it would seem that antimetabolite drugs, agents that produce their effect only when cells are actively proliferating, should be administered for prolonged periods to develop fully their antitumor effects.

Clinical studies on the effects of the prolonged administration of several antimetabolites and antibiotic compounds have been reported by us and by others.[1,12–15] These have shown that marked alteration in dose-toxicity response occurs with prolonged drug administration. The biologic effects in terms of toxicity are greatly increased when the administration of methotrexate and 5-fluoro-2′-deoxyuridine (FUDR) is prolonged; in contrast, the toxicity of 5-fluorouracil (FU), mitomycin C, and certain other antimetabolities is diminished.[16,17]

The drugs of choice employed in arterial infusion therapy are listed in Table 1. They include methotrexate (MTX), 50 mg per 24 hours, together with citrovorum factor; MTX alone; 5-fluorouracil (FU); and 5-fluoro-2′-deoxyuridine (FUDR). Other drugs currently under study include sodium 6-mercaptopurine, mitomycin C, streptonigrin and hydroxyurea.

For liver neoplasms, we perform direct intravascular introduction of the catheter at laparotomy for the following reasons: (1) Exploration of the abdominal cavity is possible, and occasionally an occult primary cancer is found which can be resected; (2) the extent of liver involvement by tumor may be directly evaluated; (3) fluorescent dye studies may be performed to ensure that the entire tumor area is receiving the arterial infusate; (4) additional catheters may be placed in anomalous hepatic arteries to assure antimetabolite distribution to entire liver, gall bladder, and portahepatic areas; and (5) it is also possible to ligate extrahepatic branches of the hepatic artery, which supply parts of the gastrointestinal tract vulnerable to the local effect of regional infusion of antimetabolite.

CONDUCT OF INFUSION

Antimetabolite infusion is usually begun immediately after catheter placement. Two methods of infusion are employed: (1) a high-volume electrical peristaltic pump delivering approximately 1000 cc per 24 hours of infusate containing the daily dose of antimetabolite. This infusion apparatus is commonly used for infusion treatments of patients in whom more than one catheter is necessary to encompass the desired area of infusion.[2] A low-volume, miniature, portable infusion pump was developed by

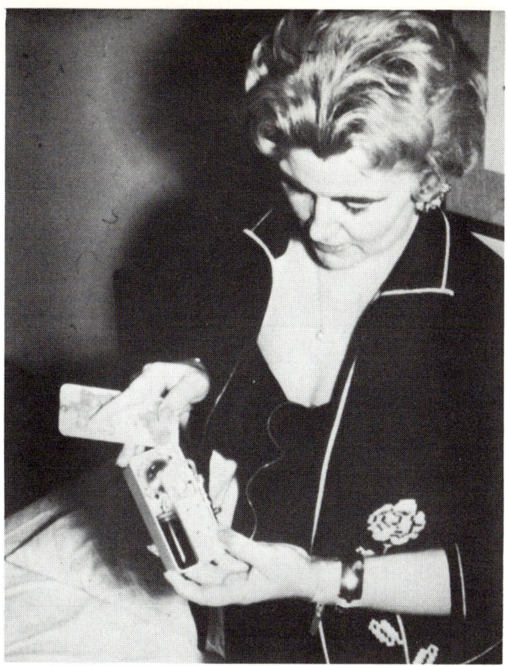

FIG. 1.—Adenocarcinoma of the liver (primary bowel cancer). An ambulatory outpatient is receiving protracted hepatic artery infusion therapy. From Sullivan,[20] with permission.

our group[18] to facilitate long-term infusion on an ambulatory, outpatient basis. This self-contained pump is carried by the patient, and has the capacity of delivering continuous, uninterrupted infusion for periods of 4 to 5 days. It delivers 5 cc of solution every 24 hours. Patients are instructed in the manner of replacing the drug-charged bags so that treatment can be continued on an outpatient basis. Clinical trials using this ambulatory infusion apparatus have been reported.[4] The apparatus, attached to the patient, is illustrated in Figure 1.

Treatment is continued for periods of 3 to 6 weeks until evidence of maximal local antimetabolic effect (i.e., local toxicity) is achieved. In liver infusions, this effect usually consists in increasing abnormality in the results of liver function tests and, at times, symptoms of anorexia and abdominal cramps. Antimetabolite treatment is then discontinued and sterile water is infused to assure patency of the arterial catheter. After recovery from local toxicity, active treatment is resumed. Courses of drug therapy alternating with periods of water infusion are continued until maximal clinical improvement has been achieved. At that time, the catheter is not removed; rather, it is ligated and permitted to remain in situ for future use. Patients are able to resume normal activity with the catheter in situ.

RESULTS OF TREATMENT

A total of 458 patients with various types of advanced but locally confined cancer, including 185 patients with primary and secondary liver neoplasms, were accepted for arterial infusion treatment, and 411 patients achieved an adequate course of therapy (Table 2). Of 352 patients for whom evaluation was suitable, partial tumor regression was noted in 188 patients and complete gross tumor regression occurred in 26 patients.

TABLE 2.—*Results of Protracted Arterial Infusion Cancer Chemotherapy*

Type of tumor	Patients catheterized	Adequate course of treatment	Suitable for objective evaluation	Objective tumor regression Partial	Complete
Head and neck cancer	134	115	90	37	25
Pelvic cancer	55	52	40	16	1
Brain neoplasms	20	16	9	4	—
Liver neoplasms	185	167	163	90	—
Other	64	61	50	41	—
Total	458	411	352	188	26

Metastatic Cancer of the Liver (Primary in Colon)

Patients with colorectal cancer admitted to study were classified according to stage of hepatic involvement, as reported by Young et al.[19] Table 3 shows the various criteria used in the study to classify our patients in the three stage categories. Life expectancy data of the three stages are also shown. Objective tumor response was defined as a decrease in liver size by greater than 50 per cent and return to normal or near-normal levels on the results of liver function tests, associated with clinical benefit. These criteria must be maintained for a period of three months or more to represent an objective response.

The results of treatment of metastatic colon and rectal cancer are shown in Table 4.

Of 182 patients who received protracted hepatic arterial infusion therapy, 164 patients achieved adequate trial. Objective response was noted in 88 (approximately 54 per cent) of these patients (Table 5). It is stated categorically that the survival of patients with hepatic metastases from colorectal cancer has been improved by regional arterial chemotherapy.

TABLE 3.—*Classification of Degree of Liver Involvement*

Classification of extent of disease	Performance status (%)*	Symptoms	Liver size	Liver function tests	Average life expectancy without treatment in months (range)
Stage III	20–40	Advanced	Massively enlarged	Highly abnormal	2.1 (0.3–3.9)
Stage II	50–70	Mild	Moderately enlarged	Abnormal	11.2 (1.6–21.8)
Stage I	80	0	±	Normal	—

* Arbitrary percentile evaluation of functional capacity.
From Sullivan,[20] with permission.

TABLE 4.—*Results of Treatment of Metastatic Liver Cancer (Primary Colon and Rectal Cancer)*

Classification of extent of disease	Patients treated (total)	Number of patients Adequate trial	Response	Average life expectancy without treatment (months)	Actual survival with treatment (months)
Stage III	30	29	18	2.1	9.4
Stage II	9	8	6	11.2	All alive on therapy*

* One patient died suddenly from causes unrelated to neoplastic growth.

TABLE 5.—*Overall Results of Protracted Hepatic Arterial Infusion Therapy*

Primary site of cancer	No. of patients infused	No. of patients having adequate trial	Objective response > 3 months	Objective response % having adequate trial
Colorectum with extrahepatic metastasis	40	35	17	48
Colorectum without extrahepatic metastasis	66	62	40	65
Gall bladder and bile ducts	18	16	9	56
Liver	8	8	3	38
Stomach	9	7	2	29
Pancreas	19	17	6	35
Breast	7	6	4	67
Miscellaneous	15	13	7	54
Total	182	164	88	54

DISCUSSION

The results of these studies demonstrate that protracted and continuous administration of several antimetabolites into the arterial blood supply of advanced, but localized, forms of cancer produces significant local antimetabolic and antitumor effects associated with practical clinical benefit in 25 to 45 per cent of the patients so treated.[20] The increased local biologic effects are attributed to the following: (1) Route of administration—the arterial route of administration may result in a higher local concentration of drug and hence a greater local antimetabolic effect. (2) The continuous, 24-hour administration of the antimetabolite may result in a continuous antimetabolic effect, and hence cells which sequentially enter an active metabolic phase may be affected by the compound, since they are continuously exposed to the agent.

The results of these studies indicate that patients with liver neoplasms have derived practical clinical benefit from this form of treatment. Indeed, in Stage III category of patients with metastatic cancer to the liver from a colorectal primary lesion, the average survival of the 11 patients who died was increased from the expected survival of 2.1 months (range, 0.3 to 3.9 months) without treatment to 9.4 months (range, 3 to 24 months). Patients with advanced hepatic decompensation and jaundice due to a diffuse intrahepatic tumor, general debility, and very abnormal results of liver function tests occasionally derive some benefit from treatment, and a few patients did show dramatic improvement. In general, such patients are poor candidates for this form of therapy.

Dose schedules of the several antimetabolite studies were explored. The recommended doses should not be exceeded to obviate early development of severe local toxicity, which would necessitate early interruption of treatment. We recommend the use of FU or FUDR initially in patients with liver neoplasms, especially if the liver alone is to be treated. We have previously reported evidence that the liver autodetoxifies certain fluorinated pyrimidines when the drugs are given by continuous infusion through the hepatic artery.[9] Thus, the remainder of the body is protected from systemic toxicity. In fact, systemic toxicity (e.g. gastrointestinal, hematologic) is virtually never seen with these compounds at these dose schedules.

The portable pump apparatus has permitted long-term infusion on an ambulatory basis and has rendered simpler and more practical protracted arterial infusion on an outpatient basis. Patients are able to return to their homes, often at remote distances, and frequently resume full activity while on treatment.

References

1. Sullivan, R. D., Miller, E. and Sykes, M. P.: Antimetabolite-metabolite combination cancer chemotherapy: Effects of intra-arterial methotrexate intramuscular citrovorum factor therapy in human cancer. Cancer 12:1248, 1959.
2. Duff, J. K., Sullivan, R. D., Miller, E., Ulm, A. H., Clarkson, B. D. and Clifford, P.: Antimetabolite-metabolite cancer chemotherapy using continuous intra-arterial methotrexate with intermittent intramuscular citrovorum factor: Method of therapy. Cancer 14:744, 1961.
3. Watkins, E., Jr. and Sullivan, R. D.: Cancer chemotherapy by prolonged arterial infusion. Surg. Gynec. Obstet. 118:3, 1964.
4. Sullivan, R. D. and Zurek, W. Z.: Protracted ambulatory infusion cancer chemotherapy by the Watkins chronometric infusor. Cancer Chemother. Rep. 37:47, 1964.
5. Sullivan, R. D.: Continuous arterial infusion cancer chemotherapy. Surg. Clin. N. Amer. 42:365, 1962.
6. Sullivan, R. D. and McPeak, C. J.: A favorable response in tongue cancer to arterial infusion chemotherapy. J.A.M.A. 179:293, 1962.
7. Sullivan, R. D., Wood, A. M., Clifford, P., Duff, J. K., Trussel, R., et al.: Continuous intra-arterial methotrexate with simultaneous, intermittent, intramuscular citrovorum factor therapy in carcinoma of the cervix. Cancer Chemother. Rep. 8:1, 1960.
8. Sullivan, R. D.: Continuous intra-arterial infusion chemotherapy of head and neck cancer. Trans. Amer. Acad. Ophthal. Otolaryng. 66:111, 1962.
9. Sullivan, R. D., Norcross, J. W. and Watkins, E., Jr.: Chemotherapy of metastatic liver cancer by prolonged hepatic artery infusion. New Eng. J. Med. 270:321, 1964.
10. Sullivan, R. D. and Zurek, W. Z.: Chemotherapy for liver cancer by protracted ambulatory infusion. J.A.M.A. 194:481, 1965.
11. Collins, V. P., Loeffler, R. K. and Tivey, H.: Observations on growth rates of human tumors. Amer. J. Roentgen. 76:988, 1956.
12. Sullivan, R. D., Miller, E., Chryssochoos, T. and Watkins, E., Jr.: Clinical effects of the continuous intravenous and intra-arterial infusion of cancer chemotherapeutic compounds. Cancer Chemother. Rep. 16:499, 1962.
13. Sullivan, R. D., Miller, E., Zurek, W. Z. and Rodriguez, F. R.: Clinical effects of prolonged (continuous) infusion of streptonigrin (NSC-45383) in advanced cancer. Cancer Chemother. Rep. 33:27, 1963.
14. Miller, E., Sullivan, R. D., Young, C. W. and Burchenal, J. H.: Clinical effects of continuous infusion of antimetabolites: Prevention of toxicity of 5-fluoro-2′-deoxyuridine by thymidine. Proc. Amer. Ass. Cancer Res. 3:251, 1961.
15. Miller, E. and Sullivan, R. D.: Alteration of biologic activity of cancer chemotherapy agents by prolonged infusion. *In* Brodsky, I. and Kahn, S. B. (Eds.): Cancer Chemotherapy. New York: Grune & Stratton, 1967.
16. Sullivan, R. D., Young, C. W., Miller, E., Glatstein, N., Clarkson, B. and Burchenal, J. H.: The clinical effects of the continuous administration of fluorinated pyrimidines (5-fluorouracil and 5-fluoro-2′-deoxyuridine). Cancer Chemother. Rep. 8:77, 1960.
17. Miller, E., Sullivan, R. D., Chryssochoos, T. and Sykes, M. P.: The clinical effects of mitomycin C by continuous intravenous administration. Cancer Chemother. Rep. 21:129, 1962.
18. Watkins, E., Jr.: Chronometric infusor: An apparatus for protracted ambulatory infusion therapy. New Eng. J. Med. 269:850, 1963.
19. Young, C. W., Ellison, R. R., Sullivan, R. D., Levick, S., Golsky, R. B. and Burchenal, J. H.: Evaluation of therapeutic response of large bowel cancer to the fluorinated pyrimidines in relation to clinical patterns. Proc. Amer. Ass. Cancer Res. 3:164, 1960.
20. Sullivan, R. D.: Clinical Cancer Chemotherapy Including Ambulatory Infusion. Springfield, Ill.: Charles C Thomas, 1970.

Hyperbaric Oxygen with Chemotherapy and Radiation Therapy in Cancer

By DONALD S. FAUST, M.D., LUTHER W. BRADY, M.D.
AND JOHN ANTONIADES, M.D.

SINCE THE EARLY 1930s radiation therapists have acknowledged the dependency of radiosensitivity on the abundance of the tumor's blood supply.[1,2] However, it was not until 1953 that this information was used in a practical sense, when Gray et al.[3] demonstrated a general relation between radiation sensitivity and tumor oxygen saturation at the time of irradiation. Other investigations[4-6] have shown that all tumors have areas of anoxic cells which are offered a degree of radioprotection by their lack of oxygen.

In the ensuing 15 years, various investigators[7-9] have applied this principle at the clinical level with the hyperbaric chamber using 1 to 4 atmospheres of absolute pressure. More than 1,000 patients have been treated with high-pressure oxygen (HPO_2) and radiation therapy administered as a combined procedure. The efficacy of HPO_2 as a radio-sensitizer of tumor tissue has become an established fact.

Because of the biochemical and cytological similarities in the mode of action of both ionizing radiation and the alkylating agents, Krementz and his coworkers[10,11] studied the effects of HN_2 on Ehrlich ascites tumor-bearing CFW mice treated in combination with HPO_2. Since their initial work, several investigators have studied the effects on animal tumors of hyperbaric oxygen combined with cancer chemotherapy. This chapter reviews the effects of hyperbaric oxygen when combined with cancer chemotherapy and also presents our experience with HPO_2 in the treatment of advanced carcinoma of the uterine cervix.

Krementz and his colleagues,[10] in their original article, demonstrated an increase in the tumoricidal effect of HN_2 when given in combination with HPO_2 at 3 atmospheres absolute pressure. His work was confirmed by Leather and Eckert,[12] DeCosse and Rogers,[13] and Kinsey.[14] Kinsey's work suggested that HPO_2 potentiated the antitumor effect of 5-FU in the treatment of S-91 melanoma in mice. Urushizaki et al.[15] have recently confirmed the effects of 5-FU and HPO_2. Working with male rats inoculated with Yoshida sarcoma ascitic fluid, they treated the animals with tritium-labeled 5-FU and mitomycin C (MMC) at 3 atmospheres absolute pressure. The animals receiving the radioactive 5-FU with HPO_2 had an increased uptake of the chemotherapeutic agent by the ascitic tumor cells as compared to the control animals treated with labeled 5-FU in air. The combination of 5-FU and HPO_2 also resulted in marked tumor inhibition as compared to the MMC and HPO_2 combination, which showed no such effect (5-FU = 5-fluorouacil).

Nathanson et al.[16] have extensively reviewed the subject of the effects of chemotherapeutic agents and HPO_2 on normal and tumor-bearing rodents. Working with

---

From the Department of Radiation Therapy and Nuclear Medicine, Hahnemann Medical College and Hospital, Philadelphia, Pennsylvania.

Supported by The Alexander and Margaret Stewart Trust; the Alperin Foundation; the Friends of the Radiation Therapy Center of the Hahnemann Medical College and Hospital; and PHS Training Grants Nos. T01-CA05185-05 and T12-CA08024-05 from the National Cancer Institute.

three groups of chemotherapeutic agents, HN2 and cyclophosphamide, actinomycin D and mitomycin C, and methotrexate and 6-mercaptopurine, they concluded that there was no specific enhancement to the drug-induced antitumor effect by the addition of hyperbaric oxygen. Back and Ambrus[17] also failed to demonstrate an enhancement to the normally expected chemotherapeutic effect by the addition of HPO_2 at 3 to 6 atmospheres absolute pressure using HN2 in treating induced tumors in Swiss mice. Marshall et al.[18] working with HN2 in treating the Walker-256 carcinosarcoma-induced tumor in rats, showed enhancement of the antitumor effect with HPO_2 but no change in the therapeutic index.

The discrepancy between the observations of various investigators using chemotherapeutic agents in combination with HPO_2 in animal tumor systems is also apparent in the human or clinical experience. To date there has been a paucity of published clinical material. Adams et al.[19] reported treating 6 patients with advanced malignancy with HN2 (0.5 to 0.6 mg/kg of body weight) in a hyperbaric chamber at 2 atmospheres absolute pressure. There were two cases of recurrent gastric carcinoma, a case of primary oat cell carcinoma of the lung with brain metastases, primary adenocarcinoma of the lung, and recurrent reticulum cell sarcoma of the stomach. The results of treatment were disappointing, and the author mentions marked bone marrow depression in the cases treated.

Kuyama[20] treated 15 cases of advanced cancer in the hyperbaric theater (walk-in chamber) at 2 atmospheres pressure at Kyoto University Hospital on a daily basis for 2 weeks. Twice a week 8 mg of mitomycin C was injected intravenously during the compression-decompression cycle. A bone marrow-sparing effect was noted in the chamber group of patients relative to the red and white cell population of the marrow. The thrombocytes were not protected in the authors' series, with thrombocytopenia being encountered. Six patients were in a terminal or preterminal state at the outset of treatment. Three became comatose and expired, with brain symptoms. The question was raised as to death secondary to metastases versus hemorrhage due to thrombocytopenia. The other 3 died of disease unrelated to brain symptomatology. The remaining 9 patients were living free of disease 2 years after the combined therapy. The specific histologic diagnoses for this group of patients are not given.

A second series of 8 cases of advanced cancer was treated by a single course of hyperbaric cancer chemotherapy with injection of bone marrow to prevent the previously encountered thrombocytopenia. Prior to treatment, 300 ml of bone marrow was withdrawn from the pelvic bone of the patient. The patients were treated in the hyperbaric theater, receiving 20 mg of mitomycin C intravenously. One hour after the injection, 100 ml of 20% thiosulfate soda was injected intravenously in a dropwise manner. This injection was followed by the injection of the patient's bone marrow in a normobaric environment. Four cases of gastric cancer and a single case of breast and caecal carcinoma were treated in this manner. A patient with retroperitoneal fibrosarcoma received both mitomycin C and Endoxan (10 mg of each drug) and a patient with lymphosarcoma received 1 mg of vincristine. At the time of this writing, all these patients were still living 1 to 2 years after initial treatment.

Hyperbaria and Radiation Therapy

In the field of HPO_2 and radiation therapy the greatest interest has centered on the treatment of squamous cell carcinoma of the head and neck and the uterine cervix. A randomized control study was initiated in the Department of Radiation Therapy at the Hahnemann Medical College in November, 1967, to treat patients with Stage III and Stage IVA carcinoma of the uterine cervix. The study was designed to answer the questions of increased tumor cure probability with HPO_2 versus the probability of damage to normal tissue (necrosis probability) when conventional radiation therapy fractionation schedules are used in combination with oxygen at 3 atmospheres absolute pressure.

Materials and Methods

Selection of cases for the control and HPO_2 groups was made on a randomized program basis. The study was designed to use identical treatment conditions and dose fractionation schedules in the control patients and in the hyperbaric groups of patients. However, after reviewing our experience in the treatment of the first 6 HPO_2 patients, it was necessary to modify our protocol and reduce the total and daily tumor dose increment by 7 per cent in the HPO_2 group. End points selected for evaluation were (1) tumor control at the site of primary lesion; (2) response and/or complication rate of normal tissues to treatment; (3) frequency and pattern of metastatic disease; and (4) patient survival.

The details of our patient pretreatment work-up, radiation therapy planning and administration (technical factors), and specific information relative to the hyperbaric chamber were presented in a previous publication.[21] Patients were thoroughly worked up and staged jointly with a member of the Department of Gynecology and, whenever possible, under general anesthesia. Pathologic confirmation was obtained on all cases and was reviewed by the Department of Pathology.

The Vickers Hyperbaric Chamber was used in the treatment of the experimental group of patients. Neither anesthesia nor premedication was used. Patients were compressed at the rate of 2 to 4 psig per minute to a level of 30 psig (3 atmospheres absolute). After compression, the patients respired 100 per cent oxygen at 30 psig for a 15-minute soaking or equilibrium period before being irradiated. The total compression-decompression cycle averaged 40 minutes and was repeated 24 times for each patient.

The 6-million volt (Varian) linear accelerator was employed for the treatment of all protocol patients. Patients in the control group received a total of 5000 rads delivered homogeneously to the pelvis at the rate of 1000 rads per week on a 4-day per week treatment schedule. An additional 1000 rads was given to the lateral pelvic (regional nodes) structures in Stage III cases. Stage IVA cases received 6000 rads homogeneously to the pelvis in 6 weeks. The HPO_2 group received 4650 rads in 5 weeks at the rate of 930 rads per week. An additional boost of 930 rads was given in the Stage III cases to the lateral pelvic structures. Stage IVA cases were carried to 5580 rads in 6 weeks to the whole pelvis. A radium placement was performed in all Stage III cases in both groups. Patients who exhibited a satisfactory response to the external therapy in the Stage IVA control and experimental group were considered for a radium placement.

Results

Since the start of the program, 34 patients have been accessioned into the study. Four additional patients were excluded because of the patient's size (350 lbs.), age or

TABLE 1.—*Cancer of the Cervix (Patients Accessioned to Study by Stage)*

	Stage IIIA	*Stage IIIB*	*Stage IVA*
HPO_2	6	6	1
Air	10	6	3

mental status, and because of the question of liver metastasis in a patient who refused liver biopsy. Two of the original 34 accepted cases were withdrawn from final statistical analysis. One patient in the control group developed distant metastases and expired prior to completion of treatment. A second patient, an extremely obese female, experienced claustrophobia during her first compression-decompression cycle in the hyperbaric chamber and refused subsequently to enter the chamber.

In the experimental group, 12 of the 13 patients were Stage III (Table 1). In the control group, 16 of the 19 patients were Stage III and the remaining three were Stage IVA. All patients in both groups had proven squamous cell carcinoma.

In the experimental group, 11 of the 13 cases were available for a 6-month follow-up (Table 2). Five patients were surviving without disease 6 to 29 months after completion of treatment. One patient, who initially presented with bilateral ureteral obstruction in a comatose condition secondary to uremia and massive vaginal bleeding, died without disease 12 months after completion of treatment. The patient had been admitted to the hospital to undergo elective surgery to correct a problem related to a vesicovaginal fistula. Her death was secondary to problems related to her surgery, and at autopsy she was found to have no residual tumor.

Of the 5 patients who expired of causes secondary to their primary disease process, 2 elderly patients died at other institutions within 2 months after completion of treatment; autopsies were not performed. Both had shown marked objective improvement in terms of primary response, but after treatment they experienced electrolyte and dehydration problems secondary to small-bowel reaction related to treatment. In one patient, extrapelvic disease developed in the left periaortic chain of nodes, which caused ureteral obstruction 1 year after treatment for her primary pelvic disease. Biopsy of the primary site revealed no evidence of recurrent disease in the pelvis. The patient expired 5 months later, with liver metastases. In the fourth patient in the group, bilateral pulmonary metastases developed, and she expired 8 months after treatment. Prior to diagnosis and treatment, she had delivered a full-term infant

TABLE 2.—*Squamous Cell Carcinoma of the Cervix: Randomized Control Study (Patient Survival 6 months to 33 months)*

	Control	(%)	HPO_2	(%)	
Stage III	4/9		5/10		Alive without disease
Stage IVA	1/3		0/1		Alive without disease
Alive without disease	5/12	(42)	5/11	(46)	
Alive with disease	1/12	(8)	0/11	(0)	
Dead without disease	1/12	(8)	1/11	(9)*	
Dead with disease	5/12	(42)	5/11	(46)	

* Proved by autopsy.

vaginally through the tumor-involved cervix. This may have produced blood-borne metastases. Marked tumor control had been noted in the pelvis. The fifth patient died at home 13 months after treatment for a Stage III lesion. The patient had done well after her treatment and was free of disease locally when last examined 6 months before her death. An autopsy was not performed.

In the control group, 12 of the 19 patients were subjected to at least a 6-month risk. Five patients survived without disease 7 to 33 months. One patient with generalized abdominal carcinomatosis was still living 17 months after treatment.

Six patients in the control group have expired, 4 with local pelvic disease. One patient expired secondary to distant metastases, with no evidence of recurrent disease in the pelvis at autopsy. The sixth patient of the group had a Stage IVA carcinoma of the cervix with bladder involvement. She expired 4 months after treatment from an acute myocardial infarction. An autopsy to determine whether she had residual disease was not performed.

Discussion

There have been no instances of toxicity or convulsions in approximately 750 compression cycles to date. Approximately one-half of the patients were treated as outpatients. Myringotomy was not performed prior to HPO_2 treatment, and serious damage to the middle ear or the drum has not been encountered.

When we compared the effects on normal tissue in the 2 groups of patients, it was immediately apparent that the morbidity was increased in the HPO_2 group. Four of the first 6 patients treated had severe bowel and treatment reactions. Severe diarrhea developed in 2 patients during treatment and maintenance intravenous fluid therapy was required. Both were elderly patients (67 and 73 years old). For the second patient, it was necessary to interrupt therapy on two separate occasions. Both patients were discharged from the hospital, only to re-experience severe diarrhea and dehydration. They expired in convalescent homes because of complications after treatment, although the exact causes of their deaths are unknown. A third and fourth patient also experienced severe bowel reactions in the form of radiation proctosigmoiditis. Colostomies were performed, and these patients did well without recurrent disease. As a result of this initial experience, the protocol was modified, and the total and daily tumor dose increment was reduced by 7 per cent in the HPO_2 group. This change was effected over a year ago, and there have been no severe bowel reactions or complications.

The question of tumor control at the primary site is difficult to answer at this stage of the study. Several patients in both groups died without histologic proof to substantiate cause of death. It has been our clinical impression that objective regression of tumor occurred earlier and at a lower tumor dose in the HPO_2 group than in the control group.

The survival statistics for both groups are similar even with a limited number of patients. As of this writing 6 of 11 patients in the HPO_2 group and 6 of 12 patients in the control group who have been followed 6 to 33 months are free of their primary disease. Although the survival results are in keeping with those reported in other centers[22-24] that use HPO_2 techniques, the limited number of cases does not permit definitive conclusions until the study has been completed. To date both control and HPO_2 groups show no significant statistical difference in a limited number of cases studied.

REFERENCES

1. Crabtree, H. G. and Cramer, W.: Action of radium on cancer cells. II. Some factors determining the susceptibility of cancer cells to radium. Proc. Roy. Soc. (Series B): Biological Sciences 113:238, 1933.
2. Mottram, J. C.: A factor of importance in the radiosensitivity of tumors. Brit. J. Radiol. 9:606, 1936.
3. Gray, L. H., Conger, A. O., Ebert, M., Hornsey, S. and Scott, O. C. A.: The concentration of oxygen dissolved in tissues at the time of irradiation as a factor in radiotherapy. Brit. J. Radiol. 26:638, 1953.
4. Thomlinson, R. H.: A comparison of fast neutrons and X-rays in relation to "oxygen effect" in experimental tumours in rats. Brit. J. Radiol. 36:89, 1963.
5. Cater, B. D. and Silver, I. A.: Quantitative measurements of oxygen tension in normal tissues and in tumours of rodents before and after radiotherapy. Acta Radiol. 53:233, 1960.
6. Powers, W. E. and Tolmach, L. J.: A multicomponent X-ray survival curve for mouse lymphosarcoma cells irradiated in vivo. Nature 197:710, 1963.
7. Churchill-Davidson, I., Sanger, C. and Thomlinson, R. H.: Oxygenation in radiotherapy. II. Clinical application. Brit. J. Radiol. 30:406, 1957.
8. van den Brenk, H. A. S., Madigan, J. P. and Kerr, R. C.: Experience with megavoltage irradiation of advanced malignant disease using high pressure oxygen. *In* Boerema, I. et al. (Eds.): Clinical application of hyperbaric oxygen. Proc. First Int. Cong. Amsterdam: Elsevier, 1964, p. 144.
9. Wildermuth, O.: The case for hyperbaric oxygen radiotherapy. J.A.M.A. 191:986, 1965.
10. Krementz, E. T., Harlin, R. and Knudson, L.: Enhancement of chemotherapy by increased tissue oxygen tension. Cancer Chemother. Rep. 10:125, 1960.
11. Krementz, E. T. and Knudson, L.: Effect of increased oxygen tension on the tumoricidal effect of nitrogen mustard. Surgery 50:266, 1961.
12. Leather, R. P. and Eckert, C.: Hyperbaric oxygenation and mechlorethamine effectiveness. Arch. Surg. 87:144, 1963.
13. DeCosse, J. J. and Rogers, L. S.: Effect of hyperbaric oxygen and cancer chemotherapy on growth of animal tumors. Surg. Forum 15:203, 1964.
14. Kinsey, D. L.: Hyperbaric oxygen and 5-fluorouracil in the treatment of experimental melanoma. Surg. Forum 15:205, 1964.
15. Urushizaki, I., Ikeda, S. and Ibayashi, J.: Experimental studies on cancer chemotherapy under hyperbaric oxygenation. Fourth Int. Cong. on Hyperbaric Medicine, 1969. Tokyo: Igaku Shoin, 1970, pp. 428–433.
16. Nathanson, L., Brown, B., Maddock, C. and Hall, T. C.: Effects of antitumor agents and hyperbaric oxygen in normal and tumor-bearing rodents. Cancer 19:1019, 1966.
17. Back, N. and Ambrus, J. L.: Effect of oxygen tension on the sensitivity of normal and tumor tissues to alkylating agents. J. Nat. Cancer Inst. 30:17, 1963.
18. Marshall, W. H., Hoppe, E. T. and Stark, F.: Effect of ambient oxygen tension on the toxicity and therapeutic effect of mechlorethamine (nitrogen mustard). Arch. Surg. 86:932, 1963.
19. Adams, J. F., Ledingham, I. M., Jackson, J. M. and Smith, G.: Combined nitrogen mustard and hyperbaric oxygen therapy in advanced malignant disease. Brit. Med. J. 1:314, 1963.
20. Kuyama, T.: Clinical experiences on cancer chemotherapy of mytomycin C at the hyperbaric theater. Fourth Int. Cong. on Hyperbaric Medicine. Tokyo: Igaku Shoin, 1970, pp. 422–427.
21. Faust, D. S., Brady, L. W., Kazem, I. and Germon, P. A.: Hybaroxia and radiation therapy in carcinoma of the cervix (Stage III and IV): A clinical trial. Fourth Int. Cong. on Hyperbaric Medicine. Tokyo: Igaku Shoin, 1970, pp. 410–414.
22. Johnson, R. J. R.: Preliminary observations and results with the use of hyperbaric oxygen and cobalt-60 teletherapy in the treatment of carcinoma of the cervix. Conf. on Radiobiology and Radiotherapy. Nat. Cancer Inst. Monographs 24:83, 1967.
23. Roulston, M. B. and Johnson, R. J. R.: Treatment of carcinoma of the cervix, Stages III and IV, using cobalt therapy and a hyperbaric oxygen chamber. J. Obstet. Gynaec. Brit. Comm. 75:1279, 1968.
24. Pizey, N. C. D. and Bullimore, J. A.: External irradiation combined with hyperbaric oxygen in the treatment of advanced cervical carcinoma. J. Obstet. Gynaec. Brit. Comm. 75:1275, 1968.

INDEX